Patient Reported Outcomes and Quality of Life in Cardiovascular Interventions

Thanos Athanasiou • Ara Darzi
Aung Ye Oo
Editors

Patient Reported Outcomes and Quality of Life in Cardiovascular Interventions

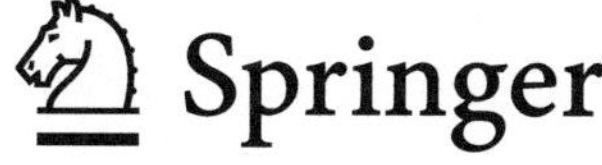

Editors
Thanos Athanasiou
Imperial College London
London, UK

Ara Darzi
Imperial College London
London, UK

Aung Ye Oo
Aortovascular Surgery
Barts Heart Centre, St Bartholomew's Hospital
London, UK

ISBN 978-3-031-09814-7 ISBN 978-3-031-09815-4 (eBook)
https://doi.org/10.1007/978-3-031-09815-4

This Springer imprint is published by the registered company Springer Nature Switzerland AG
The registered company address is: Gewerbestrasse 11, 6330 Cham, Switzerland

Preface

Over the last few decades, the combined effect of declining mortality and major morbidities after cardiovascular interventions in combination with the fact that medicine becoming more patient-centred has brought the impact on functional status of patients under the spotlight.

The ability and the time patients can resume their day-to-day activities post-intervention has been increasingly researched and considered as a key indicator of outcomes.

More often physicians are also considering the impact of the disease and the proposed interventions on patient's functional status and aspects of quality of life that are important to them.

The World Health Organization (WHO) describes QOL as "an individual's perception of their position in life in the context of the culture and value system in which they live and in relation to their goals, expectations, and standards and concerns".

In cardiovascular disease, patient-reported questionnaires help providing subjective, valid and reliable measures for QOL, and not based on physician-recognised cardiac symptoms.

QOL measures are increasingly becoming necessary to be incorporated in clinical trials due to their relevance to patients' functional status.

With the advances in percutaneous catheter interventions and with ageing population, there will undoubtedly more comparisons between such novel approaches to open cardiac surgery. The availability of valid QOL measures will assist in such comparisons to benefit what matters to the patient.

An increment in the proportion of patients above the age of 80 years presenting with cardiac disease will lead to increased demands on cardiovascular specialties.

The use of generic and disease-specific QOL instruments in randomised clinical trials (RCT) assists in quantifying the impact of cardiac intervention on patients with chronic health status.

When deciding which QOL measure to utilise, it has been suggested that concomitant use of both generic and disease-specific instruments is highly recommended and optimal. However, it has also been suggested that disease-specific QOL measures are more sensitive to change compared to generic ones in case of RCT.

There are a few limitations in the methodology in applying QOL measures in RCT. For instance, many studies utilise cross-sectional designs without baseline QOL assessment, which makes it difficult in demonstrating the efficacy of treatment. In general, the validity of QOL instruments use relies on memory recall while filling questionaries without considering physical and psychosocial adjustments over time to a chronic illness and how it is perceived. There is also significant variability in QOL instruments with some having lower sensitivity in detecting minor symptoms changes. So, it becomes challenging to accurately quantify QOL changes from interventions given the above limitations. Furthermore without a consensus in QOL use in RCT, one should be attentive to how QOL measures were defined and measured.

Recently, a Consolidated Standards of Reporting Trials Patient Reported Outcome (CONSORT PRO) has been set up to standardise QOL assessments across clinical trials and improve QOL reporting and inform clinical practice and health policy.

In clinical practice for patients undergoing emergency intervention or those critically unwell, the clinical decision making would not be affected by patient QOL scores. In comparison patients with already good pre-operative health will unlikely to have QOL benefit from surgery but will have improved survival.

Differential QOL trajectories can assist in informing patients more accurately when having discussions before surgery for their post-operative recovery. This would provide with realistic expectations when offering various interventions and an insight into functional status using generic or disease-specific QOL measures after surgery.

The importance of having accurate QOL data underpins its potential use to inform clinical practice and decision making.

To then implement PROs into clinical practice, need to consider the workflow including how they are collected, the timings, the reporting of scores and the actions that arise from it. Several RCTs have demonstrated the benefits of incorporating QOL data into routine clinical practice such as helping in discussing QOL issues without prolonging clinic and keeping patient's well-being paramount.

National databases such as the Society for Thoracic Surgeons (STS) or risk-scoring like Euroscore II provide accurate risk adjustments for common procedures and help in guiding pre-operative decision making.

The STS measures surgical outcomes including complications rates, readmissions and perioperative mortality, which are objective and easy to interpret. However, they do not reflect on what is most significant to the patient. In fact most of the post-operative complications are rare and would not be adequate for evaluating the true quality of care delivered or to compare institutions performances.

To have a better understanding of QOL measures and the outcomes associated with it, these PROs have to be assessed pre-operatively, post-operatively and also at long-term follow-up.

PROMIS provides accurate, standardised measurements of PROs. These have over 300 measures of mental, physical and social well-being that can be used for the general population or specific group like cardiac surgery.

PROMIS questionnaires have been validated for the general public and in patients with different medical conditions, so scores are obtained and compared easily across various populations.

The PROMIS is also aligned with the goals of STS PRO Task Force and the American Heart Association for exploring to incorporate PRO measures into the STS national databases. Resource use and patient-reported outcomes when added to National Databases would provide a more comprehensive perspective on quality as well as additional end points.

Incorporating PRO into National Databases will help surgeons to give more patient-centred care.

Mortality outcome is an insufficient marker for success and cardiac surgery has relied on this for too long. Operative success should not be the only criteria for providing a procedure to a patient. There is a multitude of trials that have reported improvement in QOL post-cardiac surgery and such high-quality data can be utilised for more accurate and personalised pre-operative counselling and risk stratification.

Such QOL measures can be used to benchmark in novel technologies such as transcatheter cardiac procedures and minimal access surgeries.

The use of generic and disease-specific QOL measures is a promising research field with many applications to RCT and in clinical practice.

The CONSORT PRO has been set up for assisting in adoption of validated QOL measures more routinely in trials and clinical practice. There is a lot of exciting opportunity for integrating PROs into routine clinical practice, clinical trials and national databases in cardiac surgery for optimising comparative effective research. Identifying anticipated trajectories for post-intervention recovery will assist in providing more tailored outcomes that are meaningful to patients, defining new markers for surgical success.

London, UK — Thanos Athanasiou
London, UK — Ara Darzi
London, UK — Aung Ye Oo

Contents

1 Unveiling the Concept of Minimal Clinically Important Difference (MCID) in Cardiac Surgery

Dimitrios E. Magouliotis, Grigorios Christodoulidis, Arian Arjomandi Rad, and Thanos Athanasiou

Introduction

It is crucial for surgeons and physicians to understand, identify and quantify the impact of their treatments on their patients. This need is even greater when therapies intend to improve subjective outcomes, thus increasing the complexity of assessing the clinical utility of treatment interventions [1]. However, a statistically significant change may not always represent a clinically meaningful enhancement for clinicians or patients. In this context, the smallest benefit of value to patients is called the minimal clinically important difference (MCID) [1]. In fact, the MCID concept is primarily patient-centered, thus demonstrating both the dimension of the objective clinical improvement, along with the value patients attribute to this change. The MCID has been developed to provide patient experience and clinical relevance to the reported outcomes, while defining the smallest proportion of change that an outcome should bring to be meaningful to patients [1].

The clinical importance for certain outcome measures, such as mortality or incidence of a rare complication, is intuitive, given that large multi-institutional trials are commonly needed to identify a statistical difference. Besides, other treatments may be of critical importance for patients, but might also affect health-related quality of life (HRQOL) [2]. To face this challenge, various questionnaires [3–5] have been developed, thus highlighting the urgent need for clinical interpretation of a meaningful change. These concepts are well-known and implemented in cardiac surgery, however, the application of the MCID concept remains still limited. Herein, we

Sources of financial report: The participating authors declare no sources of financial report that require acknowledgement.

Dimitrios E. Magouliotis contributed to the design of the work, the acquisition, analysis, and interpretation of data for the work, the drafting the work and revising it critically for important intellectual content, the final approval of the version to be published and is accountable for all aspects of the work.

Thanos Athanasiou, Grigorios Christodoulidis, Arian Arjomandi Rad all contributed to the conception and design of the work, the interpretation of data for the work, the revising of the work critically for important intellectual content, the final approval of the version to be published and is accountable for all aspects of the work.

Availability of Material
The data supporting the findings of the article is available upon request

D. E. Magouliotis (✉) · G. Christodoulidis
Division of Surgery and Interventional Science, Faculty of Medical Sciences, UCL, London, UK

Department of Cardiothoracic Surgery, University of Thessaly, Biopolis, Larissa, Greece
e-mail: dimitrios.magouliotis.18@ucl.ac.uk

A. A. Rad · T. Athanasiou
Department of Surgery and Cancer, Imperial College London, St Mary's Hospital, London, UK
e-mail: arian.arjomandi-rad16@imperial.ac.uk; t.athanasiou@imperial.ac.uk

T. Athanasiou et al. (eds.), *Patient Reported Outcomes and Quality of Life in Cardiovascular Interventions*,
https://doi.org/10.1007/978-3-031-09815-4_1

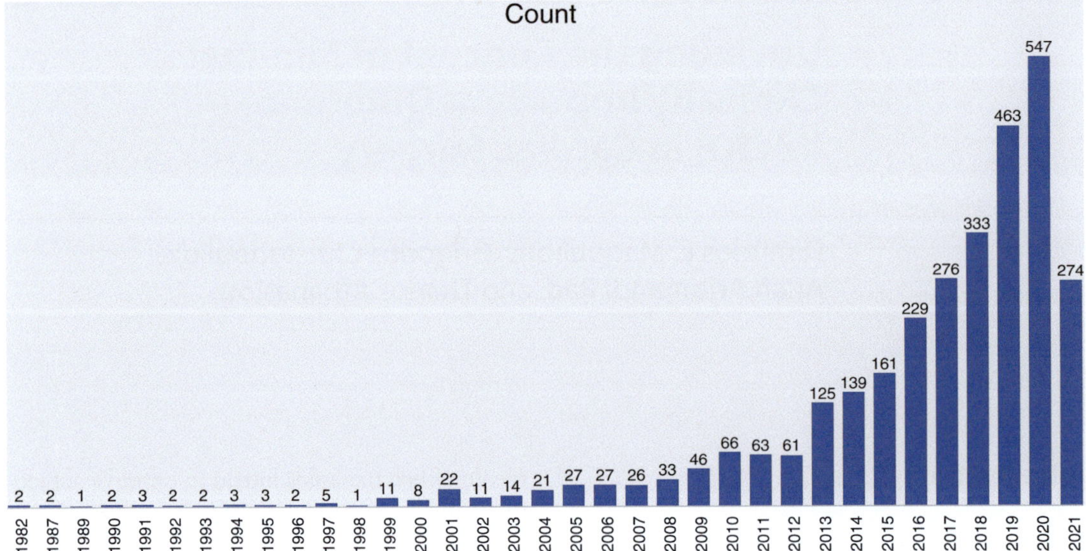

Fig. 1.1 Number of published articles per year regarding Minimal Clinically Important Difference (MCID) according to the PubMed (Medline) database

aim to unveil the potential role and value of MCID in cardiac surgery.

The Purpose of Employing the MCID

In recent years there has been an extended implementation of MCID in various medical specialties (Fig. 1.1).

The concept behind the employment and implementation of the MCID is to provide an appropriate level of clinical data interpretation regarding patient-reported changes, using a numerical scale on the basis of whether the observed change is meaningful to patients, rather than plain statistical importance. In this context, similar changes on a numerical scale may represent different levels of clinical importance in different study populations. In addition, statistical significance is directly linked to the study population size and its characteristics. In fact, when the study population is large, statistically important differences between groups might be small and clinically irrelevant [6]. Consequently, MCID methods have been developed to respond to these challenges.

Statistical and Methodological Concepts Regarding MCID

Given the different nature of the clinical questions that surgeons and physicians pose, there are several concepts of the minimum important difference (MID) including:

1. A difference demonstrating a true change within a population or an individual.
2. A change which reflects cost-effectiveness relevant for healthcare systems.
3. A meaningful difference to patients in cases that interpretation of measures is not intuitive.
4. The necessary difference regarding a prognostic factor to achieve a reduction in a clinical event within a population of study.
5. A change individuals can detect.

Moreover, these concepts affect also the determination of the size of necessary study population that should be enrolled to reliably measure a clinically important effect of an intervention. In fact, the smaller the intervention effect sought, the larger the required study sample [7]. Below we present the main methods to estimate MCID.

Distribution Methods

Distribution-based estimates are associated not only with the outcomes of interest, but also with the context in which they are implemented. For instance, they might differ in response to different interventions or populations, where the variance is homogenous [8]. These estimates rely on the statistical properties of distribution of the outcome scores, along with the variability among patients. They also identify and quantify the magnitude of change that is required to show that the change in an outcome measure is more than would be expected from chance alone [6]. Because distribution-based methods are not derived from individual patient's assessments, they probably should not be used to determine the MCID. Its logic is based on statistical reasoning, where it can only identify a minimum detectable effect, that is, an effect which is unlikely to be attributable to random measurement error. The lack of an "anchor" linking these numerical scores to assessing what is important to patients means that these methods fail to identify important and clinically meaningful outcomes for patients, as they do not include their perspective. In fact, the term MCID is sometimes replaced by "minimal detectable change" when distribution-based methods calculate the difference. For this reason, these methods are not recommended as the first line for the determination of an MCID.

Anchor-Based Methods

Certain MCIDs are employing anchor-based methodologies.

The anchor-based methods allow a comparison between a patient's situation reflected by an outcome measure and an external criterion. This external criterion is nothing more than the patient's perception. This method then compares the changes between scores with an anchor question. For example, if we use the question: "do you feel better after intervention?" as a reference to determine if the patient improved after treatment compared to baseline, based on the patient's own experience. A global pain rating scale ("much worse", "somewhat worse", "almost the same", "somewhat better", and "much better") could be used in this case to understand the patient's impression of change. The anchor question needs to be easily understandable and relevant to patients. Typical anchors may be ratings around a change in health status, presence of symptoms, disease severity, response to treatment, or prognosis of future events such as death.

Those responses that refer to a change "somewhat better" or "much better" are considered of special interest since they inform the researcher of a clinical improvement that patients have verified from their own point of view. The next would be the changes (averages) of the score in the instrument used for each answer to the anchor question in order to establish the points of interest (e.g., minimum difference for improvement or minimum difference for deterioration), often considered as the thresholds that account for the smallest change that correlates with clinical improvement.

The anchor is commonly a measure with an established MID or a patient's subjective rating of change on a 5- or 7-point scale [9]. Anchor-based methods characterize the MCID by relating the change with a numerical scale for a certain outcome. For example, patients may be asked if they felt "about the same," "a little better," or "quite better" after receiving treatment. These categorical responses are then related to the numerical measurement scale used in the study, thus "anchoring" the numerical outcome scale to the categorical assessment that is more meaningful to the patients. Another example is the MCID for the measure of functional status in the study by Hinman et al. [10], which was based on the 75th percentile of the investigated score; 75% of patients reporting an experienced benefit (the anchor) demonstrated an improvement equal to or larger than the derived MCID using this definition. This comparison between the magnitude of change in the test of interest with the known MCID of the anchor might be performed using linear or logistic regression calculations. For example, in a recent study [11] validating the Short Form-36 Health Survey (SF-36) questionnaire in cardiac surgery population, a logistic regression model was employed, to examine independent risk factors for HRQOL deterioration at 6 months post-surgery.

In cases that the anchor is a global rating of change, the rating may be given by the clinician or by the patient, but the existence of different perceptions of what constitutes a meaningful change may differ between them [12]. Furthermore, these anchor-based methods have the advantage of linking the change to a given score to the patient's perspective. Nonetheless, there are certain points that should be taken into consideration, posing certain biases. Individual patients may attribute a different value on a certain benefit (inter-patient variation) or even the same patient may attribute a different value on the same benefit (intra-patient variation) depending on the individual perceptions and circumstances [13]. Many clinical decisions with patients are balanced with potential risks of surgery during counseling. Depending on the individual patient's reflections on the potential value and risks, MCID is affected respectively.

It is important though, when constructing an anchor-based method, that the question for assessing the change is precise and easily understood. According to Copay et al. [14], four variations of the anchor-based method are identified: (1) the intra-patients score change, (2) the inter-patients score change, (3) the sensitivity-and specificity-based method, along with (4) the social comparison approach. To begin with, the intra-patient score is based on patients' rating of their improvement regarding the outcome of interest on a global scale [14]. The inter-patient approach is based on the comparison between the response of patients allocated in two adjacent levels using a global scale. The third approach employs sensitivity and specificity analyses. Sensitivity represents the proportion of patients reporting an improvement with a score exceeding the threshold value, or a true positive outcome. Specificity represents the proportion of patients reporting a deterioration, with a score lower than the threshold value or a true negative outcome. In this context, a sensitivity value of 1 would reflect that all true positives were identified, while a specificity value of 1 would demonstrate that all true negatives were identified. Receiver operating curves (ROCs) are constructed and the area under the curve (AUC) are analyzed to assess the discrimination. The AUC is determined by calculating the 95% confidence intervals and compared using nonparametric paired tests, as described by DeLong et al. [15]. Discrimination is then evaluated as poor, fair or excellent model according to the AUC value of <0.70, 0.70– 0.79 and 0.80–1.00, respectively [15]. Commonly the cut point is taken from the top left of an ROC curve, but this can vary depending on the specific situation as to how important sensitivity and/or specificity are.

The least popular approach is the fourth one. According to this method, patients compare their perceived health status with other patients' status. The MID is derived by the difference between patients assessing their status as superior or inferior, but not similar, compared to the other patients [14]. An example of this approach is provided by Redelmeier et al. [16] who employed a 6 min walk test of 54 m based on a social comparison method. In fact, patients observed other patients completing certain exercises and then compared their own physical status with them [16].

Consensus (Delphi) Methods

Consensus (also known as Delphi) methods represent a panel of experts gathered to provide independent opinions regarding of the meaning of a clinically relevant change. The opinions are revised after the panel members review all assessments, until consensus is reached, and a numerical value is provided for the MCID. An example is the MCID for the pain assessment scale used by Hinman et al. [10] that was provided by employing a Delphi method (Table 1.1).

Limitations of the MCID Methods

To begin with, distribution-based estimates are based mainly on clear statistical reasoning.

Table 1.1 Studies implementing MCID methodology in cardiac surgery

Study	Country	Year	Sample size	MCID method	Variables	Outcome
Grand et al. [11]	France	2018	326	Anchor-based	SF-36 questionnaire	Overall improvement of QoL after cardiac surgery
Blokzijl et al. [17]	Multicenter	2021	899	Anchor-based	SF-36 questionnaire	QoL improvement after aortic valve replacement
Auensen et al. [18]	Norway	2018	442	Anchor-based and Distribution-based	SF-36 and EQ-5D questionnaires	QoL improvement after aortic valve replacement

QoL Quality of Life, *SF-36* Short Form-36 Health Survey

Consequently, they might identify a minimal detectable effect, not attributed to a random measurement error [19]. In this context, the lack of an anchor linking the numeric estimates with an assessment of clinical significance limits the potential of distribution-based methods to identify clinically important outcomes for patients. On this basis, MCID might be replaced by the term "minimal detectable change" when the difference is measured using distribution-based estimates [6]. Finally, distribution-based estimates are not recommended to be employed as a first-line measure of MCID.

The main limitation of anchor-based estimates is the potential bias attributed to the choice of anchor, given that is a subjective assessment. For instance, an anchor based on patients' perception on their improvement after an intervention might produce a recall bias [19]. In this context, the validity of the anchor is important to determine a valid and reliable MCID. Furthermore, anchor-based methods might be affected by the distribution of scores within each category of the anchor. In cases of highly skewed data, the measurement of MCID might be affected by outliers. Besides, anchor-based estimates might be based on an MCID derived from a unique subgroup of patients within a particular category of the anchor, thus leading to unreliable MCID estimates.

On the other hand, consensus methods (delphi-approaches) are based on experts' opinions, rather than patients, to define the MCID. Nonetheless, expert estimates might not represent a reliable method to determine clinically important outcomes for patients.

Potential Pitfalls to Consider When Evaluating Results Based on MCIDs

A not uncommon phenomenon that has been reported in certain studies [10, 20] is the smaller observed effect compared with the predefined MCID. This phenomenon is present when the study population is appropriately selected to achieve a high probability of detecting a benefit equal to the MCID, thus identifying statistically important differences even in cases where the effect of an intervention is smaller than the MCID [19]. Another important aspect of MCIDs is the need to consider potential improvements derived from an intervention in relation to morbidity, mortality and costs. In this context, when defining a meaningful improvement from the patients' perspective it is crucial to consider all aspects of clinical care, both favorable and unfavorable.

Taking everything into consideration, there are certain alternative approaches to derive a MCID and it is crucial for the clinician/scientist/reader to know the way it was measured. As previously was commented not every MCID applies to a particular situation. In addition, the terms MID and MCID are often challenging to distinguish. To face this issue, Houchen-Wolloff et al. [21] have suggested that all MIDs should be described as such, but adding a suffix: MID-S (MID—Statistical), MID-C (MID—Clinical outcome), MID-P (MID—Patient determined). Finally, special caution should be taken when combining different MCID methods. Nonetheless, whichever methodology is chosen and employed, the MCID represents an aiding tool for the interpretation of outcomes and effects measures of interventions.

Real Life Examples of MCID Implementation in Cardiac Surgery

Following a thorough literature search, we have identified only three studies implementing the MCID concept to evaluate quality of life in cardiac surgery [11, 17, 18]. This study employed anchor-based methods to estimate MCID [11]. According to that study, a statistically significant difference was reported regarding preoperative and post-operative quality of life scores [11]. Nonetheless, this difference was below the threshold defined as a MCID [11]. A certain limitation posed in this study was that the MCID was employed in patients undergoing different cardiac surgical operations in different clinical settings [11].

A second study [17] investigated the effect of surgical aortic valve replacement on quality of life, along with the variance with age, especially for patients with a high risk of deterioration. This was an observation, multicenter cohort study conducted according to the REporting of studies Conducted using Observational Routinely collected health Data (RECORD) guidelines [22]. This study implemented the SF-36 questionnaire and used an anchor-based approach to assess the MCID regarding the post-aortic valve replacement quality of life. Based on a MCID of five points we calculated for each patient an increase (≥ 5), decrease (≤ -5) or no change in quality of life [17]. Sensitivity analyses were performed using a MCID of four points [17].

Finally, Auensen et al. [18] compared the quality of life in patients with severe aortic stenosis either operated or medically treated. In this study, the SF-36 and EQ-5D questionnaires were implemented. In fact, an anchor-based approach was used to assess the MCID regarding the SF-36 questionnaire and both an anchor-based and a distribution-based approach were followed regarding the EQ-5D questionnaire. According to the study, quality of life is improved in patients with severe aortic stenosis undergoing aortic valve replacement [18].

Conclusions

In the present study, we tried to present the basic principles of MCID. Given that cardiac surgery is associated with significant morbidity, it represents a surgical field where MCID might be a valuable tool to interpret clinical outcomes. However, it is necessary to validate different MCID methods in the cardiac surgery context.

Main Remarks

- The MCID is defined as the smallest difference in score in any domain or outcome of interest that patients can perceive as beneficial or harmful.
- It helps decisions in clinical practice emphasizing the primacy of patient's perception.
- It is a tool for the calculation of the sample size of studies
- It is a variable concept, and the different methods used for its calculation can generate differential estimates for a health situation limited in creating universally comparable or useful values of health benefit or harm perceptions.

Conflicts of Interest The participating authors declare no conflicts of interest.

Ethical Approval Does not apply.

Informed Consent Does not apply.

Acknowledgements Does not apply.

References

1. Jaeschke R, Singer J, Guyatt GH. Measurement of health status: ascertaining the minimal clinically important difference. Control Clin Trials. 1989;10(4):407–15.
2. Williams JE, Singh SJ, Sewell L, et al. Development of a self-reported Chronic Respiratory Questionnaire (CRQ-SR). Thorax. 2001;56(12):954–9.

3. Falcoz PE, Chocron S, Stoica L, et al. Open heart surgery: One-year self-assessment of quality of life and functional outcome. Ann Thorac Surg. 2003;76:1598–604.
4. Rumsfeld JS, MaWhinney S, McCarthy M Jr, et al. Health-related quality of life as a predictor of mortality following coronary artery bypass graft surgery. Participants of the department of veterans affairs cooperative study group on processes, structures, and outcomes of care in cardiac surgery. JAMA. 1999;281:1298–303.
5. Rumsfeld JS, Magid DJ, O'Brien M, et al. Changes in health-related quality of life following coronary artery bypass graft surgery. Ann Thorac Surg. 2001;72:2026–32.
6. Turner D, Schünemann HJ, Griffith LE, et al. The minimal detectable change cannot reliably replace the minimal important difference. J Clin Epidemiol. 2010;63(1):28–36.
7. Livingston EH, Elliot A, Hynan L, Cao J. Effect size estimation: a necessary component of statistical analysis. Arch Surg. 2009;144(8):706–12.
8. Troosters T. How important is a minimal difference? Eur Respir J. 2011;37(4):755–6.
9. Redelmeier DA, Lorig K. Assessing the clinical importance of symptomatic improvements. An illustration in rheumatology. Arch Intern Med. 1993;153(11):1337–42.
10. Hinman RS, McCrory P, Pirotta M, et al. Acupuncture for chronic knee pain: a randomized clinical trial. JAMA. https://doi.org/10.1001/jama.2014.12660.
11. Grand N, Bouchet JB, Zufferey P, et al. Quality of life after cardiac surgery based on the minimal clinically important difference concept, Ann Thorac Surg. 2018. https://doi.org/10.1016/j.athoracsur.2018.02.050.
12. Schunemann HJ, Guyatt GH. Commentary – goodbye M(C)ID! Hello MID, where do you come from? Health Serv Res. 2005;40(2):593–7.
13. Bellamy N, Carette S, Ford PM, et al. Osteoarthritis antirheumatic drug trials: III, setting the delta for clinical trials: results of a consensus development (Delphi) exercise. J Rheumatol. 1992;19(3):451–7.
14. Copay AG, Subach BR, Glassman SD, et al. Understanding the minimum clinically important difference: a review of concepts and methods. Spine J. 2007;7(5):541–6.
15. DeLong ER, DeLong DM, Clarke-Pearson DL. Comparing the areas under two or more correlated receiver operating characteristic curves: a nonparametric approach. Biometrics. 1988;44:837–45.
16. Redelmeier DA, Bayoumi AM, Goldstein RS, et al. Interpreting small differences in functional status: the Six Minute Walk test in chronic lung disease patients. Am J Respir Crit Care Med. 1997;155(4):1278–82.
17. Blokzijl F, Houterman S, van Straten BHM, Daeter E, Bruinsma GJBB, Dieperink W, Reneman MF, Keus F, van der Horst ICC, Mariani MA. The impact of surgical aortic valve replacement on quality of life-a multicenter study. J Thorac Cardiovasc Surg. 2021;161(4):1204–1210.e7. https://doi.org/10.1016/j.jtcvs.2019.09.184.
18. Auensen A, Hussain AI, Garratt AM, Gullestad LL, Pettersen KI. Patient-reported outcomes after referral for possible valve replacement in patients with severe aortic stenosis. Eur J Cardiothorac Surg. 2018;53:129–35.
19. McGlothlin AE, Lewis RJ. Minimal clinically important difference: defining what really matters to patients. JAMA. 2014;312(13):1342–3. https://doi.org/10.1001/jama.2014.13128.
20. Ikramuddin S, Blackstone RP, Brancatisano A, et al. Effect of reversible intermittent intra-abdominal vagal nerve blockade on morbid obesity: the ReCharge randomized clinical trial. JAMA. 2014;312(9):915–22.
21. Houchen-Wolloff L, Evans RA. Unravelling the mystery of the 'minimum important difference' using practical outcome measures in chronic respiratory disease. Chron Respir Dis. 2019;16:1479973118816491. https://doi.org/10.1177/1479973118816491.
22. Benchimol EI, Smeeth L, Guttmann A, Harron K, Moher D. The reporting of studies conducted using observational routinely-collected health data (RECORD) statement. PLoS Med. 2015;12:e1001885.

Quality of Life Following the Use of Mechanical Circulatory Support Devices

2

Antonios Kourliouros and Steven Tsui

Introduction

The therapeutic algorithm for patients in acute cardiogenic shock and for those with chronic advanced heart failure has changed over the last two decades to reflect the advances in mechanical circulatory support devices (MCSD). Extracorporeal devices provide short-term support and can be used as left ventricular assist device (LVAD), right ventricular assist device (RVAD) or biventricular assist device (BiVAD) by varying the inflow and outflow configurations of the system. For added versatility, a membrane oxygenator can be incorporated into some MCSD to provide respiratory support in addition to circulatory support. The most used means of temporary cardio-respiratory mechanical assistance is the venoarterial extracorporeal membrane oxygenation system (VA ECMO). It is most commonly established by placing an inflow cannula percutaneously through the common femoral vein, and by returning oxygenated blood via an outflow cannula in the common femoral artery (or centrally in cases of post-cardiotomy VA ECMO).

A. Kourliouros (✉)
Heart Centre, Oxford University Hospitals NHS Foundation Trust, Oxford, UK
e-mail: antonios.kourliouros@ouh.nhs.uk

S. Tsui
Royal Papworth Hospital NHS Foundation Trust, Cambridge, UK
e-mail: steven.tsui@nhs.net

Durable MCSD are implanted intrapericardially as single ventricular support, i.e. LVAD or RVAD, or as biventricular support i.e. BiVAD or total artificial heart (TAH). The inflow of durable LVADs drains from the apex of the left ventricle and the outflow graft originating from the pump is anastomosed end-to-side onto the ascending aorta. In general, durable MCSD are used to treat patients with advanced heart failure who are unlikely to survive until a donor heart is available, i.e. as a bridge to heart transplantation (BTT), or as an alternative to heart transplant for those ineligible for transplantation, i.e. as destination therapy (DT). It is now established that both extracorporeal and durable mechanical support therapies provide a survival advantage compared to conventional medical interventions. The aim of this chapter is to explore whether these invasive treatments confer a reasonable quality of life (QoL) for treated patients. In cases of acute cardiogenic shock treated with temporary MCSD, do survivors return to a reasonable QoL? For patients implanted with durable LVADs, do they experience a QoL benefit in addition to survival benefit?

Methods

A Medline (Pubmed interface) search was conducted for studies published between January 2000 and October 2020 using the following crite-

T. Athanasiou et al. (eds.), *Patient Reported Outcomes and Quality of Life in Cardiovascular Interventions*,
https://doi.org/10.1007/978-3-031-09815-4_2

ria: heart-assist devices [MeSH Term] AND (quality of life). A total of 944 articles were identified and screened according to relevance to the subject. The reference list of the studies that were critically evaluated was also screened for the inclusion of health-related QoL outcomes as endpoints. It was apparent that several publications represented longitudinal studies and included the same cohort of LVAD patients that was examined at different time points. When this occurred, the publication with the longest follow-up was selected for inclusion e.g. HeartMate 3 CE Mark Study at 2 years [1] instead of the 6-month report from the same cohort [2]. In addition, different publications used the same registry or patient group for QoL analyses where there might have been a high probability of patient overlap e.g. Interagency Registry for Mechanically Assisted Circulatory Support (INTERMACS) analysis in QoL according to implant strategy [3] versus the most recent INTERMACS database annual report [4]). The studies finally included in the review focused only on durable LVADs because, compared to RVAD and TAH, they account for over 95% of durable MCSD implanted [4].

Extracorporeal MCSD literature search was carried out within the aforementioned terms (heart-assist devices and quality of life), and by performing new searches with additional keywords: ECMO, venoarterial, extracorporeal membrane oxygenation, assisted circulation, short-term mechanical support. Only studies where the focus was on VA ECMO (and not venovenous) were included. Paediatric series were excluded because of the smaller patient numbers, the variability of extracorporeal and durable devices used, and the age-specific QoL tools for this population.

Durable Mechanical Circulatory Support

Ideally, health-related QoL ought to be disease specific. For patients with advanced heart failure, the most widely used assessment tools are the Minnesota Living with Heart Failure (MLWHF) [5] and the Kansas City Cardiomyopathy questionnaire (KCCQ) [6]. The MLWHF questionnaire comprises 21 items with a scale of 0 to 5 depending on impact of heart failure, with a maximum score of 105, signifying worst health-related QoL. The KCCQ questionnaire comprises 23 questions and with appropriate calculations it yields a range from 0 to 100 with higher scores indicating better QoL. The EuroQol 5 dimensions questionnaire (EQ-5D) and its visual analog scale (VAS) is a more generic instrument for assessment of the respondent's general health state while the Patient Health Questionnaire-9 (PHQ-9) is used to assess depression severity. The aforementioned scoring systems were used in studies assessing the effect of durable LVADs on heart failure patients spanning over a period of almost 20 years. During this time, device technology and characteristics changed significantly and we shall provide a brief overview of durable LVADs that are presented in the studies to follow for the non-specialist reader:

The first generation LVADs (e.g. HeartMate XVE) used a pulsatile flow technology, were bulkier, and their implantation included standard full sternotomy incision with an extension of the incision into the abdomen to create a pocket for the actual pump head. The second generation LVADs (e.g. HeartMate II) feature rotary-pump technology and provide continuous flow but, like their first generation counterparts an abdominal pocket had to be created. The improved flow characteristics of second generation LVADs translated into improved survival, reduction in major adverse events and reoperation rates compared with first generation LVADs [7]. Third generation devices (e.g. Heartmate 3, HeartWare HVAD) also provide continuous flow but the rotor features non-contact bearings (as opposed to mechanical bearings of the previous generation) and is suspended in blood flow. They are also smaller and the implantation does not require an abdominal pump pocket. Comparison of the third generation to the second generation LVADs at 2 years demonstrated superiority of the newer pumps both in survival rates and device-related complications [8].

One of the first studies to include QoL metrics in patients receiving durable LVADs was the randomised assessment of continuous flow (HeartMate II) against first generation devices (HeartMate XVE) [7]. With a total of 200 patients enrolled, it was apparent that both systems led to a significant improvement in QoL from baseline. The MLWHF score decreased from 75.4 to 37.4 at 3 months in the HeartMate II group and from 76.1 to 42.1 in the HeartMate XVE. Likewise, the KCCQ score improved from 27.4 at baseline to 63.4 at 3 months in the HeartMate II and from 26.5 to 56.7 in the HeartMate XVE within the same time period.

A focused assessment of QoL in patients receiving the HeartMate II LVAD as part of the BTT and DT trials (n = 655) demonstrated significant improvement at 6 months, in both the MLWHF score (38% and 52% for BTT and DT groups respectively) and KCCQ score (79% and 92% for BTT and DT groups achieved an improvement of >5 points, respectively) [9]. Sustained improved QoL was observed in patients in the DT group beyond 6 months and to the last follow-up at 24 months.

After the original publication of the HeartMate II DT trial (comparison of second generation against the first generation device) [7], QoL was assessed between the original 133 patients receiving their HMII LVAD at the outset of the trial and those half-way through (n = 281), assuming a potential change in clinical outcomes alongside the increased clinical experience of the trialists [10]. The heart failure QoL models used were MLWHF and KCCQ. An increase in QoL was observed in both the early-trial and mid-trial groups against their baseline at 6 months (KCCQ from 28 ± 18 to 70 ± 21 for the mid-trial and from 27 ± 16 to 64 ± 20 for the early-trial group). Whereas KCCQ score showed only a marginal improvement in the mid-trial vs the early-trial patients over time ($p = 0.08$), the MLWHF score was significantly improved in the mid-trial group.

The ROADMAP study was an observational comparison of end-stage heart failure patients receiving a second generation durable LVAD against optimal medical management (OMM) [11]. While acknowledging the lack of randomisation, a significant survival benefit was apparent in LVAD recipients at 24 months (70 ± 5% vs 41 ± 5%) with an improved functional assessment as measured with 6-minute walk distance. The 24-month follow up study was focused on QoL parameters as survival alone may not accurately represent the value of this intervention. Pairwise comparisons of PHQ-9 and EQ-5D VAS from baseline to 24 months were carried out for all survivors to that time-point. In the OMM group a modest increase of 8 ± 20 points in the EQ-5D score was observed against 27 ± 24 point increase in the LVAD group ($p < 0.001$). The PHQ-9 score was decreased following the LVAD by 4.6 points, which was a significant change, against 1.8 ± 6.3 point decrease in the OMM group (note that the lower the PHQ-9 score the lower the depression severity). In a sub-study of ROADMAP focusing on QoL parameters and outcomes, in patients with baseline EQ-5D VAS < 55 event free survival was significantly better with LVAD compared to their OMM counterparts (82 ± 5% vs 58 ± 7%, $p = 0.004$) [12]. Baseline EQ-5D VAS ≥ 55 was not associated with a difference in outcomes across the two different treatment arms. These findings can have important implications in the decision-making for end-stage HF patients with reasonable baseline QoL where LVAD may not exceed OMM in terms of health status improvement and that persevering with medical management may indeed be the best option in this subgroup.

Case series have included QoL in their composite outcome. When poor QoL (KCCQ < 45) was assessed among other events (e.g. death, stroke and recurrent hospitalisation) at 1 year following a durable LVAD, its occurrence was in the region of 10% [13]. With 46% of missing KCCQ follow-up assessments the contribution of QoL measurements to the poor composite outcome may have been under-represented.

One of the first studies to include QoL outcomes in patients receiving a third generation centrifugal pump (HeartWare HVAD) was the ADVANCE trial [14]. In the 140 patients where the device was implanted as BTT, QoL baseline assessment was carried out with EQ-5D VAS and KCCQ, and 6-month QoL changes was a prespecified secondary end point. The EQ-5D VAS score showed a 28 ± 25 point increase from baseline and the KCCQ a 30 ± 26 point increase, both statistically significant.

In a single-arm clinical trial of the HeartMate 3 LVAD systems with a 2-year follow up, a significant improvement in QoL was observed in patients receiving durable mechanical support against their preoperative status [1]. The investigators used the EQ-5D VAS (at 1, 3, 6, 12 and 24-month time points) which appeared in linearity with patients' objective improvement in 6-minute walk test. Mean baseline EQ-5D VAS was 48.2 and increased to 70.6 at 2 years ($p < 0.001$). The ELEVATE registry [15] succeeded the aforementioned trial, as provided QoL data for the HeartMate 3 in the post-market approval setting in a larger cohort of 482 patients (of whom 189 had EQ-5D VAS paired assessment). There was a significant improvement in QoL from 36 points at baseline to 67 by 6 months.

When variations in QoL were assessed between patients receiving the newer generation HeartMate 3 against the HeartMate II (as part of the MOMENTUM 3 clinical trial) there were no significant differences at 6 months [16]. The change from baseline score in KCCQ was 28 for the HeartMate 3 and 29 for the HeartMate II and −1 and −2 in HeartMate 3 and HeartMate II, respectively, for EQ-5D-5L (note that a negative difference in this version of EQ signifies better QoL). Serious adverse events affected EQ-5D-5L outcomes at 6 months but not KCCQ ones, which continued being significantly better from baseline across all recipients of a durable LVADs.

In the ENDURANCE clinical trial [17] and similarly to the previous study, the third generation HeartWare HVAD was compared against a the second generation HeartMate II, with QoL outcomes being a pre-specified secondary endpoint. The HVAD achieved a significant increase from baseline of 25.8 points in the KCCQ score and of 22.5 in EQ-5D VAS at three months. This trend was maintained at the last follow-up at 24 months.

The INTERMACS report provides QoL data for the largest published cohort of durable MCS patients [4]. Of the total of 18,539 patients who underwent continuous flow LVAD, 9,893 patients provided QoL data by completing the EQ-5D VAS and 7,489 the KCCQ. The main finding, which was consistent in both QoL tools, was a substantial improvement within the first 3 months post implantation (from 45 to 71 for EuroQol and from 34.5 to 63.3 for KCCQ) and a plateau of approximately 73 and 66 for up to 5 years in EQ-5D VAS and KCCQ, respectively. In this North American registry, some of the patient characteristics but more importantly the indication for LVAD support, evolved across the 11 years of analysis with patients having a more favourable preoperative risk profile with time and DT being more prevalent than BTT. Therefore, the QoL data in this study could have been influenced by the changes in patient selection and type of device used at the different time-points. The publications that report QoL following implantation specifically of third generation LVADs are included in Table 2.1, as they are

Table 2.1 Studies that include QoL data following implantation specifically of third generation durable LVADs

Author, date	Device used	Cohort	QoL instruments used	Baseline QoL	QoL at 6 months	QoL at last follow-up	Comments
Schmitto J, 2019 [1]	HeartMate 3	50 patients (43 had QoL assessment)	EQ-5D VAS	48.2	N/A	70.6, P < 0.001 (at 2 years)	CE mark trial
Gustafsson F, 2018 [15]	HeartMate 3	482 patients (253 had QoL assessment of whom 189 had paired assessment)	EQ-5D VAS	36	67	67, P < 0.001 (at 6 months)	European registry following commercial use of device

Table 2.1 (continued)

Author, date	Device used	Cohort	QoL instruments used	Baseline QoL	QoL at 6 months	QoL at last follow-up	Comments
Cowger J, 2018 [16]	HeartMate 3	153 patients	EQ-5D-5L KCCQ	11 [7–15] 40 [23–58]	Δ = −1 [−5 to 0] Δ = +28 [10 to 46]	As per previous cell, P < 0.001	Second generation LVAD cases used as a comparator—no difference in QoL between second and third generation LVAD
Rogers J, 2017 [17]	HeartWare	288 patients	EQ-5D VAS KCCQ	Numerical data not available	Δ = +22.5 at 3 months Δ = +25.8 at 3 months	Sustained improvement, absolute numbers not available	Second generation LVAD cases used as a comparator—no difference in QoL between second and third generation LVAD
Aaronson K, 2012 [14]	HeartWare	140 patients	EQ-5D VAS KCCQ	40 ± 24 35 ± 19	70 ± 20 67 ± 21	As per previous cell, P < 0.001	Control subjects from INTERMACS registry

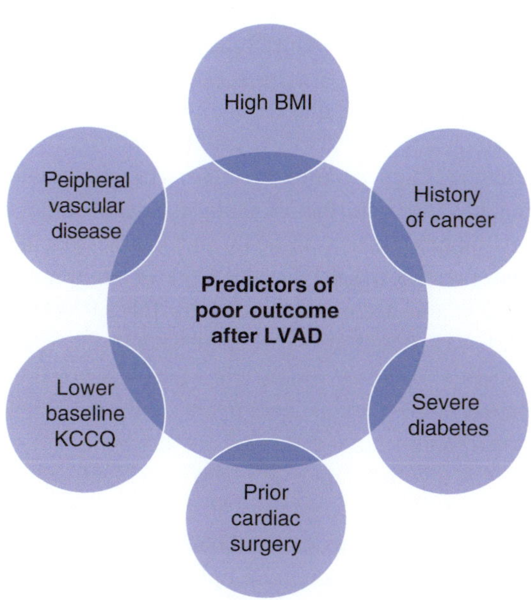

Fig. 2.1 Predictors of poor outcome following durable LVADs

more relevant to the contemporary heart failure clinician. Poor outcomes, defined as death or KCCQ < 45 at one year after LVAD implantation, have been observed in up to 30% of recipients and certain baseline predictors associated with poor outcomes have been identified [18] (Fig. 2.1).

Extracorporeal Devices

Venoarterial ECMO has been implemented by an increasing number of centres in the management of acute catastrophic cardiogenic shock, including cardiopulmonary resuscitation. Whereas crude outcomes such as mortality, cerebrovascular events, vascular complications and others can be assessed and collected with a satisfactory degree of accuracy, QoL outcome analysis is hindered by two main factors. Firstly, the acuity of the condition requiring VA ECMO precludes baseline QoL assessment; patients in shock are often agitated and occasionally intubated and ventilated. The lack of baseline health status removes the reference point for any comparisons. Secondly, post-recovery health quality may not be just the effect of the intervention, i.e. VA

ECMO, but also of the medical condition that precipitated shock e.g. a massive heart attack.

The largest study of VA ECMO patients to include QoL outcomes is the one used to create a risk stratification tool, the ENCOURAGE score [19]. Out of 138 patients who received VA ECMO for ischaemic cardiogenic shock, 65 (47%) survived and 57 contributed to QoL assessment. Short-Form health survey (SF-36) results were available after a median 32-month follow up and demonstrated inferior physical functioning and general health scores compared to age and sex matched controls. The authors concluded that when their cohort was assessed against acute MI survivors in the bibliography, with or without cardiogenic shock, their QoL outcomes compared favourably, speculating that the role of the underlying disease, rather than the MCSD therapy, was responsible for poorer QoL.

In an analysis of ECMO survivors (n = 30), which represented 40% of the original cohort, 20 eligible patients had health-related QoL assessments with the use of SF-36 and with EQ-5D-5L [20]. Compared with age-matched data, VA ECMO survivors had physical QoL in the lower normal range although none reported extreme problems and only one had experienced severe problems with physical activities.

It is established that patients in acute cardiogenic shock with INTERMACS 1 have poorer outcomes following durable LVAD implantation and VA ECMO is often used as a bridge to bridge with future consideration of LVAD, or bridge to decision following stabilisation of haemodynamics and metabolic profile. The QoL of patients with INTERMACS 1 bridged to LVAD with VA ECMO against those who received a primary LVAD was assessed in an observational study by Unai and colleagues [21]. There were no pre-implant QoL data for the VA ECMO to LVAD group due to the acuity of their condition but post-implant data between this group and the primary LVAD groups were similar. Other than the small numbers in the available QoL data in the VA ECMO to LVAD group (n = 7), a comparison of this INTERMACS 1 cohort with the primary LVAD group as a whole can be misleading because most patients in the latter group were either elective or semi-elective cases. Likewise, there is possibly a selection-bias within INTERMACS 1 patients as there was almost an equal number of those who were bridged with ECMO (n = 22) and those who had an urgent primary LVAD (n = 21).

Conclusions

In this chapter, it is apparent that durable LVAD implantation, irrespective of the indication (DT or BTT), is associated with improved QoL. Device characteristics and evolution, improvement in implantation techniques and standardised management in hospital and in the community have contributed to better outcomes, which could translate in higher patient satisfaction. Interpretation of the data from the presented studies has to be treated with caution as: (a) large observational studies where different generation durable LVADs were pooled may not be able to distinguish the effect of newer and smaller devices on QoL and (b) survivorship bias can also give falsely high longer-term satisfaction rates; those that suffered a life-changing complication or died are naturally excluded from QoL assessments.

It is imperative that LVAD implantation in the modern era also focuses on 'beyond survival' benefits. Data capture in these patients should include QoL information using validated generic instruments (such as EQ-5D) and disease-specific ones (such as MLWHF or KCCQ) for a minimum of 2 years, as recommended by INTERMACS [22]. We should also recognise that in the VAD patient's journey there is inter-relationship between the patient, caregivers, and healthcare practitioners, and that QoL assessments often require a holistic approach with novel QoL determinants that can capture well-being against the increased obligations of stakeholders [23].

Finally, the exponential uptake of VA ECMO in the management of acute cardiogenic shock (with over 25,000 cases per annum performed internationally) should translate into acceptable health-related outcomes in addition to improved survival, and future studies ought to include QoL metrics in their endpoints.

Conclusions	
1	Durable LVAD implantation leads to improved quality of life compared to baseline
2	Evolution of device technology reduced the rate of complications, which has impacted positively the quality of life of the recipients
3	Different indications for LVAD (destination therapy vs bridge to transplantation) and non-specific quality of life assessment tools hinder the extrapolation of results
4	Quality of life outcomes are often absent in large studies or form non pre-specified endpoints, introducing further bias
5	Increased uptake of LVADs as destination therapy, makes quality of life equally important to survival as a metric of their efficacy
6	The acuity of conditions requiring temporary mechanical support limits quality of life assessments against baseline within groups

References

1. Schmitto JD, Pya Y, Zimpfer D, Krabatsch T, Garbade J, Rao V, et al. Long-term evaluation of a fully magnetically levitated circulatory support device for advanced heart failure—two-year results from the HeartMate 3 CE Mark Study. Eur J Heart Fail. 2019;21:90–7. https://doi.org/10.1002/ejhf.1284.
2. Netuka I, Sood P, Pya Y, Zimpfer D, Krabatsch T, Garbade J, et al. Fully magnetically levitated left ventricular assist system for treating advanced HF: a multicenter study. J Am Coll Cardiol. 2015;66:2579–89. https://doi.org/10.1016/j.jacc.2015.09.083.
3. White-Williams C, Fazeli PL, Kirklin JK, Pamboukian SV, Grady KL. Differences in health-related quality of life by implant strategy: analyses from the interagency registry for mechanically assisted circulatory support. J Hear Lung Transplant. 2020;39:62–73. https://doi.org/10.1016/j.healun.2019.10.002.
4. Kormos RL, Cowger J, Pagani FD, Teuteberg JJ, Goldstein DJ, Jacobs JP, et al. The society of thoracic surgeons intermacs database annual report: evolving indications, outcomes, and scientific partnerships. Ann Thorac Surg. 2019;107:341–53. https://doi.org/10.1016/j.athoracsur.2018.11.011.
5. Rector TS, Cohn JN. Assessment of patient outcome with the Minnesota Living with Heart Failure questionnaire: reliability and validity during a randomized, double-blind, placebo-controlled trial of pimobendan. Am Heart J. 1992;124:1017–25. https://doi.org/10.1016/0002-8703(92)90986-6.
6. Green CP, Porter CB, Bresnahan DR, Spertus JA. Development and evaluation of the Kansas City cardiomyopathy questionnaire: a new health status measure for heart failure. J Am Coll Cardiol. 2000;35:1245–55. https://doi.org/10.1016/S0735-1097(00)00531-3.
7. Slaughter MS, Rogers JG, Milano CA, Russell SD, Conte JV, Feldman D, et al. Advanced heart failure treated with continuous-flow left ventricular assist device. N Engl J Med. 2009;361:2241–51. https://doi.org/10.1056/nejmoa0909938.
8. Mehra MR, Uriel N, Naka Y, Cleveland JC, Yuzefpolskaya M, Salerno CT, et al. A fully magnetically levitated left ventricular assist device — final report. N Engl J Med. 2019;380:1618–27. https://doi.org/10.1056/nejmoa1900486.
9. Rogers JG, Aaronson KD, Boyle AJ, Russell SD, Milano CA, Pagani FD, et al. Continuous flow left ventricular assist device improves functional capacity and quality of life of advanced heart failure patients. J Am Coll Cardiol. 2010;55:1826–34. https://doi.org/10.1016/j.jacc.2009.12.052.
10. Park SJ, Milano CA, Tatooles AJ, Rogers JG, Adamson RM, Steidley DE, et al. Outcomes in advanced heart failure patients with left ventricular assist devices for destination therapy. Circ Hear Fail. 2012;5:241–8. https://doi.org/10.1161/CIRCHEARTFAILURE.111.963991.
11. Starling RC, Estep JD, Horstmanshof DA, Milano CA, Stehlik J, Shah KB, et al. Risk assessment and comparative effectiveness of left ventricular assist device and medical management in ambulatory heart failure patients: the ROADMAP study 2-year results. JACC Hear Fail. 2017;5:518–27. https://doi.org/10.1016/j.jchf.2017.02.016.
12. Stehlik J, Estep JD, Selzman CH, Rogers JG, Spertus JA, Shah KB, et al. Patient-reported health-related quality of life is a predictor of outcomes in ambulatory heart failure patients treated with left ventricular assist device compared with medical management: results from the ROADMAP study (risk assessment and comparative effectiveness of left ventricular assist device and medical management). Circ Hear Fail. 2017;10:e003910. https://doi.org/10.1161/CIRCHEARTFAILURE.116.003910.
13. Fendler TJ, Nassif ME, Kennedy KF, Joseph SM, Silvestry SC, Ewald GA, et al. Global outcome in patients with left ventricular assist devices. Am J Cardiol. 2017;119:1069–73. https://doi.org/10.1016/j.amjcard.2016.12.014.
14. Aaronson KD, Slaughter MS, Miller LW, McGee EC, Cotts WG, Acker MA, et al. Use of an intrapericardial, continuous-flow, centrifugal pump in patients awaiting heart transplantation. Circulation. 2012;125:3191–200. https://doi.org/10.1161/CIRCULATIONAHA.111.058412.
15. Gustafsson F, Shaw S, Lavee J, Saeed D, Pya Y, Krabatsch T, et al. Six-month outcomes after treatment of advanced heart failure with a full magnetically levitated continuous flow left ventricular assist device: report from the ELEVATE registry. Eur Heart J. 2018;39:3454–60. https://doi.org/10.1093/eurheartj/ehy513.
16. Cowger JA, Naka Y, Aaronson KD, Horstmanshof D, Gulati S, Rinde-Hoffman D, et al. Quality of life and functional capacity outcomes in the MOMENTUM

3 trial at 6 months: a call for new metrics for left ventricular assist device patients. J Hear Lung Transplant. 2018;37:15–24. https://doi.org/10.1016/j.healun.2017.10.019.
17. Rogers JG, Pagani FD, Tatooles AJ, Bhat G, Slaughter MS, Birks EJ, et al. Intrapericardial left ventricular assist device for advanced heart failure. N Engl J Med. 2017;376:451–60. https://doi.org/10.1056/nejmoa1602954.
18. Arnold SV, Jones PG, Allen LA, Cohen DJ, Fendler TJ, Holtz JE, et al. Frequency of poor outcome (Death or Poor Quality of Life) after left ventricular assist device for destination therapy. Circ Hear Fail. 2016;9. https://doi.org/10.1161/CIRCHEARTFAILURE.115.002800.
19. Muller G, Flecher E, Lebreton G, Luyt CE, Trouillet JL, Bréchot N, et al. The ENCOURAGE mortality risk score and analysis of long-term outcomes after VA-ECMO for acute myocardial infarction with cardiogenic shock. Intensive Care Med. 2016;42:370–8. https://doi.org/10.1007/s00134-016-4223-9.
20. Ørbo MC, Karlsen SF, Pedersen EP, Hermansen SE, Rønning PB, Nergaard KA, et al. Health-related quality of life after extracorporeal membrane oxygenation: a single centre's experience. ESC Hear Fail. 2019;6:701–10. https://doi.org/10.1002/ehf2.12433.
21. Unai S, Yamane K, Tanaka D, Cook G, Hirose H, Cavarocchi NC, et al. Quality of life and mid-term survival of patients bridged with extracorporeal membrane oxygenation to left ventricular assist device. ASAIO J. 2017;63:273–8. https://doi.org/10.1097/MAT.0000000000000471.
22. Grady KL, Warner Stevenson L, Pagani FD, Teuteberg J, Pamboukian SV, Birks E, et al. Beyond survival: recommendations from INTERMACS for assessing function and quality of life with mechanical circulatory support. J Hear Lung Transplant. 2012;31:1158–64. https://doi.org/10.1016/j.healun.2012.08.020.
23. Ko KHK, Straker K, Dunn JL, Wrigley C. What really matters? Understanding quality of life determinants impacting ventricular assist device stakeholders. ASAIO J. 2020;66:626–36. https://doi.org/10.1097/MAT.0000000000001175.

3 What Factors Predict an Improved Quality of Life Outcome Following Coronary Artery Bypass Graft Surgery? A Systematic Review

Yusuf S. Abdullahi, Sanjay Chaubey, Roberto Casula, and Thanos Athanasiou

Aim

The aim of this study was to systematically review the literature on HRQOL following CABG surgery in all patient groups.

Introduction

Coronary artery disease (CAD) has a significant prevalence in the developed world and is considered to be one of the leading causes of premature death worldwide [1]. While it remains a key contributor to the global burden of disease, patterns show that mortality rates have directly declined in the past two decades [1]. This has been attributed to several factors—namely that the issue has been targeted holistically from a biopsychosocial perspective which has yielded this reduction [2].

Two of the leading treatments of coronary artery disease are myocardial revascularisation by means of percutaneous coronary intervention (PCI) or coronary artery bypass grafting (CABG) [3]. PCI involves arterial puncture, wire insertion and stent utilization for arterial revascularisation [4] whereas CABG is a surgical option that involves the use of autologous blood vessels (venous or arterial) to bypass distal to points of stenosis [3].

Despite being effective at relieving symptoms as well as improving survival, in recent years, there has been a shift away from CABG, with nearly half as many operations being performed in 2012 compared to 2006 [3]. In saying this it should be noted that, according to the AHA/ACC guidelines, there continues to be good evidence supporting the use of CABG, particularly in the case of left main coronary artery stenosis as well as triple vessel disease [5]. Additionally, improved perioperative care as well as surgical technique over the past 20 years has allowed this operation to be performed with an ever decreasing mortality and morbidity [3].

As the main protagonists of treatment options for this disease, clinicians treating CAD ought to approach the condition from a holistic standpoint. Indeed, the World Health Organisation's (WHO) definition of health states that health is not merely the absence of disease but encompasses domains of physical, mental and social wellbeing [6] or in other words, the (health related) quality of life (HRQOL).

Y. S. Abdullahi (✉) · T. Athanasiou
Department of Cardiothoracic Surgery, Imperial College Healthcare NHS Trust, Hammersmith Hospital, London, UK

Department of Surgery and Cancer, Imperial College London, London, UK
e-mail: y.abdullahi14@imperial.ac.uk; t.athanasiou@imperial.ac.uk

S. Chaubey · R. Casula
Department of Cardiothoracic Surgery, Imperial College Healthcare NHS Trust, Hammersmith Hospital, London, UK
e-mail: s.chaubey@nhs.net; roberto.casula@nhs.net

T. Athanasiou et al. (eds.), *Patient Reported Outcomes and Quality of Life in Cardiovascular Interventions*, https://doi.org/10.1007/978-3-031-09815-4_3

HRQOL can be defined as an "individual's perception of their position in life in the context of the culture and value systems in which they live and in relation to their goals, expectations, standards and concerns" [7]. Given the subjective measure of HRQOL, many scales exist which attempt to provide an objective numerical number to assign HRQOL. Broadly speaking, research previously conducted on HRQOL in a cardiothoracic context has generally shown that it improves post-operatively compared to baseline levels [8].

Due to the sparse amount of information available, as well as the importance of HRQOL and on-going place of CABG in myocardial revascularisation, this study aims to explore whether there is an association between CABG and improved HRQOL after surgery, as well as the potential predictors, both patient and operative, for an improved outcome.

Materials and Methods

This study was performed in accordance with guidelines for the 'Preferred Reporting Items for Systematic reviews and Meta-Analyses' (PRISMA) [8]. A systematic search was carried out using MEDLINE (1950 to date), EMBASE (1980 to date) and PsycINFO (1966 to date) databases using the following MESH terms: [coronary artery bypass grafting OR cardiac surgery] AND [health related quality of life] OR [quality of life].

Inclusion Criteria

All articles focusing on isolated CABG without concomitant cardiac procedures were generally considered. This did not necessarily exclude studies comparing CABG with PCI or medical therapy. Secondly, a variety of factors including demographics as well as operative technique were analysed to determine their effect on HRQOL. Of particular interest was the physical and mental component in HRQOL measures.

Study Quality Scoring

Quality assessment of each study was performed by attributing a quality assessment score using a modified Newcastle–Ottawa scale [9]. The scale was modified to include all 17 EuroSCORE II cardiac risk factors as well as baseline physical, social and mental health function for comparability. This is shown in Table 3.1.

Table 3.1 Criteria for quality assessment. Modified Newcastle–Ottawa scoring criteria

Quality checklist
Selection
1. Assignment for treatment—any criteria reported? (If yes, 1-star)
2. How representative was the reference group in relation to the general population undergoing CABG (If yes, 1 star, no star if the patients were selected or selection of group was not described)
3. How representative was the comparison group in relation to the general population for CABG? (If drawn from the same community as the reference group, 1-star, no star if drawn from a different source or selection of group was not described)
Comparability
Comparability variables: (1) age; (2) gender; (3) renal function; (4) extracardiac arteriopathy; (5) poor mobility; (6) previous cardiac surgery; (7) chronic lung disease; (8) active endocarditis; (9) critical preoperative state; (10) IDDM; (11) NYHA; (12) CCS IV; (13) LV function; (14) recent MI; (15) pulmonary hypertension; (16) urgency; (17) combined; (18) physical function score; (19) mental function score; (20) social function score
4. Groups comparable for 1, 2, 3, 4, 5, 6, 7, 8, 9 (If yes, 1-star was assigned for each of these. No star was assigned if the groups differed
5. Groups comparable for 10, 11, 12, 13, 14, 15, 16, 17(If yes, 1-star was assigned for each of these. No star was assigned if the two groups differed)
6. Groups comparable for 18, 19, 20 (If yes, 1-star assigned for each of these. No star was assigned if the groups differed)
Outcome assessment
7. Clearly defined outcome of interest (If yes, 1-star)
8. Follow-up (1-star if described)

IDDM insulin dependent diabetes mellitus, *MIVS* minimally invasive valve surgery, *NYHA* New York Heart Comparability includes all the EuroSCORE II risk-factors

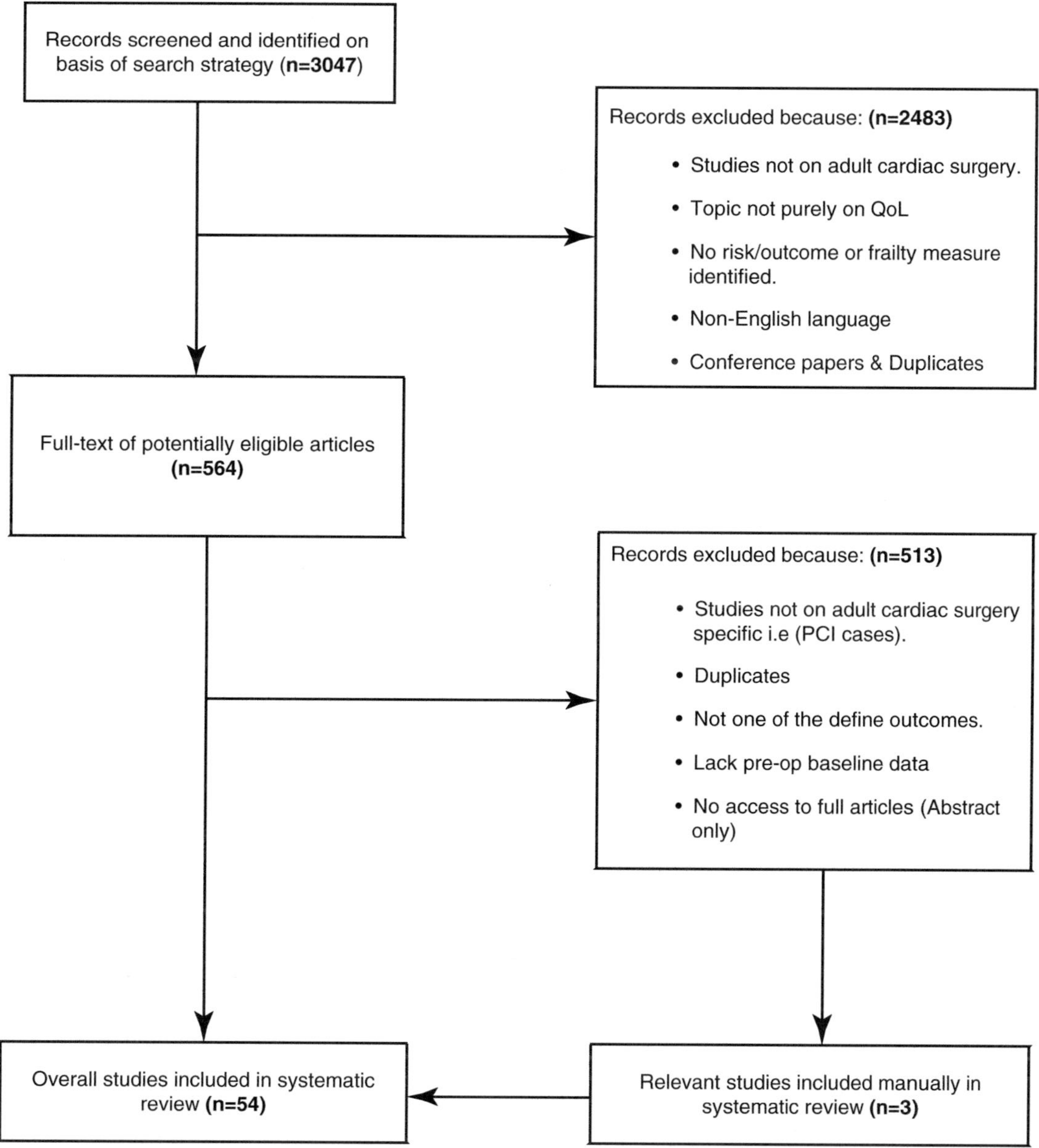

Fig. 3.1 Flow diagram of CABG QoL study selection

Results

Our literature search yielded 3047 studies (Fig. 3.1), of which 54 articles with a total patient population of 23,513 fulfilled our inclusion criteria. The data gathered from all the included studies are shown in Tables 3.2 and 3.3.

Study Design

First to note is the variability in study design. One of the incorporated studies compared CABG to best medical therapy in a randomized prospective study design. The remaining studies used CABG only as the mode of therapy, although the

Table 3.2 Multi-design studies on CABG and QoL

Author, year, Ref	Intervention	Study type	No. of patients at baseline	Age of patients	Follow-up duration (mean)	HRQOL instruments	Conclusion	Physical component improved	Quality score
Azzopardi, 2009 [10]	CABG (n = 48)	Retrospective cohort	48	66.6 (SD 9.9)	2 years	SF-36	Statistically significant improvement in 5 of the SF-36 health domains and in the physical component summary (P < 05)	Improvement in mean score of physical component from 35.2 to 43.3	**
Bjessmo, 2010 [11]	Patients undergoing CABG with ACS N = 62 Patients undergoing CABG with stable angina N = 51	Retrospective cohort study	113	Acute Coronary Syndrome: 61.7 ± 10.2 Stable Angina: 65.6 ± 8.63	10 years	SF-36	Surgical revascularization offers excellent long term QOL, comparable to that of a matched control population. No difference was found between patients with ACS or stable angina pectoris	There was no clinical significant difference in PCS after CABG for ACS or stable angina. The ACS group had a statistically significant lower PCS score than a reference population	********

Bonaros, 2009 [12]	Robot-assisted CABG. Endoscopic (n = 55) vs Sternotomy (n = 56)	Prospective cohort	120	Sternotomy 64.28 ± 7.3 Totally endo 60.28 ± 6.0	6 Months	SF-36	Endoscopic approach leads to improved physical health, shorter hospital stay and a more rapid restoration of daily activities. Conversion does not lead to QOL impairment as compared to primary sternotomy.	Physical function was significantly improved following CABG surgery for the total study population. Most prominently in the endoscopic group	*************
Covinsky, 2008 [13]	Females undergoing CAGs (n = 137) No Procedure (n = 2263)	Prospective cohort	2400	CABG 66.6 ± 0 6.9 No-Op 66.6 ± 6.8	11.5 ± 3.5 months	Duke Activity Status Index (DASI) and RAND	Following CABG surgery in postmenopausal women, on average, HRQOL is virtually identical to the pre-operative baseline. However, there is significant variability, as substantial numbers of women are significantly better or significantly worse	Difference in physical function pre vs post CABG: −0.4 (−2.2, +1.5) Statistical significance not calculated	****

(continued)

Table 3.2 (continued)

Author, year, Ref	Intervention	Study type	No. of patients at baseline	Age of patients	Follow-up duration (mean)	HRQOL instruments	Conclusion	Physical component improved	Quality score
Damgaard, 2011 [14]	Single/Double ITA + Radial grafts: 161 vs Conventional revascularisation using left ITA/ SVGs 170	Prospective cohort	329	Single/Double ITA + Radial grafts: 59 ± 8 Conventional revascularisation using left ITA/ SVGs: 59 ± 8	1 year	SF-36	Health-related quality of life up to 1 year after total arterial revascularization is equal or slightly better than results after conventional coronary surgery	For total arterial revascularization, there were not statistically significant improvements for 'physical component summary' (P = 0.09)	**********
El Baz, 2009 [15]	198 patients -> patient split between care pathway group and conventional care group not stated	Prospective cohort	198	Pathway Group: 64.93 ± 9.60 Conventional Care: 64.83 ± 10.53	6 Months	SF-36	The aims of clinical pathways—reducing LOS and costs, was not fulfilled in the study	Both groups had an improved physical function score compared to baseline, the conventional care group had a higher improvement of physical function when compared to baseline	********
Herlitz, 2009 [16]	Patients undergoing isolated CABG N = 2000	Prospective cohort	2000	62.7 (SD not stated)	15 years	The Nottingham Health Profile, the Psychological General Well-Being Index, and the Physical Activity Score	Despite an ongoing decline in HRQOL over the years, there was still an improvement in most aspects of HRQOL 15 years after CABG compared with that before surgery	A significant improvement in physical function still existed 15 years post CABG compared to baseline, despite ongoing deterioration of overall physical function	**

Hokkanen, 2014 [17]	Patients undergoing isolated CABG N = 508	Prospective cohort	508	62.3 ± 9.3	11.8 years ± 0.48	RAND-36	Despite an ongoing deterioration 12 years after the CABG, there was significant improvement in most dimensions of the HRQOL and functional capacity in comparison with the preoperative values	Physical function significantly improved post CABG, even at 12 year follow up time point. Physical function was better than that reported for general population	**
Jidéus, 2009 [18]	Sternal wound Infection n = 84 CABG group N = 42	Retrospective cohort	126	Sternal wound infection: 68.27 (46.72–81.43) CABG group 65.71 (48.58–78.83)	20 months (range 740)	SF-36	Results confirm that if the patients survive, sternal wound infection is a very serious complication concerning HRQOL. At follow up the patients who had had an infected sternal wound did not improve their HRQOL, regardless no difference in surgical technique used	Physical function for patients with sternal wound infections was below that of the normal population	****

(continued)

Table 3.2 (continued)

Author, year, Ref	Intervention	Study type	No. of patients at baseline	Age of patients	Follow-up duration (mean)	HRQOL instruments	Conclusion	Physical component improved	Quality score
Jrvinen, 2014 [19]	Patients undergoing CABG with perioperative MI N = 8 Patients undergoing CABG without perioperative MI N = 493	Prospective cohort	501	PMI: 65.4 ± 9 Non-PMI: 61.7 ± 9.3	1 year survey: Mean follow up 12.6 ± 1.2 months 12 year survey: mean follow up time 11.8 ± 0.48 years	RAND-36	Although perioperative MI has a negative impact on health-related HRQOL 1 year after CABG, this effect is only minor in the long term. Perioperative MI increases 30-day mortality but shows no effect on later mortality	Patients in both the non- and perioperative MI groups had significantly improved physical function post CABG	***********

Khoueiry, 2011 [22]	Patients undergoing Off-pump CABG N = 50	Prospective cohort	50	63.28 ± 11.20	9 months	Beck Depression Index (BDI) Beck Anxiety Index (BAI) Sheehan Disability Scale (SDS) Quality of Life Enjoyment and Satisfaction Questionnaire (Q-LES-Q)	Despite that all scores returned to or below baseline at 9 months, a high percentage of patients still had depressive symptoms and overall poor quality of life (HRQOL)	nil	**
Kołtowski, 2011 [23]	Patients undergoing isolated CABG N = 86	Prospective cohort	86	63.3 ± 8.93	5 months	EQ-5D	The quality of life significantly improves in the first 4 weeks after cardiac surgery. There is a relation between the patient's age and their reported HRQOL	nil	**
Lee, 2009 [24]	Patients undergoing CABG N = 128	Retrospective cohort (not formally stated)	162	Not stated	5 years	SF-36	study demonstrates that both anxiety and depressive symptoms are strongly implicated in determining PCS 5 years post-CABG using the SF-36	nil	*

(continued)

Table 3.2 (continued)

Author, year, Ref	Intervention	Study type	No. of patients at baseline	Age of patients	Follow-up duration (mean)	HRQOL instruments	Conclusion	Physical component improved	Quality score
Juergens, 2010 [20]	patients undergoing elective cardiac surgery CABG, heart valve surgery, or a combined procedure n = 56	Prospective cohort	56	63.6 ± 11.6	3 months	SF-12	Patients' beliefs about their illness before surgery strongly influence recovery from cardiac surgery. The results suggest that patients could benefit from pre-surgery cognitive interventions aimed at changing maladaptive illness beliefs to improve physical functioning and disability following cardiac surgery	Patients reported higher physical functioning 3 months after surgery compared to presurgery	**
Kapetanakis, 2008 [21]	Off-pump CABG N = 116 On-pump CABG N = 75	Prospective cohort	191	Off-pump CABG 68.5 (42.0 to 85.0) On-pump CABG 66.0 (39.0 to 87.0)	6 months	SF-36	no significant differences in the expected HRQOL at 6 months after either on-pump or off-pump CABG	nil	************

Lie, 2009 [25]	Isolated CABG patients receiving home based intervention program and controls N = 93 Control group N = 92	Randomised controlled trial	203	Intervention group 62 (range 39–77) Control group 62 (range 42–78)	6 months	SF-36	HRQoL after CABG improved markedly over time, but no significant or clinically important differences were found between patients receiving a home based intervention program and controls	PCS in both groups improved from baseline to 6 months following surgery, however there was no difference in PCS between intervention and control group 6 months post operation	**********
Mark, 2014 [26]	Assignment to medical therapy N = 602 Medical therapy + CABG N = 610	Randomised trial	1212	Median age of medical therapy group: 59 (53–67) Median age of CABG + medical therapy group: 60 (54–68)	36 months	The Kansas City Cardiomyopathy Questionnaire SF12 SF36 Cardiac Self-Efficacy Questionnaire EuroQol-5D	In a cohort of symptomatic high-risk patients with ischemic left ventricular dysfunction and multivessel coronary artery disease, CABG plus medical therapy produced clinically important improvements in several health status domains compared with medical therapy alone over 36 months	nil	**********

(continued)

Table 3.2 (continued)

Author, year, Ref	Intervention	Study type	No. of patients at baseline	Age of patients	Follow-up duration (mean)	HRQOL instruments	Conclusion	Physical component improved	Quality score
Markou, 2008 [27]	Group A, primary isolated CABG patients age <65 years: n = 285 group B, primary isolated CABG patients age 65—74 years: n = 210 group C, primary isolated CABG patients age 75 years: n = 73	Retrospective cohort study	568	Group A 56.9 ± 5.8 Group B 69.5 ± 2.8 Group C 77.7 ± 1.9	1 year	EuroQoL questionnaire	Elderly patients have the same improvement of their symptomatic status as younger patients However despite this improvement they have less benefit from CABG regarding to their quality of life and physical activity	For physical activity there is a statistical significant improvement for groups A and B, but the improvement is lesser in group B (mean change 0.2 vs 0.5 in group A). The improvement in PA in group C does not result in a significantly higher follow-up PA ($p = 0.744$)	*********
Merkouris, 2009 [28]	Elderly patients (age > 65) undergoing CABG N = 63	Prospective cohort study	63	72.9 ± 3.7	12 months	The MacNew Heart disease health-related quality of life questionnaire	A high proportion of the patients experienced improvement while a substantial number had exacerbations related to self confidence and dependence to others	67.9% percent of patients improved in the category 'physically restricted or limited', improvement is statistically significant, $p < 0.001$.	**

Middel, 2014 [29]	Patients scheduled for CABG N = 256	Prospective cohort study	256	64.89 ± 9.95	6 months	SF-36	There is evidence that increased symptoms of psychological distress is a strong predictor of no change-deterioration trajectories in HRQoL and that this relationship is influenced by personality trait Type D. Concluded that mediating factors, especially increased anxiety and depression, should be treated adequately in post-CABG clinical routine	Patients with and without a Type D personality showed significant improvements in PCS post CABGs, however patients with type D personality scored lower than their counterparts (both pre and post-op)	**

(continued)

Table 3.2 (continued)

Author, year, Ref	Intervention	Study type	No. of patients at baseline	Age of patients	Follow-up duration (mean)	HRQOL instruments	Conclusion	Physical component improved	Quality score
Najafi, 2012 [30]	Diabetics undergoing isolated CABG N = 113 Non-Diabetics undergoing isolated CABG N = 155	Cross-sectional study	268	Diabetics: 60.3 ± 8.4 Non-diabetics: 59.2 ± 9.4	24 h post-operatively	SF-36	An adverse relationship was found Between pre-op mental summary score and the mean of plasma glucose concentrations during 24 h after surgery. No significant association was found between pre-op physical summary score and mean of plasma glucose concentration during this time	nil	**

Najafi, 2009 [31]	Patients undergoing isolated CABG N = 283	Not formerly stated—but likely prospective cohort	283	59.8 ± 9.0	Not stated	WHOQOL-BREF questionnaire13,14	The study found that the independent physical component predictors for higher HRQOL included male gender and diabetes mellitus, while the independent psychological component predictors were male gender and high ejection fraction. Males, diabetics and patients with low education levels had higher social well-being than others	nil	*
Østergaard, 2015 [32]	Elderly patients undergoing off-pump CABG n = 61 Elderly patients undergoing on-pump CABG n = 59	Prospective cohort study	120	All patients: 75 ± 4.5 Off-pump CABG 76 ± 4.8 On-pump CABG 75 ± 4.2	8 years	SF-36	HRQoL SF-36 scores improved significantly in both groups post-operatively compared to pre-operatively. On-Pump patients had a greater social function score compared to off-pump counterparts	Physical function improved significantly between baseline and all points of follow up (3 months, 12 months, 8 years) across both groups	*******

(continued)

Table 3.2 (continued)

Author, year, Ref	Intervention	Study type	No. of patients at baseline	Age of patients	Follow-up duration (mean)	HRQOL instruments	Conclusion	Physical component improved	Quality score
Peovska, 2008 [33]	Patients with ischaemic cardiomyopathy undergoing CABG more than four viable segments N = 39 Patients with ischaemic cardiomyopathy undergoing CABG less than four viable segments N = 26	Prospective cohort study	65	56 ± 15	14 ± 4 months	Minnesota Living with Heart Failure (MLHF) scale	The presence of more than four viable segments (24% of the left ventricle) on MPI in patients with ischaemic heart failure before CABG surgery is significantly correlated with the improvement in LVEF, heart failure symptoms and quality of life post-operatively	nil	**
Peric, 2008 [34]	Patients undergoing elective CABG n = 208	Prospective cohort study	208	Male 58.2 ± 8 Females, 61.5 ± 5.6	6 months	The Nottingham Health Profile Questionnaire	The predictive factors for quality of life worsening 6 months after CABG are female gender, diabetes mellitus, low ejection fraction, and the presence of postoperative complications	Physical mobility significantly improved post-operatively (70% of patients improved)	**

Sandau, 2008 [35]	Consecutive patients undergoing CABG n = 64	Prospective cohort study	64	65.2 ± 9.3	3 months	SF-12	Patients reported improvements in HRQL measures, including two of three subjective neurocognitive measures	PCS improved from baseline (40) to 42.2 post-operatively which was statistically significant	**
Tully, 2009 [36]	Elective CABG patients n = 226	Prospective cohort study	226	62.9 ± 9.5	6 months	SF-36	Elevated depression symptoms before and after surgery showed an association with lower and worse HRQOL for vitality and social role functioning and physical and general health	Nil	**
Van Mastrigt, 2010 [37]	CABG patients undergoing short-stay intensive care (8 h intensive care) n = 201 CABG patients control subjects (overnight intensive care stay) n = 207	Randomised clinical equivalence trial	410	Control group: 62.0 ± 13.77 Short-stay intensive care group: 61.8 ± 10.67	1 year	Multidimensional index of life quality (MILQ) EQ-5D Beck Depression Inventory State-Trait Anxiety Inventory	The HRQoL of SSIC patients is similar to patients receiving care as usual	Nil	**********

(continued)

Table 3.2 (continued)

Author, year, Ref	Intervention	Study type	No. of patients at baseline	Age of patients	Follow-up duration (mean)	HRQOL instruments	Conclusion	Physical component improved	Quality score
Wagner, 2011 [38]	Patients undergoing isolated CABG, radial artery group n = 366 Patients undergoing isolated CABG, saphenous vein group n = 367	Multicentre randomised control trial	733	Saphenous Vein Group: 62 ± 8 Radial Artery group: 61 ± 8	1 year	Seattle Angina Questionnaire and Health Utility Index	Coronary artery bypass grafting with the radial artery lasts approximately 31 minutes longer than with the saphenous vein. However, costs and the quality of life were not statistically different	Nil	********

Table 3.3 RCT trial studying CABG and QoL

Author, year, Ref	Intervention	Study type	No. of patients at baseline	Follow-up duration (mean)	HRQOL instruments	Conclusion	Physical component improved	Quality score
Kaiser et al., 2004 [39]	CABG vs Medical (elderly)	RCT	CABG (n = 174) Medical (n = 127)	1 year	SF-36, DASI, RDS	CABG gave greater symptomatic relief and improvement in QoL after one year and was also associated with a higher rate of complete revascularisation	CABG better	**********
Mark et al., 2014 [26]	CABG vs Medical (High risk IHD with LV dysfunction and multivessel disease)	RCT	CABG (n = 610) Medical (602)	36 months	The Kansas City Cardiomyopathy Questionnaire, SF12, SF36 Cardiac Self-Efficacy Questionnaire EuroQol-5D	CABG plus medical therapy produced clinically important improvements in several health status domains compared with medical therapy alone over 36 months	Nil	************
Zhang et al., 2003 [40]	CABG vs PCI (SoS)	RCT	CABG (n = 500) PCI (n = 488)	1 year	SAQ	Both CABG and stent-assisted PCI dramatically improved cardiac-related health status in patients with multivessel disease at 6- and 12-month follow-up	During the first postprocedure year, patients' angina burden and physical limitations were alleviated to a greater extent with CABG	*********
Abdalla et al., 2013 [41]	CABG vs PCI (SYNTAX)	RCT	CABG (n = 897) PCI (n = 903)	1,6,12,36 and 60 months	SF-36, SAQ	Among patients with three-vessel or left main coronary artery disease, there was greater relief from angina after CABG than after PCI at 6 and 12 months	No difference in Physical component at 1 year but significantly better at 5 years in favour of CABG	************

(continued)

Table 3.3 (continued)

Author, year, Ref	Intervention	Study type	No. of patients at baseline	Follow-up duration (mean)	HRQOL instruments	Conclusion	Physical component improved	Quality score
Farkouh et al., 2012 [42]	CABG vs PCI (FREEDOM)	RCT	CABG (n = 947) PCI (n = 953)	1, 6 and 12 months. Yearly thereafter	SAQ, RDS	Between group comparisons generally favored CABG between 6 months and 2 years, but the observed differences were small. Beyond 2 years, there were no consistent differences between the 2 treatment strategies	CABG continued to demonstrate better outcomes on the physical limitations SAQ subscales through 2 to 5 years of follow-up.	***********
QoL post CABG: CABG vs OPCABG								
Noqueira et al., 2008 [43]	CABG vs OPCABG	RCT	CABG (n = 97) OPCAB (n = 105)	At baseline, six and 12 months postoperative	CCS, SF-36	Improvement in HRQoL and early return to work regardless of the technique	Male patients coped better in terms of physical functioning compared with females	*************
Tully et al., 2008 [44]	CABG vs OPCABG	RCT	CABG (n = 36) OPCAB (n = 30) Controls (n = 50)	At baseline, before discharge, 6 months postoperative	SF-36, CVLT, TMT, DigSymb, The National Adult Reading Test	OPCAB patients did not show fewer cognitive deficits or greater improvement in HRQoL than CABG patient	No difference in change in SF-36 Physical component	*************
Van Dijk et al., 2007 [45]	CABG vs OPCABG	RCT	CABG (n = 117) OPCAB (n = 123)	At baseline, three and 12 months, and 5 years postoperative	A battery of 10 neuropsychological tests, SF-36, EuroQoL	Using OPCAB instead of CABG has no effect on 5-year cognitive or HRQoL outcome after surgery	No difference in change in SF-36 Physical component	*************

Motellebzadeh et al., 2006 [46]	CABG vs OPCABG	RCT	CABG (n = 117) OPCAB (n = 123)	Six and 18 months postoperative	SF-36	OPCABG and CABG results in similar HRQoL outcome 6 and 18 months after surgery	No difference in change in SF-36 Physical component	*********
Jensen et al., 2006 [47]	CABG vs OPCABG (elderly)	RCT	CABG (n = 55) OPCAB (n = 54)	At baseline, 3 months postoperative	SF-36, MDI-scale	OPCAB and CABG improved HRQoL in elderly moderate-to-high-risk patients, but there was no clinically relevant difference in HRQoL between the groups	No difference in change in SF-36 Physical component	*************
Al Ruzzeh et al., 2006 [48]	CABG vs OPCABG	RCT	CABG (n = 84) OPCAB (84)	At baseline, 6 weeks and 6 months postoperative	A battery of 11 neuropsychological tests, WHOQOL	Using OPCAB showed a trend for better HRQoL scores compared to CABG. Better neurocognitive function was seen in patients who underwent OPCAB	No difference in change in WHOQOL Physical component	*************
Mathisen et al., 2005 [49]	CABG vs OPCABG	RCT	CABG (n = 60) OPCAB (n = 60)	At baseline, 3, 6, and 12 months postoperative	CCS, SF-36, QOLS-N, Hospital Anxiety and Depression Scale	No significant differences in HRQoL were found cross-sectionally or longitudinally	No difference in change in SF-36 Physical component	************
Puskas et al., 2004 [50]	CABG vs OPCABG	RCT	CABG (n = 99) OPCAB (n = 98)	At baseline, 4–6 weeks, 6 months and 1 year postoperative	CCS, NYHA, SF-36, EuroQoL	HRQoL at 30 days and one year after surgery was similar in CAGB and OPCAB groups	No difference in change in SF-36 Physical component	*************

(continued)

Table 3.3 (continued)

Author, year, Ref	Intervention	Study type	No. of patients at baseline	Follow-up duration (mean)	HRQOL instruments	Conclusion	Physical component improved	Quality score
Østergaard et al., 2015 [32]	CABG vs OPCABG Elderly	RCT	CABG n = 59 OPCABG n = 61	8 years	SF-36	HRQoL SF-36 scores improved significantly in both groups post-operatively compared to pre-operatively. On-Pump patients had a greater social function score compared to off-pump counterparts	Physical function improved significantly between baseline and all points of follow up (3 months, 12 months, 8 years) across both groups.	***************
Bishawi et al. 2013, [51] (ROOBY)	CABG vs OPCABG	RCT	CABG n = 1099 OPCABG n = 1104	1 year	SAQ, VR-36	low-to-moderate risk male veterans undergoing CABG surgery with off-pump versus on-pump technique had similar 3-month and 1-year HRQL outcomes	No difference in QoL measurement	*************
QoL post CABG: Further intervention								
Hirschhorn et al., 2008 [52]	CABG inpatient: physiotherapy-supervised walking program, with or without musculoskeletal and respiratory exercises	RCT	Standard PT (n = 32); Walking exercise PT (n = 31); Walking/breathing exercise PT (n = 30)	At baseline, at discharge, and four weeks after discharge	6MWA, SF-36, VC	A physiotherapy-supervised intensity walking program improves physical capacity at hospital discharge	SF-36 Physical component showed significant improvement at FU	************

Goodman et al., 2008 [53]	Enhanced risk factor prevention	RCT	CABG + enhanced risk factor prevention (n = 94); CABG only (n = 94)	At baseline, 3 and 6 months postoperative	SF-36, CROQ	Enhanced risk factor prevention (i.e., counseling, blood-pressure control, medication optimized) did not improve post-CABG HRQoL	Intervention showed significant improvement in the Physical QoL only in the SF36	************
Lie et al., 2009, [54]	Home based intervention program	RCT	CABG (n = 92) CABG/HBIP (n = 93)	At baseline, 6 weeks and 6 months postoperative	SF-36, SAQ	HRQoL improved markedly over time in both groups, but no significant effects of the HBIP were found	Compared to the general population, significant differences were found for the SF-36 subscales: role physical, role emotional and bodily pain	***********
Tranmer et al., 2004 [55]	Advanced postoperative support after CABG	RCT	Advanced postoperative support after CABG (n = 92); Usual care after CABG (n = 92)	Five weeks after discharge	SF-36, MSAS	No significant differences in HRQoL, unexpected contacts with the healthcare system, or symptom distress between groups	No difference in change in SF-36 Physical component	**********
Khatri et al., 2001 [56]	Normothermia vs Hypothermia	RCT	Normothermic CABG (n = 115); hypothermic CABG (n = 111)	At baseline, 6 weeks, and 6 months postoperative	CES-D, STAI, MOS DASI, QARS-IADL SF-36	Hypothermic conditions during CABG are associated with higher levels of emotional distress	No difference in change in SF-36 Physical component	************
Arthur et al., 2000 [57]	Multi dimensional preoperative intervention: exercise, education and social support	RCT	Enhanced intervention before CABG (n = 123); Normal intervention before CABG (n = 123)	One week before surgery, at baseline, 6 weeks, and 6 months postoperative	SF-36, ISEL, STAI, HSUQ	Enhanced intervention during the waiting period for CABG improves functional abilities and HRQoL postoperatively	Improvement in the physical component was observed	**************

(continued)

Table 3.3 (continued)

Author, year, Ref	Intervention	Study type	No. of patients at baseline	Follow-up duration (mean)	HRQOL instruments	Conclusion	Physical component improved	Quality score
Thoits et al., 2000 [58]	Supportive intervention	RCT	Peer support before and after CABG (n = 100); Controls (n = 90)	At baseline, 1, 6, and 12 months postoperative	SF-36, CES-D, SCL-90R, self-rated health assessment	Patients who received peer support in hospital at the time of CABG experienced improvements in physical and mental well-being	Improvement in the physical component was observed	***************
Namerow et al., 1999 [59]	Effect of empiric ICD post CABG in patients with an increased risk of arrhythmic cardiac death	RCT	ICD after CABG (n = 446); No ICD after CABG (n = 454)	Six months postoperative	SF-36, NYHA	Patients with ICDs had lower scores on scales measuring psychological well-being, perception of health, and emotional role functioning	Reduced physical functional component	**********
Gierszewska et al., 2018 [60]	CABG vs Hybrid (POLMIDES)	RCT	CABG (n = 102) Hybrid (n = 98)	Pre-op and 12 months	SF-36	HRQoL in patients after both modes of revascularization significantly improved after 12 months in all domains.	Obesity and Euroscore were independent predictors of the Physical component	*************
Chernyavskiy et al., 2016 [61]	CABG vs CABG+AF ablation	RCT	CABG (n = 34) CABG+PVI (n = 31) or CABG +MiniMaze (n = 30)	Pre-opo, 1 year and 2 years post-op	SF-36	Effective elimination of AF during CABG surgery improves QoL in all physical health domains of the SF-36	Patients in the CABG alone group had the lowest scores for the role-physical functioning, vitality, and social functioning domains	**************

control and intervention groups varied between each study making statistical analysis non-feasible. Population groupings by. pre-operative comorbidity, included diabetic status [30], angina status [11] and peri-operative MI [19]. The main patient demographics used as a grouping method were age [27] and gender [13]. Groupings by operative technique included on-pump vs off-pump [21, 32] and total arterial revascularisation versus saphenous vein combinations [14].

Patient ages ranged from 39 to 88.8 years and the included studies sample size ranged between 48 to 2000. The procedures undergone by these patients varied in terms of incision method and operation type; open sternotomy was noted as the preferred choice over minimal access. All studies had a follow-up period ranged from 3 months to 15 years.

Quality of Studies

Table 3.2 highlights the quality score achieved by each study according to the modified Newcastle-Ottowa scale. The scores ranged from 2 to 14, highlighting that the quality of studies was skewed negatively. This reflects the clarity in study design and outcomes reported.

HRQOL Tools

A total of 45 different health related quality of life measurement tools was applied in almost all the articles individually apart from few studies that co-applied two or more tools in their study group. Majority of the studies utilised SF-36 to assess and measure quality of life (Table 3.2).

Outcomes

Most of the studies reported improved HRQOL following CABG compared to baseline. Whilst not the focus of the studies, outcomes including in-hospital mortality, complications and prolonged length of stay were reported. However, studies failed to report on common endpoints which limited formal meta-analysis. This limited our interpretation of baseline predictors for HRQOL and a cut-off value that accurately measures CABG surgery consequences in elderly patients.

Discussion

In our present analysis, we conducted a systematic review of 54 studies assessing quality of life after coronary artery bypass graft (CABG) surgery. Whilst there was notable variability amongst the studies, our review has found that, overall, CABG surgery confers not only an improved long-term survival, but an improved physical and mental well-being as seen from a variety of scoring tools indicating a better health related quality of life (HRQOL) after CABG surgery.

In the modern era, the rise of percutaneous revascularisation over surgery makes the issue of HRQOL ever more important, and raises several questions of the overall risk gain benefit ratio, other than mortality as a single objective end point. The impact of the surgical burdens of a median sternotomy, cardiopulmonary bypass and intensive care unit stay on patients' HRQOL post-surgery in the short and longer term, especially compared to PCI, may reflect this evolution. Moreover, perhaps not unexpectedly, most of the current evidence base assesses CABG from a technical standpoint, with outcomes more-often-than not being mortality as well as traditional measures of morbidity. This is juxtaposition to the amount of literature available on the HRQOL outcomes following CABG, which is sparse; our initial search identified only 40 articles. Comparatively a crude PubMed search for 'outcomes' and 'coronary artery bypass grafts' identified thousands of articles.

Patients requiring CABG undergo a significant amount of physical and psychological stress in the perioperative process and the rehabilitation post-surgery. The impact on physical competency post sternotomy, post-surgical pain, and the psychosocial stresses associated with the recovery process, impedes gains in quality of life perceived by patients or, worse, a decline in quality of life post

CABG. Yet what our study findings suggest is that the surgical treatment of ischaemic heart disease, its symptomatic improvement and relief of myocardial ischaemia, are factors significant enough to nullify the perioperative stresses and provide an improved physical and psychosocial state for the patient owing to improved cardiopulmonary reserve. This is not without mentioning the patients' intrinsic healing potential that also makes this possible. The studies analysed cover a wide time frame, some showing improvement in HRQOL as early as 3 months, and lasting for up to 15 years. Factors affecting HQOL post CABG are presented in Fig. 3.3.

A study by Mark et al. [26] randomised 1212 patients to either CABG or medical therapy alone and found that the surgical option conferred a more significant improvement in HRQOL. This was the only study to compare CABG with such a clear control group to demonstrate significant HRQOL improvement. Being one of the larger studies in our analysis, Mark and colleagues used multiple HRQOL assessment tools to validate many of their findings and at several time points between 4 months and 3 years post-surgery. Interestingly, the authors focus on high-risk patients with impaired left ventricular function and multivessel coronary disease: patients who would be deemed higher risk for surgery, who yet still go on to have a more improved HRQOL compared to patients being offered medical therapy alone.

However, it may be that certain disease factors limit the HRQOL improvement. Peovska and colleagues [33] highlighted that choosing patients with revascularisation of viable myocardial segments (measured using myocardial perfusion scans) compared to those with more non-viable segments can confer a greater improvement in HRQOL. This was directly related to patients having a more improved LVEF, which indicates that measured success in myocardial revascularisation is crucial in ensuring patients to experience a better HRQOL after surgery.

A recent myocardial infarction (MI), which is a common indication for revascularisation, may also confound the HRQOL after surgery. This was seen in the study by Järiven et al. [19] who, using the RAND-36 questionnaire, found that the improvement in HRQOL one year after surgery was significantly less in patients who had a recent MI compared to those who did not. However, 12 years after surgery, there were no differences between the two groups, both of which showed a generalised decline in HRQOL. The study also found operative mortality to be higher in the MI group of patients, although long-term survival at 10 years was similar when compared to non-MI patients. The study by Bjessmo and Sartipy [11] reported no difference in HRQOL outcomes between MI and non-MI groups, however, the study was retrospective and patients were only assessed 10 years post-surgery, which therefore does not disagree with the Järiven study [19].

Surgical Factors

Over the years numerous studies have examined health related QoL after CABG and PCI. These comparative studies have reported a faster recovery with PCI but a long-term advantage with CABG. The majority of these studies showed higher revascularisation rates among patients treated with bare-metal stents at 5 years. However the addition of the stent did reduce the need for repeat revascularisation by about 50%, as compared to the use of balloon angioplasty alone [62].

One of the larger studies from the bare metal era was Stent or Surgery (SOS) in which patients were randomised to either CABG or stent assisted PCI. The investigators reported PCI patients with higher mortality and greater need for repeat revascularisation. They also presented important QoL information showing significant improvement in both groups at 6 and 12 months respectively. However CABG was more effective in improving QoL, angina relief, increasing physical functioning during the first year [40].

Drug coated stents led to an expanded use of PCI for patients with complex CAD. In the landmark Synergy between PCI with Taxus and Cardiac Surgery (SYNTAX) the investigators reported, after 1 year, that the primary end point (death, stroke, MI or repeat revascularisation) occurred significantly more after stenting, due in large part from greater need for repeat revascularisation [41]. Further higher rates of MI and cardiac death was reported at 5 years. Heath related QoL information collected by the investigators showed more patients were angina free at 12 months after CABG. Longer term 3 and 5 years follow up QoL data showed improvement in both PCI and CABG groups. However, compared to PCI, CABG resulted in improved angina and QoL scores at 5 years. Patients in the PCI group were more likely to be taking long term nitrates. A subgroup analysis suggested that those with the most complex CAD (highest SYNTAX score) had the greatest relief of angina with CABG along with better physical, emotional and mental scores at 5 years. Thus SYNTAX showed that surgery resulted in better QoL beyond 6 months as compared to PCI [41, 62].

In a prospective cohort study, Kapetanakis et al. [21] compared HRQOL after on-pump and off-pump CABG and found that neither surgical strategies were more beneficial than the other. They also found pre-procedure HRQOL to be similar to reported HRQOL post-surgery (time period = 6 months) between groups, adding no benefit exerted by any particular surgical strategy over the other. This contrasts to the randomized study by Ostergaard and colleagues [32], who found a more significant improvement in the social functioning subscale of the SF-36 questionnaire in on-pump patients compared to off-pump patients. They also found an improvement in five of the eight domains of SF-36 in the off-pump group, compared to eight out of the eight domains in the on-pump group.

Bonaros and colleagues [12] found that robot assisted CABG confers an even greater improvement in HRQOL when compared to conventional CABG via sternotomy. Interestingly a subgroup analysis found that, in patients planned to have robot assisted surgery who go on to have a conversion sternotomy, did not have a further impaired quality of life compared to the planned conventional sternotomy patients.

In a Scandinavian prospective study by Damgaard et al. [14], total arterial revascularisation (TAR) was compared with conventional CABG (mammary artery and vein grafts) and found a significantly greater improvement in the social functioning element of HRQOL compared to conventional surgery, as well as a non-significantly greater improvement in the physical component at one year post surgery.

Patient Factors

Many of the studies analysed patient-related predictors of poorer HRQOL performance after CABG surgery. A study by Peric et al. [34] followed 208 patients and through the use of multivariate logistic regression, identified a number of factors significantly associated with worse HRQOL 6 months after surgery, including diabetes mellitus, low preoperative ejection fraction, and female gender. This was found to influence a number of HRQOL domains, including physical, social and reports of pain. The two studies by Kapetanakis and Najafi [21, 31], respectively, also found diabetes to be an independent positive predictive factor for patients reporting a better HRQOL following CABG.

CABG has been shown in patients with diabetes, in the FREEDOM study, to result in less death, MI or stroke combined, compared to PCI. The investigators subsequently reported QoL analysis where both CABG and PCI showed improvement in angina frequency. However CABG patients had better angina scores, with respect to physical limitations the scores were higher in favour of CABG at 1 year and continued to demonstrate better outcome out to 5 years. Thus in diabetics CABG provided greater improvement in QoL as compared to PCI with drug eluting stents [41].

In the study by Markou and colleagues [27], the researchers split patients into three age groups and found the most significant improvement in HRQOL in the youngest group (age < 65) followed by the middle group (age 65–75) and an even lesser improvement in HRQOL in the third group (age > 75). This was most markedly seen in the domain of physical activity, where no significant improvement was seen in the second and third groups.

Najafi [31] also found gender to play a role, with male patients being more likely to have better physical and psychological component scores after isolated CABG than females. However, Covinsky et al. [13] focused on postmenopausal females undergoing CABG surgery and found no significant change compared to the preoperative baseline.

Post-surgical Complications

Specific attention should also be given to the impact of complications on the HRQOL outcome following surgery. Jidéus and colleagues [18] found that sternal wound infection was significant negative influence on improvement in HRQOL following surgery. Peric et al. [34] found that the occurrence of postoperative complications worsened physical and mental components of reported HRQOL outcomes 6 months after surgery. Whilst this study was not designed to assess each specific complication, significant complications affecting postoperative HRQOL included prolonged ventilation, reoperation for bleeding, sternal wound infection, pericardial effusion, arrhythmia and perioperative MI amongst others.

A protracted ICU stay after CABG surgery occurs when serious complications arise or patients have a poor baseline, leading to the need for prolonged critical care support. Some cases can remain in ICU up to a few days or even weeks. Undoubtedly this will affect the recovery period and impact the physical strength of the patient as well as the psychosocial well-being, through factors such as critical care neuropathy, malnutrition, pain, and sepsis.

Patient Health Perceptions

A small number of studies in our analysis found a crucial impact of patients' baseline mental and psychological state as well as personality traits in affecting the HRQOL outcome after cardiac surgery, albeit all studies finding an overall positive impact of CABG on HRQOL post-surgery.

In a study by Juergens et al. [20], patients received an illness perception questionnaire prior to surgery, the results of which were found to impact the variance of the HRQOL outcome post-surgery. In other words, patients' beliefs about a negative impact of their illness pre-surgery was related to poorer physical and mental component scores 3 months after surgery, suggesting a potential role for cognitive intervention prior to surgery.

The study by Khoueiry et al. [22] in off-pump CABG patients used the Beck Depression Index to identify that depression and disability initially worsen one month post-surgery but that this remarkably improves by 9 months after surgery.

Lee and colleagues found that anxiety and depression symptoms had a significantly negative impact on HRQOL improvement after surgery. A study by Middel et al. [29] took this further to identify that intrinsic personality traits possessed by patients, conferring negative affectivity and social inhibition (Type D personality), predicted failure of improvement in the physical and mental domains of the SF-36 tool 6 months after surgery. Moreover, the study concluded these findings despite patients achieving an objective improvement in known biomedical variables, including ejection fraction and relief of angina.

Limitations

Whilst our study is crucial in assessing patients' functionality after life-prolonging surgery, reviews of this nature have some important limitations to mention. First, there is heterogeneity in the tools used for measuring quality of life amongst the studies. A large portion of the studies used the short-form-36 (SF-36), which uses 36 generic questions in a number of specific domains, and a handful of studies used the EQ5D/EuroQOL. There were a few studies that used specific cardiac symptoms related questionnaires which, although different to other study tools, evaluated variables that were directly taken from validated HRQOL tools. Whilst some differences exist between these tools, the main HRQOL factors they assess are very similar. The second issue is the difficulty in taking the baseline deterioration in human HRQOL, especially in the elderly, into account. Only two studies from our cohort [16, 17] have used methods to take into account this baseline deterioration in HRQOL in the elderly. The third important factor to note is the overall positivity reported in these papers may actually reflect a publication bias. Most studies are published in surgical journals demonstrating the positive effect of CABG on quality of life, and it may be that studies reporting a negative outcome are under-reported.

Conclusions

- Variety of tools to measure QoL make comparing across studies difficult
- CABG surgery results in better long term QoL compared to PCI
- OPCABG does not significantly alter post-operative QoL
- Risk factors like diabetes, LV function, pre-op MI, gender, COPD, smoking impact post CABG QoL
- Elderly patients with time show similar improvement in QoL post CABG
- Robotic assisted/Hydrid CABG improve the short term QoL post CABG
- Post-op complication and protracted ITU stay reduces post-op CABG QoL.
- Pre-operative cognitive intervention may play a role in influencing patient factors outcome

Fig. 3.2 Conclusions

Conclusions

Summary of conclusions is presented in Fig. 3.2. There is significant evidence demonstrating that CABG improves the quality of life in physical and mental domains, as well as its established efficacy in treating angina and increasing life expectancy (Fi. Whilst factors such as minimally invasive surgery and total arterial revascularisation are positive predictors of HRQOL, post-surgical complications can worsen HRQOL outcomes. Due attention should be given to certain patient factors, and especially to patient mood and health perception, where pre-operative cognitive intervention may play a role in influencing their outcome (Fig. 3.3).

A number of Randomised Clinical Trials (RCTs) have been undertaken comparing both off and on pump CABG approaches to investigate whether any benefit was to be gained by undertaking the CABG on or off pump in regards to QoL. Neither traditional CABG techniques have been shown to be superior in respect to QoL. Also the acquired benefits are long lasting and better than that achieved with PCI.

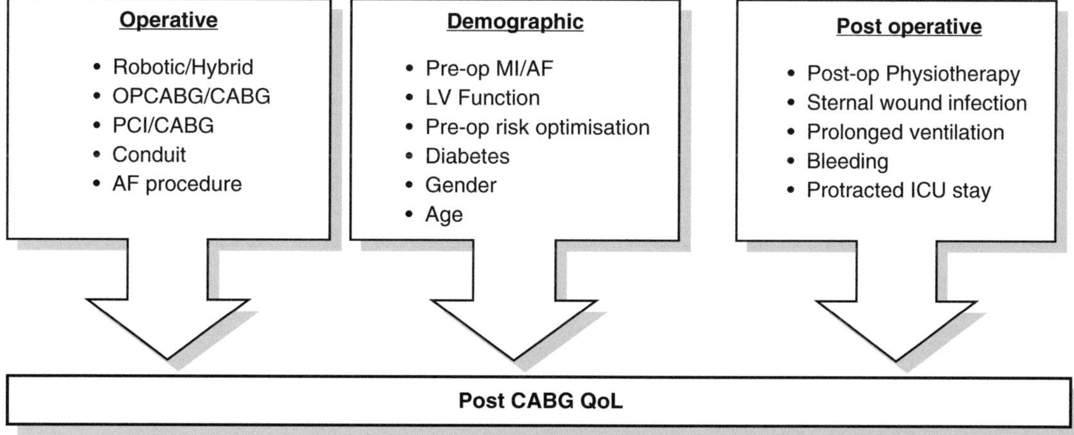

Fig. 3.3 Factors affecting HRQOL post CABG

References

1. Roth GA, Huffman MD, Moran AE, et al. Global and regional patterns in cardiovascular mortality from 1990 to 2013. Circulation. 2015;132(17):1667.
2. Jones DS, Greene JA. The decline and rise of coronary heart disease: understanding public health catastrophism. Am J Public Health. 2013;103(7):1207–18.
3. Diodato M, Chedrawy EG. Coronary artery bypass graft surgery: the past, present, and future of myocardial revascularisation. Surg Res Pract. 2014;2014:6.
4. O'Gara PT, Kushner FG, Ascheim DD, et al. 2013 ACCF/AHA guideline for the management of ST-elevation myocardial infarction. Circulation. 2013;127(4):e362.
5. Hillis LD, Smith PK, Anderson JL, et al. 2011 ACCF/AHA guideline for coronary artery bypass graft surgery. Circulation. 2011;124(23):e652.
6. International Health Conference. Constitution of the World Health Organization. 1946. Bull World Health Organ. 2002;80(12):983–4.
7. WHO. Study protocol for the World Health Organization project to develop a Quality of Life assessment instrument (WHOQOL). Qual Life Res. 1993;2(2):153–9.
8. Shan L, Saxena A, McMahon R, et al. A systematic review on the quality of life benefits after aortic valve replacement in the elderly. J Thorac Cardiovasc Surg. 2013;145(5):1173–89.
9. Wells G, Shea B, O'Connell D, et al. The Newcastle-Ottawa Scale (NOS) for assessing the quality of nonrandomised studies in meta-analyses. @ inproceedings (Wells2014TheNS).
10. Azzopardi S, Lee G. Health-related quality of life 2 years after coronary artery bypass graft surgery. J Cardiovasc Nurs. 2009;24(3):232–40.
11. Bjessmo S, Sartipy U. Quality of life ten years after surgery for Acute Coronary Syndrome or stable angina. Scand Cardiovasc J. 2010;44(1):59–64.
12. Bonaros N, Schachner T, Wiedemann D, et al. Quality of life improvement after robotically assisted coronary artery bypass grafting. Cardiology. 2009;114(1):59–66.
13. Covinsky KE, Lin F, Bittner V, et al. Health-related quality of life following coronary artery bypass graft surgery in post-menopausal women. J Gen Intern Med. 2008;23(9):1429–34.
14. Damgaard S, Lund JT, Lilleør NB, et al. Comparably improved health-related quality of life after total arterial revascularization versus conventional coronary surgery—Copenhagen arterial revascularization randomized patency and outcome trial. Eur J Cardiothorac Surg. 2011;39(4):478–83.
15. El Baz N, Middel B, Van Dijk JP, et al. Coronary artery bypass graft (CABG) surgery patients in a clinical pathway gained less in health-related quality of life as compared with patients who undergo CABG in a conventional-care plan. J Eval Clin Pract. 2009;15(3):498–505.
16. Herlitz J, Brandrup-Wognsen G, Evander MH, et al. Quality of life 15 years after coronary artery bypass grafting. Coron Artery Dis. 2009;20(6):363–9.
17. Hokkanen M, Järvinen O, Huhtalaet H, et al. A 12-year follow-up on the changes in health-related quality of life after coronary artery bypass graft surgery. Eur J Cardiothorac Surg. 2014;45(2):329–34.
18. Jidéus L, Liss A, Ståhle E. Patients with sternal wound infection after cardiac surgery do not improve their quality of life. Scand Cardiovasc J. 2009;43(3):194–200.
19. Järvinen O, Hokkanen M, Huhtala H. The long-term effect of perioperative myocardial infarction on health-related quality-of-life after coronary artery bypass grafting. Interact Cardiovasc Thorac Surg. 2014;18(5):568–73.
20. Juergens MC, Seekatz B, Moosdorf RG, Petrie KG, Rief W. Illness beliefs before cardiac surgery predict disability, quality of life, and depression 3 months later. J Psychosom Res. 2010;68(6):553–60.
21. Kapetanakis EI, Stamou SC, Petrou KR, et al. Comparison of the quality of life after conventional versus off-pump coronary artery bypass surgery. J Card Surg. 2008;23(2):120–5.
22. Khoueiry G, Flory M, Rafeh NA, et al. Depression, disability, and quality of life after off-pump coronary artery bypass grafting: a prospective 9-month follow-up study. Heart Lung. 2011;40(3):217–25.
23. Kołtowski L, Drohomirecka A, Palczewski M, Cichoń R. Short-term improvement of patients' quality of life after coronary artery bypass grafting – a prospective single-center study based on the eq-5d assessment tool. Adv Clin Exp Med. 2011;20(4).
24. Lee GA. Determinants of quality of life five years after coronary artery bypass graft surgery. Heart Lung. 2009;38(2):91–9.
25. Lie I, Arnesen H, Sandvik L, Hamilton G, Bunch EH. Health-related quality of life after coronary artery bypass grafting. The impact of a randomised controlled home-based intervention program. Qual Life Res. 2009;18(2):201–7.
26. Mark DB, Knight JD, Velazquez EJ, et al. Quality-of-life outcomes in surgical treatment of ischemic heart failure quality-of-life outcomes with coronary artery bypass graft surgery in ischemic left ventricular dysfunction: a randomized trial. Ann Intern Med. 2014;161(6):392–9.
27. Markou ALP, van der Windt A, van Swieten HA, Noyez L. Changes in quality of life, physical activity, and symptomatic status one year after myocardial revascularization for stable angina. Eur J Cardiothorac Surg. 2008;34(5):1009–15.
28. Merkouris A, Apostolakis E, Pistolas D, Papagiannaki V, Diakomopoulou E, Patriaki E. Quality of life after coronary artery bypass graft surgery in the elderly. Eur J Cardiovasc Nurs. 2009;8(1):74–81.
29. Middel B, El Baz N, Pedersen SS, et al. Decline in health-related quality of life 6 months after coronary artery bypass graft surgery: the influence of anxiety,

depression, and personality traits. J Cardiovasc Nurs. 2014;29(6):544–54.

30. Najafi M, Sheikhvatan M, Montazeri A. Blood glucose concentrations after cardiac surgery: the impact of preoperative quality of life. Int J Diabet Develop Count. 2012;32(2):93–7.
31. Najafi M, Sheikhvatan MDM, Montazeri A. Quality of life-associated factors among patients undergoing coronary artery bypass surgery as measured using the WHOQOL-BREF. Cardiovasc J Afr. 2009;20(5):284–9.
32. Østergaard B, Holbæk E, Sørensen J, et al. Health-related quality of life after off-pump compared with on-pump coronary bypass grafting among elderly high-risk patients: A randomized trial with eight years of follow-up. Eur J Cardiovasc Nurs. 2015;15(2):126–33.
33. Peovska I, Maksimovic J, Vavlukiset M, et al. Functional outcome and quality of life after coronary artery bypass surgery in patients with severe heart failure and hibernated myocardium. Nucl Med Commun. 2008;29(3):215–21.
34. Peric V, Borzanovic M, Stolic R, et al. Predictors of worsening of patients' quality of life six months after coronary artery bypass surgery. J Card Surg. 2008;23(6):648–54.
35. Sandau KE, Lindquist RA, Treat-Jacobson T, et al. Health-related quality of life and subjective neurocognitive function three months after coronary artery bypass graft surgery. Heart Lung. 2008;37(3):161–72.
36. Tully PJ, Baker RA, Turnbull DA, et al. Negative emotions and quality of life six months after cardiac surgery: the dominant role of depression not anxiety symptoms. J Behav Med. 2009;32(6):510.
37. van Mastrigt GAPG, Joore MA, Nieman FHM, et al. Health-related quality of life after fast-track treatment results from a randomized controlled clinical equivalence trial. Qual Life Res. 2010;19(5):631–42.
38. Wagner TH, Sethi G, Holman W, et al. Costs and quality of life associated with radial artery and saphenous vein cardiac bypass surgery: results from a Veterans Affairs multisite trial. Am J Surg. 2011;202(5):532–5.
39. Kaiser C. Risks and benefits of optimised medical and revascularisation therapy in elderly patients with angina ? on-treatment analysis of the TIME trial. Eur Heart J. 2004;25(12):1036–42. https://doi.org/10.1016/j.ehj.2004.02.033.
40. Zhang Z. Disease-specific health status after stent-assisted percutaneous coronary intervention and coronary artery bypass surgery: one-year results from the stent or surgery trial. Circulation. 2003;108(14):1694–700.
41. Abdallah MS. Quality of life after PCI vs CABG among patients with diabetes and multivessel coronary artery disease. JAMA. 2013;310(15):1581.
42. Farkouh ME, Domanski M, Sleeper LA, Siami FS, Dangas G, Mack M, Yang M, Cohen DJ, Rosenberg Y, Solomon SD, Desai AS. Strategies for multivessel revascularization in patients with diabetes. N Engl J Med. 2012;367(25):2375–84.
43. Nogueira CR, Hueb W, Takiuti ME, et al. Quality of life after on-pump and off-pump coronary artery bypass grafting surgery. Arq Bras Cardiol. 2008;91:217–22.
44. Tully PJ, Baker RA, Kneebone AC, et al. Neuropsychologic and quality-of-life outcomes after coronary artery bypass surgery with and without cardiopulmonary bypass: a prospective randomized trial. J Cardiothorac Vasc Anesth. 2008;22:515–21.
45. Van Dijk D, Spoor M, Hijman R, et al. Octopus Study Group. Cognitive and cardiac outcomes 5 years after offpump vs. on-pump coronary artery bypass graft surgery. JAMA. 2007;297:701–8.
46. Motallebzadeh R, Bland JM, Markus HS, et al. Healthrelated quality of life outcome after on-pump versus offpump coronary artery bypass graft surgery: a prospective randomized study. Ann Thorac Surg. 2006;82:615–9.
47. Jensen BØ, Hughes P, Rasmussen LS, et al. Healthrelated quality of life following off-pump versus on-pump coronary artery bypass grafting in elderly moderate to high-risk patients: A randomized trial. Eur J Cardiothorac Surg. 2006;30:294–9.
48. Al-Ruzzeh S, George S, Bustami M, et al. Effect of offpump coronary artery bypass surgery on clinical, angiographic, neurocognitive, and quality of life outcomes: Randomised controlled trial. BMJ. 2006;332:1365.
49. Mathisen L, Andersen MH, Hol PK, et al. Patientreported outcome after randomization to on-pump versus off-pump coronary artery surgery. Ann Thorac Surg. 2005;79:1584–9.
50. Puskas JD, Williams WH, Mahoney EM, et al. Off-pump vs conventional coronary artery bypass grafting: early and 1-year graft patency, cost, and quality-of-life outcomes: a randomized trial. JAMA. 2004;291(15):1841–9. https://doi.org/10.1001/jama.291.15.1841.
51. Bishawi M, Shroyer AL, Rumsfeld JS, Spertus JA, Baltz JH, Collins JF, Quin JA, Almassi GH, Grover FL, Hattler B. Changes in health-related quality of life in off-pump versus on-pump cardiac surgery: veterans affairs randomized on/off bypass trial. Ann Thorac Surg. 2013;95(6):1946–51.
52. Hirschhorn AD, Richards D, Mungovan SF, et al. Supervised moderate intensity exercise improves distance walked at hospital discharge following coronary artery bypass graft surgery—A randomised controlled trial. Heart Lung Circ. 2008;17:129–38.
53. Goodman H, Parsons A, Davison J, et al. A randomised controlled trial to evaluate a nurse-led programme of support and lifestyle management for patients awaiting cardiac surgery 'Fit for surgery: Fit for life' study. Eur J Cardiovasc Nurs. 2008;7:189–95.
54. Lie I, Arnesen H, Sandvik L, et al. Health-related quality of life after coronary artery bypass grafting. The impact of a randomised controlled home-based intervention program. Qual Life Res. 2009;18:201–7.
55. Tranmer JE, Parry MJ. Enhancing postoperative recovery of cardiac surgery patients: A randomized

clinical trial of an advanced practice nursing intervention. West J Nurs Res. 2004;26:515–32.

56. Khatri P, Babyak M, Croughwell ND, et al. Temperature during coronary artery bypass surgery affects quality of life. Ann Thorac Surg. 2001;71:110–6.
57. Arthur HM, Daniels C, McKelvie R, et al. Effect of a preoperative intervention on preoperative and postoperative outcomes in low-risk patients awaiting elective coronary artery bypass graft surgery. Annals of Internal Medicine, 2000;33:253–62.
58. Thoits PA, Hohmann AA, Harvey MR, et al. Similar other support for men undergoing coronary artery bypass surgery. Health Psychol. 2000;19:264–73.
59. Namerow PB, Firth BR, Heywood GM, Windle JR, Parides MK. Quality-of-life six months after CABG surgery in patients randomized to ICD versus no ICD therapy: findings from the CABG Patch Trial. Pacing Clin Electrophysiol. 1999;22(9):1305–13. https://doi.org/10.1111/j.1540-8159.1999.tb00623.x. PMID: 10527011.
60. Gierszewska K, Jaworska I, Skrzypek M, Gąsior M, Pudlo R. Quality of life in patients with coronary artery disease treated with coronary artery bypass grafting and hybrid coronary revascularization. Cardiol J. 2018;5:621–7.
61. Chernyavskiy A, Kareva Y, Pak I, Rakhmonov S, Pokushalov E, Romanov A. Quality of life after surgical ablation of persistent atrial fibrillation: a prospective evaluation. Heart Lung Circ. 2016;2016(25):378–83.
62. Cohen DJ, Van Hout B, Serruys PW, Mohr FW, Macaya C, den Heijer P, Vrakking MM, Wang K, Mahoney EM, Audi S, Leadley K, Dawkins KD, Kappetein AP. Quality of life after PCI with drug-eluting stents or coronary-artery bypass surgery. N Engl J Med. 2011;364(11):1016–26.

Thoracic Aortic Surgery

4

Matthew K. H. Tan, Omar A. Jarral, Yousuf Salmasi, Michael Sabetai, and Thanos Athanasiou

Introduction

Operations on the thoracic aorta represent a daunting challenge for even the most experienced of surgeons, requiring exceptional technical skills and a keen attention to detail for multiorgan protection. Such procedures have historically been associated with significant morbidity and mortality, but significant improvements have been observed over the last 20 years. Some specialist centres report mortality rates of less than 10% for type A dissection repair in octogenarians [1] and less than 6% paraplegia rates following thoracoabdominal aneurysm (TAA) repair [2, 3], in part due to reasons outlined in Table 4.1 [4].

In addition to morbidity and mortality, health-related quality of life (HRQoL) is increasingly recognised as an important outcome measure in recent times. Defined as a 'multi-dimensional assessment of an individual's perception of the physical, psychological and social aspects of life that can be affected by a disease process and its treatment' [5], it is necessary for the calculation and evaluation of cost-effectiveness as well as acting as a more precise indicator of patient-centred care, with significant promise to improve healthcare provision [6]—this has been recognised by the United Kingdom's Department of Health with the consolidation of efforts to collect and publish HRQoL outcomes for common procedures [7]. While not routinely collected in cardiothoracic or aortic surgery currently, HRQoL measures are still particularly important in aortic surgery for a few reasons, including: (1) Large numbers of asymptomatic patients are operated on for prognostic grounds (e.g. Marfan's syndrome), (2) Presence of rapidly evolving stent technology (e.g. thoracic endovascular aortic repair (TEVAR)) necessitating thorough assessment, and (3) Clinical situations where patient compliance is essential (e.g. two-stage aortic procedures).

This chapter therefore aims to provide readers with an overview of the available literature considering patients' HRQoL after thoracic aorta interventions. Highlights include key factors influencing both physical and mental QoL outcomes and how these may influence future clinical practice and research directions.

M. K. H. Tan (✉)
Academic Section of Vascular Surgery, Department of Surgery and Cancer, Imperial College London, Charing Cross Hospital, London, UK
e-mail: matthew.tan1@nhs.net

O. A. Jarral · Y. Salmasi · T. Athanasiou
Department of Surgery and Cancer, Imperial College London, St. Mary's Hospital, London, UK
e-mail: y.salmasi@imperial.ac.uk; t.athanasiou@imperial.ac.uk

M. Sabetai
St. Thomas' Hospital, London, UK
e-mail: michael.sabetai@gstt.nhs.uk

T. Athanasiou et al. (eds.), *Patient Reported Outcomes and Quality of Life in Cardiovascular Interventions*,
https://doi.org/10.1007/978-3-031-09815-4_4

Table 4.1 Factors contributing to reduced morbidity and mortality in aortic surgery

Physiology and anatomy	Surgical technique	Anaesthetic technique
Greater understanding of the deleterious effects of ischaemia	Right subclavian/axillary, innominate or left common carotid cannulation	Better appreciation of the impact of deep hypothermic circulatory arrest (DHCA)
Stronger appreciation of brain and spinal cord anatomy	Use of continuous and bilateral antegrade cerebral perfusion	Superior intensive care strategies to deal with multi-organ dysfunction
	Frozen elephant trunk technique reducing need for second-stage procedures	Pre-operative rehabilitation of high risk patients
	Improved risk stratification leading to less invasive hybrid strategies for appropriate patients	
	Consistent and protocol driven use of spinal cord drains in thoracoabdominal operations	
	Use of moderate rather than profound hypothermia in selected situations	

Proximal Thoracic Aorta

Aortic Root Replacement/Repair

Aortic root replacement is usually indicated for proximal aortic aneurysm or dissection, or as a concomitant procedure during intervention on the aortic valve [8]. In the current literature, 10 studies reported on outcomes after different forms of isolated aortic root replacement or repair [9–18] (Table 4.2 adapted from Jarral et al. [4]). In general, most studies showed acceptable HRQoL at follow-up, comparable to that of a healthy baseline population.

The only randomised controlled trial reported in the literature described 10-year outcomes after either homograft root replacement or the Ross procedure (pulmonary autograft) replacement for aortic valve disease [11]. In this study by El-Hamamsy et al., demonstrated better physical functioning in patients undergoing the Ross. Although this reduction may have been due to higher rates of reoperation in the homograft group, the authors also attributed the higher physical functioning and general health domain scores of patients receiving autografts to the ability of the "living" autograft root having the ability to changes in haemodynamics over the patients' life. The concept and benefits of a 'living' autograft is still debateable, with the risks of pulmonary autograft dilatation countering the advantages. The benefits of "living" tissue is supported by Franke et al. [12], a retrospective cohort study which looked at composite aortic root replacement (Bentall procedure) versus aortic valve reimplantation (David procedure). Franke et al. found HRQoL to be significantly better following the David procedure in all domains except bodily pain and social functioning. This was not seen in a study by Khaladj et al. which found no significant difference between these procedures at midterm follow-up, but this study was limited by a small cohort of only 46 patients [14]. Interestingly, Franke et al. suggested that the HRQoL benefits of the David procedure was in part due to the avoidance of anticoagulation and the mechanical heart sounds heard by patients undergoing the Bentall procedure. The latter point is supported by a study from Golczyk et al., which, using a valve-specific questionnaire, confirmed that certain mechanical aortic root prostheses were quieter than others, and patients subjectively found some conduits to be more inconvenient than others [13]. Between mechanical and bioprosthetic Bentall procedures, Lehr et al. showed no significant differences in HRQoL [15].

In a further cohort study on valve-sparing aortic root replacements, Bori Bata et al. found patients to have excellent HRQoL at mid-term follow-up, comparable to that of the normal population [10]. When comparing between younger and older patients undergoing valve-sparing aor-

Table 4.2 Studies observing aortic root replacement

Author, year of publication, study period and study type	Study intent and number of patients	Surgical centre	Patient characteristics	Pre-op HRQOL assessment	Follow-up period	HRQOL instrument used Follow-up completion rate (%)	Main findings related to HRQOL
Akhyari et al. 2009 [9] 1996–2004 Retrospective cohort study	Comparison of Ross procedure and ascending aorta replacement (n = 18) vs. mechanical composite root replacement (n = 20)	Hannover Medical School, Germany	All patients had aortic valvular disease and concomitant ascending aortic aneurysm Similar patient characteristics in both groups except Ross group had a higher proportion of patients with impaired left ventricular function.	No	Average of 38.4 months in Ross group and 49.8 months in composite group	SF-36 100%	Patients undergoing the Bentall procedure had slightly higher SF-36 scores Only statistically significant in vitality and physical functioning
Bori Bata et al. 2017 [10] 2003–2014 Prospective cohort study	Evaluating the mid-term outcomes of 88 patients with aortic root aneurysm or ascending aortic aneurysms undergoing valve-sparing aortic root replacement	Gabriel Montpied Hospital, France	All had aortic root or ascending aortic aneurysms Mean age (years): 55 ± 14 (19–77) 84% male	No	5.3 ± 3 (1–12) years	EuroQoL visual analogue scale (VAS) EuroQoL index 88%	Mean EuroQoL VAS was 83 ± 15 (30–100), mean EuroQoL index was 0.94 ± 0.12 (0.5–1) Similar HRQoL to healthy patients seen in 79% of patient cohort Valve-sparing aortic root replacement is considered to have superior HRQoL outcomes as compared to the Bentall procedure/aortic composite replacement

(continued)

Table 4.2 (continued)

Author, year of publication, study period and study type	Study intent and number of patients	Surgical centre	Patient characteristics	Pre-op HRQOL assessment	Follow-up period	HRQOL instrument used Follow-up completion rate (%)	Main findings related to HRQOL
El-Hamamsy et al. 2010 [11] 1994–2001 Prospective randomized controlled trial	Patients <69 years of age requiring AVR were randomly assigned to receive an autograft (n = 108) or homograft aortic root replacement (n = 108). Outcomes and HRQOL were measured Children and those with Marfan syndrome were excluded.	Royal Brompton and Harefield Hospitals, London, UK	Mean age (years): 39 (19–68) in homograft group, 38 (19–66) in autograft group No significant difference in comorbidities between patient groups.	No	10.2 years (± 3.2)	SF-36 73%	Median SF-36 physical functioning and general health domain scores were significantly higher in recipients of autograft aortic root replacement than in those given homograft aortic root replacement
Franke et al. 2010 [12] 1999–2005 Retrospective cohort study	Comparison in QoL between the David operation (aortic valve re-implantation, n = 76) with that of aortic composite root replacement using a mechanical prosthesis (n = 67)	University of Cologne, Germany	Mean age (years): 58 ± 14 in David group and 56 ± in composite group No significant difference in co-morbidity between patient groups, although the composite group had a significantly higher proportion of bicuspid aortic valves and aortic arch aneurysm	No	Measured 'at least 6 months after the operation was performed'	SF-36 76%	Significantly impaired in all of the SF-36 domains (apart from bodily pain and social function) for composite group compared to the David group Composite graft group significantly more compromised by prosthetic valve noise and significantly more reported feeling moderately or severely disturbed by this noise

Golczyk et al. 2010 [13] Data collection period not reported Randomised prospective cohort study	Comparison of the closing sounds of thirty patients receiving three different mechanical composite aortic root prostheses (Sorin, St. Jude and ATS)	University Hospital Berne, Switzerland	No significant difference in baseline characteristics between patients including BMI	No	At three and six months after surgery	'Valve disturbance' questionnaire and loudness of valve sounds recorded. 100%	Sound pressures at peak were lower for the ATS than for the St. Jude and Sorin composite grafts but this did not reach significance However, subjective disturbance with the ATS valves was significantly lower than the St. Jude and Sorin composite grafts
Khaladj et al. 2009 [14] 1999–2006 Retrospective cohort study	Comparison of elective composite root replacement (n = 23 of which 13 mechanical) vs. David operation (n = 23) in patients requiring aortic arch surgery using HCA and ACP with the focus on post-operative neurological outcome and QoL	Hannover Medical School, Germany	Pre-operative characteristics matched for age, gender, HCA-time and year of surgery	No	64 (6–90) months	SF-36 95%	SF-36 scores were comparable between the two groups at follow-up
Lehr et al. 2011 [15] 1998–2007 Retrospective cohort study	Early and midterm results analysis in patients undergoing aortic root replacement (Bentall): 51 mechanical and 93 biological valve conduits	The University of Alberta, Canada	Patients in the biological group were significantly older than the patients in the mechanical group (60.9 ± 13.9 vs. 47.7 ± 14.1 years) The mechanical group contained a higher proportion of males (94.1% vs. 66.7%) The biological group contained a significantly higher number of patients with hyperlipidemia, previous cardiac surgery, coronary artery disease and chronic obstructive pulmonary disease	No	40 months	EQ-5D SAD HADS 62.7%	General and disease-specific HRQoL scores were not significantly different between groups

(continued)

Table 4.2 (continued)

Author, year of publication, study period and study type	Study intent and number of patients	Surgical centre	Patient characteristics	Pre-op HRQOL assessment	Follow-up period	HRQOL instrument used / Follow-up completion rate (%)	Main findings related to HRQOL
Perrotta et al. 2010 [16] 1997–2008 Retrospective cohort study	Quality of life outcomes in patients undergoing aortic root replacement with homograft for infective endocarditis (n = 62) 31 of these patients had infective prosthetic valve endocarditis and 31 had native valve endocarditis with root abscess	University of Gothenburg, Sweden	Mean age of 57 ± 15 years and 77% were male	No	37 ± 11 months	SF-36 89%	HRQoL not significantly lower at follow-up when compared to an age- and gender-matched control group in the PCS or MCS In contrast, patients had significantly inferior results in four of the eight subscales: role-physical, general health, vitality, and mental health
Wachter et al. 2017 [17] 2007–2012 Prospective cohort study	Comparing outcomes in patients having a David procedure between minimally invasive hemisternotomy (n = 117) and conventional midline sternotomy (n = 75)	Robert Bosch Hospital, Stuttgart, Germany	Patients with the minimally invasive hemisternotomy were significantly younger (56.5 ± 13.6 vs. 64.8 ± 11.6) and had a higher proportion of males (81.2% vs. 69.3%) No significant differences in co-morbidities between groups	No	31 ± 18 months	SF-36 91%	Patients undergoing minimally invasive hemisternotomy showed non-statistically significantly higher scores in the subcategories for physical and mental health

Zacek et al. 2016 [18] 2006–2012 Cross-sectional study	Determining the QoL in patients undergoing aortic valve-sparing procedures <50 years old (n = 36), aortic valve-sparing procedure >50 years old (n = 52), the Ross procedure (n = 22), and mechanical aortic valve replacement (n = 29)	Charles University in Prague, Faculty of Medicine and Faculty Hospital, Czech Republic	Valve-sparing <50 years old: • Mean age 36.3 ± 6.1 years old • 78% male Valve-sparing >50 years old: • Mean age 59.2 ± 7.7 years old • 70% male Ross procedure: • Mean age 37.8 ± 11.9 years old • 83% male Mechanical aortic valve replacement: • Mean age 39.7 ± 7.3 years old • 69% male	No	Median 26.9 months (range 6–73 months)	SF-36 Valve-specific questionnaire 97%	Based on the SF-36, younger patients undergoing valve-sparing procedures and patients undergoing Ross procedures scored significantly better on all physical subscales and two mental subscales (vitality, social functioning) compared to older patients undergoing valve-sparing procedures and mechanical aortic valve replacements Patients undergoing valve-sparing procedures and the Ross procedures showed greater freedom from valve-related lifestyle limitations when compared to the mechanical aortic valve replacement patients (e.g. follow-up care, frequent doctor visits, blood tests, complications from implanted valve)

tic root replacements, Zacek et al. showed both younger patients undergoing valve-sparing aortic root replacements and patients undergoing the Ross procedure to have better HRQoL than older patients undergoing valve-sparing procedures and patients undergoing mechanical aortic valve replacements. In this same study, a valve-specific questionnaire was used and showed patients undergoing mechanical aortic valve replacements to have less freedom from valve-related lifestyle limitations (e.g. frequent follow-ups, blood tests etc.) [18]. In the only analysis on HRQoL outcomes following homograft replacements for endocarditis, Perrotta et al. showed follow-up HRQoL to be comparable to an age- and gender-matched population, despite more than half of their patient population experiencing prosthetic valve endocarditis with root abscess, suggesting that aggressive treatment might still be justified even in high-risk subgroups [16]. In the only study in the literature examining outcomes after minimal access root surgery, Wachter et al. examed HRQoL differences between a minimally invasive ministernotomy versus the conventional midline sternotomy for the David procedure. This analysis showed that patients undergoing minimally invasive approach showed a higher HRQoL for both physical and mental health compared to those having a median sternotomy, although this was not statistically significant at mid-term follow-up of around 3 years [17].

Other Proximal Aortic Operations

Besides aortic root replacements, HRQoL outcomes after various proximal aortic operations are also reported in six studies identified from the literature [19–24]. These procedures also resulted in generally acceptable post-operative HRQoL (Table 4.3 adapted from Jarral et al. [4]), but emergency surgery was found to be predictive of impaired long-term HRQoL and need for reoperation in patients with Marfan syndrome [22]. The use of DHCA to be predictive of impaired physical role functioning in long-term follow-up [23].

Lohse et al. (134 patients with ascending aortic aneurysms) [20] and Stalder et al. (244 patients undergoing ascending aortic operations) [23] showed that post-operative HRQoL was comparable to that of an age- and sex-matched reference population. Older age and prolonged hospital stay were also found to be risk factors for reduced physical functioning [20, 23]. Abe et al. also showed that in patients undergoing ascending aorta wrapping or graft replacement during aortic valve replacement, post-operative HRQoL was not statistically different from that of a general population as well, but this was in a small population of 40 patients only [19]. In an older study by Olsson and Thelin, patients undergoing thoracic aortic repair with either a straight Dacron graft or composite root replacement over 20 years ago had significantly lower HRQoL than a matched population [21]. This was limited by the small patient population (81 patients) and the fact that 82% of patients actually felt that their HRQoL was improved or preserved in this study, with 91% considering the operation a success. Another study by Olsson and Franco-Cereceda showed that HRQoL scores were not affected by type of proximal aortic procedure performed but was instead predicted by current symptoms and conditions experienced by patients [24]. Finally, Song et al. was the only study that observed HRQoL in patients with Marfan's syndrome, studying 194 survivors who underwent elective and emergency proximal aortic operations [22]. Emergency surgery was found to be associated with a higher incidence of chronic dissection, reoperation rate, dilated distal aorta and impaired HRQoL—the authors concluded the underlying need for early diagnosis and elective surgery based on these outcomes.

Type A Dissection Repair

Type A dissection is a surgical emergency which carries a high mortality rate in the absence of prompt surgical treatment [25]. HRQoL outcomes are reported in six studies in the current literature [26–31], results of which are found in Table 4.4 (adapted from Jarral et al. [4]).

Table 4.3 Studies observing other proximal aortic operations

Author, year of publication, study period and study type	Study intent and number of patients	Surgical centre	Patient characteristics	Pre-op HRQOL assessment	Follow-up period	HRQOL instrument used / Follow-up completion rate (%)	Main findings related to HRQOL
Abe et al. 2017 [19] 2000–2013 Prospective cohort	Outcomes in 40 consecutive patients undergoing either wrapping (n = 20) or ascending aorta replacement (n = 20) for dilated ascending aorta	Nagoya University Graduate School of Medicine, Nagoya, Japan	No significant difference in age (59.2 ± 2.3 vs. 64.5 ± 2.2 years) or gender distribution (70% male vs. 60% male) between groups	No	4.9 years (0.6–11.4)	SF-36 91.6%	No differences between groups for any of the subcategories on the SF-36 HRQoL in patients is not statistically different from the general population
Lohse et al. 2009 [20] 1999–2003 Retrospective cohort	Quality of life assessment in 134 consecutive patients with true aneurysms undergoing ascending aorta surgery: procedures consisted of interposition graft (35.9%), interposition + AVR (35.9%), David (11.2%), Bentall (9%) and Cabrol procedure in 2.2%	University of Munich, Germany	Mean age of survivors was 61.7 ± 11 years and 63.4% were men	No	36.4 ± 15.5 months	SF-36 98.7%	Post-operative HRQoL revealed physical function results significantly lower than the reference population in patients between 70–79 years of age Prolonged hospital stay (>20 days) was identified as a risk factor for a significantly reduced PCS
Olsson and Franco-Cereceda 2013 [24] Data collection period not reported Retrospective cohort study	Investigating QoL after surgical repair of the proximal aorta, comparing it to a reference population and identifying predictors of QoL in 207 patients	Karolinska Institutet, Stockholm, Sweden	Median age 57 (IQR 12) 70% male	No	Not reported	SF-36 Not reported	No significant differences in median PCS or MCS, although median scores for subgroups including physical functioning, general health, and mental health were significantly lower No significant differences between scores for patients undergoing surgery for aneurysms vs. dissection, between valve-sparing vs. mechanical/biological valve-replacements, or between types of valve replacements Exertional dyspnoea was predictive for changes in MCS and PCS, while age, exertional calf pain, and myocardial infarction only predicted for changes in PCS

(continued)

Table 4.3 (continued)

Author, year of publication, study period and study type	Study intent and number of patients	Surgical centre	Patient characteristics	Pre-op HRQOL assessment	Follow-up period	HRQOL instrument used Follow-up completion rate (%)	Main findings related to HRQOL
Olsson and Thelin 1999 [21] 1990–1995 Retrospective cohort	Assessment of QoL in survivors (n = 81) of thoracic aortic surgery In respondents: a straight Dacron vascular graft was used in 64 (81%), 12 had a composite root replacement and 3 received AVR and interposition graft. DHCA was used in 52% of cases	Uppsala University Hospital, Sweden	Mean age of 59 of whom 70% were male	No	26 months (7–76)	SF-36 General health perception questionnaire 94%	66% stated general health perception improvement post-operatively and 82% felt HRQoL improved or was preserved 91% considered the operation successful Overall quality of life in this population was significantly lower than in a matched population except for bodily pain
Song et al. 2012 [22] Marfan patients enrolled in GeneTAC registry as of March 2011 Retrospective cohort	Analysis of the long-term clinical courses of patients with Marfan syndrome who are survivors from emergency (type A dissection) vs. elective proximal aortic surgery A total of 194 patients underwent surgery of which 47 were emergencies and 147 elective operations Patients in the emergency group were more likely to have incomplete proximal aortic resection: 83% included root replacement compared with 95% of elective procedures	Multi-institutional, USA	No significant difference in age between emergency & elective group (34.9 vs. 38.0), of whom 66% were male	No	4.73 years in emergency group and 6.34 years in elective group	SF-36 and Karnofsky Performance Status score 100%	Patients in the elective group had significantly higher reported activity scores on the SF-36
Stalder et al. 2007 [23] 2001–2003 Retrospective cohort	The impact different aortic surgical procedures (n = 244) on outcome and QoL 76 patients (31.2%) underwent interposition graft to the ascending aorta, 42 (17.2%) received separate AVR and supracoronary replacement of the aorta, 86 (35.2%) received a mechanical composite graft, and 40 (16.4%) received a biologic composite graft	University Hospital Berne, Switzerland	Mean age was 60.6 ± 14.6 years and 75% were male 61.9% had true aortic aneurysm (>5 cm) and 30.7% had acute type A dissection. 58.2% underwent a procedure using DHCA	No	26.6 ± 8.8 months	SF-36 76.9%	HRQoL in all groups was comparable to an age- and sex-matched population Patients who underwent DHCA had a significant deficit in physical role functioning compared with patients of the same group operated on without DHCA

Table 4.4 Studies observing operations for type A dissection

Author, year of publication, study period and study type	Study intent and number of patients	Surgical centre	Patient characteristics	Pre-op HRQOL assessment	Follow-up period	HRQOL instrument used Follow-up completion rate (%)	Main findings related to HRQOL
Adam et al. 2018 [26] 2006–2010 Retrospective cohort	Determine HRQoL outcomes of 393 patients undergoing repair for type A aortic dissection Deep hypothermia used in 84%, with retrograde (75%) or antegrade (6%) cerebral perfusion applied 2 main procedures: • Aortic valve reconstruction (40.5%) • Aortic valve replacement with bioprosthesis (5.7%) or mechanical prosthesis (24%)	Deutsches Herzzentrum Berlin, Berlin, Germany	Mean age 59.1 ± 12.3 years 62.9% male 4 patients had Marfan's syndrome	No	51 ± 27.8 months	SF-12 Post-traumatic Diagnostic Scale (PDS) Post-traumatic Stress Scale 14 (PTSS-14) 53%	Only 188 patients filled up the SF-12 in full Lower mean PCS and MCS scores were seen compared to the population norm PCS continually declined with increasing age of patients 65 patients (31.5%) possibly had PTSD according to the PTSS-14, and 43 patients (27%) were at risk of PTSD based on the PDS criteria Trend towards more females, younger patients, unemployment and disability increasing risk of PTSD after operations

(continued)

Table 4.4 (continued)

Author, year of publication, study period and study type	Study intent and number of patients	Surgical centre	Patient characteristics	Pre-op HRQOL assessment	Follow-up period	HRQOL instrument used Follow-up completion rate (%)	Main findings related to HRQOL
Campbell-Lloyd et al. 2010 [27] 2000–2008 Retrospective cohort	Review of outcomes in 65 patients who underwent type A dissection repair. Axillary cannulation performed in 37%. HCA alone in 19%, HCA with RCP in 11% and HCA with ACP in 46 and on cross-clamp in the remaining 24%. Full root replacement in 31.7% and arch replacement in 14%.	Princess Alexandra Hospital, Australia	Mean age 61.2 ± 11.4 years 60% male 5 patients had Marfan's syndrome At presentation 59% had evidence of malperfusion	No	Mean of 26.6 months	EQ-5D 69%	Discharged patients had reasonable long-term survival and good HRQoL 90% reported minimal limitation on functional scores 48% recorded full health with an overall mean index of 0.854 (where the best possible score is 1) using the US preference weighted index score "Some" problems in only one category of the EQ-5D questionnaire was reported by 10.34% and 6.89% reported some problems in two categories Severe problems were reported in one category by a further 10.34% and nearly all were that of debilitating anxiety and/or depression

Endlich et al. 2016 [28] 1999–2006 Retrospective cohort	Determine long-term outcomes and HRQoL after type A dissection repair in 120 patients Procedures included: • Supracoronary replacement (n = 103, 85.8%) • Supracoronary replacement + subcoronary aortic valve replacement (n = 9, 7.5%) • Bentall-DeBono procedure (n = 5, 4.2%) • David procedure (n = 2, 1.7%) • Cabrol procedure (n = 1, 0.8%)	University Hospital Bonn, Bonn, Germany	Mean age 59.8 ± 12 years 70% male 2 patients with Marfan's syndrome	No	45 ± 32 months after procedure Then 46 ± 10 months after initial follow-up	SF-36 49.2%	Both PCS and MCS were significantly worse at both follow-up points when compared to the population norm PCS and MCS declined significantly between follow-up points No pre- or post-operative factors had any influence on the PCS or MCS
Ghazy et al. 2017 [29] 2007–2010 Prospective cohort	Compare post-operative HRQoL in 39 patients between management strategies for type A dissection including total arch replacement ± frozen elephant trunk procedure, isolated replacement of ascending aorta, or replacement of ascending aorta + aortic arch ± frozen elephant trunk procedure	Dresden Heart Centre, Dresden, Germany	Isolated ascending aorta replacement: mean age 62 ± 14 years, 73% male Ascending aorta + aortic arch replacement ± frozen elephant trunk procedure: mean age 62 ± 12 years, 77% male Not significantly different between groups	No	Not reported	SF-36 WHO-QOL-BREF Not reported	Bodily pain and mental health were similar to the normal population All other subcategories were non-statistically significantly lower than population normal Significantly better scores were seen on the WHO-QOL-BREF in global life quality and psychological health in patients undergoing an isolated ascending aorta replacement

(continued)

Table 4.4 (continued)

Author, year of publication, study period and study type	Study intent and number of patients	Surgical centre	Patient characteristics	Pre-op HRQOL assessment	Follow-up period	HRQOL instrument used / Follow-up completion rate (%)	Main findings related to HRQOL
Kamenskaya et al. 2019 [30] 2014–2015 Retrospective cohort	Assess HRQoL before and one year after prosthetics of the aorta for chronic type I dissection (n = 82)	National Medical Research Center of the Ministry of Health of the Russian Federation, Russia	Mean age 56.8 ± 11.5 years 75.6% male	Yes	1 year	SF-36 98.6%	Low level of HRQoL was noted pre-operatively, most impaired in physical and social functioning Post-operatively, there was a statistically significant increase in role functioning, bodily pain, vitality, social functioning, role functioning emotional, together with increase in the PCS and MCS Post-operative MCS was affected by post-operative neurological complications as well as baseline PCS and MCS while PCS was only affected by baseline PCS
Nakamura et al. 2011 [31] 2007–2010 Retrospective cohort	Impact on QoL of immediate type A dissection repair in patients with cerebral malperfusion (n = 10) Hemiarch replacement was performed in 9 and total arch replacement in 1	Kanto Medical Centre, Tokyo, Japan	Mean age of patients was 69 ± 9 years, 60% were male Pre-operative neurological symptoms were hemiplegia in 9 and motor aphasia in 1. CT confirmed evidence of cerebellar infarction in six of these patients	No	18 ± 5 months	Rankin scale Mean National Institutes of Health (NIH) stroke scale 100%	Mean NIH stroke scale improved was 5.5 ± 2.9 at presentation and improved to 1.9 ± 2.6 at discharge Mean modified Rankin score improved from 2.1 ± 1.3 at discharge to 0.8 ± 0.9 at 12 months after the surgery

Overall HRQoL of survivors following type A dissection repair was found to be acceptable in studies performed in the early half of the last decade [27, 31]. For example, Campbell-Lloyd et al. showed that in patients with cerebral malperfusion, significant improvement in overall function at long-term follow-up was seen [27]. This is supported in a more recent study by Kamenskaya et al., which showed that in a cohort of 82 patients with chronic type I dissection, HRQoL scores were improved with post-dissection repair [30], but this comparison is limited by the elective nature of these operations. Interestingly, two more recent studies on emergency operations for type A dissection by Adam et al. (210 respondents) [26] and Endlich et al. (120 patients undergoing various operations) [28] both showed significantly worse HRQoL when compared to an adjusted population, with Endlich et al. also showing decaying HRQoL over time. Ghazy et al. also showed that, while not statistically significant, patients undergoing a less aggressive procedure (ascending aorta replacement only) showed better HRQoL in all domains of the SF-36 [29]. This supports the argument for a life-saving procedure approaching the entry tear only in the acute setting [32], with further operations to manage the remaining tear further down the line [33].

Thoracoabdominal Aortic Aneurysm Repair

Thoracoabdominal aortic aneurysms (TAAs) represent a spectrum of complicated degenerative aortic disease, which is typically characterised using the Crawford classification system. While the incidence at a population level is low (estimated at 10 new cases per 100,000 person-years [34]), the potential for rupture if untreated is high, at nearly 80% [35]. Treatment for these has shifted preferentially towards endovascular options (described in the next section) due to the invasiveness of open surgery. Open surgery however still has a major role, and remains the gold standard for TAAs, especially in the elective setting for complex type 1 and 2 disease. HRQoL outcomes have been described in six studies [36–41] (Table 4.5 adapted from Jarral et al. [4]), which have all assessed HRQoL in patients undergoing elective TAA repair for various extents of TAA.

In one of the few studies to examine baseline HRQoL, Coroneos et al. showed that there was no change in HRQoL of patients at 6 and 12 months after elective open TAA repair in 80 patients. Baseline HRQoL was found to be lower than that of healthy controls prior to the operation [36]. Further studies by Crawford et al. [37], Di Luozzo et al. [38] and Eide et al. [39] also showed that, in contrast to the studies on proximal aortic surgery discussed previously, patients undergoing descending and TAA surgery have worse HRQoL compared to that of a normal population. In two studies by Ghanta et al. [40] and Zierer et al. [41], this inferior HRQoL was found to be limited to physical health, with mental and psychological components of health maintained or improved as compared to the normal population. This lower physical HRQoL may be due to baseline patient characteristics, with TAA patients usually having great burden of comorbidities (e.g. peripheral vascular disease, COPD). An alternative explanation could be due to abnormal flow patterns in the descending aorta having a complex impact on HRQoL, more so than the flow patterns in the proximal aorta. While the impact of flow patterns on HRQoL have yet to be studied, current studies have shown predictors for impaired HRQoL post-operatively to include increasing age, female gender, peripheral vascular disease, reoperations and post-operative neurological events.

Endovascular Interventions on the Thoracic Aorta

As alluded to in the previous section, endovascular options are increasingly favoured in the management of aortic disease. Four studies in the current literature have observed HRQoL outcomes in patients undergoing endovascular interventions [42–45], and the results from these studies are found in Table 4.6 (adapted from Jarral et al. [4]).

Table 4.5 Studies observing thoracoabdominal aortic aneurysm repair

Author, year of publication, study period and study type	Study intent and number of patients	Surgical centre	Patient characteristics	Pre-op HRQOL assessment	Follow-up period	HRQOL instrument used Follow-up completion rate (%)	Main findings related to HRQOL
Coroneos et al. 2009 [36] 1998–2006 Prospective cohort study	Assessment of QoL after elective open thoraco-abdominal aneurysm repair (n = 80)	Toronto and Hamilton, Ontario, Canada	Not reported specifically in group undergoing QoL assessment	Yes, but only in 56%	Measured pre-op, at 6 months and 1 year after surgery Healthy individuals recruited as control group	IIRS tool and KAS scale 44% at 1 year	No change in HRQoL at 6 and 12 months following thoracoabdominal aneurysm repair Pre-operative HRQoL was lower than that of healthy controls
Crawford et al. 2008 [37] 1987–2005 Retrospective cohort study	QoL assessed in 134 survivors of open TAA repair and compared to age-adjusted reference population	Massachusetts General Hospital, Boston, USA	Mean age of 69.5 years Male sex 619% Diabetes—6.7% Hypertension—85.1% Coronary artery disease—98.5% Urgent surgery—12.7%	No	Measured at a mean follow-up from surgery of 60 ± 38.7 months	SF-36 67%	Permanent loss of functional capacity, measured at a mean of 5 years postoperatively, occurred rarely in survivors of TAA repair HRQoL was significantly lower in TAA repair patients compared to the general population Predictors of pre-operative reduced QoL were female gender, age >75 and peripheral vascular disease Predictive factors of reduced QoL after surgery were post-operative paraplegia/CVA and re-operation TAA extent (I to IV) nor operative urgency influenced long-term HRQoL

Di Luozzo et al. 2013 [38] 2002–2008 Retrospective cohort	Retrospective review of QoL of 93 over patients over the age of 70 undergoing open repair of descending aortic aneurysm or TAAA	Mount Sinai School of Medicine, New York, USA	Mean age at operation 75 ± 4.1 years, 51% male Replacement of descending thoracic aorta in 23.7% and thoracoabdominal aorta in 76.3%.	No	4.1 years (range 1.1–7.1)	SF-36 81%	Respondents scored slightly lower than the matched US population in all HRQoL domains—these differences were not significant except in the vitality domain
Eide et al. 2005 [39] 1983–2001 Retrospective cohort	Assessment of HRQoL in long-term survivors of TAAA repair (n = 13)	University Hospital of Trondheim, Norway	Mean age at follow-up was 67.4 years (44.4–78.3) Median aneurysm diameter 7 cm Crawford classification: 4 had type 2, four had type 3 and three had type 4 One emergency presentation (rupture)	No	6.2 (range 1.3–14.1) years	SF-36 and "A Vascular specific questionnaire" 85%	SF-36 scores were generally poorer than that of the healthy population in both physical and mental dimensions but comparable in other domains Patients who had an uncomplicated postoperative course all reported general health status comparable with their pre-operative status Patients who had complicated postoperative course generally scored lower in the physical dimensions According to disease-specific questions, impotence and pain were reported as major long-term postoperative problems

(continued)

Table 4.5 (continued)

Author, year of publication, study period and study type	Study intent and number of patients	Surgical centre	Patient characteristics	Pre-op HRQOL assessment	Follow-up period	HRQOL instrument used Follow-up completion rate (%)	Main findings related to HRQOL
Ghanta et al. 2016 [40] 2004–2010 Retrospective cohort	Assess HRQoL in patients with Marfan's syndrome undergoing type II TAA repair (n = 49)	Baylor College of Medicine, Houston, TX, USA	Mean age 43 ± 12 years 65% male Concomitant aortic dissection noted—type I (n = 27, 55%) and IIIb (n = 18, 37%)	No	6.0 ± 2.5 years	SF-12v2 58.5%	Poorer PCS but better MCS than the general population
Zierer et al. 2006 [41] 1998–2003 Retrospective cohort	Quality of life assessment in patients undergoing elective thoracic aortic replacement (n = 110) Twenty-nine patients (26%) underwent ascending, 33 (30%) descending and 48 (44%) TAA aneurysm replacement	Washington University School of Medicine, USA	Mean age was 67 ± 9 years and 49% were male	No	35 ± 20 months	SF-36 84%	Psychological HRQoL at follow up was similar between the groups, but physical HRQoL was lower after thoracoabdominal aneurysm versus ascending/descending aortic aneurysms Age did not impact HRQoL, but older patients had improved psychological HRQoL Multivariate analysis identified two factors to be independent predictors of impaired late functional status at 12 months: NYHA III or IV and COPD Psychological HRQoL scores were similar to age-matched US population but physical scores were diminished

Table 4.6 Studies observing endovascular interventions on the thoracic aorta

Author, year of publication, study period and study type	Study intent and number of patients	Surgical centre	Patient characteristics	Pre-op HRQOL assessment	Follow-up period	HRQOL instrument used Follow-up completion rate (%)	Main findings related to HRQOL
Dick et al. 2008 [42] 2001–2005 Post-hoc analysis of prospective collected series	Outcome and QoL assessment after open surgical (n = 70) and endovascular (n = 52) intervention on the descending thoracic aorta	University Hospital Bern, Switzerland	Mean age was significantly higher in TEVAR patients (69 ± 10 years vs. 62 ± 15 years) as was proportion of patients undergoing emergency intervention Average aneurysm diameter significantly larger in open group (6.8 ± 1.6 cm vs 5.6 ± 1.6 cm)	No	34 ± 18 months	SF-36 and HADS questionnaire 61%	No significant different in HRQoL in all domains at follow-up when comparing open and TEVAR techniques
Kärkkäinen et al. 2019 [43] 2013–2016 Prospective cohort	Analyse changes in HRQoL for patients with pararenal aortic aneurysms (n = 57) and TAAs (n = 102) with F-BEVAR and compare these outcomes with those in the EVAR 1 trial	Mayo Clinic, Rochester, MN, USA	Overall cohort: mean age 74.8 ± 7.0 years, 70% male TAA cohort: mean age 73.8 ± 6.8 years, 70.6% male	Yes	12 months	SF-36 65%	TAAs patients had lower baseline scores than those with pararenal aortic aneurysms PCS declined 6–8 weeks after F-BEVAR and failed to return to baseline at 12 months in the TAA group Major adverse events were associated with PCS decline at 6–8 weeks but not at longer follow-up

(continued)

Table 4.6 (continued)

Author, year of publication, study period and study type	Study intent and number of patients	Surgical centre	Patient characteristics	Pre-op HRQOL assessment	Follow-up period	HRQOL instrument used Follow-up completion rate (%)	Main findings related to HRQOL
Klocker et al. 2014 [44] 1996–2014 Retrospective cohort	Report on the incidence of left arm ischemia, left arm function and QoL after TEVAR by stent grafting with and without coverage of the LSA A total of 138 patients underwent TEVAR, of who 68 had degenerative aneurysm, 38 traumatic aortic injuries and 36 type B dissection. 73 of these had LSA coverage, of which 9 had LSA revascularization	Medical University Innsbruck, Austria	Not reported specifically in group undergoing QoL assessment	No	4.1 ± 3.7 years	DASH SF-12 63%	In comparing patients with occluded vs. patent LSA, the PCS and MCS of the SF-12 and the DASH scores were comparable and the incidence of left arm ischemia is low However, during subgroup analysis, in patients with traumatic aortic injury, the PCS was superior when the LSA was patent
McBride et al. 2015 [45] 2005–2012 Retrospective cohort	Evaluation of long-term effects of LSA coverage (n = 32) vs. non-coverage (n = 50) during TEVAR on symptoms and return to normal activity in traumatic aortic injury patients	University of Texas Medical School, USA	Mean age of 46.7 ± 21.7 years (significantly lower age in LSA uncovered group)	No	3.35 ± 1.9 years	SF-12 "LSA questionnaire" Not reported	No significant difference in SF-12 physical health scores between the two groups The covered LSA group had significantly better mental health score No difference in LSA symptoms between the two groups or in ability to return to normal activities

Only one study compared HRQoL between open and endovascular interventions, performing a *post hoc* analysis on a prospectively collected database including 152 patients undergoing TEVAR or open operations. Dick et al. showed that at a mean follow-up of 34 months, post-operative HRQoL were similar between groups, despite the TEVAR group having older patients, more emergency procedures, and smaller aneurysms [42]. Kärkkäinen et al. was a recent study which observed HRQoL changes from baseline following fenestrated-branched EVAR in two groups of patients with either pararenal aortic aneurysms or TAAs [43]. All patients showed a decline in their physical HRQoL at six to eight weeks after intervention, but no decline in mental HRQoL. Interestingly, this decline persisted in the TAA group at 12 months, while that of the pararenal aneurysm group returned to baseline values. It is a common misconception that TEVAR should be associated with better HRQoL than open surgery, which may stem from extrapolation from studies on abdominal aorta stenting [46]. Kärkkäinen et al. showed lower physical component scores as compared to those obtained from the EVAR 1 trial [47], and this could be due to the anatomical and biomechanical differences innately found in the thoracic aorta. Higher shear stress, anchorage issues, reduced mechanical stability, endoleaks and other stent-related contributions may contribute to decline in HRQoL, which may explain why scores might have been comparable in the non-randomised study by Dick et al. [42].

Two studies examined the HRQoL following TEVAR with or without coverage of the left subclavian artery, showing no difference between groups for the physical component score of the SF-36 [44, 45], although McBride et al. showed significantly better mental component scores in patients who had coverage of the left subclavian artery [45]. This supports arguments for selective revascularisation based on the underlying knowledge of patients' vertebrobasilar anatomy. Both studies also used a disease-specific questionnaire in their analysis, which was not seen in other studies.

Aortic Surgery in the Elderly

Age has been identified as a predictor of mortality in some studies [48], but refuted in others [49]. It remains a controversial subject, as advanced age may be used as a preclusive criterion by referring clinicians and surgeons for major aortic surgery. In the current literature, five available studies in the literature considered HRQoL outcomes in elderly patients [1, 50–53] (Table 4.7 adapted from Jarral et al. [4]). In general, most studies found HRQoL after major aortic surgery to be generally comparable to a matched population [1, 51–53]. Kurazumi et al. for example looked at HRQoL in 47 patients greater than 80 years of age and having >6 cm arch aneurysms, showing that in the 20 patients that were operated on, HRQoL and 5-year survival were both comparable to an age- and sex-matched population [51]. Of note, this held true even in emergency surgery for type A aortic dissection. One study by Jussli-Melchers et al. compared 242 patients divided by age, showing that patients ≥70 years old had similar physical HRQoL between groups. Additionally, the mental HRQoL of the elderly group was slightly higher, but this was not statistically significant [50]. While findings of these studies should be considered together with their sample sizes and study quality, this suggests that clinicians should be positive about the long-term HRQoL outcomes in patients over the age of 80 undergoing major aortic surgery. While elderly age has been shown in the studies above to impair pre-operative HRQoL [37], it is more likely that co-morbidities have a greater role in diminishing post-operative HRQoL.

Neurological Outcomes and Cerebral Protection

Neurological complications are dreaded by patients and clinicians (in particular paraplegia), with potential impact on short- and long-term consequences. Six studies were identified in the current literature which focused on neurological outcomes and methods of cerebral protection methods in thoracic aortic interventions [54–59] (Table 4.8). In summary, prolonged DHCA peri-

Table 4.7 Studies observing aortic surgery in the elderly

Author, year of publication, study period and study type	Study intent and number of patients	Surgical centre	Patient characteristics	Pre-op HRQOL assessment	Follow-up period	HRQOL instrument used / Follow-up completion rate (%)	Main findings related to HRQOL
Jussli-Melchers et al. 2017 [50] 2004–2014 Retrospective cohort	HRQoL compared between patients <70 years old (n = 164) and patients ≥70 years old (n = 78) 1 year after surgery	University of Schleswig-Holstein, Campus Kiel, Kiel, Germany	Younger group: mean age 56 ± 10 years, 70.7% male Elderly group: mean age 76 ± 4 years, 48.7% male Presentation with cardiac tamponade higher in the elderly group	No	1 year	SF-36 91%	PCS score was similar between the groups MCS score might be slightly higher in the elderly group but not statistically significant
Kurazumi et al. 2014 [51] 2003–2012 Retrospective cohort	Quality of life assessment in 47 patients over the age of 80 referred with aortic arch pathology who ideally required surgery (>6 cm): 20 operated on and 27 treated medically (patient choice) 'Frail' individuals were excluded In the surgical cases: conventional total arch replacement in 15, debranched TEVAR in 2 and chimney TEVAR in 3	Yamaguchi University School of Medicine, Japan	Similar baseline patient characteristics between the two groups	No	31.7 ± 26.1 months	SF-36 57.1%	HRQoL was similar between those in the surgical group and those in the medical group

Oda et al. 2004 [52] 1987–1999 Retrospective cohort	Investigation in to the QoL in elderly (>65 years) following thoracic aortic surgery (n = 150) Aortic root replacement was performed in 5 (4.5%), interposition graft in 23 (20.7%), total arch replacement in 44 (39.7%), replacement of the thoracic descending aorta in 30 (27.0%) and TAA repair in 9 (8.1%)	Tohoku University, Japan	Mean age 70.6 ± 4.2 years, 38.7% were female. 39.6% of patients presented with an aortic dissection	No	62 months (range 13–167)	SF-36 74%	Some measures (physical functioning, role-physical, social functioning and role emotional) of HRQoL after thoracic aortic surgery was lower than when compared to a matched normal population, although this seemed to affect younger subgroups more Prolonged ACP time (>120 min) was associated with significantly lower scores in the dimension of role-physical in SF-36 Operative urgency, type of operation and presence of type A dissection did not influence QoL outcomes
Santini et al. 2006 [53] 1990–2004 Retrospective cohort	Clinical outcome and QoL analysis in 40 patients aged 75 and older undergoing type A dissection repair Surgical procedures were: interposition graft (85%), root replacement (12.5%) and interposition graft with AVR in 2.5%	University of Verona, Italy	Mean age was 78 ± 3 years, 52.5% were male and 22.5% had cardiogenic shock on admission	No	44 ± 38 months	RAND-36 100%	HRQoL revealed a generalized perception of independency and well-being, comparable to an age-matched population

(continued)

Table 4.7 (continued)

Author, year of publication, study period and study type	Study intent and number of patients	Surgical centre	Patient characteristics	Pre-op HRQOL assessment	Follow-up period	HRQOL instrument used / Follow-up completion rate (%)	Main findings related to HRQOL
Tang et al. 2013 [1] 2005–2011 Retrospective cohort study	Comparison of outcomes following type A dissection repair in octogenarians (n = 21) and those aged less than 80 (n = 101) Procedures consisted of 71 ascending/hemiarch replacements, 22 Bentall procedures, 2 David procedures, 4 Wheat procedures and 2 total arch replacements	Westchester Medical Centre, New York, USA	Octogenarians average age was 85 years (range 80–91). The younger group had an average age of 60 years (range 30–79 years) The two groups had similar preoperative characteristics, but the younger group experienced significantly more malperfusion and had a significantly longer DHCA time	No	17 ± 16 months in octogenarians and 20 ± 18 in the younger group	RAND-36 84%	Physical functioning was significantly better in the younger group, whereas emotional health scores were better in the octogenarian group

Table 4.8 Studies observing neurological outcomes and cerebral protection

Author, year of publication, study period and study type	Study intent and number of patients	Surgical centre	Patient characteristics	Pre-op HRQOL assessment	Follow-up period	HRQOL instrument used Follow-up completion rate (%)	Main findings related to HRQOL
Immer et al. 2004 [54] 1994–2002 Retrospective cohort study	Assessment of the impact of DHCA duration and the potential impact of ACP on mid-term QoL Total of 363 patients undergoing surgery of the thoracic aorta with DHCA. These were split in to DHCA times of <20 min, 20–29 min and ≥ 30 min for analysis ACP was used in 41 (11.3%) of cases	University Hospital Berne, Switzerland	Mean age of patients was 60.8 ± 13.3 years of whom 74% were male 167 patients had type A dissection and 187 had an aortic aneurysm	No	2.4 ± 1.2 years	SF-36 86.7%	Compared to patients with DHCA of <20 min, averaged HRQoL score was significantly decreased in patients with DHCA between 20–34 min and in >35 min Averaged HRQoL score was significantly better with the use of ACP, independent of the duration of DHCA ACP, however, improved averaged HRQoL score at each time period and allowed DHCA to be extended up to 30 min, without impairment in mid-term HRQoL DHCA >20 min resulted in significantly lower HRQoL than age and gender-matched standard population in the domains of physical functioning, social functioning and vitality HRQoL was superior in patients with thoracic aortic aneurysms as compared with patients with acute type A dissections, but this is likely to be related to the DHCA time and not the type of the disease
Immer et al. 2008 [55] 1994 onwards Retrospective cohort study	To assess the impact of continuous cerebral perfusion via the RSA on immediate outcome and QoL Total of 567 consecutive patients who underwent surgery of the aortic arch using DHCA. Divided in to three groups based on cerebral protection: 1) 387 patients had DHCA alone with pentothal, 2) 91 had selective ACP and pentothal and 3) 89 had CCP through the RSA and pentothal	University Hospital Berne, Switzerland	Pre-operative characteristics were "similar" in all three groups, although there were significantly more type A dissections in the group receiving CCP	No	2.4 ± 1.2 years	SF-36 80.0%	Average HRQoL scores up to 20 min of DHCA were similar in all three groups and comparable to age- and sex-matched standard population Average HRQoL after a DHCA time of 30–50 min with CCP through the RSA was significantly higher than with selective ACP—post-op HRQoL without CCP in this time group was significantly lower than a standardized population HR QoL limitations were mainly in the aspects of vitality and social and physical function Eight patients (20.2%) in the CCP group reported neurological symptoms of the right arm after cannulation of the right axillary artery, of which two had confirmed plexus-related dysfunction of the right arm

(continued)

Table 4.8 (continued)

Author, year of publication, study period and study type	Study intent and number of patients	Surgical centre	Patient characteristics	Pre-op HRQOL assessment	Follow-up period	HRQOL instrument used / Follow-up completion rate (%)	Main findings related to HRQOL
Kobuch et al. 2012 [56] 1998–2007 Retrospective cohort	Quality of life assessment of 79 undergoing surgery of the ascending aorta and arch with DHCA and selective ACP All patients underwent replacement of the ascending aorta, combined with hemiarch (n = 33) or total (n = 46) arch replacement	University Medical Centre Regensburg, Germany	Mean age of 59 ± 12 years, 71% male 65% of patients had acute aortic dissection and 34% with aortic aneurysm 71% of operations were performed on an emergent basis 11% of patients underwent a redo procedure Arterial cannulation was via the central aorta in 57%, the femoral in 19% and the RSA in 24%	No	28 (9–109) months	SIP questionnaire 82%	HRQoL after surgery with selective ACP was "excellent in the long-term"
Krähenbühl et al. 2008 [57] 1996–2005 Retrospective cohort	Assessment of the influence of TND (confusion, delirium and agitation with a GCS of <13) on short- and long-term outcome in 917 patients who underwent surgery of the ascending aorta and proximal arch	University Hospital Berne, Switzerland	290 (31.9%) patients had type A dissection and 617 had an aortic aneurysm. In 547 patients (60.3%) the distal anastomosis was performed using DHCA	No	27 ± 14 months	SF-36 82%	Patients with TND showed a significantly impaired HRQoL in all aspects except that of bodily pain when compared to those with no post-operative TND In patients which did not suffer from TND, the results of the SF-36 in all eight domains were within the reported range of age- and gender-matched population

Krähenbühl et al. 2010 [58] 2004–2007 Retrospective cohort	Comparison of three different cerebral protection techniques on QoL: DHCA alone (n = 12), SACP (n = 133) vs. RAACP (n = 118) vs. RAACCP (n = 29) Total of 292 patients included who underwent surgery of the thoracic aorta using DHCA	University Hospital Berne, Switzerland	Mean age was 64 ± 10.6 years and 69.8% were male. 60.2% were operated on electively and 38% presented with type A dissection Patient characteristics were similar in all groups. Bentall was performed in 43.5% and supracoronary repair in 56.5% Patients receiving RAACP and RAACCP comprised of significantly more emergency cases with significantly longer DHCA and CPB duration	No	23.2 ± 15 months	SF-36 100%	HRQoL was similar in all four groups for duration of DHCA up to 20 min and were within the reported range of age- and sex-matched standard population For DHCA >40 min, bilateral perfusion provided superior midterm HRQoL results and these patients still remained comparable to an age- and gender-matched standard population
Stewart et al. 2018 [59] 2007–2011 Prospective cohort	Comparison between patients undergoing thoracic aortic surgery with hypothermic circulatory arrest (n = 30) vs. patients undergoing coronary artery surgery without hypothermic circulatory arrest (n = 31)	Helsinki University Hospital, Helsinki, Finland	Thoracic aortic surgery: • Median age 62 years old (range 30–75) • 73% male Coronary artery surgery: • Median age 64 years old (range 37–80) • 81% male Those in the coronary artery surgery group had higher rates of smoking history and diabetes, but had a lower EuroSCORE I	No	Median 6.8 years (range 5–8) for thoracic aortic surgery group Median 6.3 years (range 4.6–7.8) for coronary artery surgery group	RAND-36 88% for thoracic aortic surgery 59% for coronary artery surgery	All scores were similar between groups and comparable to national reference population with chronic health conditions

ods and post-operative neurological injury predicted impaired HRQoL. Advanced cerebral protection methods (e.g. bilateral selective antegrade cerebral perfusion) improved HRQoL at follow-up.

Krähenbühl et al. looked at the impact of temporary neurological dysfunction (TND; confusion, delirium or agitation) on HRQoL post-operatively. In 917 patients undergoing proximal aortic surgery, 9.8% of patients suffered from TND which resulted in significant impairment of HRQoL in all domains excluding bodily pain. Patients without TND were shown to have comparable HRQoL to the normal population. TND was predicted by older age, pre-operative haemodynamic compromise and the use of DHCA [57]. Prolonged use of DHCA was also associated with poor post-operative HRQoL in two other studies [54, 55], but this was mitigated with various DHCA protection strategies (i.e. selective antegrade cerebral perfusion [54, 58], right axillary antegrade cerebral perfusion [58], right axillary perfusion with an additional catheter in the left carotid artery [58], right subclavian artery continuous cerebral perfusion [55]). Immer et al. for example showed that in 363 consecutive patients having proximal aortic surgery and prolonged DHCA (defined as >20 min), HRQoL at follow-up was impaired compared to a normal population [54]. However, this impairment was not seen when the cerebral perfusion strategies were applied in further studies, with superior mid-term HRQoL which was comparable to the normal population associated with the use of right subclavian cannulation (with continuous and bilateral cerebral protection) [55, 58].

These findings relating neurological outcomes and cerebral protection to mid- and long-term HRQoL are not surprising. Animal models have shown that 11% of brain activity still remains even when temperatures are decreased to 8 °C, suggesting that if DHCA alone is used, there still remains the possibility of incomplete protection and consequent diffuse brain injury [54]. With the addition of ACP in other animal models, reduced apoptosis in the hippocampus and preserved oxygen tension has been reported [60–62]. While the current evidence suggests that right axillary cannulation with bilateral continuous cerebral protection appears to be the most effective means of cerebral protection, this must be considered in the context of a high incidence of right arm dysfunction (up to 20%) and brachial plexus injury (estimated around 2%) [55].

Discussion

HRQoL has become increasingly important in thoracic aortic surgery, with increased appreciation of the differences between patient-centred outcomes and traditional surgical perceptions of what is important [63]. This was recently recognised in a review describing key aspects of HRQoL and patient-reported outcomes measures, including patients being the best judges of the impact of interventions on their symptoms and daily function, provision of a shared clinical decision-making framework, and in the improvement of quality and safety [64]. This is particularly important in patients with a high pre-operative HRQoL, with studies in related fields of cardiac surgery [65, 66] showing ceiling effects, suggesting that patients with good HRQoL have little to gain but much to lose with respect to their quality of life.

This chapter has outlined the literature regarding HRQoL after interventions on the thoracic aorta. Most studies, as detailed above, confirm that HRQoL after major surgery (both elective and emergency interventions, as well as in elderly patients) is acceptable and is often comparable to that of a general population. A summary framework shows contributory factors that may impair HRQoL in thoracic aortic surgery (Fig. 4.1). This analysis must however be interpreted with recognition of the limitations detailed below. Suggestions for future research are also discussed further in this section.

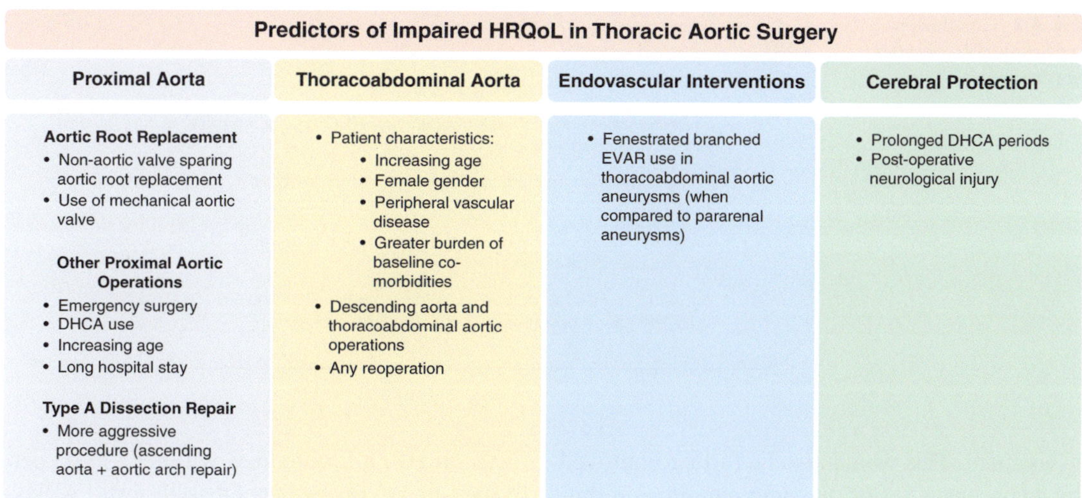

Fig. 4.1 Predictors of poor HRQoL in aortic surgery

Study Limitations

In the current literature, majority of studies are retrospective and only one contains an element of randomisation. Differences in baseline demographics and patient characteristics, as highlighted in the tables where identified, is largely due to this observational design in most studies and the lack of experimental methodology. As previously mentioned, patients with thoracic aortic disease tend to have a significant number of co-morbidities, and the lack of randomisation leads to heterogeneity seen in the current literature. Additionally, while the overall follow-up completion rate was generally high, only two studies reported baseline HRQoL. Together with the lack of uniformity of instruments used and the variety of timepoints used for follow-up, comparisons of outcomes was challenging. This may be improved with initiatives promoting pre- and post-intervention HRQoL collection—the United Kingdom's Department of Health has started routine collection for a selection of operations which unfortunately does not include thoracic aorta surgery [7], while the Netherlands has started a national initiative termed '*Meetbaar Beter*' to encourage cardiothoracic centres to collect pre- and post-operative HRQoL [67]. Finally, bias may be an issue given that patients with poor HRQoL are unlikely to respond to surveys, leading to falsely elevated HRQoL results. Institutions may also contribute to the bias with increased efforts to publish and present positive findings—notably, a number of studies in the literature originate from the same institution.

Suggestions for Future Research

HRQoL outcomes are not a new reporting instrument in the literature—one of the first studies to publish on these outcomes was available over 40 years ago [68]. Despite this, few randomised controlled trials report such outcomes, with the current literature reviewed in this chapter still only including one randomised trial [11]. Future research into thoracic aortic interventions should include elements of randomisation. As for instrument selection, while most studies use generic instruments (e.g. SF-36, RAND-36) that are frequently used in all areas of medicine and surgery, there is still no consensus as to which instrument is best for data collection in aortic surgery. Additionally, while a number of disease-specific instruments were used in the current studies, future data collection would be facilitated by a standardised aortic specific common instrument. This standardisation should also be extended to a uniform reporting standard of baseline and post-operative (at predefined timepoints) HRQoL

Chapter Conclusions:

- HRQoL after aortic surgery is satisfactory
- Even in elderly and high-risk populations, HRQoL is comparable to healthy age- and sex-matched individuals
- Aortic surgery should aim to preserve, if not improve, HRQoL especially in elective scenarios where patients are largely asymptomatic
- Available literature on HRQoL in aortic surgery is currently lacking, especially with regards to randomised trials
- Focusing on HRQoL outcomes in future trials will be required to allow for evidence-based policymaking and resource allocation

Fig. 4.2 Conclusions regarding HRQoL after aortic surgery

assessment. This would also be further improved by a consensus set of outcome measures in thoracic aortic surgery such as those already available through the International Consortium for Health Outcomes Measurement for coronary artery disease and heart failure [69]. Innovation may take the form of correlating HRQoL to patient activity as measured by wrist-worn accelerometers [70, 71] or biomechanical parameters such as aortic blood flow, shear wall stress and pulse wave velocity [72–74].

Conclusions

HRQoL after aortic surgery is generally satisfactory and found to be at similar levels (even in elderly and high-risk populations) to healthy age- and sex-matched patients (Fig. 4.2). Baseline characteristics of patients with descending thoracic aortic disease tend to be poorer, which may be secondary to the multitude of co-morbidities they usually have. Patients undergoing emergency operations for type A dissections also often appear to have poorer HRQoL when compared to matched populations. Aortic surgery should aim to preserve or improve HRQoL, especially in elective operations where a good number of patients are asymptomatic, and patients will need to be made aware of HRQoL outcomes as part of the consent process. Despite increasing interest in HRQoL as an outcome measure in aortic surgery, there is still only one prospective randomised trial in the current literature which studies HRQoL outcomes. Further trials with a focus on HRQoL outcomes will need to be performed to advise evidence-based aortic policymaking and resource allocation in the future.

References

1. Tang GH, Malekan R, Cindy JY, Kai M, Lansman SL, Spielvogel D. Surgery for acute type A aortic dissection in octogenarians is justified. Elsevier; 2013.
2. Isselbacher EM. Thoracic and abdominal aortic aneurysms. Circulation. 2005;111(6):816–28.
3. Black JH, Cambria RP. Current results of open surgical repair of descending thoracic aortic aneurysms. J Vasc Surg. 2006;43(2):A6–11.
4. Jarral OA, Kidher E, Patel VM, Nguyen B, Pepper J, Athanasiou T. Quality of life after intervention on the thoracic aorta. Eur J Cardiothorac Surg. 2016;49(2):369–89.
5. Baig K, Harling L, Papanikitas J, Attaran S, Ashrafian H, Casula R, et al. Does coronary artery bypass grafting improve quality of life in elderly patients? Interact Cardiovasc Thorac Surg. 2013;17(3):542–53.
6. Black N. Patient reported outcome measures could help transform healthcare. BMJ. 2013;346:f167.
7. Guidance on the routine collection of Patient Reported Outcome Measures (PROMs). 28.
8. Ramanath VS, Oh JK, Sundt TM, Eagle KA. Acute aortic syndromes and thoracic aortic aneurysm. Mayo Clin Proc. 2009;84(5):465–81.
9. Akhyari P, Bara C, Kofidis T, Khaladj N, Haverich A, Klima U. Aortic root and ascending aortic replacement. Int Heart J. 2009;50(1):47–57.
10. Bori Bata A-K, D'Ostrevy N, Pereira B, Geoffroy E, Dauphin N, Eljezi V, et al. Valve-sparing aortic root replacement-midterm outcomes and quality of life. Cardiovasc Diagn Ther. 2017;7(6):572–80.
11. El-Hamamsy I, Eryigit Z, Stevens L-M, Sarang Z, George R, Clark L, et al. Long-term outcomes after autograft versus homograft aortic root replacement in adults with aortic valve disease: a randomised controlled trial. Lancet. 2010;376(9740):524–31.

12. Franke UF, Isecke A, Nagib R, Breuer M, Wippermann J, Tigges-Limmer K, et al. Quality of life after aortic root surgery: reimplantation technique versus composite replacement. Ann Thorac Surg. 2010;90(6):1869–75.
13. Golczyk K, Kompis M, Englberger L, Carrel TP, Stalder M. Heart valve sound of various mechanical composite grafts, and the impact on patients' quality of life. J Heart Valve Dis. 2010;19(2):228–32.
14. Khaladj N, Ismail I, Shrestha M, Peterss S, Pichlmaier M, Kallenbach K, et al. Aortic root surgery in combination with hypothermic circulatory arrest: preserve or replace the aortic valve in the context of postoperative neurological outcome? A case match comparison. Interact Cardiovasc Thorac Surg. 2009;9(2):246–50.
15. Lehr EJ, Wang PZT, Oreopoulos A, Kanji H, Norris C, Macarthur R. Midterm outcomes and quality of life of aortic root replacement: mechanical vs biological conduits. Can J Cardiol. 2011;27(2):262.e15–20.
16. Perrotta S, Aljassim O, Jeppsson A, Bech-Hanssen O, Svensson G. Survival and quality of life after aortic root replacement with homografts in acute endocarditis. Ann Thorac Surg. 2010;90(6):1862–7.
17. Wachter K, Franke UFW, Yadav R, Nagib R, Ursulescu A, Ahad S, et al. Feasibility and clinical outcome after minimally invasive valve-sparing aortic root replacement. Interact Cardiovasc Thorac Surg. 2017;24(3):377–83.
18. Zacek P, Holubec T, Vobornik M, Dominik J, Takkenberg J, Harrer J, et al. Quality of life after aortic valve repair is similar to Ross patients and superior to mechanical valve replacement: a cross-sectional study. BMC Cardiovasc Disord. 2016;2(16):63.
19. Abe T, Terazawa S, Ito H, Tokuda Y, Fujimoto K, Mutsuga M, et al. Clinical outcomes and quality of life after surgery for dilated ascending aorta at the time of aortic valve replacement; wrapping versus graft replacement. Nagoya J Med Sci. 2017;79(4):443–51.
20. Lohse F, Lang N, Schiller W, Roell W, Dewald O, Preusse C-J, et al. Quality of life after replacement of the ascending aorta in patients with true aneurysms. Tex Heart Inst J. 2009;36(2):104–10.
21. Olsson C, Thelin S. Quality of life in survivors of thoracic aortic surgery. Ann Thorac Surg. 1999;67(5):1262–7.
22. Song HK, Kindem M, Bavaria JE, Dietz HC, Milewicz DM, Devereux RB, et al. Long-term implications of emergency versus elective proximal aortic surgery in patients with Marfan syndrome in the Genetically Triggered Thoracic Aortic Aneurysms and Cardiovascular Conditions Consortium Registry. J Thorac Cardiovasc Surg. 2012;143(2):282–6.
23. Stalder M, Staffelbach S, Immer FF, Englberger L, Berdat PA, Eckstein FS, et al. Aortic root replacement does not affect outcome and quality of life. Ann Thorac Surg. 2007;84(3):775–80. Discussion 780–1.
24. Olsson C, Franco-Cereceda A. Health-related quality of life in thoracic aortic disease: part II. After surgery on the proximal (root, ascending, arch) aorta. Aorta Stamford Conn. 2013;1(3):162–70.
25. Hagan PG, Nienaber CA, Isselbacher EM, Bruckman D, Karavite DJ, Russman PL, et al. The International Registry of Acute Aortic Dissection (IRAD): new insights into an old disease. JAMA. 2000;283(7):897–903.
26. Adam U, Habazettl H, Graefe K, Kuppe H, Wundram M, Kurz SD. Health-related quality of life of patients after surgery for acute Type A aortic dissection. Interact Cardiovasc Thorac Surg. 2018;27(1):48–53.
27. Campbell-Lloyd AJ, Mundy J, Pinto N, Wood A, Beller E, Strahan S, et al. Contemporary results following surgical repair of acute type A aortic dissection (AAAD): a single centre experience. Heart Lung Circ. 2010;19(11):665–72.
28. Endlich M, Hamiko M, Gestrich C, Probst C, Mellert F, Winkler K, et al. Long-term outcome and quality of life in aortic type A dissection survivors. Thorac Cardiovasc Surg. 2016;64(2):91–9.
29. Ghazy T, Eraqi M, Mahlmann A, Hegelmann H, Matschke K, Kappert U, et al. Quality of life after surgery for stanford type a aortic dissection: influences of different operative strategies. Heart Surg Forum. 2017;20(3):E102–6.
30. Kamenskaya O, Klinkova A, Loginova I, Chernyavskiy A, Sirota D, Lomivorotov VV, et al. Health-related quality of life one year after surgical treatment of the type I chronic aortic dissection. Int Angiol J Int Union Angiol. 2019;38(1):46–53.
31. Nakamura Y, Tagusari O, Ichikawa Y, Morita A. Impact of immediate aortic repair on early and midterm neurologic status in patients with acute type a aortic dissection complicated by cerebral malperfusion. Ann Thorac Surg. 2011;92(1):336–8.
32. Myrmel T, Trimarchi S, Rampoldi V. Cardiovascular surgery in the initial treatment of aortic dissection and acute aortic syndromes. In: Eagle KA, Baliga RR, Isselbacher EM, Nienaber CA, editors. Aortic dissection and related syndromes [Internet]. Boston, MA: Springer US; 2007 [cited 2020 Jan 27]. p. 167–90. (Developments in Cardiovascular Medicine). Available from: https://doi.org/10.1007/978-0-387-36001-0_9.
33. Uchida N, Katayama K, Takahashi S, Sueda T. Endovascular stent grafting of the downstream aorta after complete arch replacement using the frozen elephant trunk technique for acute type A aortic dissection. Eur J Cardiothorac Surg. 2013;43(1):196.
34. Clouse WD, Hallett JW, Schaff HV, Gayari MM, Ilstrup DM, Melton LJ. Improved prognosis of thoracic aortic aneurysms: a population-based study. JAMA. 1998;280(22):1926–9.
35. Frederick JR, Woo YJ. Thoracoabdominal aortic aneurysm. Ann Cardiothorac Surg. 2012;1(3):277–85.
36. Coroneos CJ, Mastracci TM, Barlas S, Cinà CS. The effect of thoracoabdominal aneurysm repair on quality of life. J Vasc Surg. 2009;50(2):251–5.
37. Crawford RS, Pedraza JD, Chung TK, Corey M, Conrad MF, Cambria RP. Functional outcome after thoracoabdominal aneurysm repair. J Vasc Surg. 2008;48(4):828–35.

38. Di Luozzo G, Shirali AS, Varghese R, Lin H-M, Weiss AJ, Bischoff MS, et al. Quality of life and survival of septuagenarians and octogenarians after repair of descending and thoracoabdominal aortic aneurysms. J Thorac Cardiovasc Surg. 2013;145(2):378–84.
39. Eide TMO, Romundstad P, Klepstad P, Myhre HO. Health-related quality of life in long term-survivors of thoracoabdominal aortic aneurysm repair. J Vasc Nurs. 2005;23(3):88–94.
40. Ghanta RK, Green SY, Price MD, Arredondo CC, Wainwright D, Preventza O, et al. Midterm survival and quality of life after extent ii thoracoabdominal aortic repair in Marfan syndrome. Ann Thorac Surg. 2016;101(4):1402–9. Discussion 1409.
41. Zierer A, Melby SJ, Lubahn JG, Sicard GA, Damiano RJ, Moon MR. Elective surgery for thoracic aortic aneurysms: late functional status and quality of life. Ann Thorac Surg. 2006;82(2):573–8.
42. Dick F, Hinder D, Immer FF, Hirzel C, Carrel TP, Schmidli J. Outcome and quality of life after surgical and endovascular treatment of descending aortic lesions. Ann Thorac Surg. 2008;85(5):1605–12.
43. Kärkkäinen JM, Sandri G d A, Tenorio ER, Macedo TA, Hofer J, Gloviczki P, et al. Prospective assessment of health-related quality of life after endovascular repair of pararenal and thoracoabdominal aortic aneurysms using fenestrated-branched endografts. J Vasc Surg. 2019;69(5):1356–66.
44. Klocker J, Koell A, Erlmeier M, Goebel G, Jaschke W, Fraedrich G. Ischemia and functional status of the left arm and quality of life after left subclavian artery coverage during stent grafting of thoracic aortic diseases. J Vasc Surg. 2014;60(1):64–9.
45. McBride CL, Dubose JJ, Miller CC, Perlick AP, Charlton-Ouw KM, Estrera AL, et al. Intentional left subclavian artery coverage during thoracic endovascular aortic repair for traumatic aortic injury. J Vasc Surg. 2015;61(1):73–9.
46. Ouriel K, Greenberg RK. Endovascular treatment of thoracic aortic aneurysms. J Card Surg. 2003;18(5):455–63.
47. Patel R, Sweeting MJ, Powell JT, Greenhalgh RM. Endovascular versus open repair of abdominal aortic aneurysm in 15-years' follow-up of the UK endovascular aneurysm repair trial 1 (EVAR trial 1): a randomised controlled trial. Lancet. 2016;388(10058):2366–74.
48. Rampoldi V, Trimarchi S, Eagle KA, Nienaber CA, Oh JK, Bossone E, et al. Simple risk models to predict surgical mortality in acute type A aortic dissection: the International Registry of Acute Aortic Dissection score. Ann Thorac Surg. 2007;83(1):55–61.
49. Shah PJ, Estrera AL, Miller CC, Lee T-Y, Irani AD, Meada R, et al. Analysis of ascending and transverse aortic arch repair in octogenarians. Ann Thorac Surg. 2008;86(3):774–9.
50. Jussli-Melchers J, Panholzer B, Friedrich C, Broch O, Renner J, Schöttler J, et al. Long-term outcome and quality of life following emergency surgery for acute aortic dissection type A: a comparison between young and elderly adults. Eur J Cardiothorac Surg. 2017;51(3):465–71.
51. Kurazumi H, Mikamo A, Kudo T, Suzuki R, Takahashi M, Shirasawa B, et al. Aortic arch surgery in octogenarians: is it justified? Eur J Cardiothorac Surg. 2014;46(4):672–7.
52. Oda K, Hata M, Kawatsu S, Adachi O, Yamaya K, Saiki Y, et al. Quality of life in elderly patients following thoracic aortic surgery. Jpn J Thorac Cardiovasc Surg. 2004;52(11):515–23.
53. Santini F, Montalbano G, Messina A, D'Onofrio A, Casali G, Viscardi F, et al. Survival and quality of life after repair of acute type A aortic dissection in patients aged 75 years and older justify intervention. Eur J Cardiothorac Surg. 2006;29(3):386–91.
54. Immer FF, Lippeck C, Barmettler H, Berdat PA, Eckstein FS, Kipfer B, et al. Surgery for aortic and peripheral vascular disease-improvement of quality of life after surgery on the thoracic aorta: effect of antegrade cerebral perfusion and short duration of deep hypothermic. Circulation. 2004;110(11):II250.
55. Immer FF, Moser B, Krähenbühl ES, Englberger L, Stalder M, Eckstein FS, et al. Arterial access through the right subclavian artery in surgery of the aortic arch improves neurologic outcome and mid-term quality of life. Ann Thorac Surg. 2008;85(5):1614–8. Discussion 1618.
56. Kobuch R, Schelker E, Schmid C, Hirt S, Amann M, Diez C. Quality of life following surgery of ascending aorta and aortic arch with selective antegrade cerebral perfusion. Thorac Cardiovasc Surg. 2012;60(8):496–500.
57. Krähenbühl ES, Immer FF, Stalder M, Englberger L, Eckstein FS, Carrel TP. Temporary neurological dysfunction after surgery of the thoracic aorta: a predictor of poor outcome and impaired quality of life. Eur J Cardiothorac Surg. 2008;33(6):1025–9.
58. Krähenbühl ES, Clément M, Reineke D, Czerny M, Stalder M, Aymard T, et al. Antegrade cerebral protection in thoracic aortic surgery: lessons from the past decade. Eur J Cardiothorac Surg. 2010;38(1):46–51.
59. Stewart JA, Ilkka VH, Jokinen JJ, Vakkuri AP, Suojaranta RT, Wennervirta J, et al. Long-term survival and quality of life after hypothermic circulatory arrest in aortic surgery. Scand J Surg. 2018;107(4):322–8.
60. Zhao R, Cui Q, Yu S-Q, Sun G-C, Wang H-B, Jin Z-X, et al. Antegrade cerebral perfusion during deep hypothermia circulatory arrest attenuates the apoptosis of neurons in porcine hippocampus. Heart Surg Forum. 2009 Aug;12(4):E219–24.
61. Salazar JD, Coleman RD, Griffith S, McNeil JD, Steigelman M, Young H, et al. Selective cerebral perfusion: real-time evidence of brain oxygen and energy metabolism preservation. Ann Thorac Surg. 2009;88(1):162–9.
62. Salazar J, Coleman R, Griffith S, McNeil J, Young H, Calhoon J, et al. Brain preservation with selective cerebral perfusion for operations requiring cir-

culatory arrest: protection at 25 degrees C is similar to 18 degrees C with shorter operating times. Eur J Cardiothorac Surg. 2009;36(3):524–31.
63. Korteland NM, Kluin J, Klautz RJM, Roos-Hesselink JW, Versteegh MIM, Bogers AJJC, et al. Cardiologist and cardiac surgeon view on decision-making in prosthetic aortic valve selection: does profession matter? Neth Heart J. 2014;22(7):336–43.
64. Williams K, Sansoni J, Morris D, Grootemaat P, Thompson C. Patient-reported outcome measures. 91.
65. Kurfirst V, Mokráček A, Krupauerová M, Čanádyová J, Bulava A, Pešl L, et al. Health-related quality of life after cardiac surgery – the effects of age, preoperative conditions and postoperative complications. J Cardiothorac Surg. 2014;9(1):46.
66. Koch CG, Khandwala F, Estafanous FG, Loop FD, Blackstone EH. Impact of prosthesis–patient size on functional recovery after aortic valve replacement. Circulation. 2005;111(24):3221–9.
67. de Heer F, Gökalp AL, Kluin J, Takkenberg JJM. Measuring what matters to the patient: health related quality of life after aortic valve and thoracic aortic surgery. Gen Thorac Cardiovasc Surg. 2019 Jan;67(1):37–43.
68. Ross JK, Diwell AE, Marsh J, Monro JL, Barker DJ. Wessex cardiac surgery follow-up survey: the quality of life after operation. Thorax. 1978;33(1):3–9.
69. McNamara RL, Spatz ES, Kelley TA, Stowell CJ, Beltrame J, Heidenreich P, et al. Standardized outcome measurement for patients with coronary artery disease: consensus from the international consortium for health outcomes measurement (ICHOM). J Am Heart Assoc. 2015;4(5):e001767.
70. Tan MKH, Wong JKL, Bakrania K, Abdullahi Y, Harling L, Casula R, et al. Can activity monitors predict outcomes in patients with heart failure? A systematic review. Eur Heart J Qual Care Clin Outcomes. 2019;5(1):11–21.
71. Rowlands AV, Olds TS, Hillsdon M, Pulsford R, Hurst TL, Eston RG, et al. Assessing sedentary behavior with the GENEActiv: introducing the sedentary sphere. Med Sci Sports Exerc. 2014;46(6):1235–47.
72. Jarral OA, Tan MKH, Salmasi MY, Pirola S, Pepper JR, O'Regan DP, et al. Phase-contrast magnetic resonance imaging and computational fluid dynamics assessment of thoracic aorta blood flow: a literature review. Eur J Cardiothorac Surg [Internet]. [cited 2020 Jan 28]. Available from: https://academic.oup.com/ejcts/advance-article/doi/10.1093/ejcts/ezz280/5602446.
73. Kidher E, Cheng Z, Jarral OA, O'Regan DP, Xu XY, Athanasiou T. In-vivo assessment of the morphology and hemodynamic functions of the BioValsalva™ composite valve-conduit graft using cardiac magnetic resonance imaging and computational modelling technology. J Cardiothorac Surg. 2014;9:193.
74. Kidher E, Harling L, Nihoyannopoulos P, Shenker N, Ashrafian H, Francis DP, et al. High aortic pulse wave velocity is associated with poor quality of life in surgical aortic valve stenosis patients. Interact Cardiovasc Thorac Surg. 2014;19(2):189–97.

5 Patient Reported Outcomes and Quality of Life following Heart Transplantation

Alex Jacob Poovathoor, Jason Ali, and Marius Berman

Introduction

It is well-established that heart transplantation is the gold-standard treatment for eligible patients with end-stage heart failure. The survival benefit over medical management and durable LVADs has been demonstrated in multiple studies [1–4]. The main challenge of this life-saving treatment is the availability of donor organs, leading to prolonged waiting times on the list, often with significant deterioration of symptoms, and even demise. In the UK, 10% of non-urgent patients will die on the waiting list in 2 years and only 17% will be transplanted [5]. For those that receive an organ, the average waiting time is 1.6 years [5].

A. J. Poovathoor (✉)
University of Cambridge, Cambridge, UK

Department of Cardiothoracic Surgery, Royal Papworth Hospital NHS Foundation Trust, Cambridge, UK

J. Ali · M. Berman
Department of Cardiothoracic Surgery, Royal Papworth Hospital NHS Foundation Trust, Cambridge, UK
e-mail: jason.ali@nhs.net; marius.berman@nhs.net

For those who receive a heart transplant, along with prolongation in life-expectancy one should recognize a significant improvement is heart-failure related symptoms and quality of life. The survival prognosis for heart transplantation is 12.5 years, and the 1-year conditional survival is 14.8 years, so the gap between outcomes from cardiac transplantation and natural history is notable [6]. The survival over 1 and 5 years of heart transplants between 1982 and 2013 was 82% and 69%, respectively [6]. Heart transplantation is a remarkably successful operation, and there is a significant improvement prognostically. Not only this, death in association with heart transplantation is continually decreasing. The survival for 1-year survivors between 2002 and 2009 was 12.5 years, now increased to 14.8 years [6].

However, post-transplant management is a multidisciplinary journey with the patient in the center that involves life-long pharmacological treatment, blood tests, biopsies etc., which can have an impact in the physical and mental well-being of the recipient and overall QoL. In this chapter we sought to examine QoL parameters using established tools in assessing the effect of heart transplantation against patients' pre-transplant status but also against other patient groups, including LVAD recipients.

T. Athanasiou et al. (eds.), *Patient Reported Outcomes and Quality of Life in Cardiovascular Interventions*, https://doi.org/10.1007/978-3-031-09815-4_5

Methods

Literature Search

A literature search was performed in the PubMed database with the following terms: ((((((((((((((patient reported outcomes) OR (prom)) OR (quality of life)) OR (QoL)) OR (SF-36)) OR (short form 36)) OR (HRQoL)) OR (health related quality of life)) OR (EQ5D)) OR (euroqol 5d)) OR (Minnesota Living with Heart Failure Questionnaire)) OR (MLHFQ)) OR (Kansas City Cardiomyopathy Questionnaire)) OR (KCCQ)) OR (Quality of Life Index cardiac version)) OR (WHOQOL-BREF)) AND ((((cardiac transplant) OR (heart transplant)) OR (heart failure surgery)) OR (end-stage heart failure surgery)).

Date of search: 15-12-2020.

Study Selection

Exclusion of studies that are: non- English, paediatric cohorts; focusing mainly on depression without a holistic approach to QoL; combining heart transplant with other organ transplants without differentiating the outcomes; and using QoL tools that are not holistic in approach.

Study Classification

From the studies we identified as eligible, we subsequently carried out classification and critical appraisal based on the comparative arms as follows:

1. ***comparative studies: vs LVADs control group***. Patients implanted with a bridge to transplant left ventricular assist device compared to HTx recipients. Table 5.1.
2. ***comparative studies: vs medical therapy control group***. Patients stabilized on best medical therapy compared to HTx recipients. Table 5.2.
3. ***comparative studies: vs waiting-list control group*** . Patients on the transplant waiting-list compared to recipients. Table 5.3.
4. ***longitudinal studies: pre-operation and post-operation intervals***. Assessing baseline quality of life with heart failure, then at intervals post-operatively. Table 5.4.
5. ***longitudinal studies: post—operation intervals only***. Studies that focused on outcomes at post-operative intervals only. Table 5.5.
6. ***longitudinal studies: long-term follow-up***. studies that focused on outcomes in long-term survivors (defined as >5 years). Table 5.6.

Refer to Fig. 5.1 for a comparison of four heart-failure-specific quality of life instruments commonly used in the selected studies.

Results

Comparative Studies

vs. LVADs

Grady et al. [7] conducted a longitudinal, multi-site study comparing paired QoL data of 40 LVAD patients at 3 months post-LVAD-implantation vs 3 months post-HTx. Patients after HTx were found to be more satisfied with their lives and with their health and functioning. Furthermore, an improvement in mobility, self-care ability, physical ability and overall functional ability was observed from 3 months post-LVAD-implantation to 3 months post-HTx. However, self-care stress and hospital/clinic-related stress were seen to be lower in the post-LVAD period.

As compared to Grady et al's study, which used patients implanted with LVADs as a bridge-to-transplant and following them longitudinally to post-HTx, Jakovljevic et al. [8] compared the QoL in LVAD and HTx recipients using two separate cohorts. This LVAD bridge-to-destination group comprised of 14 patients, and was compared to 12 post-HTx patients. Physical activity and QoL were assessed at 4 to 6 weeks (baseline)

Table 5.1 *Comparative studies: vs LVAD control group*. Patients implanted with a bridge to transplant left ventricular assist device compared to HTx recipients

Study	Title	Country	Study intent and number of patients	HRQOL instrument used	QoL scores (figures given as HTx vs. LVAD)	Main findings related to HRQOL
Jakovljevic et al. (2014) [8]	Effect of Left Ventricular Assist Device Implantation and Heart Transplantation on Habitual Physical Activity and Quality of Life	United Kingdom	Short- and long-term effects of bridge to transplant LVAD implantation and HTx on physical activity and QoL. $n = 40$ (+14 healthy subjects)	MLHFQ	39 ± 5 vs. 57 ± 7 (3 Mo post-Tx/LVAD) 30 ± 6 vs. 63 ± 7 (6 Mo post-Tx/LVAD) 29 ± 7 vs. 60 ± 5 (12 Mo post-Tx/LVAD)	LVAD implantation and HTx increased daily physical activity by 60% and 52%. level of activity unchanged at 3, 6, and 12 months. QoL improved in LVAD implantation and HTx groups but unchanged afterward. HTx higher activity level vs. LVAD implantation - associated with better QoL
Grady et al. (2003) [7]	Change in Quality of Life From After Left Ventricular Assist Device Implantation to After Heart Transplantation	United States of America	Compare QOL of patients listed for HTx with bridge to transplant LVAD at 3 months after LVAD implantation vs. 3 months after HTx. $n = 40$	QLI	**Life Satisfaction** = 0.79 ± 0.13 vs. 0.75 ± 0.12 ($p = 0.01$) **Health and Functioning** = 0.78 ± 0.16 vs. 0.68 ± 0.17 (p = 0.0003)	Patients more satisfied with lives overall and health and functioning at 3 months post-HTx vs. post-LVAD implant. Mobility, self-care ability, physical ability and overall functional ability improved from 3 months after LVAD implant to 3 months after HTx. Work/school/financial stress lower post-HTx vs post-LVAD implant
Emin et al. (2016) [9]	Quality of life of advanced chronic heart failure: medical care, mechanical circulatory support and transplantation	United Kingdom	QoL in patients assessed for HTx, listed for HTx on medical therapy, supported with bridge to transplant LVAD and patients after HTx. $n = 386$	KCCQ EQ-5D	**KCCQ domains** **Symptom stability** = 54.7 ± 21.6 vs. 60.9 ± 21.7 **Self-efficacy** = 93.4 ± 15.0 vs. 93.8 ± 11.1 **Symptom frequency** = 77.1 ± 26.3 vs. 68.5 ± 25.3 **Symptom burden** = 77.8 ± 25.1 vs. 69.5 ± 25.5 **Total symptom score** = 77.5 ± 25.1 vs. 69.0 ± 24.7 **Physical limitation** = 75.4 ± 31.1 vs. 56.5 ± 25.9 **Clinical summary score** = 76.6 ± 26.1 vs. 62.6 ± 23.8 **QoL** = 71.4 ± 28.5 vs. 44.1 ± 23.2 **Social limitation** = 67.0 ± 34.2 vs. 41.6 ± 27.0 **Overall summary score** = 73.0 ± 27.2 vs. 52.6 ± 22.0 **EQ-5D index score** = 0.74 ± 0.27 vs. 0.58 ± 0.26	Best QoL in recipients; EQ-5D scores highest in recipients

HTx: Heart Transplant; LVAD: Left Ventricular Assist Device

Table 5.2 *Comparative studies: vs medical therapy control group*. Patients stabilized on best medical therapy compared to HTx recipients

Study	Title	Country	Study intent and number of patients	HRQOL instrument used	QoL scores (figure given as HTx vs. medical therapy)	Main findings related to HRQOL
Evangelista et al. (2005) [13]	Two-year follow-up of quality of life in patients referred for heart transplant	United States of America	Comparative effects of HTx or medical treatment on HRQOL. $n = 77$	SF 12	**Physical health** = 35.2 (32.4–44.6 IQR) vs. 46.9 (37.7–56.7 IQR) **Mental health** = 41.9 (38.8–51.2 IQR) vs. 49.2 (49.2–57.8 IQR)	Physical health score significantly improved over time in all patients; changes in mental health were minimal. Although all patients continued to have low HRQOL scores at the time of follow-up, medically stable patients had higher mental health scores and less depressive symptoms
Emin et al. (2016) [9]	Quality of life of advanced chronic heart failure: medical care, mechanical circulatory support and transplantation	United Kingdom	QoL in patients assessed for HTx, listed for HTx on medical therapy, supported with bridge to transplant LVAD and patients after HTx. $n = 386$	KCCQ EQ-5D	**KCCQ domains** **Symptom stability** = 54.7 ± 21.6 vs. 33.9 ± 23.8 **Self-efficacy** = 93.4 ± 15.0 vs. 79.5 ± 18.7 **Symptom frequency** = 77.1 ± 26.3 vs. 43.5 ± 22.5 **Symptom burden** = 77.8 ± 25.1 vs. 47.9 ± 20.7 **Total symptom score** = 77.5 ± 25.1 vs. 45.7 ± 20.6 **Physical limitation** = 75.4 ± 31.1 vs. 34.7 ± 25.8 **Clinical summary score** = 76.6 ± 26.1 vs. 40.2 ± 22.0 QoL = 71.4 ± 28.5 vs. 24.4 ± 20.4 **Social limitation** = 67.0 ± 34.2 vs. 27.3 ± 27.2 **Overall summary score** = 73.0 ± 27.2 vs. 33.3 ± 21.1 **EQ-5D index score** = 0.74 ± 0.27 vs. 0.44 ± 0.27	Highest QoL in recipients. EQ-5D scores highest in recipients

Walden et al. (1994) [46]	Extended comparison of quality of life between stable heart failure patients and heart transplant recipients		QOL at the time of transplantation evaluation and again after 41 months in patients stabilized with medical therapy and recipients. $n = 31$	3 questionnaires		Psychologic adaptation, and perceived functional capability improved in transplant recipients. More weakness after surgery in recipients - major symptom that limited activities. No significant differences in QOL changes over time between medical therapy group and recipients at 41 months. QOL for medical therapy group may not be different from recipients
Jakovljevic et al. (2014) [8]	Effect of Left Ventricular Assist Device Implantation and Heart Transplantation on Habitual Physical Activity and Quality of Life	United Kingdom	Short- and long-term effects of LVAD implantation and HTx on physical activity and QoL. $n = 40$ (+14 healthy subjects)	MLHFQ	39 ± 5 vs. 74 ± 4	LVAD implantation and HTx increased daily physical activity by 60% and 52%. level of activity unchanged at 3, 6, and 12 months. QoL improved in LVAD implantation and HTx groups but unchanged afterward. HTx higher activity level vs LVAD implantation - associated with better QoL

Table 5.3 *Comparative studies: vs waiting-list control group.* Patients on the transplant waiting-list compared to recipients

Study	Title	Country	Study intent and number of patients	HRQOL instrument used	QoL scores (figures given as HTx vs wait-list)	Main findings related to HRQOL
Mantovani et al. (2017) [15]	Comparison of quality of life between patients on the waiting list and heart transplant recipients	Brazil	Compare QOL between wait-listed patients and recipients. $n = 56$	SF-36	**Physical functioning** = 9.5 vs. 32.1 **Role-physical** = 22.6 vs. 29.6 **Bodily pain** = 18.2 vs. 29.1 **General health** = 9.1 vs. 32.2 **Vitality** = 14.9 vs. 31.1 **Social functioning** = 17.6 vs. 30.0 **Role-emotional** = 24.8 vs. 29.2 **Mental health** = 24.6 vs. 29.2	Significant difference between two groups in the QOL score and four dimensions. Mean rank = 16.9 in wait-listed patients, = 30.7 in transplant recipients. Lowest scores for general health and highest scores for role-emotional in wait-listed patients. Highest scores for general health and the lowest scores for bodily pain in recipients
Emin et al. (2016) [9]	Quality of life of advanced chronic heart failure: medical care, mechanical circulatory support and transplantation	United Kingdom	QoL in patients assessed for HTx, listed for HTx on medical therapy, supported with bridge to transplant LVAD and patients after HTx. $n = 386$	KCCQ EQ-5D	**KCCQ domains** **Symptom stability** = 54.7 ± 21.6 vs. 47.8 ± 29.5 **Self-efficacy** = 93.4 ± 15.0 vs. 74.2 ± 22.2 **Symptom frequency** = 77.1 ± 26.3 vs. 45.5 ± 26.8 **Symptom burden** = 77.8 ± 25.1 vs. 48.5 ± 25.5 **Total symptom score** = 77.5 ± 25.1 vs. 47.0 ± 24.9 **Physical limitation** = 75.4 ± 31.1 vs. 43.3 ± 26.7 **Clinical summary score** = 76.6 ± 26.1 vs. 45.0 ± 23.5 QoL = 71.4 ± 28.5 vs. 27.0 ± 22.1 **Social limitation** = 67.0 ± 34.2 vs. 23.7 ± 23.4 **Overall summary score** = 73.0 ± 27.2 vs. 35.5 ± 21.5 **EQ-5D index score** = 0.74 ± 0.27 vs. 0.50 ± 0.30	Best QoL in recipients. EQ-5D scores highest in patients after HTx

Table 5.3 (continued)

Study	Title	Country	Study intent and number of patients	HRQOL instrument used	QoL scores (figures given as HTx vs wait-list)	Main findings related to HRQOL
Evangelista et al. (2004) [14]	Functional Status and Perceived Control Influence Quality of Life in Female Heart Transplant Recipients	United States of America	Describe and compare QOL and psychologic well-being of recipients and waiting list candidates, correlates of QOL in female recipients. $n = 100$	MLHFQ (lower score denotes higher QoL)	**LHFQ total** = 28.0 ± 26.4 vs. 52.3 ± 26.1 ($p = 0.000$) **Physical** = 11.3 ± 11.2 vs. 19.9 ± 12.1 ($p = 0.000$) **Emotional** = 7.5 ± 8.2 vs. 12.8 ± 7.8 ($p = 0.001$)	Overall QOL scores higher in recipients than candidates. Higher physical and emotional health for recipients compared with candidates. Functional status, depression and perceived control significant correlates of QOL among female recipients, accounted for 49% variance in overall QOL
Evangelista et al. (2005) [13]	Two-year follow-up of quality of life in patients referred for heart transplant	United States of America	Comparative effects of surgical or medical treatment on HRQOL. $n = 77$	SF 12	**Physical health** = 35.2 (32.4–44.6 IQR) vs. 40.4 (26.9–54.0 IQR) Mental health = 47.6 (36.758.8 IQR) vs. 42.4 (38.6–53.0 IQR)	Physical health score significantly improved over time in all patients, changes in mental health were minimal. Although all patients continued to have low HRQoL scores at the time of follow-up, medically stable patients had higher mental health scores and less depressive symptoms

Table 5.4 *Longitudinal studies: pre-operation and post-operation intervals*. Assessing baseline quality of life with heart failure, then at intervals post-operatively

Study	Title	Study intent and number of patients	HRQOL instrument used	QoL scores	Main findings related to HRQOL
Wu et al. (2019) [24]	Quality of life, demoralization syndrome and health-related lifestyle in cardiac transplant recipients—a longitudinal study in Taiwan	Compare different post-transplant times of recipients in terms of QOL, demoralization syndrome and health-related lifestyle, predictors of quality of life. $n = 99$	SF-12	**Group 1 (<1 year post-Tx)** **PCS** = 38.83 ± 7.65 (*baseline*) vs. 44.54 ± 7.93 (*3 Mo*) vs 45.18 ± 7.69 (*6 Mo*) vs. 48.15 ± 7.59 (*12 Mo*) **MCS** = 48.89 ± 9.59 (*baseline*) vs. 49.98 ± 7.70 (*3 Mo*) vs. 48.15 ± 8.25 (*6 Mo*) vs. 49.27 ± 7.58 (*12 Mo*) **Group 2 (1–3 years post-Tx)** **PCS** = 46.70 ± 8.43 (*baseline*) vs. 46.55 ± 8.40 (*3 Mo*) vs. 46.91 ± 8.43 (*6 Mo*) vs. 44.62 ± 8.67 (*12 Mo*) **MCS** = 46.35 ± 8.19 (*baseline*) vs. 45.29 ± 13.05 (*3 Mo*) vs. 48.16 ± 8.21 (*6 Mo*) vs. 49.30 ± 9.66 (*12 Mo*) **Group 3 (>3 years post-Tx)** **PCS** = 45.75 ± 8.93 (*baseline*) vs. 45.10 ± 9.28 (*3 Mo*) vs. 44.54 ± 9.62 (*6 Mo*) vs. 46.73 ± 8.43 (*12 Mo*) **MCS** = 47.92 ± 9.44 (*baseline*) vs. 49.98 ± 8.15 (*3 Mo*) vs. 50.93 ± 8.87 (*6 Mo*) vs. 50.39 ± 8.82 (*12 Mo*)	Fewer than half had good QOL, one-third had demoralization syndrome. Demoralization syndrome combined with post-transplant time, age, use of mechanical circulatory support during hospitalization and stress status accounted for 35.2% of PCS. Demoralization syndrome combined with age and religion accounted for 40.3% of MCS
Czyżewski et al. (2014) [23]	Comparative analysis of the quality of life for patients prior to and after heart transplantation	Quality of life of patients before and after HTx, $n = 63$	authors' questionnaire (Scale of 1 to 5)	**Physical** = 2.079 ± 0.79 (*Pre-Tx*) vs. 4.10 ± 0.39 (*Post-Tx*) **Mental** = 2.56 ± 0.98 (*Pre-Tx*) vs. 3.92 ± 0.75 (*Post-Tx*)	QOL pre-HTx = 3.16 ± 1.47, post-HTx = 7.60 ± 1.21. After HTx people consider their physical health better. Positive correlation between the assessment of QoL and that of physical and mental health

Shih et al. (2003) [37]	Changes in Health-Related Quality of Life and Working Competence Before and After Heart Transplantation: One-Year Follow-Up in Taiwan	Relationships between the changes in the HRQoL and working capacity (WC), changes in various aspects of physical well being related to HRQoL and WC in the first year. $n = 10$	interviewed x7 (QoL %)	31.25 ± 18.08 (*Pre-Tx*) vs. 60.00 ± 16.04 (*Post-Tx ICU transition*) vs. 64.38 ± 14.99 (*1 day pre-discharge*) vs. 68.75 ± 14.58 (*1 Mo post-discharge*) vs. 72.50 ± 7.07 (*3 Mo post-discharge*) vs. 72.50 ± 11.65 (*6 Mo post-discharge*) vs. 71.25 ± 11.26 (*12 Mo post-discharge*)	Correlation in the changes of perceived HRQoL between the preoperative and each postoperative stage. HRQoL in the postdischarge-12th month stage reached 2.29 times preoperative scores
Martín-Rodríguez et al. (2008) [21]	Health-Related Quality of Life Evolution in Patients After Heart Transplantation	Evolution of HRQOL during the first year. $n = 13$	SF 36 interview	**Physical functioning** = 21.92 (*Pre-Tx*) vs. 51.92 (*3 Mo*) vs. 75.00 (*6 Mo*) vs. 69.61 (12 Mo) **Role Limitations Due to Physical Problems** = 0 (*Pre-Tx*) vs. 33.84 (*3 Mo*) vs. 57.69 (*6 Mo*) vs. 53.84 (*12 Mo*) **Body Pain** = 77.11 (*Pre-Tx*) vs. 76.15 (*3 Mo*) vs. 91.53 (*6 Mo*) vs. 77.88 (*12 Mo*) **General Health** = 24.23 (*Pre-Tx*) vs. 29.23 (*3 Mo*) vs. 43.07 (*6 Mo*) vs. 77.88 (*12 Mo*) **Vitality** = 14.61 (*Pre-Tx*) vs. 45.76 (*3 Mo*) vs. 65.84 (*6 Mo*) vs. 53.84 (*12 Mo*) **Social Functioning Role Limitations Due to Emotional Problems** = 20.78 (*Pre-Tx*) vs. 47.94 (*3 Mo*) vs. 66.66 (*6 Mo*) vs. 51.27 (*12 Mo*) **Mental Health** = 47.07 (*Pre-Tx*) vs. 60.92 (*3 Mo*) vs. 73.53 (*6 Mo*) vs. 63.69 (*12 Mo*)	Progressive improvement in physical, psychologic, and social areas post-HTx, HRQoL stable at 6 months
O'Brien et al. (1987) [38]	Measuring the effectiveness of heart transplant programmes: quality of life data and their relationship to survival analysis	Examine relationship between the survival and QoL. $n = 1036$	NHP (mean rank score)	**Energy** = 27.21 (*pre-Tx*) vs. 18.00 (*3 Mo*) **Pain** = 24.65 (*pre-Tx*) vs. 12.25 (*3 Mo*) **Emotional reactions** = 31.22 (*pre-Tx*) vs. 5.90 (*3 Mo*) **Sleep** = 30.71(*pre-Tx*) vs. 11.05 (*3 Mo*) **Social isolation** = 23.86 (*pre-Tx*) vs. 3.88 (*3 Mo*) **Physical mobility** = 32.29 (*pre-Tx*) vs. 5.50 (*3 Mo*)	Large and rapid change in health status post-HTx; absence of spontaneous improvement prior to transplant and gradual deterioration post-transplant. NHP scores relate closely to clinical categorization. Pre-Tx NHP scores may be useful prognostic indicator for post-Tx survival

(continued)

Table 5.4 (continued)

Study	Title	Study intent and number of patients	HRQOL instrument used	QoL scores	Main findings related to HRQOL
Karapolat et al. (2007) [22]	The relationship between depressive symptoms and anxiety and quality of life and functional capacity in heart transplant patients	Relationship between depressive symptoms and anxiety with QoL and functional capacity. *n* = 34	SF-36	**Physical function** = 35.00 ± 25.68 (*pre-Tx*) vs. 68.52 ± 22.65 (*post-Tx*) **Physical role** = 27.68 ± 36.34 (*pre-Tx*) vs. 65.37 ± 36.35 (*post-Tx*) **Bodily pain** = 40.15 ± 21.62 (*pre-Tx*) vs. 63.00 ± 24.03 (*post-Tx*) **General health** = 40.67 ± 19.57 (*pre-Tx*) vs. 66.11 ± 19.35 (*post-Tx*) **Vitality** = 50.00 ± 16.76 (*pre-Tx*) vs. 71.67 ± 20.05 (*post-Tx*) **Social function** = 44.63 ± 28.12 (*pre-Tx*) vs. 71.04 ± 31.37 (*post-Tx*) **Emotional role** = 18.49 ± 26.67 (*pre-Tx*) vs. 68.85 ± 35.82 (*post-Tx*) **Mental Health** = 59.41 ± 20.89 (*pre-Tx*) vs. 72.30 ± 18.31 (*post-Tx*)	Negative correlation between BDI and subgroups on SF36. Significant improvements noted in all subgroups on the SF36 after the HTx
Evangelista et al. (2005) [13]	Two-year follow-up of quality of life in patients referred for heart transplant	Comparative effects of surgical or medical treatment on HRQoL. *n* = 77	SF 12	**Physical health** = 30.3 (20.1–35.8 IQR) (*pre-Tx*) vs. 35.2 (32.4–44.6 IQR) (*post-Tx*) **Mental health** = 47.6 (36.7–58.8 IQR) (*pre-Tx*) vs. 41.9 (38.8–51.2 IQR) (*post-Tx*)	Physical health score significantly improved over time in all patients, changes in mental health were minimal. Although all patients continued to have low HRQOL scores at the time of follow-up, medically stable patients had higher mental health scores and less depressive symptoms
Jakovljevic et al. (2014) [8]	Effect of Left Ventricular Assist Device Implantation and Heart Transplantation on Habitual Physical Activity and Quality of Life	Short- and long-term effects of LVAD implantation and HTx on physical activity and QoL. *n* = 40 (+14 healthy subjects)	MLHFQ	72 ± 8 (*pre-Tx*) vs. 39 ± 5 (*3 Mo*) vs. 30 ± 6 (*6 Mo*) vs. 29 ± 7 (*12 Mo*)	LVAD implantation and HTx increased daily physical activity by 60% and 52%. level of activity unchanged at 3, 6, and 12 months. QoL improved in LVAD implantation and HTx groups but unchanged afterward. HTx higher activity level vs. LVAD implantation—associated with better QoL

SF 12: Short Form 12; SF 36: Short Form 36; NHP: Nottingham Health Profile; MLHFQ: Minnesota Living with Heart Failure Questionnaire; PCS: Physical Component Score; MCS: Mental Component Score; Mo: month; Tx: transplant

Table 5.5 *Longitudinal studies: post—operation intervals only*. Studies that focused on outcomes at post-operative intervals only

Study	Title	Country	Study intent and number of patients	HRQOL instrument used	QoL scores	Main findings related to HRQOL
Trevizan et al. (2017) [28]	Quality of Life, Depression, Anxiety and Coping Strategies after Heart Transplantation	Brazil	Mental disorders and symptoms, such as depression and anxiety, quality of life and coping strategies in the post-surgical situation. $n = 33$	WHOQOL-BREF	**Physical** = 59.09 (*female*) vs. 65.75 (*male*) **Psychological** = 60.23 (*female*) vs. 75.57 (*male*) **Social Relations** = 64.39 (*female*) vs. 72.35 (*male*) **Environment** = 62.22 (*female*) vs. 69.89 (*male*) **Total** = 61.63 (*female*) vs. 71.01 (*male*)	Perception of quality of life considered good in all domains
Delgado et al. (2015) [25]	Health-related quality of life, social support, and caregiver burden between six and 120 months after heart transplantation: a Spanish multicenter cross-sectional study	Spain	Clinical and functional status, HRQoL, social support, and caregiver burden were analyzed in adult transplant recipients living with one functioning graft. $n = 303$	KCCQ EQ-5D	**KCCQ** **Symptom frequency** = 87.82 ± 2.25 (*6 Mo*) vs. 89.00 ± 2.21 (*12 Mo*) vs. 90.34 ± 2.10 (*36 Mo*) **Symptom stability** = 60.10 ± 2.68 (*6 Mo*) vs. 54.39 ± 2.18 (*12 Mo*) vs. 54.92 ± 2.24 (*36 Mo*) **Impact of symptoms** = 88 94 ± 2.26 (*6 Mo*) vs. 90.92 ± 1.88 (*12 Mo*) vs. 93.43 ± 1.73 (*36 Mo*) **Global symptoms** = 78.95 ± 1.63 (*6 Mo*) vs. 78.01 ± 1.47 (*12 Mo*) vs. 79.57 ± 1.45 (*36 Mo*) **Quality of life** = 77.72 ± 2 99 (*6 Mo*) vs. 79.82 ± 2.73 (*12 Mo*) vs. 88.57 ± 1.59 (*36 Mo*) **Social limitation** = 81.09 ± 3.23 (*6 Mo*) vs. 84.65 ± 2.76 (*12 Mo*) vs. 9[illegible].57 ± 2.05 (*36 Mo*) **Physical limitation** = 83.83 ± 2.68 (*6 Mo*) vs. 84.12 ± 2.80 (*12 Mo*) vs. 88.57 ± 2.51 (*36 Mo*) **Self-efficacy** = 87.50 ± 2.85 (*6 Mo*) vs. 85.31 ± 2.22 (*12 Mo*) vs. 89.39 ± 1.97 (*36 Mo*) **Overall status summary** = 80.46 ± 2.16 (*6 Mo*) vs. 81.65 ± 1.92 (*12 Mo*) vs. 87.05 ± 1.30 (*36 Mo*) **Clinical summary score** = 81.39 ± 1.80 (*6 Mo*) vs. 81.06 ± 1.77 (*12 Mo*) vs. 84.11 ± 1.54 (*36 Mo*) **EQ-5D utility index** = 0.8[illegible] ± 0.03 (*6 Mo*) vs. 0.82 ± 0.03 (*12 Mo*) vs. 0.85 ± 0.03 (*36 Mo*) **EQ-5D VAS** = 79.04 ± 2.0[illegible] (*6 Mo*) vs. 76.35 ± 2.18 (*12 Mo*) vs. 79.48 ± 1.68 (*36 Mo*)	Reasonable HRQoL, social support, and caregiver burden levels found at all time points, slight decrease in HRQoL recorded at 120 months. Complications, comorbidities, and hospitalizations were associated with HRQoL
Milaniak et al. (2014) [29]	Psychological Predictors (Personal Recourses) of Quality of Life for Heart Transplant Recipients	Poland	Subjective QoL of patients, relationship between personal resources and QoL. $n = 121$	WHOQOL-BREF	**Physical** = 13.035 ± 1.549 **Psychological** = 13.046 ± 1.100 **Social relationship** = 15.044 ± 2.404 **Environment** = 14.159 ± 2.437 **Total QoL** = 13.75 ± 1.44	The patients gained an average level of QOL (13.75). Positive relationship between the QOL in all its domains and personal resources: a sense of coherence, optimism, self-efficacy, and strategies for coping, planning, and positive revaluing

(continued)

Table 5.5 (continued)

Study	Title	Country	Study intent and number of patients	HRQOL instrument used	QoL scores	Main findings related to HRQOL
Evangelista et al. (2003) [39]	Hope, Mood States and Quality of Life in Female Heart Transplant Recipients	United States of America	Levels of hope, mood states and QoL, relationships between these variables and demographics, predictors of QoL in female recipients. $n = 50$	SF-12	**PCS** = 37.91 ± 8.57 **MCS** = 41.64 ± 12.59	Low levels of QOL as reflected in their low PCS and MCS scores. Strong positive association between hope, mood states and MCS. Age, hope and depression accounted for 69% of the variance in the MCS
Streiff et al. (2001) [40]	The Effects of Rejection Episodes, Obesity, and Osteopenia on Functional Performance and Health-Related Quality of Life After Heart Transplantation	United States of America	Correlate pre- and postoperative clinical parameters and events with HRQoL and functional performance (FP). $n = 70$	SF-36	Not given	HRQoL improves significantly in these patients post-HTx and is related to FP
Aguiar et al. (2011) [30]	Quality of Life of Patients that Had a Heart Transplant: Application of Whoqol-Bref Scale	Brazil	Evaluate the QoL of HTx patients by using a standardized scale. $n = 55$	WHOQOL-BREF	**% of patients satisfied with regards to:** **Physical** = 62.8% (*male*) vs. 58.3% (*female*) **Psychological** = 65.1% (*male*) vs. 58.3% (*female*) **Social relations** = 53.5 (*male*) vs. 100% (*female*) **Environment** = 65.1% (*male*) vs. 83.3% (*female*)	Patients are satisfied with their quality of life in all domains. Patients dissatisfed were few and did not represent a statistically significant value. Need for greater attention to negative feelings
Jokinen et al. (2010) [41]	Association between gastrointestinal symptoms and health-related quality of life after heart transplantation	Finland	Association between GI symptoms and HRQoL. $n = 167$	SF-36	Not given	Higher or equal SF-36 scores compared to general population: physical functioning; role-physical, bodily pain; general health; vitality; social functioning; role-emotional; and mental health. The prevalence of troublesome GI symptoms per GSRS dimension was 53.9% for diarrhea, 91.0% for indigestion, 60.6% for constipation, 73.4% for abdominal pain, 46.4% for reflux and 95.8% for any GI symptom. Diabetes contributed to diarrhea, use of prednisolone to indigestion and increased age to constipation

Saeed et al. (2008) [26]	Health-related Quality of Life After Cardiac Transplantation: Results of a UK National Survey With Norm-based Comparisons	United Kingdom	Descriptive analyses of HRQoL and norm-based comparisons. $n = 323$	SF-36 EQ-5D	**SF-36 domains** **Physical functioning** = 65.01 (58.5–71.5) **Role-physical** = 44.61 (34.5–54.8) **Bodily pain** = 42.32 (40.2–44.4) **General health** = 57.92 (53.9–62.0) **Vitality** = 54.32 (48.8–59.8) **Social functioning** = 71.02 (64.9–77.0) **Role emotional** = 65.43 (55.7–75.0) **Mental health** = 72.104 (67.7–76.5) **EQ-5D tariff** = 0.70 (0.64–0.75) **EQ-5D VAS** = 69.92 (65.6–74.3)	66% and 28% reported much better and somewhat better health. No deterioration in general health reported at 3 and 5 years. Norm-based comparisons suggested poorer HRQOL and all SF 36 dimensions except mental health
Karapolat et al. (2008) [42]	The effect of functional performance, respiratory function and osteopenia on the quality of life after heart transplantation	Turkey	Effect of functional performance, respiratory function, and osteopenia on QOL. $n = 31$	SF-36	not given	Significant relationship between pVO2 and physical function and the physical role scores. Significant relationship found between scores on the respiratory function tests and physical and social function scores. No significant relationship found between osteopenia and SF36 scores
Hummel et al. (2001) [27]	Quality of Life After Heart and Heart–Lung Transplantation	Germany	Physical and emotional condition after the first hospital discharge, quality of life 2 to 7 years after heart and heart-lung transplantation. $n = 369$	SF-36	**Physical functioning** = 58.29 ± 2.10 **Role-physical** = 45.38 ± 3.32 **Bodily pain** = 64.00 ± 2.26 **General health** = 58.29 ± 2.10 **Vitality** = 51.25 ± 1.54 **Social functioning** = 72.04 ± 1.92 **Role emotional** = 69.22 ± 3.19 **Mental health** = 58.11 ± 1.17	After Tx patients estimated their personal status positively, despite impaired physical capabilities. 2–7 years post-Tx family relationships remained stable, significant impairments in the physical functioning and the physical role, only minor impairments of normal activities compared to healthy population. Compared to heart failure control group, improvement of the quality of life after heart transplantation concerning particularly the vitality, mental health, general health perception, and bodily pain. Low proportion of patients went back to full-time employment

Table 5.5 (continued)

Study	Title	Country	Study intent and number of patients	HRQOL instrument used	QoL scores	Main findings related to HRQOL
Jones et al. (1992) [43]	Longitudinal study of quality of life and psychological adjustment after cardiac transplantation	Australia	psychological adjustment and QOL over time. $n = 27$	NHP		Well-being scores improved after Tx; did not deteriorate over time. No significant correlations found between psychological measures and medical/demographic data
Wu et al. (2019) [24]	Quality of life, demoralization syndrome and health-related lifestyle in cardiac transplant recipients – a longitudinal study in Taiwan	Taiwan	Compare different post-transplant times of recipients in terms of QoL, demoralization syndrome and health-related lifestyle, predictors of quality of life. $n = 99$	SF-12	**PCS** = 38.83 ± 7.65 **MCS** = 48.89 ± 9.59	Fewer than half had good QOL, one-third had demoralization syndrome. Demoralization syndrome combined with post-transplant time, age, use of mechanical circulatory support during hospitalization and stress status accounted for 35.2% of PCS. Demoralization syndrome combined with age and religion accounted for 40.3% of MCS

WHOQOL-BREF: World Health Organisation Quality of Life Brief Version; KCCQ: Kansas City Cardiomyopathy Questionnaire; EQ-5D: EuroQol-5D; EQ-5D VAS: EQ-5D Visual Analogue Scale; FP: Functional Performance; GI: Gastrointestinal; GSRS: Gastrointestinal Symptom Rating Scale

Table 5.6 *Longitudinal studies: long-term follow-up*. studies that focused on outcomes in long-term survivors (defined as >5 years)

Study	Title	Country	Study intent and number of patients	HRQOL instrument used	QoL scores	Main findings related to HRQOL
Grady et al. (2007) [44]	Patterns and Predictors of Quality of Life at 5–10 Years after Heart Transplantation	United States of America	Predictors of QoL 5–10 years after HTx. $n = 555$	QLI – Cardiac Version IV	Not given	High levels of satisfaction with QOL at 5 to 10 years, stable over 5-year period. Predictors of satisfaction with overall QOL = primarily psychosocial variables, predictors of satisfaction with QOL related to health and functioning = symptom distress, physical function and psychosocial variables
Martinelli et al. (2007) [18]	Getting Old With a New Heart: Impact of Age on Depression and Quality of Life in Long-term Heart Transplant Recipients	Italy	Role of age on depression and QoL in long-term HTx recipients still alive at more than 10 years. $n = 137$	SF-36	**MCS** = 48.75 ± 10.2 (young), 48.47 ± 10.1 (old) **PCS** = 46.88 ± 10.2 (young), 40.81 ± 10.6 (old)	Mental Component Summary did not differ between young and old subjects. Physical Component Summary higher in younger subjects
Aravot et al. (2000) [17]	Functional Status and Quality of Life of Heart Transplant Recipients Surviving Beyond 5 Years	Israel	Functional status and QoL of survivors 5 years +. $n = 10$	interview (working status, daily walk routine, pain or discomfort, immunosuppression complications, sex life, and satisfaction with regard to quality of life)	**No of patients experiencing:** **Discomfort** = 2 **Dizziness and headaches** = 1 **Joint pains** = 1 **Complications of immunosuppression** = 5 (skin infection = 1, Kaposi ssarcoma = 1, hirsutism = 1, gum hypertrophy = 1, renal failure = 1) **Dissatisfaction with sex life** = 2 **Dissatisfaction with functional status and QoL** = 2	Despite discomfort and complications with immunosuppression, vast majority of patients maintain good physical activity and working ability. They enjoy good family and sex life, indicating high degree of satisfaction with the transplant and their current status and quality of life

(continued)

Table 5.6 (continued)

Study	Title	Country	Study intent and number of patients	HRQOL instrument used	QoL scores	Main findings related to HRQOL
Salyer et al. (2003) [31]	Lifestyle and Quality of Life in Long- Term Cardiac Transplant Recipients	United States of America	Long-term recipients' perceptions of barriers to health-promoting behaviors, ability to manage their health, health-promoting lifestyle, health status and QoL; predictors of QoL. $n = 93$	QLI–Cardiac Version.	**Life satisfaction** = 0.79 ± 0.13 **Family life** = 0.84 ± 0.15 **Psychosocial/spiritual** = 0.81 ± 0.15 **Socioeconomic factors** = 0.79 ± 0.15 **Health and functioning** = 0.77 ± 0.14	Rated their health as good and moderately satisfied with life. Predictors of better perceptions of QOL = less education, longer time since transplant, ischemic etiology of heart failure, fewer barriers, higher perceived health competence and a health-promoting lifestyle
Barr et al. (2003) [45]	Determinants of Quality of Life Changes Among Long-term Cardiac Transplant Survivors: Results From Longitudinal Data	United States of America	Factors that affect differences in QoL among recipients; individual changes in QoL during 1-year period. 569 participants	LSI TCI	**LSI** = 77.4 ± 16.8 **TCI** = 70.9 ± 14.5	The number of comorbidities, treatment non-compliance, and several adverse effects were associated with low QOL. Waiting to take medications and taking less medication because of lifestyle restrictions were associated with decreases in QOL over time. Hair loss, changes in face shape, and decreased sexual interest or ability had the largest adverse effects on QOL changes
Politi et al. (2004) [19]	Ten Years of "Extended" Life: Quality of Life Among Heart Transplantation Survivors	Italy	Health status and QoL of survivors with associated predictors 10 years after HTx. $n = 122$	SF36	**PCS** = 44.6 (95% CI 42.7–46.4) **MCS** = 48.6 (95% CI 46.8–50.5)	Mental QOL of patients at 10 years similar to general population. Physical QoL worse among patients when compared with general population, predictors including older age, being married, the presence of complications, and impaired renal function

Grady et al. (2005) [16]	Predictors of Quality of Life at 5 to 6 Years After Heart Transplantation	United States of America	Describe QOL; identify differences in QOL by age, sex, and race; and identify predictors of QOL at 5 to 6 years after HTx. $n = 231$	QLI	**Life satisfaction** = 0.86 ± 0.12 **Family** = 0.91 ± 0.12 **Socioeconomic** = 0.86 ± 0.13 **Psychological/ spiritual** = 0.85 ± 0.15 **Health and functioning** = 0.84 ± 0.13	Patient satisfaction with all areas of life high at 5 to 6 years. Patients who were ≥ 60 years were more satisfied with QOL than patients <60 years. At 5 to 6 years after heart transplantation, almost 80% of variance in QOL was explained by psychological, physical, social, clinical, and demographic variables
Fusar-Poli et al. (2005) [32]	Depression and Quality of Life in Patients Living 10 to 18 Years Beyond Heart Transplantation	Italy	Factors that influence long-term QOL outcomes, depression on perceived health status, $n = 137$	SF-36	**PCS** = 45.5 (95% CI: 43.76–47.34) **MCS** = 48.62 (95% CI: 46.98–50.40)	Rated their health as good and only the physical QoL (PCS) was impaired when compared with general population. 32% of patients experienced mood depressive symptoms in the long term after transplantation, indicating a low perceived QoL
Galeone et al. (2014) [20]	Clinical outcome and quality of life of patients surviving 20 years or longer after heart transplantation	France	Outcome and QoL in ≥20 years survivors. $n = 131$	SF-36	**PCS** = 57 ± 23 **MCS** = 58 ± 21	Mean physical and mental scores were 57 ± 23 and 58 ± 21. Sixteen per cent of heart recipients survived ≥20 years with good ventricular performance and QoL

(continued)

Table 5.6 (continued)

Study	Title	Country	Study intent and number of patients	HRQOL instrument used	QoL scores	Main findings related to HRQOL
Delgado et al. (2015) [25]	Health-related quality of life, social support, and caregiver burden between six and 120 months after heart transplantation: a Spanish multicenter cross-sectional study	Spain	Clinical and functional status, HRQoL, social support, and caregiver burden were analyzed in adult transplant recipients living with one functioning graft. $n = 303$	KCCQ EQ-5D	**KCCQ** **Symptom frequency** = 87.74 ± 2.50 (5 years) vs. 83.43 ± 2.69 (10 years) **Symptom stability** = 54.17 ± 2.16 (5 years) vs. 59.62 ± 2.61 (10 years) **Impact of symptoms** = 88.17 ± 2.26 (5 years) vs. 82.44 ± 2.77 (10 years) **Global symptoms** = 76.83 ± 1.86 (5 years) vs. 75.16 ± 2.07 (10 years) **Quality of life** = 85.35 ± 2.39 (5 years) vs. 80.51 ± 2.40 (10 years) **Social limitation** = 81.18 ± 3.09 (5 years) vs. 78.74 ± 2.88 (10 years) **Physical limitation** = 83.05 ± 3.23 (5 years) vs. 78.35 ± 2.80 (10 years) **Self-efficacy** = 84.68 ± 2.10 (5 years) vs. 84.42 ± 2.59 (10 years) **Overall status summary** = 81.60 ± 2.14 (5 years) vs. 78.27 ± 1.94 (10 years) **Clinical summary score** = 79.94 ± 2.19(5 years) vs. 76.79 ± 1.89 (10 years) **EQ-5D utility index** = = 0.86 ± 0.02 (5 years) vs. 0.75 ± 0.03 (10 years) **EQ-5D VAS** = 75.34 2.43 (5 years) vs. 68.31 2.46 (10 years)	Reasonable HRQoL, social support, and caregiver burden levels found at all time points, slight decrease in HRQoL recorded at 120 months. Complications, comorbidities, and hospitalizations were associated with HRQoL

QLI-Cardiac Version IV: Quality of Life Index-Cardiac Version IV; LSI: Life Satisfaction Index; TCI: Temperament and Character Inventory; CI: Confidence Interval

Instrument, author	Number of items	Domains	Scoring
Minnesota Living with Heart Failure Questionnaire (MLHFQ)	21	Physical	**Total score** (sum of scores from individual items (6-point Likert Scale 0 to 5))
		Emotional	Range 0 to 105.
Rector et al 1987(34)			Higher scores = poorer quality of life
Quality of Life Index–Cardiac Version IV (QLI - cardiac version IV)	36	Health and functioning	Scores from part 1 (levels of satisfaction) and part 2 (levels of importance) combined
		Social and economic	Higher scores = higher satisfaction and importance
Ferrans and Powers 1985(35)		Psychological/spiritual	
		Family and relationships	
Kansas City Cardiomyopathy Questionnaire	23	Symptom frequency	**Total symptom score** (symptom frequency + symptom burden)
(KCCQ)		Symptom burden	**Clinical summary score** (symptom frequency + symptom burden + physical limitation)
Green et al. 2000(36)		Symptom stability	**Overall summary score** (symptom + physical limitations + social limitations + quality of life)
		Physical limitations	0-to-100-point scale
		Social limitations	Lower scores = more severe symptoms and/or limitations
		Quality of life Self-efficacy	Scores of 100 = no symptoms, no limitations, and excellent quality of life

Fig. 5.1 A comparison of four heart-failure-specific quality of life instruments commonly used in the selected studies

and 3, 6, and 12 months. Baseline physical activity was impaired in all groups, and baseline QoL was not significantly different among the LVAD and HTx cohorts. Although the study observed a significant improvement in both physical activity and QoL in both LVAD and HTx groups from baseline to 3 months, at any point in time the HTx group demonstrated higher activity level and QoL. Beyond 3 months, physical activity and QoL remain unchanged and inferior to that of healthy participants.

Emin et al. [9] performed a cross-sectional survey of four groups: patients assessed for HTx; patients listed for HTx on medical therapy; patients supported with LVAD; and patients after HTx. 82 LVAD patients and 82 post-HTx patients completed the KCCQ and EQ-5D questionnaires. Patients after HTx scored the highest for both the KCCQ overall summary score (73.0 vs. 52.6) and EQ-5D mean (0.74 vs. 0.58).

The ongoing SUSTAIN-IT trial (Sustaining Quality of Life of the Aged: Heart Transplant or Mechanical Support?) [10] seeks to compare health-related quality of life outcomes in 60–80 year old heart failure patients, who receive a heart transplant or are implanted with a destination therapy mechanical circulatory support. The trial utilizes a prospective, longitudinal design, and assesses HRQoL from baseline to 2 years post-operatively. The trial's primary aim is to establish whether mechanical circulatory support devices offer non-inferior benefits to HRQoL as compared to HTx.

Unlike patients in need for organs such as lungs or liver where there is no alternative, patients with end-stage heart failure can have a durable LVAD, which is shown to provide a survival benefit against medical management [11] and equipoise against marginal organ recipients [12]. In this chapter we have demonstrated that while HTx still seems to confer an overall improved QoL vs durable LVADs, those receiving LVADs still had an improved QoL compared to baseline and comparable to HTx.

vs. Medical Therapy

Evangelista et al. [13] performed a longitudinal study assessing 77 patients referred for HTx evaluation, to examine the "effects of time and treatment status on changes in HRQOL scores". Assessment using the Short Form-12 questionnaire was conducted at baseline, and at a 2 year follow-up. The follow-up identified 3 groups of patients: HTx recipients, HTx candidates, and medically stable patients who were not eligible for HTx. Results show a temporal improvement in physical health and depression scores in all groups; there was not much difference in mental health. Furthermore, despite all groups displaying impaired QoL at follow-up, medically stable patients had greater mental health scores and less depressive symptoms than the other groups.

Emin et al's [9] cross-sectional survey of HTx recipients and medical therapy recipients (among other groups) showed HTx recipients to have the greatest QoL scores in both the KCCQ and EQ-5D surveys.

vs. Waiting-List

Evangelista et al. [14] compared 2 groups of women controlled for age and functional status using the MLHFQ; group 1 were HTx recipients (n = 50) and group 2 were candidates on a transplant waiting list (n = 50). QoL was higher among the recipient cohort than the candidates, the scores being 28.0 and 56.3 respectively (lower scores denoting higher QoL). Moreover, physical and emotional health was higher for the recipient cohort.

Similarly, Mantovani et al. [15] performed a cross-sectional study of 47 HTx recipients and 9 wait-list patients. A significant difference between the two cohorts was seen in the overall QoL score (recipients = 30.7 mean rank; wait-list = 16.9) and in the four dimensions. The wait-list group had the lowest scores for general health and the highest for role-emotional. Whereas the transplant recipients reported the highest scores for general health and the lowest for bodily pain.

Emin et al. found similar results to these studies: patients listed for HTx had lower QoL scores than HTx recipients in both the KCCQ and EQ-5D surveys.

Longitudinal Studies

Of the long-term follow-up studies reviewed, they can be further sub-classified into immediate-, mid-, and extreme- long-term follow-up. Immediate long-term is defined as 5–10 years post-HTx, mid-long-term as >10 years, and extreme long-term as >20 years. The issue of survivorship bias is particularly relevant when reviewing long-term follow-up studies, as only those who survive and those without major complications will contribute to QoL assessments.

Immediate Long-Term Follow-Up (5–10 Years Post-HTx)

Grady et al. [16] studied a non-random sample of 231 patients who were 5 to 6 years post-HTx. Patients reported a high level of satisfaction with life overall and with the following specific areas of life: family, socioeconomic, psychological/spiritual and health and functioning. Moreover, these areas were reported to be very important from the Quality of Life Index proportional scores. When asked "whether they would make the same decision of having heart transplant surgery again, knowing what they knew 5 to 6 years later", 87% of responses were "definitely yes", 8% "probably yes", 3% "not sure", and 1% "probably no".

Aravot et al. [17] reviewed the QoL of their first ten patients surviving beyond 5 years. The interview included questions regarding working status, daily walk routine, pain or discomfort, complications of immunosuppression, sex life, and satisfaction with their QoL. It was found that half of patients reported side effects of the immunosuppressive regimen, and that of these 3 patients needed secondary treatment. These were chronic dialysis, radiotherapy for Kaposi sarcoma and gum resections. Aravot et al. found that 90% were married, 60% employed and 90% walk several kilometres daily. Those in employment stressed their "satisfaction in being able to contribute and not feel like a burden to society and their loved ones".

Mid Long-Term Follow-Up (10–20 Years Post-HTx)

Martinelli et al. [18] studied 137 consecutive patients surviving more than 10 years post-HTx, aiming to examine the role of age on QoL in this cohort of long-term survivors. They found that the SF-36 MCS was not significantly different between the young (<70 years) and old patients (≥70 years). However, the PCS was found to be greater in the young patients. The authors identify that "age per se does not represent a major limiting factor when considering candidates for this procedure, at least with regard to the issue of psychologic distress".

Politi et al. [19] also examined the long-term QoL of 276 patients surviving at 10 years in a cross-sectional study. It was found that mental QoL of 10 year survivors were similar to that of the general population. In contrast, the physical QoL was inferior to that of the general population. Predictors included older age, being married, the presence of complications, and impaired renal function.

Extreme Long-Term Follow-Up (>20 years Post-HTx)

The longest term follow up reviewed was that done by Galeone (2014) [20]. The quality of life in eight hundred and twenty-seven patients surviving ≥20 years with a single graft was retrospectively assessed. Mean physical and mental scores were 57 ± 23 and 58 ± 21, respectively. These scores were significantly lower than that of patients surviving <20 years, perhaps reflecting the lower comorbidity and age in the latter cohort. The mean scores of each SF-36 domain were also lower in norm-based comparisons to the general French population.

Discussion

Challenges in QOL Assessment in Transplant

The follow up period varied widely between the studies, the earliest after transplant being the post-Tx ICU transition phase. Of course the studies are assessing quality of life in survivors as mortality is an issue when studying heart failure therapies. The longest follow up period was of survivors 20 years+ incorporating 131 subjects.

Some studies break down the QOL of scores into their separate physical and mental domains, while others only provide a summary score. Therefore, separate analysis of the physical and mental components can only incorporate the former group of studies. A further challenge is that even this group of studies use a diverse range of tools, so that one must be careful in the comparison of alike domains from different questionnaires (refer Fig. 5.1). For example, the following domains all describe the physical wellbeing: 'physical *functioning'* in SF-12 and -36; vs 'physical *mobility*' in NHP; vs 'physical *limitation'* in KCCQ. The words 'functioning', 'mobility' and 'limitation' all relate to physical wellbeing but are subtly different.

Finally, the control groups varied widely. Some studies used the baseline QOL in pre-transplant patients with heart failure as the comparison group. Other used a separate cohort of patients implanted with LVAD, stabilised on medical therapy or on the waiting list as the comparison group. Some studies do not have a comparison group at all. These studies can still be useful as norm-based comparisons can be made to the general population.

Baseline QOL in Pre-transplant Patients

The baseline physical component in those with heart failure is significantly more impaired than the mental component in all of the Short Form questionnaire studies (all values expressed as physical functioning score vs mental health score: Mantovani et al. (2017) 9.5 vs. 24.6 [15], Martín-Rodríguez et al. (2008) 21.92 vs. 47.07 [21], Karapolat et al. (2007) 35.00 vs. 59.41 [22], Evangelista et al. (2005) 30.3 vs. 47.6 [13]. The study using the MLHFQ instrument [14] (11.3 vs. 7.5—note lower score denotes higher QOL) and an authors' questionnaire [23] (2.079 vs. 2.56) both agree with this discrepancy in mental and physical domains.

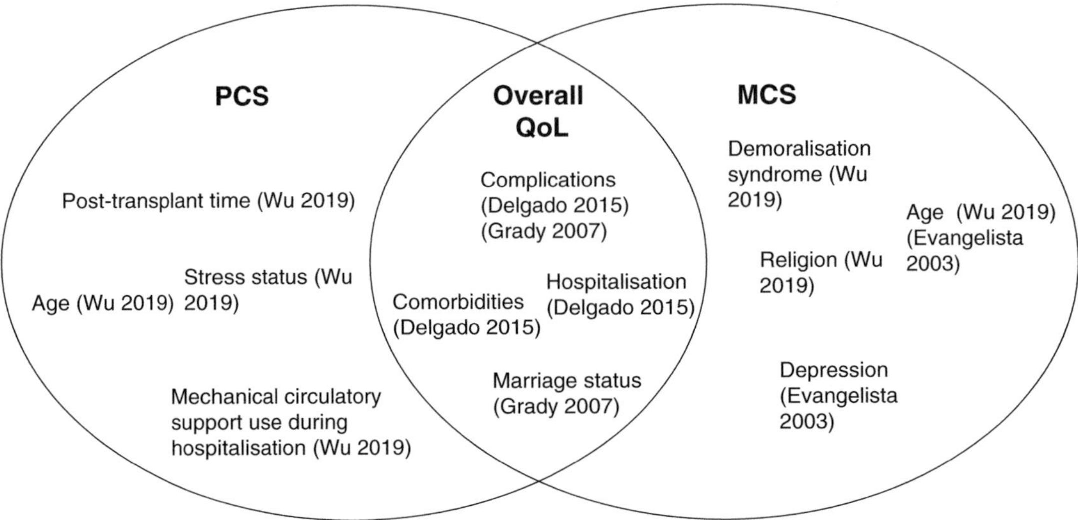

Fig. 5.2 Predictors of QoL, PCS and MCS. *PCS* Physical Component Score. *MCS* Mental Component Score

Regardless, both physical and mental scores are severely impaired compared to the general population.

Physical Activity Post-transplant

Using the Short Form 12 and 36 instruments, a rapid improvement in the physical component is seen within the first year after transplant, then after 1 year it seems to remain steady. Wu et al. [24] studied 3 groups of patients: group1 < 1 year post-Tx; group 2 1–3 years post-Tx; and group 3 > 3 years post-Tx. Group 1 patients' PCS scores rapidly improved from pre-Tx (38.83) to 3 months post-Tx (44.54) to 6 months (45.18) to 12 months (48.15). Comparatively groups 2 and 3, who were 1 year + post-Tx, did not show such a temporal improvement, and sometimes even a slight decrease. Martín-Rodriguez [21] corroborates with the immediate improvement in physical score (21.92 pre-Tx to 51.92 3 months to 75.00 6 months to 69.61 12 months). Unfortunately this study does not follow the cohort beyond 1 year to ascertain corroboration with Wu et al's findings. However, another study [25] disagrees with Wu et al's study finding of the stasis in physical score beyond 1 year as it showed persistent improvement up to 3 years – although it must be noted that this study used the KCCQ form with its physical limitation domain and not the Short Form questionnaire.

In all studies it appears that the greatest step in improvement occurs between pre-Tx and 3 months post-Tx, which is to be expected considering the severely impaired baseline physical domain in heart failure patients.

The predictors of the physical component of quality of life as identified in the selected studies include: post-transplant time, mechanical circulatory support during hospitalisation, stress status and age (refer to Fig. 5.2).

Mental Well-Being Post-transplant

In direct contrast to the physical component which showed an immediate improvement within the first year post-Tx, the mental component did not exhibit this improvement but stayed steady within the first year (group 1: 48.89 baseline vs. 49.98 3 months vs. 48.15 6 months vs. 49.27 12 months) [24]. However, again unlike the physical component (which slowed down in its improvement after 1 year), the mental component showed a steady improvement after 1 year. Groups 2 (1–3 years post-Tx): 45.29 to 48.16 to 49.30, and finally reaching 50.39 in group 3 (>3 years post-Tx)).

Perhaps this is because the physical component is severely impaired pre-Tx as compared to the mental component, and so the benefits of transplantation is seen more in the physical component first.

The predictors of the mental component of quality of life as identified in the selected studies include: religion, depression, demoralisation syndrome and age (refer to Fig. 5.2).

This 'reversal of changes' between the physical and mental components show that transplantation has benefits in both domains, albeit that the mental benefits can be expected to be more delayed. However this is not a reason for discouragement, as the baseline mental scores are relatively high to begin with, and while an immediate improvement is not seen, a depreciation is not observed either. Furthermore, this can be of some reassurance to patients that a long-term improvement in their mental wellbeing can be expected even if it is not immediately experienced.

While the physical domain was consistently more impaired than the mental domain before transplant in the Short Form questionnaires, following transplant the difference in the scores are much less, and the gap progressively diminishes the longer after transplant [13, 21, 22, 24, 26, 27]. This observation is also seen in the WHOQOL-BREF studies [28–30] and the Quality of Life Index studies [16, 31]. Moreover, it appears that this phenomena is maintained into the long term beyond 5 years, as unanimously seen in the long term studies [18–20, 32].

This may be explained by the 'reversal of changes' postulated earlier, as the physical scores rapidly improve in the immediate aftermath of transplant and close the gap between the two domains. After one year, the changes in physical scores wean and the mental gradually improves. This hypothesis would suggest that the longest surviving patients would have near-equal physical and mental scores. Indeed, the longest-term study is of ≥20 years survivors by Galeone et al. [20], showing similar physical and mental scores - 57 and 58, respectively. Of course, as mortality is an issue when studying heart transplantation outcomes, there is not sufficient data for the extreme long-term, and any conclusions must be cautiously drawn.

Forsberg [33] proposes a framework for improving adaptation in heart transplant patients. It is suggested that endeavoring for control and predictability results in reducing the patient's ability to adjust, thereby prolonging the transition period. The importance given to self management support is identified as problematic. Furthermore, the importance of conditioning patients to adjust to their new situation is stressed: "instead of relying on unrealistic expectations, they can focus on accepting their situation and the unknown, as well as on what can be achieved".

Key Conclusions

1. There is a significant impairment in the physical domain in baseline heart failure patient pre-Tx.
2. There is a significant difference in the physical and mental components pre-Tx, the physical being worse.
3. "Reversal of Changes": Immediately post-Tx there is a rapid improvement in physical wellbeing and no change in mental wellbeing. Longer term there is no change in physical wellbeing and a gradual improvement in mental wellbeing.
4. Less discrepancy between physical and mental component scores post-Tx. This is maintained in the longer term and scores equalizes in the extreme long term.

References

1. Lala A, Rowland JC, Ferket BS, Gelijns AC, Bagiella E, Pinney SP, et al. Strategies of Wait-listing for Heart Transplant vs Durable Mechanical Circulatory Support Alone for Patients With Advanced Heart Failure. JAMA Cardiol. 2020;5(6):652–9.
2. Aissaoui N, Morshuis M, Maoulida H, Salem J-E, Lebreton G, Brunn M, et al. Management of end-stage heart failure patients with or without ventricular assist device: an observational comparison of clinical and economic outcomes†. Eur J Cardiothorac Surg. 2018;53(1):170–7.
3. Long EF, Swain GW, Mangi AA. Comparative survival and cost-effectiveness of advanced therapies for end-stage heart failure. Circ Heart Fail. 2014;7(3):470–8.
4. Lim E, Ali Z, Ali A, Motalleb-Zadeh R, Jackson C, Ong SL, et al. Comparison of survival by allocation

to medical therapy, surgery, or heart transplantation for ischemic advanced heart failure. J Heart Lung Transplant. 2005;24(8):983–9.

5. NHS Blood and Transplant. Annual Report on Cardiothoracic Organ Transplantation; 2020. p. 25.
6. Khush KK, Cherikh WS, Chambers DC, Harhay MO, Hayes D, Hsich E, et al. The International Thoracic Organ Transplant Registry of the International Society for Heart and Lung Transplantation: Thirty-sixth adult heart transplantation report - 2019; focus theme: Donor and recipient size match. J Heart Lung Transplant. 2019;38(10):1056–66.
7. Grady KL, Meyer PM, Dressler D, White-Williams C, Kaan A, Mattea A, et al. Change in quality of life from after left ventricular assist device implantation to after heart transplantation. J Heart Lung Transplant. 2003;22(11):1254–67.
8. Jakovljevic DG, McDiarmid A, Hallsworth K, Seferovic PM, Ninkovic VM, Parry G, et al. Effect of left ventricular assist device implantation and heart transplantation on habitual physical activity and quality of life. Am J Cardiol. 2014;114(1):88–93.
9. Emin A, Rogers CA, Banner NR, Steering Group, UK. Cardiothoracic Transplant Audit. Quality of life of advanced chronic heart failure: medical care, mechanical circulatory support and transplantation. Eur J Cardio-Thorac Surg. 2016;50(2):269–73.
10. Grady K. SUSTAIN-IT: Sustaining Quality of Life of the Aged: Heart Transplant or Mechanical Support? [Internet]. clinicaltrials.gov; 2021 Nov [cited 2021 Nov 25]. Report No.: NCT02568930. Available from: https://clinicaltrials.gov/ct2/show/NCT02568930
11. Shah KB, Starling RC, Rogers JG, Horstmanshof DA, Long JW, Kasirajan V, et al. Left ventricular assist devices versus medical management in ambulatory heart failure patients: An analysis of INTERMACS Profiles 4 and 5 to 7 from the ROADMAP study. J Heart Lung Transplant. 2018;37(6):706–14.
12. Schumer EM, Ising MS, Trivedi JR, Slaughter MS, Cheng A. Early Outcomes With Marginal Donor Hearts Compared With Left Ventricular Assist Device Support in Patients With Advanced Heart Failure. Ann Thorac Surg. 2015;100(2):522–7.
13. Evangelista LS, Dracup K, Moser DK, Westlake C, Erickson V, Hamilton MA, et al. Two-year follow-up of quality of life in patients referred for heart transplant. Heart Lung J Crit Care. 2005;34(3):187–93.
14. Evangelista LS, Moser D, Dracup K, Doering L, Kobashigawa J. Functional status and perceived control influence quality of life in female heart transplant recipients. J Heart Lung Transplant. 2004;23(3):360–7.
15. Mantovani VM, Silveira CB, Lima LL, Orlandin L, Rabelo-Silva ER, Moraes MA. Comparison of quality of life between patients on the waiting list and heart transplant recipients. Rev Gaucha Enferm. 2017;37(4):e53280.
16. Grady KL, Naftel DC, White-Williams C, Bellg AJ, Young JB, Pelegrin D, et al. Predictors of quality of life at 5 to 6 years after heart transplantation. J Heart Lung Transplant. 2005;24(9):1431–9.
17. Aravot D, Berman M, Ben-Gal T, Sahar G, Vidne B. Functional status and quality of life of heart transplant recipients surviving beyond 5 years. Transplant Proc. 2000;32(4):731–2.
18. Martinelli V, Fusar-Poli P, Emanuele E, Klersy C, Campana C, Barale F, et al. Getting old with a new heart: impact of age on depression and quality of life in long-term heart transplant recipients. J Heart Lung Transplant. 2007;26(5):544–8.
19. Politi P, Piccinelli M, Fusar-Poli P, Poli PF, Klersy C, Campana C, et al. Ten years of 'extended' life: quality of life among heart transplantation survivors. Transplantation. 2004;78(2):257–63.
20. Galeone A, Kirsch M, Barreda E, Fernandez F, Vaissier E, Pavie A, et al. Clinical outcome and quality of life of patients surviving 20 years or longer after heart transplantation. Transpl Int. 2014;27(6):576–82.
21. Martín-Rodríguez A, Pérez-San-Gregorio MA, Díaz-Domínguez R, Pérez-Bernal J. Health-related quality of life evolution in patients after heart transplantation. Transplant Proc. 2008;40(9):3037–8.
22. Karapolat H, Eyigor S, Durmaz B, Yagdi T, Nalbantgil S, Karakula S. The relationship between depressive symptoms and anxiety and quality of life and functional capacity in heart transplant patients. Clin Res Cardiol. 2007;96(9):593–9.
23. Czyżewski Ł, Torba K, Jasińska M, Religa G. Comparative analysis of the quality of life for patients prior to and after heart transplantation. Ann Transplant. 2014;17(19):288–94.
24. Wu Y-C, Tung H-H, Wei J. Quality of life, demoralization syndrome and health-related lifestyle in cardiac transplant recipients - a longitudinal study in Taiwan. Eur J Cardiovasc Nurs. 2019;18(2):149–62.
25. Delgado JF, Almenar L, González-Vilchez F, Arizón JM, Gómez M, Fuente L, et al. Health-related quality of life, social support, and caregiver burden between six and 120 months after heart transplantation: a Spanish multicenter cross-sectional study. Clin Transpl. 2015;29(9):771–80.
26. Saeed I, Rogers C, Murday A. Steering Group of the UK Cardiothoracic Transplant Audit. Health-related quality of life after cardiac transplantation: results of a UK National Survey with Norm-based Comparisons. J Heart Lung Transplant. 2008;27(6):675–81.
27. Hummel M, Michauk I, Hetzer R, Fuhrmann B. Quality of life after heart and heart-lung transplantation. Transplant Proc. 2001;33(7–8):3546–8.
28. Trevizan FB, MCOS M, YLW S, CMW R. Quality of Life, Depression, Anxiety and Coping Strategies after Heart Transplantation. Braz J Cardiovasc Surg. 2017;32(3):162–70.
29. Milaniak I, Wilczek-Rużyczka E, Przybyłowski P, Wierzbicki K, Siwińska J, Sadowski J. Psychological predictors (personal recourses) of quality of life for heart transplant recipients. Transplant Proc. 2014;46(8):2839–43.

30. de Aguiar MIF, Farias DR, Pinheiro ML, Chaves ES, Rolim ILTP, de Almeida PC. Quality of life of patients that had a heart transplant: application of Whoqol-Bref scale. Arq Bras Cardiol. 2011;96(1):60–8.
31. Salyer J, Flattery MP, Joyner PL, Elswick RK. Lifestyle and quality of life in long-term cardiac transplant recipients. J Heart Lung Transplant. 2003;22(3):309–21.
32. Fusar-Poli P, Martinelli V, Klersy C, Campana C, Callegari A, Barale F, et al. Depression and quality of life in patients living 10 to 18 years beyond heart transplantation. J Heart Lung Transplant. 2005;24(12):2269–78.
33. Adaptation after heart transplantation: A framework for the future. Available from: https://www.openaccessgovernment.org/adaptation-after-heart-transplantation-a-framework-for-the-future/101548/
34. Delcroix M, Lang I, Pepke-Zaba J, Jansa P, D'Armini AM, Snijder R, et al. Long-Term Outcome of Patients With Chronic Thromboembolic Pulmonary Hypertension: Results From an International Prospective Registry. Circulation. 2016;133(9):859–71.
35. Ferrans CE, Powers MJ. Quality of life index: development and psychometric properties. ANS Adv Nurs Sci. 1985;8(1):15–24.
36. Green CP, Porter CB, Bresnahan DR, Spertus JA. Development and evaluation of the Kansas City Cardiomyopathy Questionnaire: a new health status measure for heart failure. J Am Coll Cardiol. 2000;35(5):1245–55.
37. Shih FJ, Tsao CI, Ko WJ, Chou NK, Hsu RB, Chen YS, et al. Changes in health-related quality of life and working competence before and after heart transplantation: one-year follow-up in Taiwan. Transplant Proc. 2003;35(1):466–71.
38. O'Brien BJ, Buxton MJ, Ferguson BA. Measuring the effectiveness of heart transplant programmes: quality of life data and their relationship to survival analysis. J Chronic Dis. 1987;40(Suppl 1):137S–58S.
39. Evangelista LS, Doering LV, Dracup K, Vassilakis ME, Kobashigawa J. Hope, mood states and quality of life in female heart transplant recipients. J Heart Lung Transplant. 2003;22(6):681–6.
40. Streiff N, Feurer I, Speroff T, Davis SF, Butler J, Chomsky D, et al. The effects of rejection episodes, obesity, and osteopenia on functional performance and health-related quality of life after heart transplantation. Transplant Proc. 2001;33(7–8):3533–5.
41. Jokinen JJ, Hämmäinen P, Lemström KB, Lommi J, Sipponen J, Harjula ALJ. Association between gastrointestinal symptoms and health-related quality of life after heart transplantation. J Heart Lung Transplant. 2010;29(12):1388–94.
42. Karapolat H, Eyigor S, Durmaz B, Nalbantgil S, Yagdi T, Zoghi M. The effect of functional performance, respiratory function and osteopenia on the quality of life after heart transplantation. Int J Cardiol. 2008;124(3):381–3.
43. Jones BM, Taylor F, Downs K, Spratt P. Longitudinal study of quality of life and psychological adjustment after cardiac transplantation. Med J Aust. 1992;157(1):24–6.
44. Grady KL, Naftel DC, Kobashigawa J, Chait J, Young JB, Pelegrin D, et al. Patterns and predictors of quality of life at 5 to 10 years after heart transplantation. J Heart Lung Transplant. 2007;26(5):535–43.
45. Barr ML, Schenkel FA, Van Kirk A, Halbert RJ, Helderman JH, Hricik DE, et al. Determinants of quality of life changes among long-term cardiac transplant survivors: results from longitudinal data. J Heart Lung Transplant. 2003;22(10):1157–67.
46. Walden JA, Stevenson LW, Dracup K, Hook JF, Moser DK, Hamilton M, et al. Extended comparison of quality of life between stable heart failure patients and heart transplant recipients. J Heart Lung Transplant. 1994;13(6):1109–18.
47. Tackmann E, Dettmer S. Health-related quality of life in adult heart-transplant recipients-a systematic review. Herz. 2020;45(5):475–82.
48. Stubber C, Kirkman M. The experiences of adult heart, lung, and heart-lung transplantation recipients: A systematic review of qualitative research evidence. PLoS One. 2020;15(11):e0241570.
49. Sarasa MM, Olano-Lizarraga M. Exploring the experience of living with a heart transplant: a systematic review of the literature. An Sist Sanit Navar. 2019;42(3):309–24.
50. Conway A, Schadewaldt V, Clark R, Ski C, Thompson DR, Doering L. The psychological experiences of adult heart transplant recipients: a systematic review and meta-summary of qualitative findings. Heart Lung J Crit Care. 2013;42(6):449–55.

QOL and PROMS Following Transcatheter Aortic Valve Implantation

6

M. Monteagudo-Vela, V. Panoulas, and G. Krasopoulos

Introduction

Aortic stenosis (AS) is an insidious disease with high mortality after the onset of the symptoms and with an incidence that increases logarithmically after the sixth decade of life [1]. As life expectancy has substantially increased over the past twenty years, (AS) has become the most frequent valvular heart disease [2]. Surgical aortic valve replacement (sAVR) was until recently, the only invasive treatment option with conservative/palliative therapies being the only alternative for patients who could not have surgery [3].

sAVR is the gold standard therapy for symptomatic aortic stenosis with proven capacity to alleviate symptoms, improve quality of life and increase survival [4] and with durability that extends beyond 15 years [5]. The National Adult Cardiac Surgery Audit (NACSA) published in 2020 presented all cardiac surgical activity levels and trends in the United Kingdom, over the past 3 years (1st April 2016 to 31st March 2019) [6]. In this report sAVR was found to be the second most commonly cardiac operation performed in the UK after coronary artery bypass surgery, with a mortality rate of 0.9% for patients under 75 years of age, and 1.2% for those over 75 years. However, there are many patients that, due to coexisting comorbidities, high frailty index or advanced age (>80 years), do not qualify for sAVR due to very high peri-procedural surgical risk [7].

The significant increase in life expectancy that our society has been experiencing over the past couple of decades, and the association of AS and ageing has generated an ever-expanding population of very elderly with significant restrictions in their quality of life due to AS [8]. Since 2002 when the first procedure of transcutaneous aortic valve implantation (TAVI) was performed [9], TAVI has rapidly evolved as the alternative invasive procedure that could be offered to patients with severe AS. As the procedural risk of TAVI decreases thanks to technical improvements to the valve-implants and delivery systems, this technique has emerged and established itself as the invasive treatment option of choice for patients who have been deemed inoperable [10], for those at high surgical risk due to high frailty

M. Monteagudo-Vela
Department of Cardiothoracic Surgery, Oxford University Hospitals NHS Foundation Trust, Oxford, UK
e-mail: maria.monteagudo-vela@ouh.nhs.uk

V. Panoulas
Department of Cardiology, Royal Brompton and Harefield NHS Foundation Trust, London, UK
e-mail: v.panoulas@rbht.nhs.uk

G. Krasopoulos (✉)
Department of Cardiothoracic Surgery, Oxford University Hospitals NHS Foundation Trust, Oxford, UK

Department of Cardiothoracic Surgery, Oxford University Hospitals NHS Foundation Trust & University of Oxford, Oxford, UK
e-mail: george.krasopoulos@ouh.nhs.uk

T. Athanasiou et al. (eds.), *Patient Reported Outcomes and Quality of Life in Cardiovascular Interventions*,
https://doi.org/10.1007/978-3-031-09815-4_6

index or co-morbidities [11] or those at intermediate or low surgical risk in their ninth or tenth decade of life [12, 13].

Even though both, sAVR and TAVI, are effective invasive treatment options for the management of symptomatic AS, capable of substantially improving survival at short and mid-term (up to 7 years) [14], sAVR remains the only option with known durable long-term results that extend beyond 10 years [15]. In the modern era, durability and long-term outcomes are equally important to quality of life (QoL) for many patients suffering from AS and plays a significant part in their decision-making process.

In 2018/19 the numbers of TAVI cases in the UK (5197) overtook isolated sAVR (5091) [6], a trend that has been observed in other European countries such as Germany [16, 17]. So much in UK but also internationally, the total number of all procedures for aortic valve disease continued to increase over the past 5 years [6], probably due to a combination of high prevalence of the disease attributed to an ageing population and the availability of an alternative interventional option like TAVI.

This chapter is set out to review and analyse all currently available published information related to QoL following sAVR or TAVI as treatment for AS that include QoL in their endpoints. We will attempt to provide a comprehensive understanding of the currently available tools in assessing QoL in patients treated for AS, summarise available knowledge in order to assist patients and clinicians in their decision-making process.

Summary of Interventions (Surgical, Endovascular/Minimally Invasive) for Aortic Stenosis

Surgical aortic valve replacement (SAVR) and transcatheter aortic valve implantation (TAVI) are the mainstays of treatment for severe aortic stenosis (AS).

Transcatheter aortic valve implantation (TAVI) is a minimally invasive procedure that entails different approaches of implanting a biological prosthetic valve, within a usually calcified native aortic valve. TAVI can be performed under local anaesthesia and sedation or under general anaesthesia. These techniques are based in gaining arterial access, either percutaneously or with a surgical cut down. The most common access to deliver the valve is via the femoral arteries (over 90% in most major registries), followed by trans-carotid and trans-subclavian/trans-axillary. Trans-apical and trans-aortic are fading as options, due to their more invasive nature. Trans-caval access is also used in select centres, however its generalizability has been questioned due to its complexity. The TAVI valve is mounted onto a stent, and it is advanced to the heart using specialised intravascular equipment, known as delivery systems. The diseased native aortic valve is stretched open and the new bioprosthetic valve is implanted within the old diseased (usually stenotic) native aortic valve of the patient. The majority of commercially available valves are either balloon expandable or self-expanding and come with a skirt, aiming to improve sealing and reduce paravalvular leaks [13, 18].

Surgical aortic valve replacement is carried out under general anaesthesia. sAVR is performed with the help of cardiopulmonary bypass machine. The heart is arrested in order to access the aortic valve and replace it. Although the traditional approach is a median sternotomy, modern techniques of minimally invasive approaches with smaller incisions can minimise the trauma to the patient, reduce complications and accelerate the postoperative recovery [19] (Fig. 6.1). sAVR has the capacity to fully replace the diseased aortic valve and it can treat native aortic valves that suffer from both stenosis and insufficiency. Under the generic terminology of sAVR come a number of different procedures, with choices of different prosthesis that are ranging from biological valves to homografts, mechanical valves or even preserving the patient's own aortic valve and repairing it. Stented biological and mechanical valves are the most widely used valves currently and they need to be sutured onto the patient's aortic valve annulus. Sutureless bioprostheses represent a contemporary option for sAVR and offer the possibility of replacing the

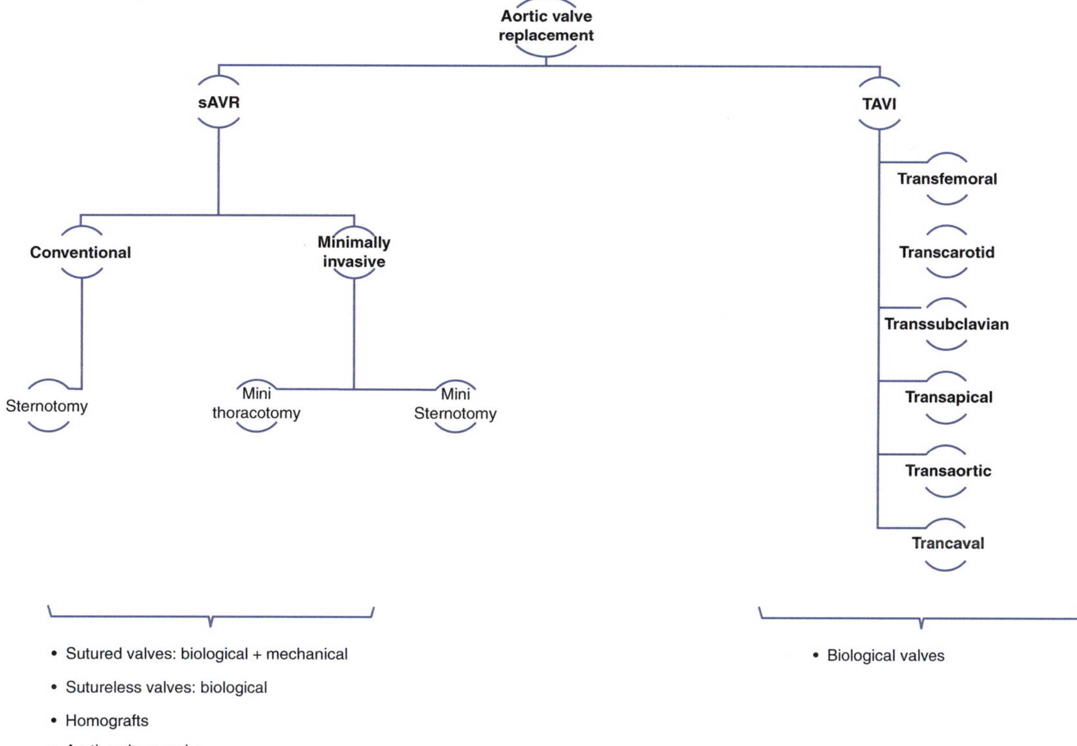

Fig. 6.1 Summary of interventions for aortic valve replacement

diseased native aortic valve without the need of having to suture the implant onto the heart. When sutureless technology is combined with conventional or minimally invasive sAVR, can offer further advantages in reducing perioperative exposure of patients to risk, augment patients' recovery and positively influence post-procedural QoL [20, 21].

Analysis of the Utility of Different QOL Tool

There are plenty of quality-of-life tools available to analyse health related issues. These are multidimensional assessment instruments and are designed to assess patient's subjective health perception, related to a procedure or a condition [22]. These questionnaires integrate both physical/functional and emotional dimensions and some of them include social dimensions as well. The aim is to convert qualitative information into quantitative data and generate a score that can universalize and compare differences.

Methods

After Entrez, PubMed, MEDLINE, Scopus and Google Scholar were searched using the MeSH terms 'Quality of life' AND 'TAVI', we identified 159 articles referred to Quality of life in patients after TAVI procedures and 15 were finally included into the review.

Within the included articles, health status was assessed at different time points depending on the study (pre-procedural and 1, 2, 3-, 6-, 12- and 24-months post-procedural). Health-related Quality of Life questionnaires used in this review were the Kansas City Cardiomyopathy Questionnaire, the Short Form-12, the Short Form-36, the EuroQol-5D and 3D and the Minnesota Living with Heart Failure Questionnaire.

These questionnaires investigate several dimensions and grade them to different levels, in order to target the answer and link them, as best as possible, with the age group and personal expectations of the cohort of patients included at each study. However, none of them are age specific or age weighted, and this could potentially lead to bias, as expectations and perceptions related to QoL differ greatly amongst different age groups. The diversity among the different QoL questionnaires used makes it difficult to compare outcomes, summarise or meta-analyse reported outcomes.

The Minnesota Living with Heart Failure Questionnaire (MLHFQ) score is widely used for heart failure patients, has well-documented validity, reliability, and sensitivity, and is also validated in patients referred for valvular surgery [23]. However, despite its proven validity in physical and emotional subscales in patients with HF, it lacks social dimension, which is particularly important when QoL is assessed in a cohort of elderly TAVI patients [24].

EQ-5D-3L and EQ-5D-5L questionnaires, introduced by the EuroQol Group in 1990 and 2009, are comprised of five dimensions, as explained in Table 6.1. In the latest EQ-5D-3L, the number of levels of perceived problems per dimension was changed from 3 to 5, increasing the sensitivity and reducing the ceiling effect caused by the big gap between "severe and extreme problems", mostly enhancing the assessment of the mobility dimension of the questionnaire.

The Short Form 36 Health Survey Questionnaire (SF-36) has been widely used in cardiac patient populations. Its complexity however (36 items, covering eight domains of health (Table 6.1) [25]), makes it difficult to implement, as it has a considerable burden upon both patients and investigators. The SF-12 was derived from the larger SF-36, and the physical and mental summary scores obtained from the SF-12 correlate highly with those calculated using the original, longer questionnaire (Table 6.2).

The Kansas City Cardiomyopathy Questionnaire (KCCQ) has 23 items. It is designed and validated to evaluate self-reported, disease-specific health status in patients with heart failure. The analysed domains include symptoms, physical limitation, social limitation, self-efficacy and knowledge, and quality-of-life. The KCCQ summary scores have previously been reported to correlate well with New NYHA classification for shortness of breath and has shown to independently predict mortality and health care costs in heart failure populations [26].

Discussion

In this chapter we reviewed and analysed contemporaneous information related to QoL following treatment for AS after TAVI. Our goal was to identify the most common tools used to assess quality of life and summarise this knowledge to improve decision-making process for both patients and clinicians, while we can identify areas of potential future research opportunities.

As life expectancy increases and TAVI is offered as treatment option to patients in their eighth but mainly in their ninth and tenth decade of life, quality of life assessment has fundamental implications in the decision-making process for this particular group of patients [27]. sAVR can be offered as a treatment option to all ages, it has a wider range of therapeutic profiles, has a lower overall cost to healthcare systems [23] and it has a well-documented and established durability that extends well beyond 15 years.

In recent years, TAVI has been widely accepted and recognised as a safe and effective treatment for severe aortic stenosis in patients that are inoperable, those with high frailty index or the ones with very high risk for sAVR. TAVI indications have recently been expanded to intermediate and low risk groups, but this is normally reserved for patients in the eighth, ninth or 10thdecade of their life. Despite sufficient favourable outcome data in short- and mid-term follow up for TAVI, there is a clear paucity of data with regards to long-term quality of life and valve durability beyond 7 years [28].

In 1966 Elkinton described quality of life as 'not just the absence of death but life with the

Table 6.1 Quality of life questionnaires

Questionnaire	Dimensions studied	Advantages	Disadvantages
MLHFQ	Physical and emotional	Short and easy	Lack of social dimension
EQ-5D-3L	Mobility, self-care, usual activities, pain/discomfort, anxiety/depression		Ceiling effect due to number of levels perceived
EQ-5D-5L	Mobility, self-care, usual activities, pain/discomfort, anxiety/depression	Two levels more to increase sensitivity	
SF-36	Limitations in: – Physical activities – Social activities – Usual role activities (physical/emotional related) – Bodily pain – General mental health – Vitality – General health perceptions	More responsive with musculoskeletal disorders [25]	– 36-items making it tedious – Physical component and a mental component: difficult to interpret
SF-12	Shorter version of SF-36 questionnaire with good correlation in the physical and mental summary scores with the larger version described above		
KCCQ	Physical function, symptoms, social function, self-efficacy and knowledge, and quality of life	Correlates with New NYHA class and predicts mortality and health care costs in heart failure populations [26]	

MLHFQ: Minnesota Living with Heart Failure Questionnaire; SF-12: Short Form 12 Health Survey Questionnaire; SF-36: Short Form 36 Health Survey Questionnaire; EQ-5D-3L: EuroQol 3 L questionnaire; EQ-5D-5L: EuroQol 5 L questionnaire; KCCQ: Kansas City Cardiomyopathy Questionnaire

Table 6.2 Summary of relevant studies

Study	Period	Patients (included/total)	Procedures & mean age	Questionnaire	Follow-up	Conclusions	Limitations/critics
RANDOMIZED TRIALS TAVI vs sAVR							
Mack et al. [13] Transcatheter Aortic-Valve Replacement with a Balloon Expandable Valve in Low-Risk Patients	2016–2017	950/1000	496 TAVI (73.3yo) 454 sAVR (73.6 yo)	**KCCQ**	1–12 months	– TAVI had more rapid improvements in QoL at 30 days but no differences seen at 1 year	– More patients in the surgery group than in the TAVI group withdrew from the trial – Missing data from the KCCQ
Makkar et al. [32] Five-Year Outcomes of Transcatheter or Surgical Aortic-Valve Replacement Results From the PARTNER 2 Randomized Clinical Trial	Recruitment: 2011–2013 Follow up: Up to 2016–2018	2032	Data available at 5 y: – TAVI 920 (91.0%) – sAVR 831 (81.4%)	**KCCQ**	Baseline-1-12-24-36-48-60 months	– Both TAVI and sAVR led to improvements in health status at 5 years	– sAVR patients having more extensive procedures than isolated AVR – QoL in the surgical cohort was also assessing complex operations other than isolated sAVR – More reinterventions, rehospitalizations, and paravalvular leaks in the TAVI cohort at 5 year
Baron et al. [41] Health Status Benefits of Transcatheter vs Surgical Aortic Valve Replacement in Patients With Severe Aortic Stenosis at Intermediate Surgical Risk: Results From the PARTNER 2 Randomized Clinical Trial	2011–2013	2032	1011 TAVI (81.5 yo) 1021 sAVR (81.7 yo)	**KCCQ** **EQ-5D** **SF-36**	Baseline-1-12-24 months	– QoL improved significantly with both TAVI and sAVR through 2 years of follow up – Early improvement was greater for TAVIs via transfemoral access (borderline significance)	– sAVR patients having more extensive procedures than isolated AVR – QoL in the surgical cohort was also assessing complex operations other than isolated sAVR

Adams et al. [42] Transcatheter Aortic-Valve Replacement with a Self-Expanding Prosthesis	2011–2012	795/871	394 TAVI (83.2 yo) 401 sAVR (83.5 yo)	**KCCQ** **SF-12**	1–12 months	– QoL was non-inferior with TAVI	More patients declined surgery post randomisation
Reynolds et al. [40] Health-Related Quality of Life After Transcatheter or Surgical Aortic Valve Replacement in High-Risk Patients With Severe Aortic Stenosis	2007–2009	628/699	446 Transfemoral (83.8 yo) 182 sAVR (82.6 yo)	**KCCQ** **EQ-5D** **SF-12**	1–6-12 months	– Improvement between baseline and 1 year after either TAVR or sAVR – TF was associated with a short-term advantage compared with surgery	– PATNER trial was not blinded – Very early experience with TA
Non-RANDOMIZED TRIALS TAVI							
Carroll et al. [44] STS-ACC TVT Registry of Transcatheter Aortic Valve Replacement	2011–2019	59,130/276316	High risk: 81 yo Intermediate risk: 80 yo Low risk: 75 yo	**KCCQ**	Baseline-1-12 months	– Patients stratified by surgical risk – Improvement in QoL at 30 days that was sustained over 1 year follow-up	– Retrospective registry – Attrition bias: analysis on results from only 20% of the cohort
Stańska et al. [37] Improvement of quality-of-life following transcatheter aortic valve implantation in the elderly: a multi-centre study based on the Polish national TAVI registry	POL-TAVI registry 2017	184	Transfemoral: 167 Transapical: 17 84 yo	**EQ-5D-3L**	Baseline-1 m	– QoL increased in one-month follow-up – TAVI procedure helps to improve QoL – Adequate for octogenarians and nonagenarians	– Multi-centre – Short/early results – No mortality reported

(continued)

Table 6.2 (continued)

Study	Period	Patients (included/total)	Procedures & mean age	Questionnaire	Follow-up	Conclusions	Limitations/critics
Lauck et al. [45] Very Early Changes in Quality of Life After Transcatheter Aortic Valve Replacement: Results From the 3 M TAVR Trial	2015–2017	358/411	Transfemoral 84 yo	**KCCQ** **SF-12**	2 weeks-1-12 months	– Disease-specific and generic health status improved substantially within the first 2 weeks. – Only minimal further improvement thereafter	
Zelis et al. [39] Survival and quality of life after transcatheter aortic valve implantation relative to the general population	2013–2017	5498	Transfemoral Transapical Transaortic Divided in 3 groups ages: >80, 80–65, <65	**SF-36 (isolated questions)**	Baseline-12 months	– >80 y have similar survival and QoL compared to general population – <80 y worse survival and QoL compared to the general population	– QoL analysis was not based on full questionnaires but isolated questions
Tokarek et al. [46] Assessment of Quality of Life in Patients After Surgical and Transcatheter Aortic Valve Replacement	2011–2013	173	TAVI: 39 (80 yo) sAVR: 134 (69.5 yo) (surgical includes mini thoracotomy, mini sternotomy, and sternotomy)	**MLHFQ** **EQ-5D-3L** – Mobility – Self-care – Usual activities – Pain/ discomfort – Anxiety/ depression	Perioperative 12 month 24 month	– QoL is maintained up to 12 months post-TAVI and sAVR but only improves at 2 year after sAVR – TAVI adequate in population with limited life expectancy	– Mental status not assessed – No mortality reported – Significant mean age difference between groups
Murray et al. [33] Life beyond 5 Years after TAVI: Patients' Perceived Health Status and Long-Term Outcome after Transcatheter Aortic Valve Implantation	2006–2012	103 alive at 5 year (452 TAVIs in that period)	Transfemoral: 68 Transapical: 35 80.1 ± 7.9 yo	**EQ-5D-5L**	5 years	– In H mortality: 9.2% – PPM: 12.6% – 64.7% were in NYHA III/IV, compared to 67.0% prior to TAVI – 22.8% were alive at a median FU of 7 year	– No baseline analysis – No improvement in NYHA class – High mortality – Attrition bias (77% drop off)

Lange et al. [34] Quality of Life After Transcatheter Aortic Valve Replacement: Prospective Data from GARY (German Aortic Valve Registry)	2011	2288/3875	Transcatheter: 1626 (81.1 yo) Transapical: 662 (80.3 yo)	**EQ-5D-5L**	Baseline-12 months	– Improvements in QoL, (mobility and usual activities) – Higher in the transcatheter TAVI as compared to the transapical TAVI group	– Prospective observational study – Attrition bias (30% drop off)
Kala et al. [47] Quality of life after transcatheter aortic valve implantation and surgical replacement in high-risk elderly patients	June 2009–Dec 2010	45	Transfemoral: 15 Transapical: 15 sAVR: 15	**EQ-5D-3L**	1–2–3–12 months	– Improved NYHA and general health in TAVI and positive trend in sAVR	– Small cohort – sAVR have a better baseline QoL
Gonçalves et al. [35] Quality of life improvement at midterm follow-up after transcatheter aortic valve implantation	April 2009–April 2010	74/74	Transfemoral:49 Transapical: 25 81.6 ± 8 yo	**MLHFQ**	6.5 months	– Improved NYHA and MLHFQ – Less improvement in QoL if PVD	– Small cohort. – 30 days mortality 9.5% – 6.5 month mortality: 20% – Attrition bias (28% drop off)
Krane et al. [36] Quality of life among patients undergoing transcatheter aortic valve implantation	Nov 2007 Dec 2008	99/164	Transfemoral:73 Transapical: 26 82 yo (57–94)	**SF-36**	3 months	– Improved physical function, bodily pain, general health, vitality – No changes in mental health – Worse role & emotional dimensions	– 30 days mortality 10.1% – Small cohort – Attrition bias (40% drop off)

MLHFQ: Minnesota Living with Heart Failure Questionnaire; **SF-12**: Short Form 12 Health Survey Questionnaire; **SF-36**: Short Form 36 Health Survey Questionnaire; **EQ-5D-3L**: EuroQol 3L questionnaire; **EQ-5D-5L**: EuroQol 5L questionnaire; **KCCQ**: Kansas City Cardiomyopathy Questionnaire

vibrant quality that was associated with the vigour of youth' [29]. In this sense, recent studies [30] not only focus on clinical outcomes but also on health status pre- and post-procedure in order to clarify indications, decision-making process and to judge outcomes (Fig. 6.2).

Our analysis has shown that TAVI, when performed via the transfemoral access, has a short-term advantage over surgery in improving QoL within the first month following the procedure. However, there is no difference in QoL for patients treated with either TAVI or sAVR after the first year following the procedure. Even though improvements in QoL are sustained in sAVR treated patients up to 10 years [15], this remains largely unknown for TAVI patients beyond 2 years, with only two studies reporting QoL results at 5 years; one with an attrition bias of 77% [31] and another, with higher incidences of paravalvular leaks, valve related reinterventions and rehospitalizations in the TAVI cohort [32].

Most of the studies reviewed have not stratified their patients by age groups. The questionnaires were not age-weighted, which makes it difficult to quantify and compare answers not only between studies but also between age groups in each study. This is an important factor if the published results are to be extrapolated and used to expand TAVI into younger age groups, using the recently published results on intermediate- and low-risk patients.

TAVI Registries Reporting on QoL

The majority of the studies contribute very limited data on long-term complication rates and hospital readmissions following TAVI. Most studies are reporting outcomes on the procedure survivors,

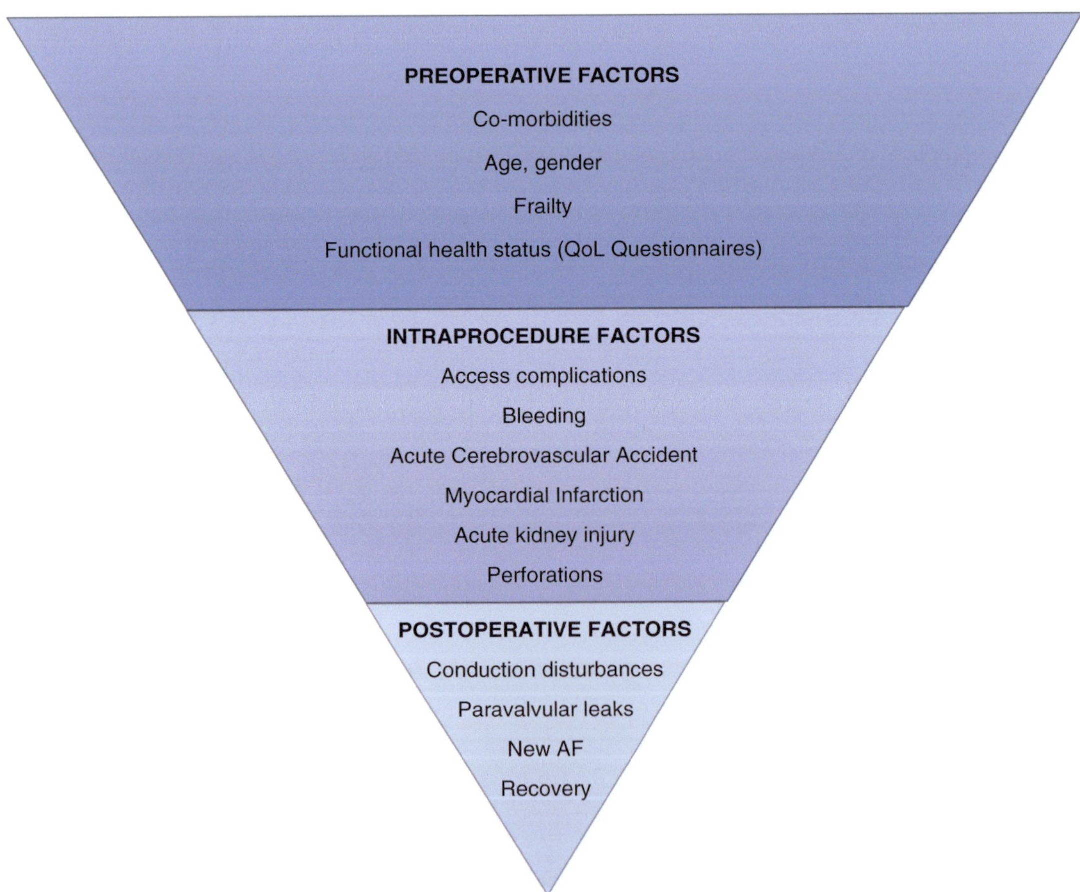

Fig. 6.2 Predictors of poor quality of life in TAVI population

with a large number of studies having well over 20% attrition rate, adding a significant bias in their QoL analysis. As an example, the study from Murray et al. [33] published QoL data from a cohort of 452 TAVI patients with a very high attrition rate (only 22.7% of patients alive at 5-years). With such an attrition rate it is rather difficult to derive any meaningful long-term QoL conclusions from this study, especially given the fact that there was no baseline assessment of the 22.7% of patients analysed and reported upon. In the large study from the GARY registry, transfemoral TAVI was associated with more pronounced improvement of QoL when compared to transapical TAVI. However, there is a considerable selection bias in this comparison [34] and the transapical as an approach in performing TAVIs has largely fallen off favour in the current years.

The studies by Gonçalves [35] et al. and Krane [36] et al. showed an improvement of QoL in early follow-up but they both had a very high reported mortality at follow-up. Stanska et al. [37] showed improvement in QoL at the early post procedural period (1 month) and concluded based on this that TAVI is an adequate treatment for octogenarians and nonagenarians.

TAVI has clearly proven useful in patients at their ninth and tenth decade of life, where sAVR is associated with higher mortality and morbidity. While younger patients have particular expectations including lower tolerance of complications and hospital stay, elderly people often express their preference for quality of life over quantity, and therefore the consequences of health status after TAVI procedure could be even more important than survival in this age group [38]. In this sense, Krane et al. highlight the importance of an improvement in QoL after TAVI, especially with regards to patients' satisfaction and procedure-related perception [36].

TAVI vs. General Population

In the study by Zelis et al. an age and gender subgroup was propensity matched to a similar cohort of people from the general population. Their survival and QoL were compared. They concluded that TAVI patients aged 80 or older have a similar long-term survival and a comparable QoL as the age-matched general population cohort. However, patients under 80 had a worse survival and QoL when compared to the general population [39]. This could imply a worsening QoL with time, reflecting possible issues with valve durability, other associated diseases or even medically induced, post-TAVI related problems like paravalvular leaks, pacemaker, and prosthetic valve endocarditis.

TAVI vs. sAVR Short and Intermediate Term Outcomes – Results from Randomised Controlled Trials (Industry Supported Studies)

Reynolds et al. [40] studied the PARTNER-1 trial population and described a health status improvement between baseline and 1-year after either TAVI or sAVR, in high-risk patients with severe AS. The benefit in early QoL improvement was only seen in the transfemoral access.

PARTNER-2 trial reported a significant improvement of the health status on intermediate risk patients [12] for both TAVI and sAVR, at 2-years [41] and 5-years [32] follow up. An early (30 days) health status improvement of borderline significance was observed with TAVI, amongst patients treated via transfemoral access [41]. QoL after TAVI however, was compared to QoL from mixed population of patients, all under the umbrella of sAVR, 10% of which had extensive cardiac procedures (sAVR with mostly concomitant CABG but also concomitant root replacement, root enlargement, and mitral valve procedures). At 5 years there was no difference in QoL between TAVI and sAVR despite more reinterventions, rehospitalizations, and paravalvular leaks in the TAVI cohort.

In the PARTNER-3 trial by Mack et al. [13], patients who underwent TAVI had more rapid improvements in the NYHA class, 6-min walk-test distance, and KCCQ score than those who underwent surgery. However, at 1 year, the differences vanished for both NYHA class and KCCQ scores and the analysis was performed accepting the fact that more patients in the surgery group than in the TAVI group withdrew from the trial and that there were missing data from the KCCQ.

Similar non-inferiority QoL improvement was reported by Adams et al., at 1 year after TAVI when compared to sAVR [42] with a large number of patients having declined surgery post randomisations.

With this review we have exposed the need for further, better-structured research into the field of QoL after TAVI, with bigger cohorts and longer follow-ups. Further research might need to also evaluate the influence that procedure-related complications (stroke, need for permanent pacemaker, vascular complications, residual paravalvular aortic regurgitation or mismatch and prosthesis durability) have upon QoL for patients who have TAVI as treatment of their underlying aortic valve disease.

Delivering treatment to patients with severe aortic stenosis irrespective of durability or QoL but primarily based on general service capacity, speed, and pressure in treating life threatening conditions like severe AS [37] when the health system is under stress can be an option, as we are currently experiencing with the COVID-19 pandemic. There is an ongoing debate whether TAVI should be offered for patients who in normal, non-pandemic setting would have undergone sAVR, in order to release resources and help hospitals allocate help where needed. TAVI patients have normally shorter procedural times, limited use of intensive care beds at a period of crisis and shorter hospital stay when resources are limited [13, 43]. This can lead to improve patient satisfaction and early resolution of symptoms but unspecified and uncharted long-term consequences for the patients and the health service alike.

Conclusions

Quality of life plays a crucial role in the decision-making process for health-related procedures like TAVI and sAVR. TAVI can offer a faster improvement in QoL when compared to sAVR but there is no difference to the QoL at intermediate 2 and 5-year follow-up. Further research is required using standardise tools to further evaluate QoL and durability of TAVI procedures in younger populations, providing this is ethically acceptable, given the excellent and long-term outcomes currently available and supporting sAVR (Fig. 6.3).

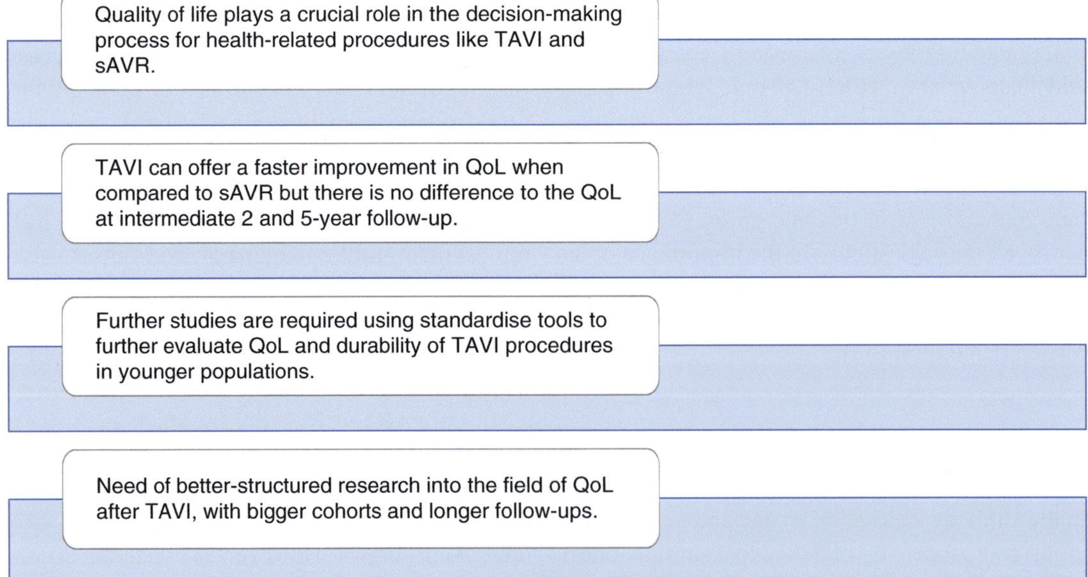

Fig. 6.3 Highlighted conclusions

References

1. Bhatia N, et al. Aortic valve disease in the older adult. J Geriatr Cardiol. 2016;13(12):941–4.
2. Carabello BA, Paulus WJ. Aortic stenosis. Lancet. 2009;373(9667):956–66.
3. Vahanian A, et al. Guidelines on the management of valvular heart disease: The Task Force on the Management of Valvular Heart Disease of the European Society of Cardiology. Eur Heart J. 2007;28(2):230–68.
4. O'Brien SM, et al. The Society of Thoracic Surgeons 2008 cardiac surgery risk models: part 2--isolated valve surgery. Ann Thorac Surg. 2009;88(1 Suppl):S23–42.
5. Fatima B, et al. Durability Data for Bioprosthetic Surgical Aortic Valve: A Systematic Review. JAMA Cardiol. 2019;4(1):71–80.
6. NATIONAL ADULT CARDIAC SURGERY AUDIT (NACSA). 2020. Available from: https://www.nicor.org.uk/wp-content/uploads/2020/12/National-Adult-Cardiac-Surgery-Audit-NACSA-FINAL.pdf.
7. Alexander KP, et al. Outcomes of cardiac surgery in patients > or = 80 years: results from the National Cardiovascular Network. J Am Coll Cardiol. 2000;35(3):731–8.
8. Bouma BJ, et al. To operate or not on elderly patients with aortic stenosis: the decision and its consequences. Heart. 1999;82(2):143–8.
9. Cribier A, et al. Percutaneous transcatheter implantation of an aortic valve prosthesis for calcific aortic stenosis: first human case description. Circulation. 2002;106(24):3006–8.
10. Leon MB, et al. Transcatheter aortic-valve implantation for aortic stenosis in patients who cannot undergo surgery. N Engl J Med. 2010;363(17):1597–607.
11. Otto CM, et al. 2020 ACC/AHA Guideline for the Management of Patients With Valvular Heart Disease: Executive Summary: A Report of the American College of Cardiology/American Heart Association Joint Committee on Clinical Practice Guidelines. Circulation. 2021;143(5):e35–71.
12. Leon MB, et al. Transcatheter or Surgical Aortic-Valve Replacement in Intermediate-Risk Patients. N Engl J Med. 2016;374(17):1609–20.
13. Mack MJ, et al. Transcatheter Aortic-Valve Replacement with a Balloon-Expandable Valve in Low-Risk Patients. N Engl J Med. 2019;380(18):1695–705.
14. Brennan JM, et al. Long-term survival after aortic valve replacement among high-risk elderly patients in the United States: insights from the Society of Thoracic Surgeons Adult Cardiac Surgery Database, 1991 to 2007. Circulation. 2012;126(13):1621–9.
15. Petersen J, et al. Long-Term Outcome and Quality of Life After Biological Aortic Valve Replacement in Nonelderly Adults. Ann Thorac Surg. 2021;111(1):142–9.
16. Gaede L, et al. Transvascular transcatheter aortic valve implantation in 2017. Clin Res Cardiol. 2020;109(3):303–14.
17. Hamm CW, Beyersdorf F. GARY-The Largest Registry of Aortic Stenosis Treatment Worldwide. Eur Heart J. 2020;41(6):733–5.
18. Popma JJ, et al. Transcatheter Aortic-Valve Replacement with a Self-Expanding Valve in Low-Risk Patients. N Engl J Med. 2019;380(18):1706–15.
19. Miceli A, et al. Minimally invasive aortic valve replacement with a sutureless valve through a right anterior mini-thoracotomy versus transcatheter aortic valve implantation in high-risk patients. Eur J Cardiothorac Surg. 2016;49(3):960–5.
20. Benetti FJ, et al. Minimally invasive aortic valve replacement. J Thorac Cardiovasc Surg. 1997;113(4):806–7.
21. Gundry SR, et al. Facile minimally invasive cardiac surgery via ministernotomy. Ann Thorac Surg. 1998;65(4):1100–4.
22. Deutsch MA, et al. Beyond adding years to life: health-related quality-of-life and functional outcomes in patients with severe aortic valve stenosis at high surgical risk undergoing transcatheter aortic valve replacement. Curr Cardiol Rev. 2013;9(4):281–94.
23. Supino PG, et al. Acceptability and psychometric properties of the Minnesota Living With Heart Failure Questionnaire among patients undergoing heart valve surgery: validation and comparison with SF-36. J Card Fail. 2009;15(3):267–77.
24. Bilbao A, et al. The Minnesota living with heart failure questionnaire: comparison of different factor structures. Health Qual Life Outcomes. 2016;14:23.
25. Beaton DE, Hogg-Johnson S, Bombardier C. Evaluating changes in health status: reliability and responsiveness of five generic health status measures in workers with musculoskeletal disorders. J Clin Epidemiol. 1997;50(1):79–93.
26. Green CP, et al. Development and evaluation of the Kansas City Cardiomyopathy Questionnaire: a new health status measure for heart failure. J Am Coll Cardiol. 2000;35(5):1245–55.
27. Watt M, et al. Cost-effectiveness of transcatheter aortic valve replacement in patients ineligible for conventional aortic valve replacement. Heart. 2012;98(5):370–6.
28. Avanzas P, et al. Long-term Follow-up of Patients With Severe Aortic Stenosis Treated With a Self-expanding Prosthesis. Rev Esp Cardiol (Engl Ed). 2017;70(4):247–53.
29. Elkinton JR. Medicine and the quality of life. Ann Intern Med. 1966;64(3):711–4.
30. O'Sullivan CJ, Wenaweser P. Can We Predict Quality of Life and Survival After Transcatheter Aortic Valve Replacement? Circ Cardiovasc Interv. 2015;8(12):e003347.
31. Huynh K. Interventional cardiology: 6-year follow-up of TAVI patients. Nat Rev Cardiol. 2015;12(4):195.

32. Makkar RR, et al. Five-Year Outcomes of Transcatheter or Surgical Aortic-Valve Replacement. N Engl J Med. 2020;382(9):799–809.
33. Murray MK, et al. Life beyond 5 Years after TAVI: Patients' Perceived Health Status and Long-Term Outcome after Transcatheter Aortic Valve Implantation. J Interv Cardiol. 2019;2019:4292987.
34. Lange R, et al. Quality of Life After Transcatheter Aortic Valve Replacement: Prospective Data From GARY (German Aortic Valve Registry). JACC Cardiovasc Interv. 2016;9(24):2541–54.
35. Goncalves A, et al. Quality of life improvement at midterm follow-up after transcatheter aortic valve implantation. Int J Cardiol. 2013;162(2):117–22.
36. Krane M, et al. Quality of life among patients undergoing transcatheter aortic valve implantation. Am Heart J. 2010;160(3):451–7.
37. Stanska A, et al. Improvement of quality of life following transcatheter aortic valve implantation in the elderly: a multi-centre study based on the Polish national TAVI registry. Kardiol Pol. 2017;75(1):13–20.
38. Bowling A, Ebrahim S. Measuring patients' preferences for treatment and perceptions of risk. Qual Health Care. 2001;10(Suppl 1):i2–8.
39. Zelis JM, et al. Survival and quality of life after transcatheter aortic valve implantation relative to the general population. Int J Cardiol Heart Vasc. 2020;28:100536.
40. Reynolds MR, et al. Health-related quality of life after transcatheter or surgical aortic valve replacement in high-risk patients with severe aortic stenosis: results from the PARTNER (Placement of AoRTic TraNscathetER Valve) Trial (Cohort A). J Am Coll Cardiol. 2012;60(6):548–58.
41. Baron SJ, et al. Health Status Benefits of Transcatheter vs Surgical Aortic Valve Replacement in Patients With Severe Aortic Stenosis at Intermediate Surgical Risk: Results From the PARTNER 2 Randomized Clinical Trial. JAMA Cardiol. 2017;2(8):837–45.
42. Adams DH, Popma JJ, Reardon MJ. Transcatheter aortic-valve replacement with a self-expanding prosthesis. N Engl J Med. 2014;371(10):967–8.
43. Sanchez C, e.a., Comparison of Year-Over-Year U.S. Hospital Costs Between Transcatheter Aortic Valve Replacement (TAVR) and Surgical Aortic Valve Replacement (SAVR). J Am Coll Cardiol. 2019;74:13.
44. Carroll JD, et al. STS-ACC TVT Registry of Transcatheter Aortic Valve Replacement. J Am Coll Cardiol. 2020;76(21):2492–516.
45. Lauck SB, et al. Very Early Changes in Quality of Life After Transcatheter Aortic Valve Replacement: Results From the 3M TAVR Trial. Cardiovasc Revasc Med. 2020;21(12):1573–8.
46. Tokarek T, et al. Assessment of quality of life in patients after surgical and transcatheter aortic valve replacement. Catheter Cardiovasc Interv. 2016;88(3):E80–8.
47. Kala P, et al. Quality of life after transcatheter aortic valve implantation and surgical replacement in high-risk elderly patients. Biomed Pap Med Fac Univ Palacky Olomouc Czech Repub. 2013;157(1):75–80.

7 Patient-Reported Quality of Life After Stand-Alone and Concomitant Arrhythmia Surgery: A Systematic Review and Meta-Analysis

Bart Maesen, Claudia A. J. van der Heijden, Elham Bidar, Rein Vos, Thanos Athanasiou, and Jos G. Maessen

Abbreviation

AF	Atrial fibrillation
AFEQT	AF Effect on QualiTy-of-life Questionnaire
AFSS	AF Symptom and Severity score
AV	Aortic valve
CABG	Coronary artery bypass graft
C-cap	Cardiff cardiac ablation prom
CCS-SAF	Canadian Cardiovascular Society Severity of AF
CFAE	Complex fractionated atrial Electrograms
CTI	Cavotricuspid isthmus
CVA	Cerebrovascular accident
EHRA	European Heart Rhythm Association
EQ-5D	Euroqol 5d
GP	Ganglionated plexi
Hrqol	Health related quality of life
LA	Left atrial
LAA	LA appendage
LM	Ligament of Marshall
MFI	Multidimensional fatigue inventory
MV	Mitral valve
Prom	Patient recorded outcome
PVI	Pulmonary vein isolation
QOL	Quality of life
RCT	Randomized controlled trial
RF	Radiofrequency
SCV	Superior caval vein
SE	Standard error
SF-12	Short Form 12

Bart Maesen and Claudia A. J. van der Heijden contributed equally with all other contributors.

B. Maesen (✉) · E. Bidar · J. G. Maessen
Department of Cardiothoracic Surgery, Maastricht University Medical Centre, Maastricht, The Netherlands

Cardiovascular Research Institute Maastricht, Maastricht, The Netherlands
e-mail: b.maesen@mumc.nl; elham.bidar@mumc.nl; j.g.maessen@mumc.nl

C. A. J. van der Heijden
Department of Cardiothoracic Surgery, Maastricht University Medical Centre, Maastricht, The Netherlands
e-mail: claudia.vander.heijden@mumc.nl

R. Vos
Department of Methodology and Statistics, Maastricht University, Maastricht, The Netherlands
e-mail: rein.vos@maastrichtuniversity.nl

T. Athanasiou
Department of Cardiothoracic Surgery, Imperial College London, St Mary's Hospital, London, UK
e-mail: t.athanasiou@imperial.ac.uk

T. Athanasiou et al. (eds.), *Patient Reported Outcomes and Quality of Life in Cardiovascular Interventions*,
https://doi.org/10.1007/978-3-031-09815-4_7

SF-36	Short Form 36	TV	Tricuspid valve
SMD	Standardized mean difference	Vas-score	Visual analogue scale
SR	Sinus rhythm	VATS	Visual assisted thoracoscopic surgery
SSQ	Symptom and Severity Questionnaire		

Highlighted Conclusions

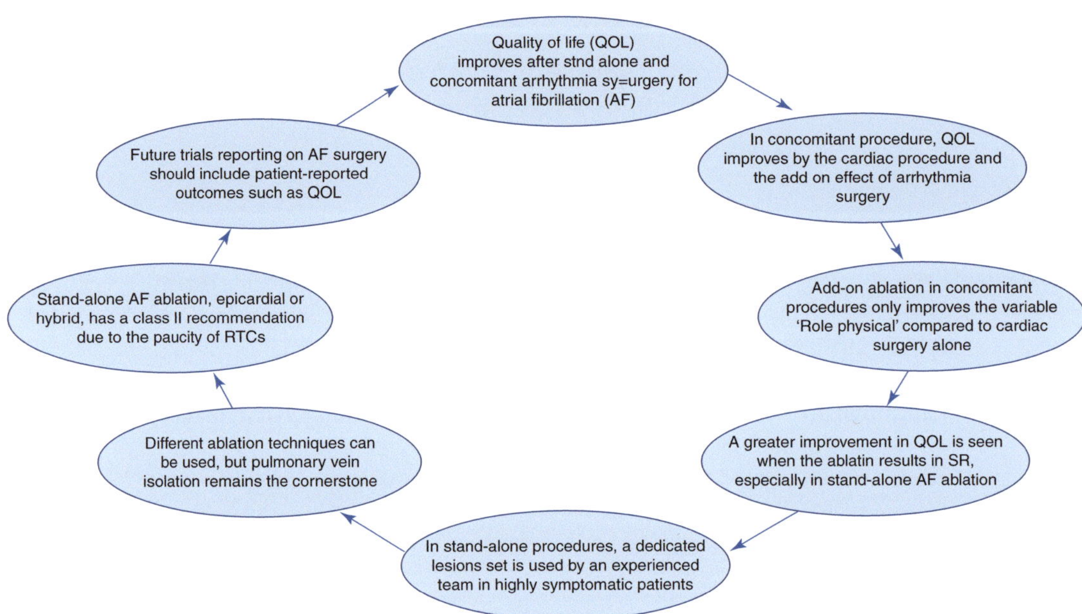

Introduction

Historically, the emergence of a surgical treatment for heart rhythm disorders was mainly triggered by ventricular arrhythmias and with the first successful surgical interruption of the bundle of Kent in a patient with the Wolff-Parkinson-White syndrome [1], arrhythmia surgery got off to a great start. Notwithstanding the above, today most surgical arrhythmia procedures are focussed on the management of supraventricular arrhythmias [2]. Surgical ablation of atrial fibrillation (AF) can be either done in conjunction with other cardiac procedures as a concomitant procedure or on itself as a standalone procedure. Concomitant AF surgery is often performed with cardiopulmonary bypass via sternotomy or right anterolateral mini-thoracotomy, but recently also left thoracoscopic ablation in combination with minimal invasive direct coronary artery bypassing on the beating heart has been reported [3, 4]. Although standalone procedures are often performed via bilateral thoracoscopy, unilateral thoracoscopic and subxiphoid techniques have been successfully introduced [5–7]. This progression in minimally invasiveness of surgical ablation approaches is important as it can be expected that the reduction in complications and postoperative pain by limiting surgery to one side will lead to further improvement in QOL.

Although one-year success of arrhythmia surgery for AF has long been defined as freedom from any supraventricular tachyarrhythmia, the evaluation of other endpoints, such as patient-reported quality of life (QOL), have become increasingly important in recent years [8]. Despite the fact that the measurement of QOL is potentially limited by a treatment expectancy bias, it represents an important endpoint for ablation studies [9]. Be that as it may, studies specifically evaluating the effect of standalone or add-on arrhythmia surgery on QOL are scarce. Moreover, the reported outcomes are often heterogeneous as not all studies use the same ablation strategy to treat the arrhythmia.

In this systematic review and meta-analysis, we summarized current evidence on QOL at baseline and one year after both stand-alone and concomitant arrhythmia surgery for AF. Since the guidelines for AF define success of rhythm outcome after surgical ablation for AF after one year, we chose to evaluate the improvement in QOL as well after one year, along with the rhythm outcome.

Patients and Methods

Literature Search

This systematic review and meta-analysis was written according to PRISMA standards [10]. A systematic literature search was conducted with free terms in the PubMed and Cochrane databases. Forwards and backwards search were also performed to screen for further eligible papers.

PubMed

((((((((((((((((((((patient recorded outcome measures) OR prom) OR patient recorded outcomes) OR QoL) OR quality of life) OR SF-36) OR short form 36) OR hrqol) OR health related quality of life) OR EQ5D) OR EQ-5D) OR euroqol 5d) OR c-cap questionnaire) OR cardiff cardiac ablation prom) OR vas-score) OR visual analogue scale) OR MFI-20 questionnaire) OR multidimensional fatigue inventory) OR afeqt) OR atrial fibrillation effect on quality of life) AND ((((((((((((((((((Arrhythmia surgery) OR arrhythmia ablation) OR Surgical ablation) OR Thoracoscopic ablation) OR Totally thoracoscopic maze) OR TT maze) OR Cox maze) OR Maze procedure) OR mini maze) OR Minimally invasive surgical ablation) OR VATS) OR VATS ablation) OR video assisted thoracoscopic surgery) OR Hybrid ablation) OR Hybrid procedure) OR Hybrid approach) OR Epicardial-endocardial procedure) OR Epicardial-endocardial ablation) OR Epicardial-endocardial approach)) AND ((((((atrial fibrillation) OR paroxysmal) OR persistent) OR longstanding-persistent). Date search: 06/07/2021.

Cochrane

((((((((((patient recorded outcome measures) OR prom) OR patient recorded outcomes) OR QoL) OR quality of life) OR SF-36) OR short form 36) OR hrqol) OR health related quality of life) AND ((((((((((((((((((Arrhythmia surgery) OR arrhythmia ablation) OR Surgical ablation) OR Thoracoscopic ablation) OR Totally thoracoscopic maze) OR TT maze) OR Cox maze) OR Maze procedure) OR mini maze) OR Minimally invasive surgical ablation) OR VATS) OR VATS ablation) OR video assisted thoracoscopic surgery) OR Hybrid ablation) OR Hybrid procedure) OR Hybrid approach) OR Epicardial endocardial procedure) OR Epicardial-endocardial ablation) OR Epicardial-endocardial approach)) AND ((((((atrial fibrillation) OR paroxysmal) OR persistent) OR longstanding-persistent). Date search:07/07/2021.

Study Selection and Risk of Bias

All identified studies were screened based on their title and abstract, and full text when necessary, by two independent reviewers (C.H. and B.M.). All English articles reporting on QOL using any validated questionnaire for evaluating QOL after arrhythmia surgery in patients with AF, both stand-alone and concomitant, were found eligible. In all observational studies and non-randomized clinical trials, the methodological quality was assessed with use of the ROBINS-I tool [11]. In articles reporting on randomized controlled trials (RCTs), the risk of bias was assessed using the Cochrane Checklist [12].

Endpoints

The primary endpoint was defined as the standardized mean difference (SMD) in QOL variables assessed one year after arrhythmia surgery compared to baseline scores, using the Short-Form 36 (SF-36) QOL questionnaire. As secondary endpoints, differences in the improvement of QOL between patients who were in sinus rhythm (SR) or in AF after 12 months of follow-up were determined for standalone procedures and differences between patients who did and did not receive add-on ablation for concomitant procedures. Furthermore, other QOL questionnaires that address different aspects of QOL, such as disease specific tools for AF, were evaluated as well.

Statistical Analysis

The metric 'standardized mean difference (μ)' (rho = 0) was used to analyse continuous QOL changes, comparing one year outcomes with baseline scores, per variable of the SF-36 QOL questionnaire [13]. Additional meta-regression was performed using rhythm outcome and add-on arrhythmia surgery after 12 months of follow up as covariate. All statistical values were computed with a 95% confidence interval in a random-effects model and the two-tailed *P*-value threshold for statistical significance was set at 0.05.

Weighted means (μ) of continuous baseline characteristics were computed using the metric 'TX Mean', whereas 'Untransformed Proportions', defined as the count of successes in the sample divided by the size of that sample, were used for mean frequencies [14]. The latter metric was also used to analyse the percentage of patients that was in SR after 12 months of follow-up. Due to the relatively low complication rate, the metric 'Freeman–Tukey Double Arcsine Proportion' was used to analyse the incidence of peri-operative complications following arrhythmia surgery.

Inter-study heterogeneity was tested and visualized in forest plots per variable of the SF-36 QOL questionnaire. A statistical P value <0.10 and/or $I^2 > 50\%$ was used as cut-off point for significant heterogeneity. All statistical analyses were performed using Meta-Analyst for Mac software (2009) [14] (version Beta 1.0). Furthermore, publication bias was tested using funnel plots made in Excel, where the SMD was plotted against the standard error (SE) of that study. The variance was calculated after transforming Cohen's d to Hedges' g by correcting for sample size and standard deviation per study [15].

Results

Study Selection

After exclusion based on title, abstract and full text reading, 12 out of 2.482 studies from the literature search in PubMed were included in our systematic review. The Cochrane database did not identify any additional studies for the analysis, since the only 4 eligible studies had already been found in the PubMed database [16–19]. Reasons for exclusion were overlapping patient populations, studies who presented their data other than mean ± standard deviation or descriptive studies [4, 20–38]. No studies could be supplemented by manually screening the reference and cited lists of included studies. Of the 12 included articles, only 9 were included in our meta-analysis due to reporting on the QOL using at least the SF-36 questionnaire [16–19, 39–43]. The other 3 studies reported on different tools for measuring QOL, such as AFSS, EuroQol, Short-Form 12, MFI, CCS-SAF, SSQ or AFEQT [44–46] (Fig. 7.1a, b, Table 7.1).

Risk of Bias

The risk of bias in most of the RCT's was estimated to be medium to low, mostly due to unclear reporting of blinding of patients and/or researchers during follow-up [16, 17, 44]. For the observational studies and nonrandomized trials, risk of bias was estimated to be medium high. Confounding due to missing baseline characteristics or marked differences in important predictors

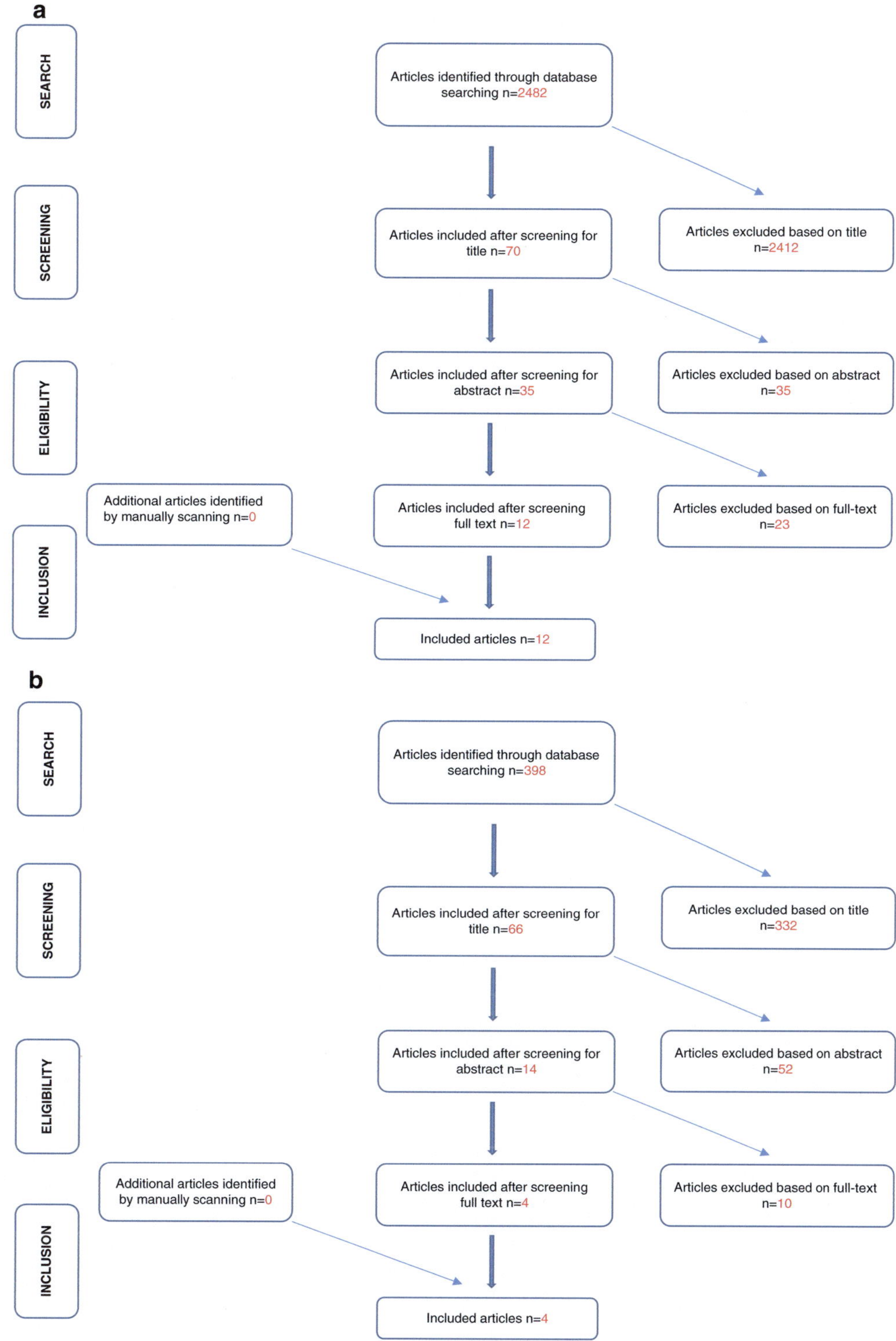

Fig. 7.1 Study flow diagram. (**a**): PubMed search. (**b**): Cochrane search

Table 7.1 Overview of included studies in this systematic review

Study	Year	Title	Country	Score system quality of life
Al-Jazairi et al.	2019	Hybrid atrial fibrillation ablation in patients with persistent atrial fibrillation or failed catheter ablation	The Netherlands	SF-36, Toronto AFSS, EHRA
Bagge et al.	2009	Epicardial off-pump pulmonary vein isolation and vagal denervation improve long-term outcome and quality of life in patients with atrial fibrillation	Sweden	SF-36, SSQ
Buist et al.	2019	Quality of life after catheter and minimally invasive surgical ablation of paroxysmal and early persistent atrial fibrillation: results from the SCALAF trial	The Netherlands	SF-36, EHRA
Driessen et al.	2017	Quality of life improves after thoracoscopic surgical ablation of advanced atrial fibrillation: Results of the Atrial Fibrillation Ablation and Autonomic Modulation via Thoracoscopic Surgery (AFACT) study	The Netherlands	SF-36
Gehi et al.	2013	Hybrid epicardial-endocardial ablation using a pericardioscopic technique for the treatment of atrial fibrillation	United States of America	CCS-SAF
Gillinov et al.	2015	Surgical ablation of atrial fibrillation during mitral-valve surgery	United States of America	AFSS, SF-12
Joshibayev et al.	2016	Early and long-term outcomes and quality of life after concomitant mitral valve surgery. Left atrial size reduction. and radiofrequency surgical ablation of atrial fibrillation	Kazakhstan	SF-36
Lonnerholm et al.	2000	Effects of the maze operation on health-related quality of life in patients with atrial fibrillation	Sweden	SF-36
Lundberg et al.	2008	Long-term health-related quality of life after maze surgery for atrial fibrillation	Sweden	SF-36
Osmancik et al.	2019	Improvement in the quality of life of patients with persistent or long-standing persistent atrial fibrillation after hybrid ablation	Czech-Republic	AFEQT, EuroQol
van Breugel et al.	2010	A prospective randomized multicentre comparison on health-related quality of life: the value of add-on arrhythmia surgery in patients with paroxysmal, permanent or persistent atrial fibrillation undergoing valvular and/or coronary bypass surgery	The Netherlands	SF-36, EuroQol, MFI
von Oppell et al.	2009	Mitral valve surgery plus concomitant atrial fibrillation ablation is superior to mitral valve surgery alone with an intensive rhythm control strategy	United Kingdom	SF-36

SF-36: Short Form 36; AFSS: Atrial Fibrillation Symptom and Severity score; EHRA: European Heart Rhythm Association; SSQ: Symptom and Severity Questionnaire; CCS-SAF; Canadian Cardiovascular Society (CCS) Severity of Atrial Fibrillation; SF-12: Short Form 12; AFEQT: Atrial Fibrillation Effect on QualiTy-of-Life; MFI; Multidimensional Fatigue Index

of the procedure's success (e.g. type and duration of AF) between groups could not be ruled out in the studies by Joshibayev et al. [41] and Lundberg et al. [43]. Selection bias based on the inclusion of patients with serious comorbidities was present in the studies of Gehi et al. [45] and Joshibayev et al. [41]. Other factors contributing to the increased risk of bias were missing QOL data due to substantial loss of follow-up in the study by Bagge et al. [40] and Gehi et al. [45], and the lack of continuous heart rhythm monitoring in the studies by Joshibayev et al. [41] and Lonnerholm et al. [42].

Furthermore, funnel plots where the SMD was plotted against the SE of Hedges'g of that study showed that publication bias cannot be ruled out in this review. Due to marked variance of the included studies, scattering of results unequally along the x-axis occurred. Moreover, the forest plots illustrated that statistical heterogeneity, and thus inter-study variance, per QOL variable measured by the SF-36 was marked.

Table 7.2 Baseline characteristics of studies reporting on cardiac arrhythmia surgery and quality of life using the Short-Form-36 questionnaire

Characteristics (n = 545)	Reported on number of patients: n (%)	Adjusted mean (95% CI)
Age (years)	453 (83)	59.8 years (56.5–63.0)
AF duration (months)	316 (58)	53.0 months (5.0–101.0)
CVA (%)	466 (86)	8.0% (5.6–10.5)
Female (%)	545 (100)	30.6% (23.6–37.6)
Hypertension (%)	491 (90)	32.7% (22.1–43.2)
LA diameter (mm)	369 (68)	49.2 mm (43.8–54.6)
LVEF (%)	395 (72)	52.3% (50.0–54.5)
Type of AF		
Paroxysmal (%)	520 (95)	27.6% (12.5–42.8)
Persistent (%)	520 (95)	29.8% (11.8–47.9)
Longstanding-persistent (%)	520 (95)	41.9% (4.6–79.3)

Data are presented as number of patients (n) and the percentage (%) of the total group at baseline. The adjusted means or proportions followed by the 95% confidence interval were calculated using the metric 'TX Mean' or 'Untransformed Proportion' respectively in a binary random-effects model. AF: atrial fibrillation; CVA: cerebrovascular accident; LA: left atrial; LVEF: left ventricular ejection fraction

Study Population

Most studies reported on arrhythmia surgery performed in the Netherlands [16–18, 39], followed by Sweden [40, 42, 43], the United States of America [44, 45], Czech Republic [46], the United Kingdom [19] and Kazakhstan [41]. In total, 545 patients in 9 studies were included in the analysis as they reported on QOL using (at least) the SF-36 questionnaire (Table 7.2). Most patients were men (69.4%), mean age was 60 years, mean duration of AF was 53 months, 8.0% had a history with cerebrovascular accident (CVA) and the mean left atrial (LA) diameter was 49.2 mm. Most patients had longstanding-persistent AF (41.9%), followed by persistent (29.8%) and paroxysmal AF (27.6%).

Arrhythmia Surgery

The technique by which arrhythmia surgery was performed differed between the twelve studies (Table 7.3). In most of the studies, the LAA was addressed, either by surgically excision, clipping or stapling. Furthermore, there were three studies that reported on thoracoscopic beating-heart AF ablation [16, 17, 40]. Two studies reported on single-stage and 1 on staged hybrid ablation [39, 45, 46]. Of the remaining studies, five reported on concomitant AF ablation, in most of them a Cox-Maze-III or -IV procedure was performed, and one study used an alternative overlapping PVI technique. While different techniques were used, all studies performed PVI with or without extra lesions (Table 7.4). Five studies ablated the roof and inferior lines as well to create the so called 'box lesion', while van Breugel only added a roof line [18]. Four studies ablated the RA free wall, a line to the mitral annulus and 3 ablated the posterior LA wall.

Table 7.3 Surgical characteristics per study including type of cardiac surgery performed, left atrial appendage procedure, energy source, concomitant surgery

Study	Arrhythmia surgery			LAA	Energy source	Concomitant surgery
	Minimally invasive (off-pump)	Hybrid	Cox-Maze III/IV			
Al-Jazairi et al.	–	Single Stage	–	Occlusion (Atriclip 30%)	Bipolar RF	–
Bagge et al.	Thoracoscopic	–	–	Excised (stapler, 76%)	Bipolar RF	–
Buist et al.	Thoracoscopic	–	–	Ligation (endoloop, 100%)	Bipolar RF	–
Driessen et al.	Thoracoscopic	–	–	Excised (stapler, 100%)	Bipolar RF	–
Gehi et al.	–	Single Stage	–	–	Unipolar RF	–
Gillinov et al.	–	–	NS	Excised or excluded (100%)	Cryoenergy, uni- & bipolar RF	AV replacement $n = 14$ CABG $n = 21$ MV repair $n = 79$ MV replacement $n = 54$ Other $n = 16$
Joshibayev and Bolatbekov et al.	–	–	Cox-Maze IV	LA sealing (55%)	Unipolar RF	MV repair $n = 12$ MV replacement $n = 42$
Lonnerholm et al.	–	–	Cox-Maze III	100%	Cut and sew	Atrial septum defect closure $n = 1$ CABG $n = 3$ Septal myectomy $n = 1$ TV repair $n = 1$
Lundberg et al.	–	–	Cox-Maze III	100%	Cut and sew	CABG $n = 2$ Atrial septal defect closure $n = 1$ MV repair $n = 5$
Osmancik et al.	–	Staged, right sided	–	Occlusion (Atriclip, 64%)	Uni/Bipolar RF	–
van Breugel et al.	–	–	–	Resection (100%)	Bipolar RF	CABG $n = 18$ Valve replacement $n = 32$ CABG + valve replacement $n = 10$ Other $n = 5$
von Oppell et al.	–	–	Cox-Maze IV	Excised (100%)	Bipolar RF	AV replacement $n = 7$ CABG $n = 10$ MV repair $n = 8$ MV replacement $n = 16$ TV repair $n = 13$

AV: aortic valve; CABG: coronary artery bypass graft; LAA: left atrial appendage; MV: mitral valve; NS: non specified; RF: radiofrequency; TV: tricuspid valve.

Table 7.4 Lesion set per study

Study	Lesion set														
	PVI	Box	SCV to ICV	CS	TV	RA free wall	Mitral annulus	Posterior LA	CTI	CFAE	Bi-atrial maze	LA reduction	GP	LM	Roof line
Al-Jazairi et al.	X	X	X						X	X					
Bagge et al.	X												X	X	
Buist et al.	X														
Driessen et al.	X	X													
Gehi et al.	X							X							
Gillinov et al.	X ($n = 67$)										X ($n = 66$)				
Joshibayev and Bolatbekov et al.	X	X	X	X	X	X	X					X			
Lonnerholm et al.	X					X	X	X							
Lundberg et al.	X					X	X	X							
Osmancik et al.	X	X													
van Breugel et al.	X														X
von Oppell et al.	X	X	X	X	X	X	X								

CTI: cavotricuspid isthmus; CFAE: complex fractionated atrial electrograms; GP: ganglionated plexi; LA: left atrial; LM: Ligament of Marshall; PVI: pulmonary vein isolation; SCV: superior caval vein; TV: tricuspid valve

Three studies ablated the connection between the superior and inferior caval vein and two ablated the coronary sinus and the tricuspid valve. Six studies ablated either an additional cavotricuspid isthmus line, CFAE, ganglionated plexi or the ligament of Marshall, or performed a bi-atrial maze or LA reduction. These marked differences in techniques and lesion sets have led to marked clinical heterogeneity in this review and meta-analysis.

Primary Endpoint: QOL Following Stand-Alone Arrhythmia Surgery

Most studies (9 out of 12) reported on QOL using (at least) the SF-36 questionnaire, where SF-36 scores one year after arrhythmia surgery could be compared with baseline scores [16–19, 35, 39–41, 43]. Overall, QOL improved across all variables incorporated in the SF-36 tool (e.g. physical functioning, bodily pain, role physical, general health, role emotional, vitality, social functioning and mental health). Moreover, the incidence of perioperative complications was low for all studies (Tables 7.5 and 7.6).

Interestingly, studies with higher success percentages in terms of rhythm outcome (SR after one year) also showed greater QOL improvements across all variables. (Figs. 7.2 and 7.3). Moreover, meta-regression based on rhythm outcome in the two studies by Al-Jazairi et al. and Driessen et al., who divided outcomes into two groups based on rhythm outcome, showed that following cardiac surgery the QOL scores of both SR and AF patients improved. Moreover, patients who were in SR showed significantly greater improvements in QOL compared to baseline concerning physical functioning, physical role, general health and social functioning, than those who experienced recurrent AF [17, 39]. The other variables, including bodily pain, role emotional, vitality and mental health, also showed better outcomes for those in SR compared to those in AF, however non-significant (Table 7.7).

Primary Endpoint for Concomitant Procedures

Furthermore, 3 of the 9 included studies performed an extra analysis on comparing QOL outcomes of patients receiving cardiac surgery with and without add-on arrhythmia surgery for AF (add-on surgical AF ablation vs. control group) [18, 19, 41]. While van Breugel et al. and von Oppell et al. randomized their patients between the two groups, the study by Joshibayev and Bolatbekov et al. did not [18, 19, 41]. As such, their patients undergoing add-on arrhythmia surgery had a higher rate of longstanding-persistent AF ($p = 0.02$), greater LA size ($p = 0.004$), lower LVEF ($p = 0.03$) and a longer AF duration ($p = 0.05$) compared to the control group. Yet this study showed the most improvement in QOL across all variables. Von Oppell et al. showed an improvement in five out of eight variables in the add-on arrhythmia group compared to their control group, but van Breugel et al. only reported a significant improvement in the variable bodily pain compared to the control group. We performed a meta-regression of the 3 abovementioned studies to evaluate the overall effect of add-on ablation concomitant with cardiac surgery on the QOL. This analysis showed that adding arrhythmia surgery to cardiac surgery as a concomitant procedure overall only leads to a significant improvement in the variable 'Role physical' at one year after the procedure (Table 7.8).

Follow-up

Of the 505 patients who completed the follow-up and reported on QOL using the SF-36 questionnaire, 73.8% (62.5–85.0) was in SR after 12 months. The type of rhythm monitoring differed across studies; most studies used a 24-h Holter, followed by 72-h Holter, while only one study used continuous monitoring and two used a 12-leads ECG for arrhythmia detection (Table 7.9).

Table 7.5 Quality of life scores per Short-Form 36 variable per study at baseline and one year after cardiac arrhythmia surgery

	Physical functioning		Role physical		Bodily pain		General health		Role emotional		Vitality		Social functioning		Mental health	
Study	Baseline	1 year	Baseline	1 year	Baseline	1 year	Baseline	1 year	Baseline	1 year	Baseline	1 year	Baseline	1 year	Baseline	1 year
Al-Jazairi et al. SR	60 ± 27	84 ± 19	43 ± 46	81 ± 36	89 ± 20	91 ± 18	56 ± 20	69 ± 22	76 ± 35	93 ± 19	49 ± 22	72 ± 18	73 ± 25	92 ± 13	74 ± 16	85 ± 14
Al-Jazairi et al. AF	59 ± 23	75 ± 18	20 ± 37	45 ± 42	87 ± 19	86 ± 15	60 ± 20	61 ± 23	83 ± 30	80 ± 42	60 ± 22	64 ± 17	66 ± 26	81 ± 19	80 ± 13	82 ± 16
Bagge et al.	64 ± 27	82 ± 21	32 ± 38	58 ± 44	70 ± 31	74 ± 26	52 ± 21	64 ± 24	49 ± 44	74 ± 38	41 ± 23	59 ± 29	64 ± 27	82 ± 21	68 ± 22	79 ± 20
Buist et al.	64 ± 24	79 ± 17	46 ± 48	78 ± 32	68 ± 28	85 ± 22	51 ± 19	67 ± 13	71 ± 44	87 ± 32	44 ± 22	65 ± 11	64 ± 32	88 ± 19	75 ± 19	86 ± 11
Driessen et al. SR	68 ± 25	85 ± 18	37 ± 42	75 ± 37	81 ± 22	81 ± 23	63 ± 19	71 ± 20	75 ± 41	86 ± 30	51 ± 20	64 ± 19	69 ± 24	85 ± 20	73 ± 17	81 ± 16
Driessen et al. AF	62 ± 26	69 ± 25	39 ± 44	54 ± 42	83 ± 21	79 ± 23	57 ± 20	54 ± 20	66 ± 44	80 ± 35	45 ± 24	56 ± 21	63 ± 26	71 ± 23	70 ± 19	75 ± 17
Joshibayev and Bolatbekov et al.	20 ± 7	84 ± 22	38 ± 13	81 ± 17	29 ± 23	79 ± 5	39 ± 7	89 ± 21	41 ± 23	89 ± 22	44 ± 12	88 ± 31	39 ± 7	84 ± 21	39 ± 7	89 ± 29
Lonnerholm et al.	57 ± 26	91 ± 11	17 ± 34	85 ± 23	70 ± 30	83 ± 26	56 ± 16	84 ± 19	37 ± 43	87 ± 32	41 ± 19	81 ± 17	59 ± 24	92 ± 18	65 ± 18	86 ± 17
Lundberg et al.	61 ± 18	83 ± 17	30 ± 38	69 ± 41	74 ± 27	86 ± 22	56 ± 20	77 ± 17	42 ± 42	73 ± 41	39 ± 20	65 ± 24	64 ± 25	85 ± 20	66 ± 21	80 ± 17
van Breugel et al.	50 ± 24	68 ± 23	24 ± 35	53 ± 40	76 ± 25	78 ± 23	53 ± 20	56 ± 18	68 ± 43	72 ± 36	51 ± 22	61 ± 17	67 ± 25	80 ± 19	70 ± 20	78 ± 13
von Oppel et al.	42 ± 26	62 ± 32	14 ± 26	55 ± 47	66 ± 34	70 ± 28	58 ± 24	67 ± 25	51 ± 43	56 ± 8	32 ± 23	53 ± 27	56 ± 37	69 ± 34	71 ± 20	74 ± 23

Data are presented as mean ± standard deviation. SR: sinus rhythm; AF: atrial fibrillation.

Table 7.6 Peri-operative major and minor complications of all patients reporting on quality of life using the SF-36 questionnaire

Complications	Number of patients per complication (total patients n = 545)	Adjusted mean% (95% CI)
Bleeding: reoperation	*n* = 16	2.0% (0.9–3.2)
Bleeding: transfusion	*n* = 15	1.8% (0.5–3.0)
Conversion to sternotomy	*n* = 7	1.5% (0.2–3.5)
Haemodynamic instability/cardiac failure	*n* = 0	0.5% (−0.1–1.1)
Mortality <30 days	*n* = 8	1.7% (0.6–2.8)
Myocardial infarction	*n* = 7	0.8% (−0.1–1.6)
Pacemaker implantation	*n* = 14	2.0% (0.8–3.1)
Pericarditis	*n* = 6	1.3% (0.4–2.2)
Phrenic nerve palsy	*n* = 5	1.1% (0.2–2.0)
Pleural effusion	*n* = 11	1.8% (0.7–2.9)
Pneumonia	*n* = 7	1.6% (0.5–2.6)
Pneumothorax	*n* = 8	1.4% (0.4–2.4)
Renal failure	*n* = 0	0.5% (−0.1–1.1)
Respiratory failure (requiring intubation)	*n* = 0	0.5% (−0.1–1.1)
Stroke/TIA	*n* = 3	0.8% (0.0–1.6)
Tamponade	*n* = 1	0.7% (0.0–1.5)

Data are presented as the total number of patients of all cardiac arrhythmia surgery studies per complication, followed by the adjusted mean of proportion and the 95% CI in a binary random-effects model. Statistical test peri-operative complications: one-arm meta-regression 'Freeman-Tukey Double Arcsine Proportion'. CI: confidence interval; SR: sinus rhythm; TIA: transient ischemic attack

Secondary Endpoint: QOL Sub-Analyses Using Other Questionnaires

Of the 12 studies, 7 reported on QOL using questionnaires other than the SF-36, including both general health questionnaires as well as disease specific questionnaires. Gillinov et al. reported declined AF related symptom severity as well as symptom frequency scores one year after surgery using the AFSS questionnaire [44]. They also found that, by using the SF-12, mainly physical related improvements were seen, while mental scores remained rather the same. While Al-Jazairi et al. used both the Toronto AFSS and EHRA questionnaires [39], Bagge et al. used the EHRA and SSQ to investigate the improvement in AF related symptoms [40]. Both studies concluded that lower scores (meaning less AF symptoms) were seen one year after arrhythmia surgery, especially for those who were still in SR. Gehi used the CCS-SAF to investigate AF related symptoms and reported consistent outcomes, where those in SR had almost no AF specific symptoms anymore [45]. Van Breugel et al. measured different elements of fatigue incorporated in the MFI [18]. It turned out that fatigue related symptoms declined after 6 and 12 months compared to baseline. Osmancik et al. evaluated the effect of AF on QOL using the AFEQT questionnaire in patients with SR, pAF and persAF [46]. While all three groups showed an improvement in QOL after one year, scores from the SR group increased the most. Finally, Osmancik et al. and van Breugel et al. reported on the EuroQol [18, 46]. While the descriptive part decreased significantly for the SR group in the study by Osmancik et al., this was not the case in the study by van Breugel et al. The visual analogue scale however did improve in both studies, independently of rhythm outcome (Tables 7.10, 7.11, 7.12, 7.13, 7.14).

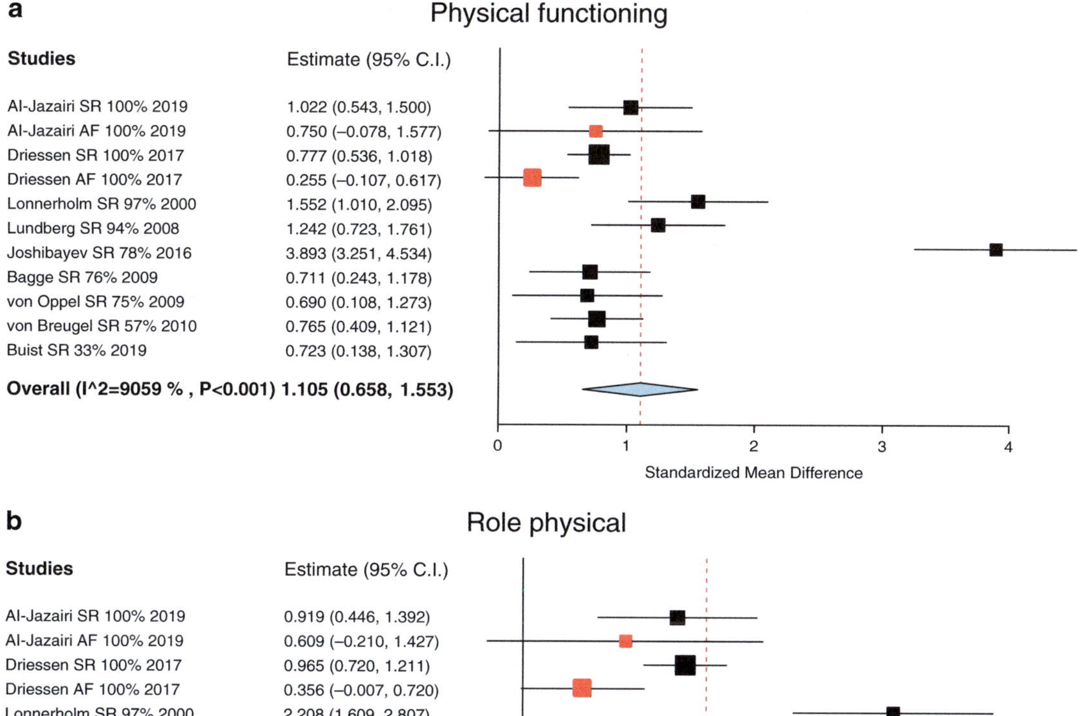

Fig. 7.2 Forest plots showing the changes per Short-Form 36 quality of life variable after 12 months' follow-up, expressed by the standardized mean difference. The weight given to each study is illustrated by the size of the square box, the point effect estimate by its mid-point and the degree of variance per study by the horizontal line through the box. A greater horizontal line indicates a greater 95% confidence interval for the effect estimates. Red boxes are studies where all patients were still in AF after 12 months. The overall effect estimate is represented by the diamante shape. (**a**). Physical functioning. Heterogeneity: $\tau^2 = 0.503$, $Q(\text{df} = 10) = 106.286$, $P < 0.001$, $I^2 = 90.6\%$. (**b**). Role physical. Heterogeneity: $\tau^2 = 0.354$, $Q(\text{df} = 10) = 78.169$, $P < 0.001$, $I^2 = 87.2\%$. (**c**). Bodily pain. Heterogeneity: $\tau^2 = 0.482$, $Q(\text{df} = 10) = 111.276$, $P < 0.001$, $I^2 = 91.0\%$. (**d**). General health. Heterogeneity: $\tau^2 = 0.577$, $Q(\text{df} = 10) = 125.791$, $P < 0.001$, $I^2 = 92.0\%$. (**e**). Role emotional. Heterogeneity: $\tau^2 = 0.265$, $Q(\text{df} = 10) = 65.670$, $P < 0.001$, $I^2 = 84.7\%$. (**f**). Vitality. Heterogeneity: $\tau^2 = 0.215$, $Q(\text{df} = 10) = 52.832$, $P < 0.001$, $I^2 = 81.1\%$. (**g**). Social functioning. Heterogeneity: $\tau^2 = 0.327$, $Q(\text{df} = 10) = 75.008$, $P < 0.001$, $I^2 = 86.7\%$. (**h**). Mental health. Heterogeneity: $\tau^2 = 0.253$, $Q(\text{df} = 10) = 62.246$, $P < 0.001$, $I^2 = 83.9\%$. SR: sinus rhythm; AF: atrial fibrillation

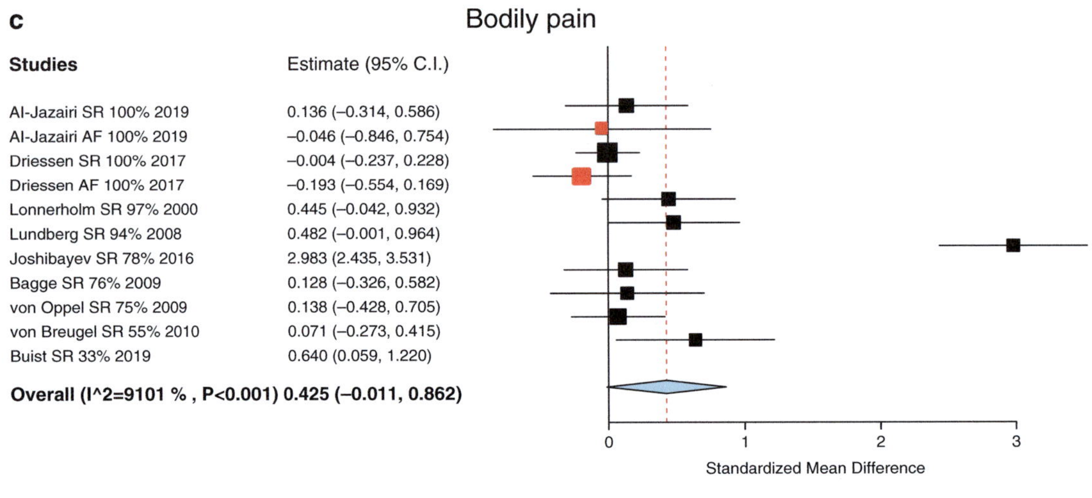

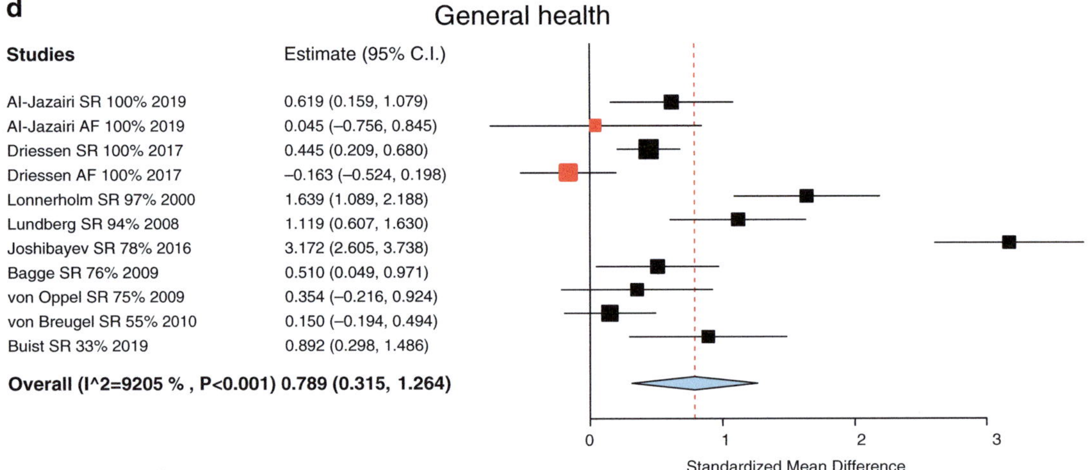

Fig. 7.2 (continued)

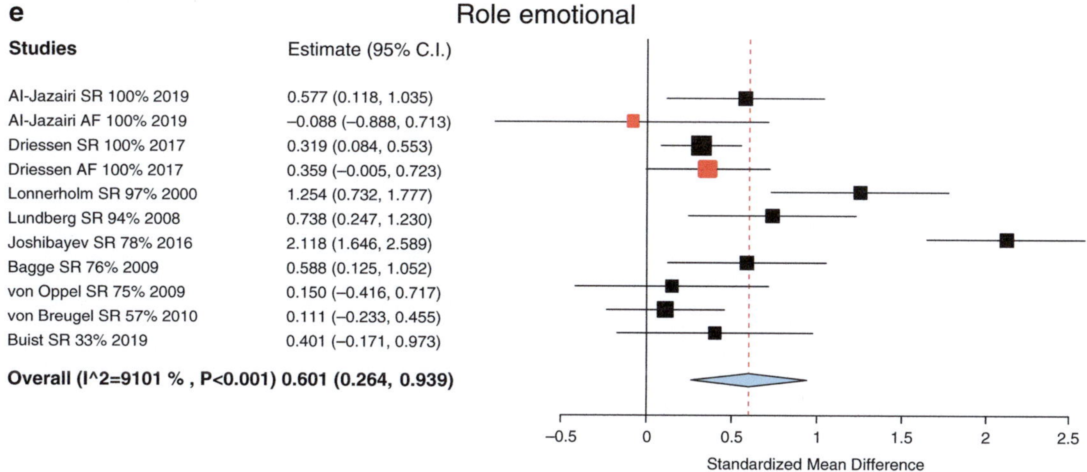

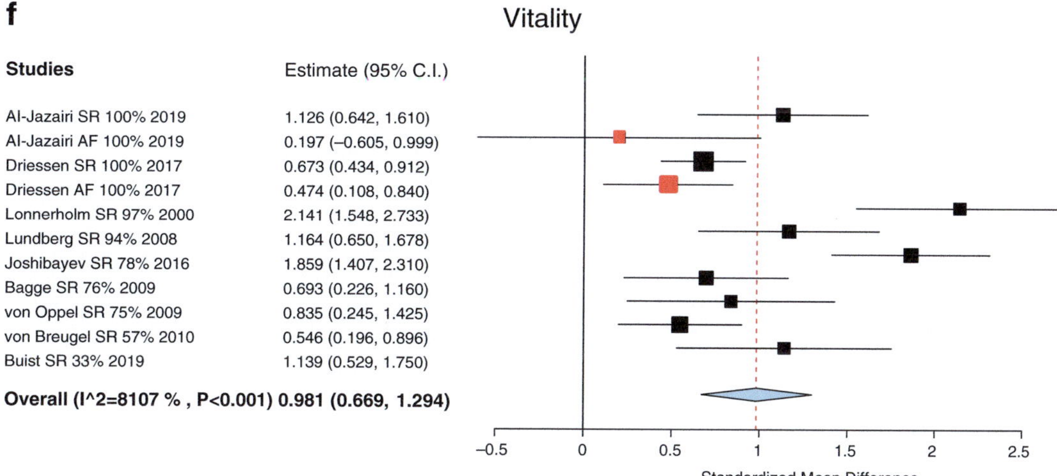

Fig. 7.2 (continued)

g Social functioning

Studies	Estimate (95% C.I.)
Al-Jazairi SR 100% 2019	0.963 (0.488, 1.438)
Al-Jazairi AF 100% 2019	0.627 (–0.193, 1.446)
Driessen SR 100% 2017	0.711 (0.471, 0.951)
Driessen AF 100% 2017	0.300 (–0.062, 0.663)
Lonnerholm SR 97% 2000	1.479 (0.941, 2.016)
Lundberg SR 94% 2008	0.917 (0.417, 1.417)
Joshibayev SR 78% 2016	2.855 (2.319, 1.178)
Bagge SR 76% 2009	0.711 (0.243, 1.178)
von Oppel SR 75% 2009	0.362 (–0.208, 0.933)
von Breugel SR 57% 2010	0.580 (0.229, 0.931)
Buist SR 33% 2019	0.868 (0.276, 1.461)
Overall (I^2=8667 % , P<0.001)	**0.935 (0.565, 1.306)**

h Mental health

Studies	Estimate (95% C.I.)
Al-Jazairi SR 100% 2019	0.746 (0.281, 1.211)
Al-Jazairi AF 100% 2019	0.135 (–0.666, 0.936)
Driessen SR 100% 2017	0.501 (0.265, 0.737)
Driessen AF 100% 2017	0.265 (–0.097, 0.628)
Lonnerholm SR 97% 2000	1.167 (0.650, 1.684)
Lundberg SR 94% 2008	0.724 (0.234, 1.215)
Joshibayev SR 78% 2016	2.353 (1.863, 2.844)
Bagge SR 76% 2009	0.493 (0.032, 0.953)
von Oppel SR 75% 2009	0.147 (–0.419, 0.714)
von Breugel SR 57% 2010	0.477 (0.128, 0.826)
Buist SR 33% 2019	0.679 (0.096, 1.261)
Overall (I^2=8393 % , P<0.001)	**0.704 (0.373, 1.036)**

Fig. 7.2 (continued)

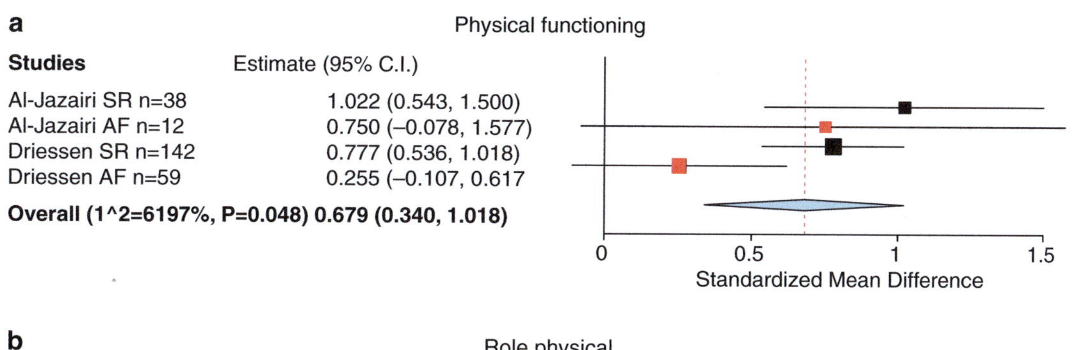

Fig. 7.3 Forest plots showing the changes per Short-Form 36 quality of life variable after 12 months' follow-up, expressed by the standardized mean difference, comparing studies with 100% sinus rhythm (black box) with 100% atrial fibrillation (red box) after 12 months' follow-up. The weight given to each study is illustrated by the size of the square box, the point effect estimate by its mid-point and the degree of variance per study by the horizontal line through the box. A greater horizontal line indicates a greater 95% confidence interval for the effect estimates. Red boxes are studies where all patients had AF after 12 months. The overall effect estimate is represented by the diamante shape. (**a**). Physical functioning. Heterogeneity: $\tau^2 = 0.069$, $Q(\text{df} = 3) = 7.888$, $P = 0.048$, $I^2 = 62.0\%$. (**b**). Role physical. Heterogeneity: $\tau^2 = 0.069$, $Q(\text{df} = 3) = 7.887$, $P = 0.048$, $I^2 = 62.0\%$. (**c**). Bodily pain. $\tau^2 = 0.000$, $Q(\text{df} = 3) = 1.345$, $P = 0.718$, $I^2 = 0\%$. (**d**). General health. Heterogeneity: $\tau^2 = 0.095$, $\chi(\text{df} = 3) = 9.990$, $P = 0.019$, $I^2 = 70.0\%$. (**e**). Role emotional. Heterogeneity: $\tau^2 = 0.000$, $Q(\text{df} = 3) = 2.155$, $P = 0.541$, $I^2 = 0\%$. (**f**). Vitality. $\tau^2 = 0.040$, $Q(\text{df} = 3) = 5.842$, $P = 0.120$, $I^2 = 48.7\%$. (**g**). Social functioning. Heterogeneity: $\tau^2 = 0.035$, $Q(\text{df} = 3) = 5.476$, $P = 0.140$, $I^2 = 45.2\%$. (**h**). Mental health. Heterogeneity: $\tau^2 = 0.004$, $Q(\text{df} = 3) = 3.306$, $P = 0.347$, $I^2 = 9.3\%$. AF: atrial fibrillation; SR: sinus rhythm

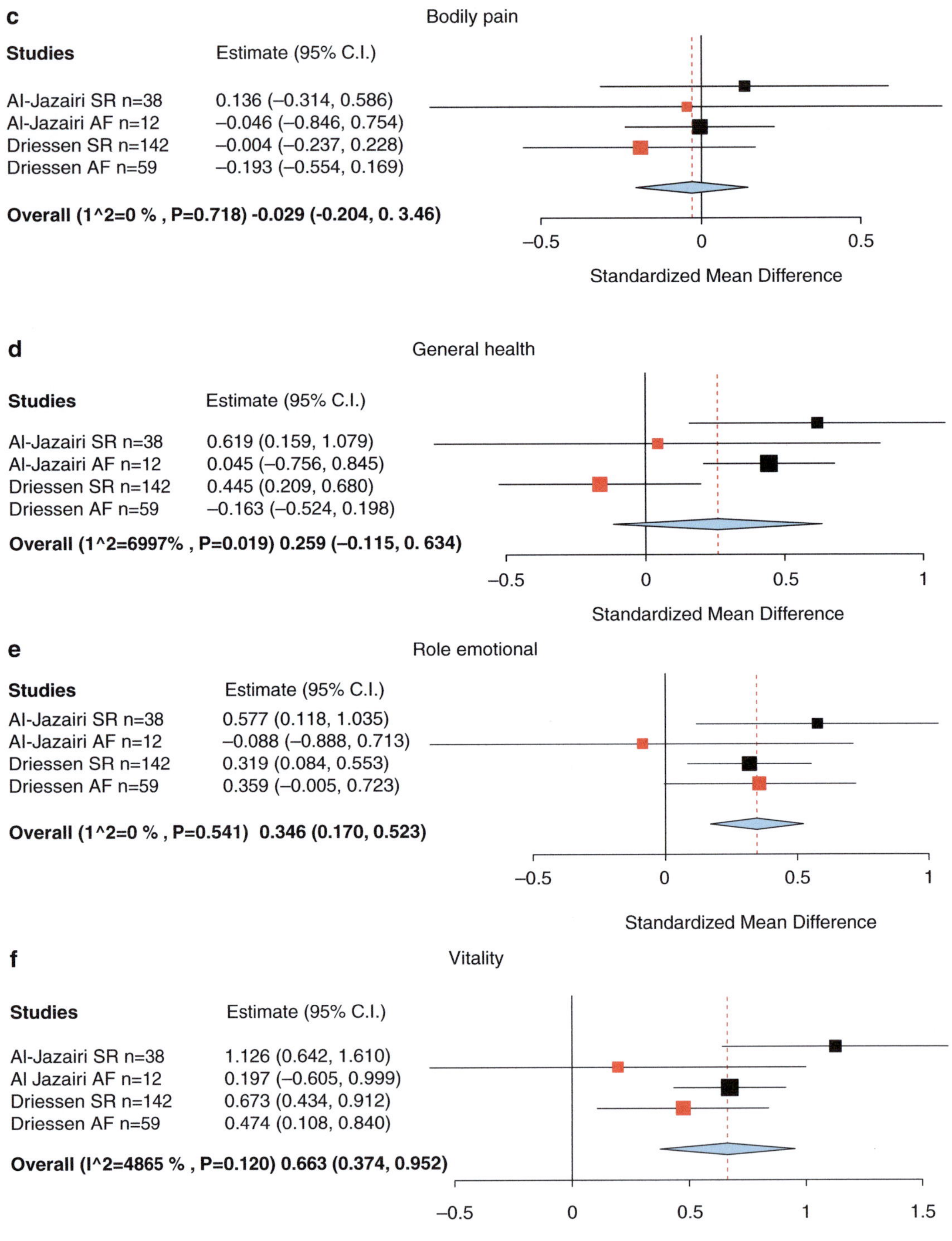

Fig. 7.3 (continued)

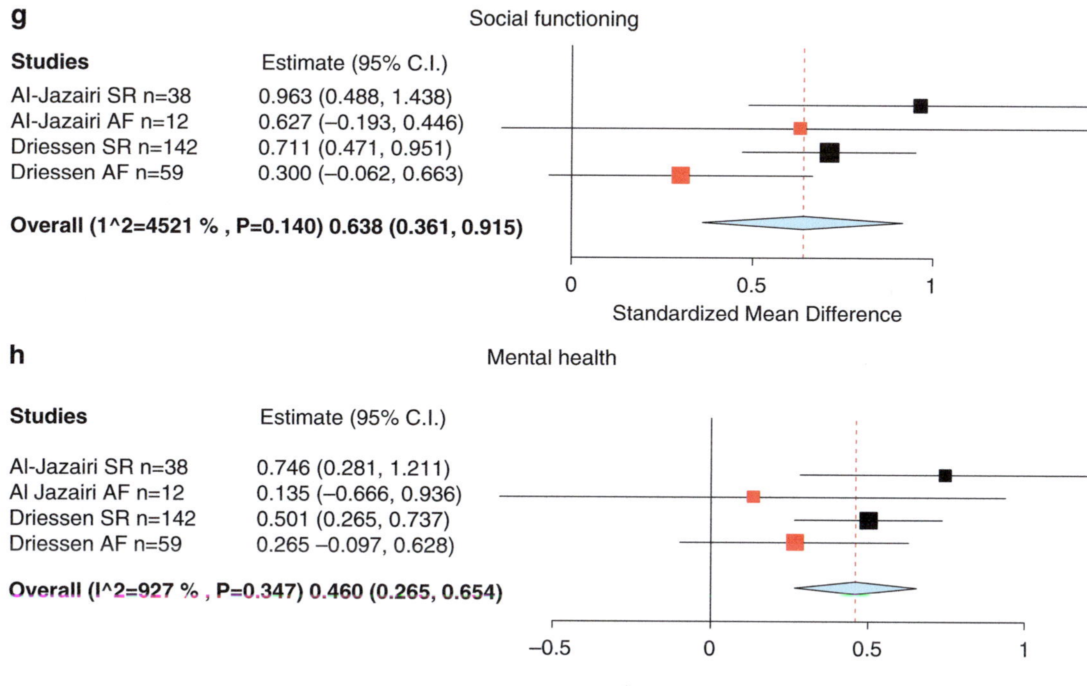

Fig. 7.3 (continued)

Table 7.7 Changes in SF-36 quality of life variables based on rhythm outcome after 12 months of follow-up

SF-36 variable	SR 12 months		AF 12 months		*P*-Value
	Adjusted mean	95% CI	Adjusted mean	95% CI	
Physical functioning	0.8	(0.6–1.0)	0.3	(0.0–0.7)	0.015
Role physical	1.0	(0.7–1.2)	0.4	(0.1–0.7)	0.006
Bodily pain	0.0	(−0.2–0.2)	−0.2	(−0.5–0.2)	0.331
General health	0.5	(0.3–0.7)	−0.1	(−0.5–0.2)	0.002
Role emotional	0.4	(0.2–0.6)	0.3	(0.0–0.6)	0.654
Vitality	0.8	(0.5–1.0)	0.4	(0.1–0.8)	0.096
Social functioning	0.8	(0.5–1.0)	0.4	(0.0–0.7)	0.043
Mental health	0.6	(0.3–0.8)	0.2	(−0.1–0.6)	0.123

Data are presented as adjusted mean between QOL scores after 12 months versus baseline scores, followed by the 95% CI. *P*-value of the meta-regression was computed using the metric 'Standardized mean difference' in a binary random-effects model using rhythm outcome after 12 month's follow-up as covariate factor. AF: atrial fibrillation; CI: confidence interval; SF: Short-Form 36; SR: sinus rhythm

Table 7.8 Changes in SF-36 quality of life variables comparing cardiac surgery with and without (control group) add-on surgical AF ablation

Study	SF-36 variable	Add-on surgical AF ablation		Control group		*P*-Value
		Baseline	1 year	Baseline	1 year	
Joshibayev and Bolatbekov et al.		***n* = 54**	***n* = 54**	***n* = 93**	***n* = 93**	
	Physical functioning	20.0 ± 7.0	84.0 ± 22.0	38.0 ± 12.0	49.0 ± 7.0	<0.001
	Role physical	38.0 ± 13.0	81.0 ± 17.0	44.0 ± 9.0	47.0 ± 9.0	<0.001
	Bodily pain	29.0 ± 23.0	79.0 ± 5.0	53.0 ± 11.0	51.0 ± 6.0	<0.001
	General health	39.0 ± 7.0	89.0 ± 21.0	51.0 ± 5.0	54.0 ± 6.0	<0.001
	Vitality	44.0 ± 12.0	88.0 ± 31.0	49.0 ± 5.0	60.0 ± 5.0	<0.001
	Social functioning	39.0 ± 7.0	84.0 ± 21.0	33.0 ± 11.0	51.0 ± 17.0	<0.001
	Role emotional	41.0 ± 23.0	89.0 ± 22.0	61.0 ± 11.0	50.0 ± 7.0	<0.001
	Mental health	39.0 ± 7.0	89.0 ± 29.0	55.0 ± 13.0	59.0 ± 9.0	<0.001
van Breugel et al.		***n* = 65**	***n* = 65**	***n* = 67**	***n* = 67**	
	Physical functioning	50.2 ± 24.1	68.4 ± 23.2	50.1 ± 24.2	61.2 ± 23.9	0.143
	Role physical	23.5 ± 35.3	53.2 ± 39.7	42.9 ± 42.1	47.9 ± 38.1	0.295
	Bodily pain	76.0 ± 25.0	77.7 ± 22.6	72.3 ± 24.6	72.8 ± 21.9	0.032
	General health	53.2 ± 19.7	56.0 ± 18.2	60.2 ± 17.4	54.9 ± 17.4	0.458
	Vitality	50.5 ± 22.4	61.4 ± 17.0	51.3 ± 21.8	60.0 ± 17.8	0.246
	Social functioning	66.9 ± 25.2	80.0 ± 19.3	67.0 ± 25.8	76.2 ± 24.7	0.410
	Role emotional	67.7 ± 42.9	72.1 ± 35.7	69.2 ± 42.0	69.5 ± 36.6	0.157
	Mental health	69.6 ± 20.0	77.7 ± 13.0	72.0 ± 22.0	74.0 ± 17.5	0.300
von Oppell et al.		***n* = 24**	***n* = 24**	***n* = 25**	***n* = 25**	
	Physical functioning	41.5 ± 25.6	61.8 ± 31.9	41.4 ± 29.3	80.3 ± 20.3	<0.001
	Role physical	13.5 ± 25.5	54.5 ± 47.3	23.0 ± 38.1	58.8 ± 44.6	<0.001
	Bodily pain	65.7 ± 34.2	70.1 ± 28.1	80.7 ± 27.3	92.2 ± 12.8	NS
	General health	58.2 ± 23.9	67.0 ± 25.0	55.1 ± 23.3	78.3 ± 16.8	<0.001
	Vitality	31.9 ± 23.0	53.0 ± 26.2	30.2 ± 30.5	62.5 ± 19.9	<0.001
	Social functioning	55.7 ± 36.9	68.8 ± 34.2	57.5 ± 29.8	88.8 ± 17.6	<0.001
	Role emotional	51.4 ± 42.8	56.1 ± 47.6	58.7 ± 43.3	86.7 ± 33.2	NS
	Mental health	70.8 ± 19.8	74.0 ± 22.8	76.8 ± 17.4	84.4 ± 17.1	NS
Overall change		**Adjusted mean (95% CI)**		**Adjusted mean (95% CI)**		***P*-Value**
	Physical functioning	1.8 (0.1–3.4)		1.0 (0.5–1.4)		0.403
	Role physical	1.5 (0.5–2.6)		0.3 (0.1–0.5)		0.037
	Bodily pain	1.1 (−0.5–2.6)		0.0 (−0.3–0.3)		0.230
	General health	1.2 (−0.3–2.8)		0.4 (−0.2–1.1)		0.371
	Vitality	1.1 (0.4–1.7)		1.3 (0.4–2.1)		0.704
	Social functioning	1.3 (−0.0–2.5)		0.9 (0.4–1.4)		0.654
	Role emotional	0.8 (−0.3–1.8)		−0.2 (−1.1–0.7)		0.178
	Mental health	1.0 (−0.1–2.1)		0.3 (0.1–0.5)		0.203

Data are presented as mean ± standard deviation or adjusted mean between QOL scores after 12 months versus baseline scores, followed by the 95% CI. NS: non-significant. SF: Short-Form 36. AF: atrial fibrillation. CI: confidence interval. P-value of the meta-regression was computed using the metric 'Standardized mean difference' in a binary random-effects model using add-on surgery as covariate factor

Table 7.9 Follow-up of patients reporting on quality of life using the Short Form-36 questionnaire. The follow-up duration is followed by the number of patients at one-year follow-up, the percentage of patients that was in SR direct after surgery, after three, six and twelve months and how heart rhythm was monitored

Total SR after 12 months of follow-up (n = 505)	Adjusted mean (95% CI)						
	73.8% (62.5–85.0)						
Study	Follow-up duration (months)	Patients at 1 year follow-up (n)	% SR post-operative	% SR 3 months	% SR 6 months	% SR 12 months	Rhythm monitoring
Al-Jazairi et al.	12	50	–	–	–	76	72-h Holter
Bagge et al.	12	33	–	–	–	76	24-h Holter
Buist et al.	12	23	–	–	–	33	ILR
Driessen et al.	12	201	–	–	–	71	24-h Holter
Joshibayev and Bolatbekov et al.	12	54	63	38	72	78	12-lead ECG
Lonnerholm et al.	12	25	97	–	–	–	12-lead ECG
Lundberg et al.	12	34	–	–	–	94	24-h Holter
van Breugel et al.	12	65	–	–	–	57	24-h Holter
von Oppel et al.	12	24		50	–	75	24-h Holter

CI: confidence interval; ILR: implanted rhythm monitoring; SR: sinus rhythm

Table 7.10 QOL scores measured by Atrial Fibrillation Symptom and Severity Score (AFSS) and Short-Form 12 (SF-12)

	Symptom severity score		Symptom frequency score		SF-12 Physical		SF-12 Mental	
Study	Baseline	1 year	Baseline	1 year	Baseline	1 year	Baseline	1 year
Gillinov et al. (n = 124)	4.7 ± 2.8	3.6 ± 2.5	8.3 ± 2.7	4.4 ± 3.7	38.4 ± 8.0	44.3 ± 9.0	48.1 ± 8.8	48.0 ± 6.3

Data are presented as mean ± standard deviation

Table 7.11 QOL scores measured by Toronto AFSS at baseline and European Heart Rhythm Association score of atrial fibrillation (EHRA) after 12 months of follow-up

	Palpitations		Dyspnoea de repos		Dyspnoea d'effort		Fatigue at rest		Fatigue at physical activity		Dizziness		Chest pain		EHRA	
Study	Baseline	1 year	Baseline	1 year	Baseline	1 year	Baseline	1 year	Baseline	1 year	Baseline	1 year	Baseline	1 year	Baseline	1 year
Al-Jazairi et al. SR ($n = 38$)	2.0 ± 1.9	0.4 ± 0.7	1.4 ± 1.4	0.3 ± 0.6	2.6 ± 1.5	1.1 ± 1.1	2.0 ± 1.3	0.8 ± 0.9	2.2 ± 1.4	1.0 ± 1.1	1.4 ± 1.2	0.5 ± 0.8	0.6 ± 1.1	0.1 ± 0.4	2.5 ± 0.6	2.0 ± 0.0
Al-Jazairi et al. AF ($n = 12$)	1.9 ± 1.9	1.1 ± 1.3	1.5 ± 1.1	1.1 ± 1.3	2.6 ± 1.6	1.9 ± 1.5	2.2 ± 1.2	1.2 ± 1.3	2.5 ± 1.2	1.7 ± 1.3	0.7 ± 1.1	1. 3 ± 1.6	0.7 ± 0.8	0.7 ± 0.8	2.5 ± 0.5	1.8 ± 0.4
Buist et al. ($n = 23$)	–	–	–	–	–	–	–	–	–	–	–	–	–	–	2.7 ± 0.9	1.5 ± 0.5

Data are presented as mean ± standard deviation. SR: sinus rhythm; AF: atrial fibrillation

Table 7.12 QOL scores measured by Symptom Status Questionnaire (SSQ)

Study	Overall		Palpitations		Fatigue		Dizziness		Lack of energy		Dyspnoea	
	Baseline	1 year	Baseline	1 year	Baseline	1 year	Baseline	1 year	Baseline	1 year	Baseline	1 year
Bagge et al. ($n = 33$)	15.2 ± 4.0	10.7 ± 4.8	2.6 ± 1.5	2.2 ± 1.2	3.6 ± 1.3	2.2 ± 1.4	2.1 ± 1.3	1.8 ± 1.2	3.9 ± 1.2	2.5 ± 1.4	2.9 ± 1.3	2.0 ± 1.2
Bagge et al. SR ($n = 25$)	15.8 ± 4.7	10.2 ± 5.0	–	–	–	–	–	–	–	–	–	–
Bagge et al. AF ($n = 8$)	15.0 ± 1.6	13.4 ± 3.2	–	–	–	–	–	–	–	–	–	–

Data are presented as mean ± standard deviation. SR: sinus rhythm; AF: atrial fibrillation

Table 7.13 QOL scores measured by Atrial Fibrillation Effect on Quality-of-Life (AFEQT), Canadian Cardiovascular Society Severity of Atrial Fibrillation (CCS-SAF) and EuroQoL

						EuroQoL			
	AFEQT		CCS-SAF			EQ-5D		EQ-VAS	
Study	Baseline	1 year	Baseline	6 months	1 year	Baseline	1 year	Baseline	1 year
Gehi et al. SR (n = 63)	–	–	2.8 ± 0.5	0.0 ± 0.0	0.0 ± 0.0	–	–	–	–
Gehi et al. AF (n = 63)	–	–	2.6 ± 1.1	0.3 ± 0.4	0.5 ± 0.8	–	–	–	–
Osmancik et al. SR (n = 52)	59.9 ± 19.4	91.4 ± 10.8	–	–	–	7.9 ± 2.6	6.6 ± 1.9	63.6 ± 19.11	79.3 ± 16.9
Osmancik et al. pAF (n = 16)	58.8 ± 19.0	81.5 ± 14.1	–	–	–	7.1 ± 2.1	8.1 ± 3.1	64.7 ± 21.1	70.0 ± 23.9
Osmancik et al. persAF (n = 7)	44.6 ± 7.5	47.4 ± 5.5	–	–	–	8.7 ± 2.8	8.9 ± 3.1	60.7 ± 12.4	64.3 ± 18.4
van Breugel et al. (n = 65)	–	–	–	–	–	5.2 ± 1.1	6.5 ± 1.5	61.5 ± 19.2	71.1 ± 15.5

Data are presented as mean ± standard deviation. SR: sinus rhythm; AF: atrial fibrillation

Table 7.14 QOL scores measured by Multidimensional Fatigue Inventory (MFI)

	General fatigue			Physical fatigue			Reduced activity			Reduced motivation			Mental fatigue		
Study	Baseline	6 months	1 year	Baseline	6 months	1 year	Baseline	6 months	1 year	Baseline	6 months	1 year	Baseline	6 months	1 year
van Breugel et al. ($n = 65$)	3.6 ± 1.1	2.6 ± 1.1	2.9 ± 1.0	3.6 ± 1.2	2.6 ± 1.1	2.7 ± 1.0	3.3 ± 1.2	2.6 ± 1.1	2.7 ± 1.1	2.6 ± 1.1	2.1 ± 0.9	2.2 ± 0.8	2.2 ± 1.0	2.1 ± 0.9	2.1 ± 1.0

Data are presented as mean ± standard deviation

Discussion

To the best of our knowledge, this is the first systematic review and meta-analysis that summarizes the effect of arrhythmia surgery for AF on patient reported quality of life (QOL). Overall, arrhythmia surgery leads to an improvement in QOL in patients with AF. This improvement seems to be related to the success of the procedure, because the improvement in QOL is higher in studies who reported a higher rate of SR after 12 months of follow-up. This is especially true for patients undergoing standalone AF surgery and less in patients undergoing concomitant AF surgery.

In 1991, drs. Cox and Schuessler designed the Cox-Maze procedure after extensive epicardial mapping studies [47]. The surgical technique is based on an anatomical approach to prevent macro reentrant circuits in both atria without blocking the atrial activation front. Although new surgical tools and alternative surgical approaches were developed, the basic concept of the procedure did not change and still forms the basis of present-day concomitant AF surgery. Even though the procedure has been shown to be very effective in restoring SR [48] and concomitant AF surgery had a class I indication in 2017 [49], it was recently downgraded to a class IIa indication [8]. A potential reason is that the add-on of AF surgery does not result in improved QOL nor reduced stroke and mortality at 1 year follow-up [8].

Overall Effect on QOL Following Arrhythmia Surgery for AF

In this meta-analysis, there was an improvement in QOL after cardiac surgery with concomitant AF ablation compared to baseline. However, it is difficult to distinguish between the effect of the cardiac surgical procedure itself and the effect of the add-on arrhythmia surgery on the improvement in QOL. When the results are plotted in relation to the success rate of the arrhythmia surgery in terms of SR after 12 months, the forest plots (Figs. 7.1 and 7.2) suggest that the improvement in QOL is higher in the studies that report a higher freedom of AF. Of course, these results should be interpreted with caution. First, the type of surgical lesions is not consistent between the different studies. While a large variability of lesion sets was performed, at least all studies performed PVI, which represents the cornerstone for AF ablation [50]. Furthermore, in 10 out of 12 studies the LAA was electrically isolated in at least half of their patients. In the BELIEF trial, isolation of the LAA lowered the incidence of AF without increasing the periprocedural complication rate [51]. As such, isolation of the LAA prevents the propagation of triggers that originate from the LAA to the left atrium and by substrate reduction [51]. Moreover, the overall reported stroke incidence in the present study was low (0.8%). As the LAA is considered the main source of thromboembolism in AF, oral anticoagulation and other techniques such as isolating the LAA are key in stroke prevention in AF patients, which may contribute to an improved QOL [52]. Secondly, follow-up was conducted with different monitoring devices. While using continuous monitoring devices is the most reliable way to keep track of (asymptomatic) palpitations, this was only used by two studies. Thirdly, no data on AAD use was given, though most of the included patients in this analysis had longstanding-persistent AF (41.9%) and treatment with AADs seems to be less efficient in this patient population for rhythm control and symptom management [53]. Moreover, for the study of Lonnerholm, the reported percentage of patients in SR in the forest plot represents the outcome directly after surgery, while in the other studies it represents the outcome after 12 months [35]. Nevertheless, it seems that the improvement in QOL is related to the outcome of the AF ablation.

Primary Endpoint: Concomitant AF Surgery and QOL

The analysis of the 3 studies that compared cardiac surgery with and without add-on arrhythmia surgery failed to show an overall improvement in

QOL between the patients that did and did not undergo add-on arrhythmia surgery [19, 37, 41]. While QOL scores after one year were improved compared to baseline for both the add-on and stand-alone arrhythmia group, differences were insignificant. These differences between the studies regarding the improvement in QOL is very obvious, suggesting that even if there is an effect of add-on arrhythmia on QOL for concomitant procedures, it is not very strong. Joshibayev and Bolatbekov et al. reported a very strong improvement in QOL, but this study did not randomize between both arms and therefore it cannot be excluded that there was a selection bias in the patients that received arrhythmia surgery [41]. Furthermore, it is surprising that there was almost no improvement in QOL between baseline and 12 months follow-up in the control group, despite the fact that all patients in the control group underwent mitral valve (MV) surgery. The other 2 studies were randomized, but only the study of von Oppel found an increase in QOL in several parameters, while in the study of van Breugel, only the SF-36 parameter 'Bodily pain' improved [19, 37]. In both studies, patients received CABG or aortic or mitral valve procedures concomitant to ablation. Interestingly, the study by Grady et al. further examined the improvement of health-related QOL using the SF-36 between patients undergoing different isolated cardiac procedures [54]. At baseline, patients with MV disease had a better physical component summary (PCS), but lower mental component summary (MCS) than patients undergoing aortic valve (AV) surgery, CABG or a Maze procedure. Three and six months after surgery, PCS scores improved reliably in all groups compared to baseline, except for patients who underwent MV surgery, probably due to their healthier preoperative scores and receiving early intervention. Furthermore, a strong trend was seen for better PCS scores of CABG patients than for AV patients. For changes in MCS scores, the improvement was faster for patients undergoing a Maze procedure compared with the other groups, and patients undergoing MV surgery did not show a clinically important improvement after three months.

Primary Endpoint: Standalone AF Surgery and QOL

In standalone AF surgery, the effect of arrhythmia surgery on QOL can be better evaluated, since there is no other surgical procedure that can act as a confounding factor. All studies evaluating QOL using the SF-36 questionnaire in standalone AF surgery showed an increase in QOL at 12 months compared to baseline [16, 17, 39, 40, 45, 46]. It must be noted that patients who are referred for an isolated surgical ablation for AF are highly symptomatic and undergo a surgical intervention as a last resort treatment. Accordingly, they usually have a worse QOL at baseline compared to the general population. As such, it is not unexpected that a rapid and significant improvement in QOL follows after a successful surgical ablation, returning patients to SR. [54] Furthermore, 2 studies specifically compared the improvement in QOL between patients who were in SR and patients who were in AF 12 months after the procedure [17, 39]. Both studies showed that the improvement in QOL was greater if surgical AF ablation resulted in SR. As such, it can be concluded that successful standalone arrhythmia surgery does result in an improvement in QOL. Despite this increase and the fact that standalone surgical AF ablation, epicardial or in a hybrid setting, is associated with higher success rates compared to catheter ablation [55, 56], it remains to have a class II recommendation due to the paucity of RCT's [8, 9].

Techniques and Lesion Sets in Concomitant and Stand-Alone AF Ablation

The inconsistency in the type of lesions performed during concomitant arrhythmia surgery makes it difficult and challenging to compare the different studies. For example, the studies of Gillinov et al., Joshibayev and Bolatbekov et al. and von Oppell et al. included a variety of lesions and a mixture of unipolar and bipolar radio frequent energy. This stands in contrast with the studies evaluating standalone AF surgery, that adhere more to a fixed ablation protocol. As such, it can be concluded that arrhythmia surgery does result in an improvement in QOL, but it requires a dedicated lesion set. Finally, a potential reason for the greater improvement in QOL after stand-alone AF than concomitant arrhythmia surgery is that stand-alone AF surgery is performed by a dedicated team, while concomitant AF surgery is also performed by surgeons without the extensive experience in AF ablation.

Limitations

This study contains some limitations. Ideally, we aimed to compare the improvements in QOL outcomes obtained by RCT's in our meta-analysis. Unfortunately, solely 2 studies have evaluated this outcome in an RCT. Due to this gap in literature, we worked with pre- and post-surgical QOL values in our meta-analysis of studies using the SF-36 questionnaire and performed a sub-study based on rhythm outcome after one year. Furthermore, since there is no golden standard for measuring QOL following arrhythmia surgery for AF, the included studies have used a variety of questionnaires to estimate the effect of ablation surgery on QOL. While being an important endpoint for ablation studies, QOL remains a rather subjective endpoint and comes along with (at least some) expectation bias. As such, the placebo effect of undergoing surgery as rhythm therapy was most likely present in at least some degree for all patients. In this meta-analysis, risk of bias due to other factors such as selection, confounding factors and publication was present as well. Moreover, marked differences between lesion sets between the studies was present. As such, not only statistical but also clinical heterogeneity was present in this study and results about the effectiveness of arrhythmia surgery and the improvement in QOL should be interpreted with caution. Lastly, the analyses in this study were based on a specific subgroup of highly symptomatic patients, which is especially true for patients undergoing stand-alone surgical ablation for AF. As such, these papers reflect only a small subset of all AF patients and thus the findings of improved QOL in this group should not be used as an endorsement for surgery for less symptomatic AF patients.

Conclusion

Overall, arrhythmia surgery does result in an improvement in QOL in patients with AF when a dedicated lesion set is used. This effect seems to be related to the outcome in terms of SR after 1 year, both in concomitant as in standalone AF ablation. However, studies evaluating QOL following arrhythmia surgery are scarce and analysis based on small, heterogenic, single-arm studies in a random-effects model hinders drawing definite conclusions. Therefore, future trials reporting on AF surgery, both concomitant and standalone, should include the evaluation of patient reported outcomes such as QOL.

Acknowledgments We acknowledge the authors of the included studies for their cooperation in providing the required additional data.

Conflict of Interest Bart Maesen is consultant for Atricure and Medtronic.

Source of Funding None.

References

1. Cobb FR, Blumenschein SD, Sealy WC, Boineau JP, Wagner GS, Wallace AG. Successful surgical interruption of the bundle of Kent in a patient with Wolff-Parkinson-White syndrome. Circulation Dec. 1968;38:1018–29.
2. Cox JL. Cardiac surgery for arrhythmias. Heart Rhythm. 2004;1:85c–101c.
3. Maesen B, La Meir M, Luermans J, Segers P. A minimally invasive all-in-one approach for patients with left anterior descending artery disease and atrial fibrillation. Eur J Cardiothorac Surg. 2020;57:803–5.
4. Ad N, Henry L, Friehling T, Wish M, Holmes SD. Minimally invasive stand-alone Cox-maze procedure for patients with nonparoxysmal atrial fibrillation. Ann Thorac Surg. 2013;96:792–9.

5. Maesen B, La Meir M. Unilateral Left-sided Thoracoscopic Ablation of Atrial Fibrillation. Ann Thorac Surg Mar. 2020;110(1):e63–6.
6. Luo X, Li B, Zhang D, Zhu J, Qi L, Tang Y. Efficacy and safety of the convergent atrial fibrillation procedure: a meta-analysis of observational studies. Interact Cardiovasc Thorac Surg. 2019;28:169–76.
7. Fleerakkers J, Hofman FN, van Putte BP. Totally thoracoscopic ablation: a unilateral right-sided approach. Eur J Cardiothorac Surg. 2020;58(5):1088–90.
8. Hindricks G, Potpara T, Dagres N, et al. ESC Guidelines for the diagnosis and management of atrial fibrillation developed in collaboration with the European Association of Cardio-Thoracic Surgery (EACTS). Eur Heart J Aug. 2020;29:2020.
9. Calkins H, Hindricks G, Cappato R, et al. 2017 HRS/EHRA/ECAS/APHRS/SOLAECE expert consensus statement on catheter and surgical ablation of atrial fibrillation: Executive summary. Europace. 2018;20:157–208.
10. Beller EM, Glasziou PP, Altman DG, Hopewell S, Bastian H, Chalmers I, Gøtzsche PC, Lasserson T, Tovey D. Group PfA. PRISMA for abstracts: reporting systematic reviews in journal and conference abstracts. PLoS Med. 2013;10:e1001419.
11. Sterne JA, Hernán MA, Reeves BC, Savović J, Berkman ND, Viswanathan M, Henry D, Altman DG, Ansari MT, Boutron I, et al. ROBINS-I: a tool for assessing risk of bias in non-randomised studies of interventions. BMJ. 2016;355:i4919.
12. Deeks JJ, Higgins J, Altman DG, Green S. Cochrane handbook for systematic reviews of interventions version 5.1. 0 (updated March 2011). The Cochrane Collaboration; 2011. p. 20112.
13. Smith LJW, Beretvas SN. Estimation of the standardized mean difference for repeated measures designs. J Mod Appl Stat Methods. 2009;8:27.
14. Wallace BC, Schmid CH, Lau J, Trikalinos TA. Meta-Analyst: software for meta-analysis of binary, continuous and diagnostic data. BMC Med Res Methodol. 2009;9:80.
15. Borenstein M, Hedges LV, JPT H, Rothstein H. Introduction to meta-analysis 2011. Hoboken, New Jersey: John Wiley & Sons; 2021.
16. Buist TJ, Adiyaman A, Beukema RJ, Smit JJJ, Delnoy PPH, Hemels ME, Sie HT, Misier ARR, Elvan A. Quality of life after catheter and minimally invasive surgical ablation of paroxysmal and early persistent atrial fibrillation: results from the SCALAF trial. Clin Res Cardiol. 2020;109(2):215–24.
17. Driessen AH, Berger WR, Bierhuizen MF, Piersma FR, van den Berg NW, Neefs J, Krul SP, van Boven WP, de Groot JR. Quality of life improves after thoracoscopic surgical ablation of advanced atrial fibrillation: Results of the Atrial Fibrillation Ablation and Autonomic Modulation via Thoracoscopic Surgery (AFACT) study. J Thorac Cardiovasc Surg. 2018;155:972–80.
18. van Breugel HN, Nieman F, Accord RE, Van Mastrigt G, Nijs JF, Severens J, Vrakking R, Maessen J. A Prospective Randomized Multicenter Comparison on Health-Related Quality of Life: The Value of Add-On Arrhythmia Surgery in Patients with Paroxysmal, Permanent or Persistent Atrial Fibrillation Undergoing Valvular and/or Coronary Bypass Surgery. J Cardiovasc Electrophysiol. 2010;21:511–20.
19. von Oppell UO, Masani N, O'Callaghan P, Wheeler R, Dimitrakakis G, Schiffelers S. Mitral valve surgery plus concomitant atrial fibrillation ablation is superior to mitral valve surgery alone with an intensive rhythm control strategy. Eur J Cardiothorac Surg. 2009;35:641–50.
20. Ad N, Henry L, Hunt S, Holmes SD. The outcome of the Cox Maze procedure in patients with previous percutaneous catheter ablation to treat atrial fibrillation. Ann Thorac Surg. 2011;91:1371–7.
21. Ad N, Henry L, Hunt S. The impact of surgical ablation in patients with low ejection fraction, heart failure, and atrial fibrillation. Eur J Cardiothorac Surg. 2011;40:70–6.
22. Ad N, Henry L, Hunt S. The concomitant cryosurgical Cox-Maze procedure using Argon based cryoprobes: 12 month results. J Cardiovasc Surg. 2011;52:593–9.
23. Ad N, Henry LL, Holmes SD, Hunt SL. The impact of surgical ablation for atrial fibrillation in high-risk patients. Ann Thorac Surg. 2012;93:1897–904.
24. Ad N, Henry L, Hunt S, Holmes SD. Do we increase the operative risk by adding the Cox Maze III procedure to aortic valve replacement and coronary artery bypass surgery? J Thorac Cardiovasc Surg. 2012;143:936–44.
25. Ad N, Henry L, Holmes SD, Stone LE, Hunt S. The association between early atrial arrhythmia and long-term return to sinus rhythm for patients following the Cox maze procedure for atrial fibrillation. Eur J Cardiothorac Surg. 2013;44:295–301.
26. Ad N, Henry L, Hunt S, Holmes S, Halpin L. Results of the Cox-Maze III/IV procedure in patients over 75 years old who present for cardiac surgery with a history of atrial fibrillation. J Cardiovasc Surg. 2013;54:281–8.
27. Ad N, Holmes SD, Massimiano PS, Pritchard G, Stone LE, Henry L. The effect of the Cox-maze procedure for atrial fibrillation concomitant to mitral and tricuspid valve surgery. J Thorac Cardiovasc Surg. 2013;146:1426–35.
28. Ad N, Holmes SD, Pritchard G, Shuman DJ. Association of operative risk with the outcome of concomitant Cox Maze procedure: a comparison of results across risk groups. J Thorac Cardiovasc Surg. 2014;148:3027–33.
29. Ad N, Holmes SD, Friehling T. Minimally invasive stand-alone Cox maze procedure for persistent and long-standing persistent atrial fibrillation: perioperative safety and 5-year outcomes. Circ Arrhythm Electrophysiol. 2017;10:e005352.

30. Forlani S, De Paulis R, Wolf LG, Greco R, Polisca P, Moscarelli M, Chiariello L. Conversion to sinus rhythm by ablation improves quality of life in patients submitted to mitral valve surgery. Ann Thorac Surg. 2006;81:863–7.
31. Henry L, Hunt S, Holmes SD, Martin LM, Ad N. Are there gender differences in outcomes after the Cox-Maze procedure for atrial fibrillation? Innovations. 2013;8:190–8.
32. Holmes SD, Fornaresio LM, Shuman DJ, Pritchard G, Ad N. Health-Related Quality of Life After Minimally Invasive Cardiac Surgery. Innovations. 2016;11:128–33.
33. Jessurun ER, van Hemel NM, Defauw JA, Stofmeel MA, Kelder JC, Brutel de la Rivière A, Ernst JM. Results of maze surgery for lone paroxysmal atrial fibrillation. Circulation. 2000;101:1559–67.
34. Jessurun E, Van Hemel N, Defauw J, De La Riviere AB. A randomized study of combining maze surgery for atrial fibrillation with mitral valve surgery. J Cardiovasc Surg. 2003;44:9.
35. Lönnerholm S, Blomström P, Nilsson L, Blomström-Lundqvist C. A high quality of life is maintained late after Maze III surgery for atrial fibrillation. Eur J Cardiothorac Surg. 2009;36:558–62.
36. Massimiano PS, Yanagawa B, Henry L, Holmes SD, Pritchard G, Ad N. Minimally invasive fibrillating heart surgery: a safe and effective approach for mitral valve and surgical ablation for atrial fibrillation. Ann Thorac Surg. 2013;96:520–7.
37. van Breugel HN, Parise O, Nieman FH, Accord RE, Lucà F, Lozekoot P, Kumar N, van Mastrigt GA, Nijs JF, Vrakking R. Does sinus rhythm conversion after cardiac surgery affect postoperative health-related quality of life? J Cardiothorac Surg. 2016;11:75.
38. Yanagawa B, Holmes SD, Henry L, Hunt S, Ad N. Outcome of concomitant Cox-maze III procedure using an argon-based cryosurgical system: a single-center experience with 250 patients. Ann Thorac Surg. 2013;95:1633–9.
39. Al-Jazairi M, Rienstra M, Klinkenberg T, Mariani M, Van Gelder I, Blaauw Y. Hybrid atrial fibrillation ablation in patients with persistent atrial fibrillation or failed catheter ablation. Neth Hear J. 2019;27:142–51.
40. Bagge L, Blomström P, Nilsson L, Einarsson GM, Jidéus L, Blomström-Lundqvist C. Epicardial off-pump pulmonary vein isolation and vagal denervation improve long-term outcome and quality of life in patients with atrial fibrillation. J Thorac Cardiovasc Surg. 2009;137:1265–71.
41. Joshibayev S, Bolatbekov B. Early and long-term outcomes and quality of life after concomitant mitral valve surgery, left atrial size reduction, and radiofrequency surgical ablation of atrial fibrillation. Anatol J Cardiol. 2016;16:797.
42. Lönnerholm S, Blomstrom P, Nilsson L, Oxelbark S, Jideus L, Blomstrom-Lundqvist C. Effects of the maze operation on health-related quality of life in patients with atrial fibrillation. Circulation. 2000;101:2607–11.
43. Lundberg C, Albåge A, Carnlöf C, Kennebäck G. Long-term health-related quality of life after maze surgery for atrial fibrillation. Ann Thorac Surg. 2008;86:1878–82.
44. Gillinov AM, Gelijns AC, Parides MK, DeRose JJ Jr, Moskowitz AJ, Voisine P, Ailawadi G, Bouchard D, Smith PK, Mack MJ. Surgical ablation of atrial fibrillation during mitral-valve surgery. N Engl J Med. 2015;372:1399–409.
45. Gehi AK, Mounsey JP, Pursell I, Landers M, Boyce K, Chung EH, Schwartz J, Walker TJ, Guise K, Kiser AC. Hybrid epicardial-endocardial ablation using a pericardioscopic technique for the treatment of atrial fibrillation. Heart Rhythm. 2013;10:22–8.
46. Osmancik P, Budera P, Talavera D, Herman D, Vesela J, Prochazkova R, Rizov V, Kacer P. Improvement in the quality of life of patients with persistent or long-standing persistent atrial fibrillation after hybrid ablation. J Interv Card Electrophysiol. 2020;57(3):435–42. https://doi.org/10.1007/s10840-019-00546-7. Epub 2019 Apr 17. PMID: 31001766.
47. Cox JL, Schuessler RB, D'Agostino HJ Jr, Stone CM, Chang BC, Cain ME, Corr PB, Boineau JP. The surgical treatment of atrial fibrillation. III. Development of a definitive surgical procedure. J Thorac Cardiovasc Surg. 1991;101:569–83.
48. Weimar T, Schena S, Bailey MS, Maniar HS, Schuessler RB, Cox JL, Damiano RJ Jr. The cox-maze procedure for lone atrial fibrillation: a single-center experience over 2 decades. Circ Arrhythm Electrophysiol. 2012;5:8–14.
49. Calkins H, Hindricks G, Cappato R, et al. 2017 HRS/EHRA/ECAS/APHRS/SOLAECE expert consensus statement on catheter and surgical ablation of atrial fibrillation: executive summary. J Interv Card Electrophysiol. 2017;50:1–55.
50. Maesen B, Van-Loo I, Pison L, La-Meir M. Surgical ablation of atrial fibrillation: is electrical isolation of the pulmonary veins a must? J Atr Fibrillation. 2016;9:1426.
51. Chernyavskiy A, Kareva Y, Pak I, Rakhmonov S, Pokushalov E, Romanov A. Quality of life after surgical ablation of persistent atrial fibrillation: a prospective evaluation. Heart Lung Circ. 2016;25:378–83.
52. van Laar C, Verberkmoes NJ, van Es HW, Lewalter T, Dunnington G, Stark S, Longoria J, Hofman FH, Pierce CM, Kotecha D. Thoracoscopic left atrial appendage clipping: a multicenter cohort analysis. JACC Clin Electrophysiol. 2018;4:893–901.
53. Hindricks G, Potpara T, Dagres N, Arbelo E, Bax JJ, Blomström-Lundqvist C, Boriani G, Castella M, Dan G-A, Dilaveris PE. 2020 ESC Guidelines for the diagnosis and management of atrial fibrillation developed in collaboration with the European Association for Cardio-Thoracic Surgery (EACTS) The Task

Force for the diagnosis and management of atrial fibrillation of the European Society of Cardiology (ESC) Developed with the special contribution of the European Heart Rhythm Association (EHRA) of the ESC. Eur Heart J. 2021;42:373–498.

54. Grady KL, Lee R, Subačius H, Malaisrie SC, McGee EC Jr, Kruse J, Goldberger JJ, McCarthy PM. Improvements in health-related quality of life before and after isolated cardiac operations. Ann Thorac Surg. 2011;91:777–83.

55. Phan K, Phan S, Thiagalingam A, Medi C, Yan TD. Thoracoscopic surgical ablation versus catheter ablation for atrial fibrillation. Eur J Cardiothorac Surg Apr. 2016;49:1044–51.

56. van der Heijden CAJ, Vroomen M, Luermans JG, Vos R, Crijns H, Gelsomino S, La Meir M, Pison L, Maesen B. Hybrid versus catheter ablation in patients with persistent and longstanding persistent atrial fibrillation: a systematic review and meta-analysisdagger. Eur J Cardiothorac Surg. 2019;56:433–43.

8 Transcatheter Mitral Valve Procedures

Matthew K. H. Tan and Omar A. Jarral

Introduction

Increasingly, emphasis has been placed on health-related quality of life (HRQoL) as a measure of outcome in surgery. Defined as a "multi -dimensional assessment of an individual's perception of the physical, psychological, and social aspects of life that can be affected by a disease process and its treatment", it provides a more nuanced look at the outcomes following surgery when compared to crude mortality and morbidity rates. It is also necessary for the calculation and evaluation of cost-effectiveness as well as acting as a more precise indicator of patient-centred care, with significant promise to improve healthcare provision [1] – this has been recognised by the United Kingdom's Department of Health with the consolidation of efforts to collect and publish HRQoL outcomes for common procedures [2].

While not routinely collected in cardiothoracic or valve surgery currently, this concept is particularly applicable to intervention on the mitral valve (MV), including transcatheter MV procedures, for a few reasons. Firstly, AHA/ACC and ESC/EACTS guidelines recommend early intervention on severe degenerative mitral regurgitation (MR) even if patients are asymptomatic [3–5]. Measurement and maintenance of pre-operative HRQoL is therefore essential in maintaining the confidence of patients and referring cardiologists. Secondly, transcatheter MV procedures are rapidly evolving and require robust assessment prior to widespread use. Knowledge of HRQoL outcomes in these new technologies will benefit both clinicians and patients in their decision-making.

This chapter aims to provide readers with a comprehensive systematic review of all available literature detailing HRQoL outcomes in patients undergoing transcatheter MV interventions. This chapter will also make recommendations for clinical practice and future research.

MitraClip Implantation

The MitraClip, as its name suggests, is a clip that grasps the anterior and posterior leaflets of the mitral valve, creating a "double orifice" valve that reduces the extent of regurgitation. In the current literature on transcatheter MV interventions, the majority of studies (n = 20) reported on MitraClip implantation (Table 8.1 adapted from Tan *et al.* [6–26]), the largest group of studies on a single device. All showed significant HRQoL improvements post-implantation. Three studies

M. K. H. Tan (✉)
Academic Section of Vascular Surgery, Department of Surgery and Cancer, Imperial College London, Charing Cross Hospital, London, UK
e-mail: matthew.tan1@nhs.net

O. A. Jarral
Department of Surgery and Cancer, Imperial College London, St. Mary's Hospital, London, UK

T. Athanasiou et al. (eds.), *Patient Reported Outcomes and Quality of Life in Cardiovascular Interventions*, https://doi.org/10.1007/978-3-031-09815-4_8

Table 8.1 Mitraclip

Author, publication year, study period, study type, and centre	Study intent and no. of patients	Patient characteristics	Follow-up duration / Time points at which HRQoL was measured	HRQoL instrument used / Follow-up completion rate	Main findings related to HRQoL
Arnold et al. 2019 [7] Data collection period not reported Randomised controlled trial Multicentre	Determine the health status outcomes of patients with HF and secondary MR treated with MitraClip versus standard care 302 patients with MitraClip repair Compared against 312 patients who underwent standard care	MitraClip group: mean age 71.7 ± 11.8 years, 66.6% male Standard care group: mean age 72.7 ± 10.6 years, 61.8% male	2 years Pre-op, 1 month, 6 months, 12 months and 24 months post-op	KCCQ SF-36 35.3% at 24 months	All patients had poor baseline HRQoL with mean KCCQ overall summary score of 52.4 ± 23.0 HRQoL remained unchanged for the standard care group, but improved significantly for the MitraClip group at 1 month MitraClip group also showed significantly higher SF-36 scores at each follow-up time point when compared to the standard care group
Buzzatti et al. 2015 [8] September 2008–April 2014 Retrospective cohort study San Raffaele Scientific Institute, Milan, Italy	Comparing outcomes between MitraClip repair and conventional surgical repair and replacement in octogenarian patients 25 patients selected for MitraClip repair Compared against 35 retrospectively selected patients from the same time period, $n = 29$ for repair and $n = 6$ for replacement	MitraClip group: mean age 84.5 ± 3.2 years, 68% NYHA III/IV, logistic EuroScore 19.4%, STS morbidity and mortality 25.9 ± 10.0% Conventional surgery group: mean age 81.9 ± 2.0 years, 37% NYHA III/IV, logistic EuroScore 8.4%, STS morbidity and mortality 18.7 ± 5.8%	MitraClip group: 1.8 ± 1.3 years Conventional surgery group: 2.5 ± 1.5 years Pre-op, no specific time point for post-op	SF-36 100%	In MitraClip group, SF-36 score significantly improved for physical but not significantly changed for mental scores No baseline data available for conventional surgery group, but had similar post-operative SF-36 scores to the MitraClip group
Edelman et al. 2014 [9] March 2011–March 2013 Prospective cohort study Sir Charles Gairdner Hospital, Australia	Reporting the clinical, quality of life, and echocardiographic results of MitraClip use in 25 patients	Mean age 74.1 ± 9.1 years, 72% male, 84% NYHA class III/IV	6 months Pre-op and at day 1, 30 and 6 months post-op	6 Domain Australian Quality of Life index MLHFQ Not reported	Significant improvement in MLHFQ score over time from baseline AQoL-6D showed significant improvement in independence, mental, and coping at 30 days and 6 months

Feldman et al. 2011 [31] September 2005–November 2008 Randomised controlled trial Multicentre (37 centres)	Assessing effectiveness and safety of percutaneous repair using MitraClip for MR 279 patients with grade 3+/4+ MR split in 2:1 ratio:Percutaneous repair (n = 184)Conventional surgery (n = 95)	Percutaneous repair: mean age 67.3 ± 12.8 years, 62% male, 52% NYHA class III/IV Surgery: mean age 65.7 ± 12.9 years, 66% male, 47% NYHA class III/IV	12 months Pre-op, 30 days and 12 months post-op	SF-36 71.1% at 12 months (192 responses from 270 included patients in 12 month analysis)	Undergoing conventional surgery was associated with a transient decrease in quality of life at 30 days Patients' quality of life improved from baseline to 12 months in both study groups
Franzen et al. 2011 [11] September 2008–March 2010 Retrospective cohort study Multicentre	Assessing feasibility, short-term durability, and clinical outcomes of MitraClip therapy in patients with end-stage heart failure and severely reduced LV ejection fraction 50 patients	Mean age 70 ± 11 years, 76% male, 100% NYHA class III/IV Logistic EuroSCORE 34 ± 21% All had functional mitral regurgitation	6 months Pre-op, 6 months post-op	MLHFQ 40%	Significant MLHFQ score reduction
Glower et al. 2014 [12] EVEREST II HRR: 2007–2008 EVERST II REALISM HR: 2009-present Prospective cohort study Multicentre	Reporting 12 month treatment outcomes in high-risk patients treated with percutaneous MV edge-to-edge repair 351 patients who have completed 12 months follow-up	Mean age of 75.7 ± 10.5 years, 61.0% male, NYHA class III/IV 84.9% Mean STS-predicted mortality risk of 11.3 ± 7.7%	12 months Pre-op, 12 months post-op	SF-36 70.5%	HRQoL improved from baseline
Hellhammer et al. 2015 [13] Data collection period not reported Retrospective cross-sectional study Heart Centre Dusseldorf	Assessing safety and efficacy of MitraClip repair in patients with and without anaemia 80 patients: n = 41 with anaemia, n = 39 without anaemia	Anaemia group: mean age 76 ± 9.7 years, 68.3% male, logistic EuroSCORE 21.5 ± 18.6%, 92.7% NYHA III/IV No anaemia group: 70 ± 11.3, 66.7% male, logistic EuroSCORE 18.5 ± 6.0%, 89.7% NYHA III/IV	– Pre-op, and no specific time point for post-op	MLHFQ Not reported	HRQoL was improved in all patients, with no significant difference in the magnitude of change between both groups

(continued)

Table 8.1 (continued)

Author, publication year, study period, study type, and centre	Study intent and no. of patients	Patient characteristics	Follow-up duration Time points at which HRQoL was measured	HRQoL instrument used Follow-up completion rate	Main findings related to HRQoL
Krawczyk-Ożóg et al. 2018 [14] January 2016 to January 2017 Prospective cohort study University Hospital, Krakow, Poland	Evaluate clinical and HRQoL outcomes in patients with severe secondary MR undergoing MitraClip or conservative treatment 33 patients: *n* = 10 treated with MitraClip, *n* = 23 undergoing conservative treatment	MitraClip group: mean age 71.8 ± 7.8 years, EuroSCORE II 3.9 ± 1.7%, 90.0% NYHA III/IV Conservative group: mean age 73.0 ± 11.5 years, EuroSCORE II 6.2 ± 3.8%, 91.3% NYHA III/IV	8.0 ± 2.3 months Pre-op, and no specific time point for post-op	EQ-5D SF-12v2 Not reported	Significant improvement in the HRQoL in the MitraClip group while no significant changes were seen in the conservative treatment group Higher scores seen in the MitraClip group in physical functioning and PCS on the SF-12v2
Lim et al. 2014 [15] 2003–2012 Retrospective cohort study Multicentre	Evaluate treatment of MR in patients at prohibitive surgical risk with transcatheter mitral valve repair 141 patients (127 retrospectively identified)	Mean age 82.4 ± 8.7 years, 55.1% male All patients had STS predicted risk of mortality for MV replacement ≥8% 86.6% NYHA class III/IV at baseline	At 30 days and 12 months Pre-op, 1, 6 and 12 months post-op	SF-36 Not reported	PCS scores improved by ~6 points from baseline MCS scores improved by ~3 at 30 days and ~ 5–6 points thereafter from baseline All score improvements indicate a minimum clinical important difference Post-transcatheter MV repair scores approximated population norms for adults ≥75 years
Maisano et al. 2013 [16] April 2009–April 2011 Non-randomised post-approval study (Phase IV clinical trial) Multicentre (14 centres)	Report on early and mid-term outcomes of post-approval study of MitraClip 567 patients (from 3 different studies) with significant MR	ACCESS-EU patients: mean age 73.7 ± 9.6 years, 63.8% male EVEREST II randomised controlled trial patients: mean age 67.3 ± 12.8 years, 62.5% male EVEREST II High Risk Study patients: mean age 76.7 ± 9.8 years, 62.8% male Baseline mean logistic EuroSCORE of 23.0 ± 18.3	12 months Pre-op, 6 and 12 months post-op	MLHFQ 56.3% at 12 months	Significant MLHFQ score improvement

Metze et al. 2017 May 2014–June 2016 Prospective cohort study Heart Centre of the University of Cologne, Cologne, Germany	Investigate the impact of frailty on outcomes in patients undergoing the MitraClip procedure 213 patients underwent the MitraClip procedure, 97 considered frail	Frail cohort: mean age 79 ± 7 years, 50.5% male, logEuroSCORE 20.5% Non-frail cohort: mean age 76 ± 9 years, 62.9% male, log EuroSCORE 15.4%	6 weeks	SF-36 MLHFQ	Frail patients had similar improvements in SF-36 scores to non-frail patients, but significantly greater improvement in MLHFQ scores
			Pre-op, 6 weeks post-op	79.8%	
Neuss et al. 2013 [18] March 2009–November 2012 Prospective cohort study Heart Centre Brandenburg, Bernau, Germany	Determine selection criteria for MitraClip implantation in patients with severe congestive heart failure 157 patients All had EuroSCORE >20 and symptomatic MR grade >2+	Mean age 74 ± 10 years, 67% male, 100% NYHA class III/IV 43% patients had logistic EuroSCORE of >20 and were considered very high-risk patients for surgery	6 months: 111 patients 12 months: 68 patients	MLHFQ	Improvement in MLHFQ scores, which were persistent after 12 months
			Pre-op, 6 and 12 months post-op	27.8%	
Reichenspurner et al. 2013 [19] October 2008–April 2011 Post-approval study (ACCESS-EU Phase I) Multicentre (14 centres)	Describe 12 months outcomes with MitraClip treatment in 117 patients with degenerative MR	Mean age 75.6 ± 12.1 years, 49.6% male, 74% NYHA class III/IV Mean logistic EuroSCORE: 15.5 ± 13.3% In high-risk group (*n* = 33): mean age 81.2 ± 5.2 years, 45.5% male, 96.9% NYHA class III/IV In low-risk group (*n* = 84): mean age 73.4 ± 13.3 years, 51.2% male, 64.7% NYHA class III/IV	12 months	MLHFQ	Scores were significantly improved at 12 months
			Pre-op, 6 and 12 months post-op	45.4%	
Rudolph et al. 2011 [20] September 2008–March 2010 Prospective cohort study University Medical Center Hamburg-Eppendorf, Germany	Assess outcomes of 104 patients at prohibitive surgical risk undergoing MitraClip therapy	Mean age 74 ± 9 years, 62% male Characteristics were significantly different from patients in the EVEREST II trial	Median of 359 days	MLHFQ	MLHFQ score improved significantly, comparable with results reported in MV surgery
			Pre-op, 6 and 12 months post-op	55.3%	

(continued)

Table 8.1 (continued)

Author, publication year, study period, study type, and centre	Study intent and no. of patients	Patient characteristics	Follow-up duration Time points at which HRQoL was measured	HRQoL instrument used Follow-up completion rate	Main findings related to HRQoL
Rudolph et al. 2014 [21] Enrolled patients in the German MV registry up till 18 November 2013 Prospective cohort study Multicentre (21 centres) inclusion of patients Analysis done at the Stiftung für Herzinfarktforschung (IHF), Heart Center Ludwigshafen	Evaluate feasibility, safety, and outcomes of MitraClip therapy in high perioperative risk patients as compared to stable clinical patients as assessed by NYHA class 803 patients separated into groups based on NYHA class	NYHA I/II (n = 88): mean age 75.0 years, 64.8% male NYHA III (n = 572): mean age 76.0 years, 58.9% male NYHA IV (n = 143): mean age 75.0 years, 65% male Mean logistical EuroSCORE of 20.0 for NYHA III patients and 23.0 for NYHA IV patients	Scheduled at 30 days, and 1, 3, and 5 years Pre-op and 30 days post-op	EQol-D5 100%	NYHA IV patients had the worst QOL at 30 days follow-up, but showed significant improvement in score
Taramasso et al. 2014 [22] October 2008–July 2013 Retrospective cohort study San Raffaele University Hospital, Milan, Italy	Reporting midterm clinical and echocardiographic results of MitraClip therapy for symptomatic high-risk or elderly patients with degenerative MR 48 consecutive high-risk patients	Mean age 78.5 ± 10.8 years, 54% male, logistic EuroSCORE 15.7 ± 12.2%, STS-PROM 12 ± 10%, 60.5% NYHA III, 10.5% NYHA IV 56.6% (n = 27) patients were ≥ 80 years, with significant EuroSCORE differences between the stratified groups<80 years: 12.1 ± 18.5% ≥80 years: 18.5 ± 12%	Median follow-up 16 months Pre-op, 1 year post-op	MLHFQ SF-36 Not reported	At baseline, patients aged 80 years or more had a worse perceived HRQoL Significant improvement in MLHFQ and SF-36 scores postoperatively
Terhoeven et al. 2019 [23] 2014–2016 Pre-post-interventional controlled trial University of Heidelberg, Heidelberg, Germany	Assess the impact of MitraClip on psychological and cognitive functioning compared to pre-intervention in 40 patients	Median age 73 years, 52.5% male, STS-score 5.16, EF 35 ± 15%	6 weeks Pre-op and 6 weeks post-op	SF-36 100%	Psychological wellbeing and physical wellbeing improved post-MitraClip treatment

Ussia et al. 2012 [24] October 2008–January 2011 Prospective cohort study Ferrarotto Hospital, University of Catania, Italy	Evaluate HRQoL changes following percutaneous repair of MR with the MitraClip system in patients with high surgical risk 39 patients with MR ≥3+	Mean age 72 ± 11 years, 82.1% male 25 patients presented with functional disease, 14 patients had organic degenerative MR Logistic EuroSCORE: 20 ± 6%	6 months Pre-op, 6 months post-op	SF-12v2 100%	Clear improvement to physical functioning, role physical, general health, vitality, social functioning, role emotional, and mental health Only bodily pain did not show significant improvement, paper suggests reason as co-morbidities not related to mitral valve disease At 6 months, improvement in physical and mental components was higher in group of patients with functional MR than patients with degenerative MR
Van den Branden et al. 2012 [25] January 2009–November 2010 Prospective cohort study St. Antonius Hospital, Nieuwegein, the Netherlands	Assess feasibility and safety of percutaneous edge-to-edge repair in high-risk patient population 52 patients	Mean age 73.2 ± 10.1 years, 69.2% male Logistic EuroSCORE: 27.1 ± 17.0%	6 months Pre-op, 6 months post-op	MLHFQ 95.7%	HRQoL score significantly improved
Whitlow et al. 2012 [26] Data collection period not reported Retrospective cohort study Multicentre	Evaluate safety and efficacy of MitraClip in high-risk patients with significant MR 78 high-risk patients with 36 patients in concurrent comparator group	High-risk group: mean age 76.7 ± 9.8 years, 62.8% male, all with history of congestive heart failure, STS risk score 14.2 ± 8.2% Comparator group: mean age 77.2 ± 13.0 years, 50.0% male, STS risk score 14.9 ± 8.5% 46 patients had malcoaptation of leaflets secondary to leaflet restriction and LV dilation Remaining 32 patients had leaflet pathology consistent with degenerative disease	1 year Pre-op, 30 days, and 12 months post-op	SF-36 91.7% at 12 months	HRQoL improved in majority of patients with both PCS and MCS improving from baseline to 12 months

compared MitraClip to conventional surgery [8, 10, 20] while two studies compared this device to conservative management [7, 14].

Studies Comparing Against Conventional Surgery

Buzzatti et al. compared conventional MV surgery in 35 retrospectively selected patients to 25 octogenarian patients who underwent MitraClip implantation [8]. Importantly, this older patient population showed significantly improved SF-36 physical scores but failed to show improvement in the mental components. On comparing with the conventional surgery group, both groups had similar post-operative physical and mental HRQoL scores. Due to the lack of baseline measurement in the conventional surgery group, it was not possible to compare HRQoL improvements between groups. This finding was supported by Rudolph et al., which observed significant improvement in MLHFQ scores in 104 patients with prohibitive surgical risk [20]. In a randomised controlled trial by Feldman et al., the MitraClip was compared to conventional surgery, showing HRQoL improvements in both groups [10]. Patients undergoing conventional procedures experienced a transient decrease in HRQoL 30-days post-surgery attributed to the invasive nature of the surgeries. In patients with life expectancy less than a year or two, this finding is likely to support the argument for percutaneous therapy.

Studies Comparing Against Conservative Management

Both studies from Arnold et al. and Krawczyk-Ożóg et al. showed that patients with MR secondary to HF treated conservatively had no difference in HRQoL at all follow-up timepoints [7, 14]. In contrast, patients treated with the MitraClip showed improvements in HRQoL post-operatively. Arnold et al. showed incrementally higher SF-36 scores at each timepoint, with early 1-month improvements sustained till the end of the 2-year follow-up period [7]. This was echoed in Krawczyk-Ożóg et al. which showed significant improvement in EQ-5D and SF-12v2 scores at follow-up, although the specific time of HRQoL measurement was not stated [14].

Studies Considering High-Risk or Frail Patients

A number of studies considered patients who were undergoing MitraClip implantation who were elderly, frail or of prohibitive surgical risk [9, 12, 15, 17, 20, 21, 24–26]. Edelman et al. was an early small cohort study looking at the use of MitraClip in 25 high-risk patients, showing improvements in MLHFQ and AQoL-6D scores from baseline [9]. This was also seen in a larger cohort study by Rudolph et al., 803 patients divided into groups based on NYHA functional class [21]. Baseline HRQoL varied between classes, with worsening HRQoL with increasing heart failure severity and class IV patients having the worst baseline EQ-5D scores. Although patients with class IV heart failure were also shown to have the worst HRQoL at 30-days post-MitraClip implantation, this was still significantly improved from baseline. Similarly, in a cohort study by Neuss et al., 157 very high-risk patients (all EuroSCORE >20) with severe heart failure showed persistent improvements in MLHFQ scores at 1-year post-MitraClip implantation. This HRQoL improvement was also shown in the EVEREST II trials performed by Glower et al., which studied a patient population with a significant proportion of patients in NYHA class III/IV [12]. In another prospective study in a high-risk population, Ussia et al. found significant improvement in all SF-12 components except for bodily pain [24]. Lim et al. evaluated treatment of MR in 141 patients at prohibitive surgical risk, finding improvements in both PCS and MCS of the SF-36 [15], and echoed in cohort studies by Van den Branden et al. [25] and Whitlow et al. [26]. This was also the case in a cohort study from Rudolph et al., which showed MLHFQ scores improving significantly in patients at prohibitive surgical risk. Again, scores improvements were comparable with those reported in MV surgery [20]. Finally, a post-approval study by Reichenspurner *et al.* considered the use of the MitraClip in both high-risk and low-risk groups of patients with degenerative MR. While overall HRQoL scores in the patient population improved at 12-months follow-up, the study unfortunately failed to determine if there was any significant differences between the improvements seen in either group [19].

Interestingly, a more recent study by Metze et al. showed while frail patients had similar improvements in SF-36 scores to non-frail patients after undergoing the MitraClip procedure, these frail patients showed significantly greater improvement MLHFQ scores. This suggests that patients previously considered unfit for conventional surgery should not only be considered for percutaneous therapy but might indeed benefit more from interventional therapies than fitter candidates, at least from a HRQoL point of view. This is also true for elderly candidates – while baseline HRQoL is worse with increasing age [22], HRQoL improvements are significant post-MitraClip intervention [15, 22] and comparable to population norms for the elderly population [15].

Miscellaneous Studies

The impact of anaemia was considered in a study by Hellhammer et al., which compared 41 anaemic patients to 39 patients without anaemia. While HRQoL improved in both groups, no significant difference was seen between the improvements in HRQoL between the groups [13]. Terhoeven et al. specifically observed the impact of MitraClip on the psychological and cognitive functioning of 40 patients using the SF-36, showing improved mental wellbeing post-MitraClip implantation [23].

Cardioband Implantation

The Cardioband Mitral system is a transcatheter device that aims to reduce annular reduction and thus reduce functional MR. Through deploying between 12 to 17 anchors around the mitral annulus, the Cardioband implant is affixed around the annulus. The implant is then used to cinch the diameter of the mitral annulus, improving the coaptation of the cusps and decreasing MR severity. Two prospective cohort studies reported outcomes on Cardioband implantation (Table 8.2)

Table 8.2 Cardioband

Author, publication year, study period, and study type	Study intent and no. of patients	Patient characteristics	Follow-up duration Time points at which HRQoL was measured	HRQoL instrument used Follow-up completion rate	Main findings related to HRQoL
Messika-Zeitoun et al. 2018 [27] 2013–2016 Prospective cohort study Multicentre (11 centres)	Reporting 1-year outcomes of patients undergoing the Cardioband (Edwards Lifesciences, Irvine, California) system 60 patients	Mean age 72 ± 7 years, 72% male, 87% NYHA III/IV, EuroSCORE II 7 ± 6%, STS-score 5 ± 6%	1 year Pre-op, 6 months and 12 months post-op	MLHFQ 65.0% at 12-months	MLHFQ scores improved at 6-months and maintained improvement at 12-months post-operatively
Nickenig et al. 2016 [28] February 2013–October 2014 Prospective cohort study Multicentre (5 centres)	Determine the safety and efficacy of the Cardioband (Edwards Lifesciences, Irvine, California) system 31 patients	Mean age 71.8 ± 6.9 years, 83.9% male, 97% NYHA III/IV, EuroSCORE II 8.6 ± 5.9%	6 months Pre-op, 6 months post-op	MLHFQ 91.7%	MLHFQ scores improved from baseline (38.2 ± 21) at the 6-month follow-up (18.1 ± 10.9)

[27, 28]. Nickenig et al. showed that MLHFQ scores improved from baseline at 6-month follow-up [28]. This was also seen in a more recent 1-year follow-up study by Messika-Zeitoun et al., with improvement of MLHFQ scores at 6-months. This improvement was sustained at 12-months post-operatively [27].

Carillon Mitral Contour Device

The Carillon Mitral Contour system is a right-heart transcatheter MV repair system designed for patients with functional MR. It is deployed and positioned within the coronary sinus or great cardiac vein, with the double-anchor designed to apply pressure onto the mitral annulus and improve the coaptation of the cusps by this modification of the annulus' shape. Three studies reported outcomes from the use of this device (Table 8.3 adapted from Tan et al. [6, 29, 31]).

Schofer et al. used the device as a therapeutic adjunct to standard care and showed 6-month post-intervention KCCQ scores to be significantly improved from baseline. In this score, the patient portion of the global assessment score was significantly improved in the majority of the 30 patients studied [29]. This was supported by the functional assessment of 14 patients after Carillon device implantation by Wołoszyn et al. [31]. KCCQ scores were improved at 1-month, comparable to the improvement seen by Schofer *et al.* [29]. This is likely due to the significant reduction in MR observed. A third study by

Table 8.3 Carillon Mitral Contour System

Author, publication year, study period, and study type	Study intent and no. of patients	Patient characteristics	Follow-up duration Time points at which HRQoL was measured	HRQoL instrument used Follow-up completion rate	Main findings related to HRQoL
Schofer et al. 2009 [29] Data collection period not reported Prospective cohort study (AMADEUS) Multicentre	Evaluation of novel coronary sinus-based mitral annuloplasty device as a therapeutic adjunct to standard medical care Mitral annuloplasty achieved in 30 patients (out of 48 enrolled) using the Carillon Mitral Contour System	Implanted patients ($n = 30$): mean age 64 ± 9 years, 87% male Nonimplanted patients ($n = 18$): mean age 65 ± 15 years, 78% male	6 months Pre-op, 1 and 6 months post-op	KCCQ Patient component of the global assessment 89.3% (25/28 survivors) for KCCQ 92.9% (26/28 survivors at 6 months) for global assessment	KCCQ Overall Summary Score was significantly improved between baseline and 6 months 84% patients reported some degree of improvement between baseline and 6 months in the patient portion of the global assessment score
Siminiak et al. 2012 [30] Data collection period not reported Non-randomised controlled trial (TITAN study) Multicentre (7 centres)	Determine percutaneous mitral annuloplasty (Carillon Mitral Contour System) effectiveness in reducing functional MR with long-term clinical benefit 53 patients 36 permanent implantations 17 recaptured device	Permanent implant group ($n = 36$): mean age 62.37 ± 12.67 years, 75% male Recaptured group ($n = 17$): mean age 62.59 ± 13.11 years, 82.4% male	12 months Pre-op, 1, 6, and 12 months post-op	KCCQ 81.6% at 12 months	Significantly higher HRQoL change in permanent implant group compared to recaptured group at 12 months follow-up

Table 8.3 (continued)

Author, publication year, study period, and study type	Study intent and no. of patients	Patient characteristics	Follow-up duration / Time points at which HRQoL was measured	HRQoL instrument used / Follow-up completion rate	Main findings related to HRQoL
Wołoszyn et al. 2011 [31] Data collection period not reported Prospective cohort study Poznan University of Medical Sciences, Poznan, Poland	Functional assessment of 14 patients who had undergone mitral annuloplasty using the Carillon Mitral Contour System	Mean age 61.1 ± 1.9 years, 78.6% male All had MR grade of 2–4	1 month Pre-op, 1 month post-op	KCCQ 92.9%	Mean HRQoL score improved

Siminiak et al. observed the effectiveness of the Carillon system in improving functional MR. This study compared patients with permanent implants to those who had recaptured devices, and those with the permanent implants had higher HRQoL at 1-year follow-up [30].

Studies Including Other Percutaneous MV Interventions

Four studies reported outcomes from other percutaneous MV interventions (Table 8.4 adapted from Tan *et al.* [6, 32–35]). In a cohort study using the PASCAL repair system, Lim *et al.* showed early improvements in KCCQ and EQ-5D scores [33]. HRQoL improvements were seen in a study by Sorajja et al. which used a novel Tendyne prothesis, the only device designed to be an implanted MV valve replacement [35]. One study by MacHaalany et al. on the Viacor percutaneous transvenous mitral annuloplasty device was stopped prematurely after perioperative complications and mortality, observing no significant HRQOL benefits [34].

Finally, in a registry study using patients undergoing any transcatheter intervention from the Society of Thoracic Surgeons/American College of Cardiology Transcatheter Valve Therapy Registry, Arnold et al. looked at the changes in KCCQ scores at 30-day and 1-year post-intervention [32]. This registry study confirms the findings of the individual studies described in this chapter—HRQoL shows early improvement at 30-days and this improvement is maintained till 1-year follow-up. This study also performed a multivariate analysis of risk factors for lower HRQoL post-intervention, showing atrial fibrillation, permanent pacemakers, severe lung disease, long-term home oxygen therapy, and lower baseline HRQoL scores to be associated with poorer HRQoL at early follow-up.

Discussion

This chapter provides a comprehensive overview of the current state of literature detailing HRQoL after percutaneous MV interventions, with predictors of poor HRQoL after such interventions summarised in Fig. 8.1. There is an increasing burden of MV disease with an ageing population [36] and this population is usually deemed to be of high surgical risk and unable to withstand the stresses of invasive surgery. Indeed, up to 50% are declined for conventional MVr or MVR [37, 38]. Thus, there is increasing requirements for less invasive therapeutic approaches, with development of multiple transcatheter or percutaneous devices to meet this demand.

Table 8.4 Other Percutaneous MV Intervention

Author, publication year, study period, and study type	Study intent and no. of patients	Patient characteristics	Follow-up duration	HRQoL instrument used	Main findings related to HRQoL
			Time points at which HRQoL was measured	Follow-up completion rate	
Arnold et al. 2018 [32] November 2013–March 2017 Prospective cohort study Multicentre (217 centres)	Examine health status outcomes in transcatheter mitral valve repair (device used not specified) patients and the factors associated with improvement 4226 patients at 30-days, 1124 patients at 1-year	30 days cohort: median age 81 years, 53.2% male, median STS-score 5.7% 1 year cohort: median age 82 years, 53.2% male, median STS-score 5.5%	1 year	KCCQ	KCCQ overall summary score significantly increased from 41.9 baseline to 66.7 at 30 days, with scores remaining stable until 1-year follow-up Multivariate analysis revealed atrial fibrillation, permanent pacemakers, severe lung disease, home oxygen, and lower baseline KCCQ scores to be associated with lower 30-day scores
			Pre-op, and 30 days and 12 months post-op	69.3% at 30 days 47.4% at 1 year	
Lim et al. 2019 [33] June 2017 – September 2018 Prospective cohort study Multicentre (14 centres)	Describe early outcomes following the use of the PASCAL repair system (Edwards Lifesciences, Irvine, California) for MR 62 patients	Mean age 76.5 ± 8.8 years, 62.9% male	30 days	KCCQ EQ-5D	KCCQ and EQ-5D scores improved with intervention
			Pre-op and 30 days post-op	96.8% KCCQ 91.9% EQ-5D	
MacHaalany et al. 2013 [34] October 2008–September 2010 Non-randomised controlled trial Multicentre	Evaluate effectiveness of permanent percutaneous transvenous mitral annuloplasty (Viacor device) in reducing MR43 patients recruited, with 30 patients implanted	Mean age 71.6 ± 11.0 years, 63% male	Mean follow-up 5.8 ± 3.8 months	MLHFQEQ-5D	No consistent improvement in HRQoL was documented
			Pre-op and 1, 3, 6 and 12 months post-op	10.0% at 12-months	
Sorajja et al. 2019 [35] November 2014–November 2017 Prospective cohort study Multicentre	Analysis of the first 100 patients treated with a novel prosthesis (Tendyne prosthesis, Abbott Structural, Santa Clara, California)	Mean age 75.4 ± 8.1 years, 69% male, 66% NYHA III/IV, STS-PROM 7.8 ± 5.7%	12 months	KCCQ	KCCQ scores increased significantly with improvements occurring from 1-month post-op KCCQ improved by ≥5 points in 81.3% and ≥10 points in 73.4% of survivors
			Pre-op, 1, 3, 6, and 12 months post-op	87.5% at 12 months	

Fig. 8.1 Predictors of poor HRQoL after transcatheter mitral valve interventions

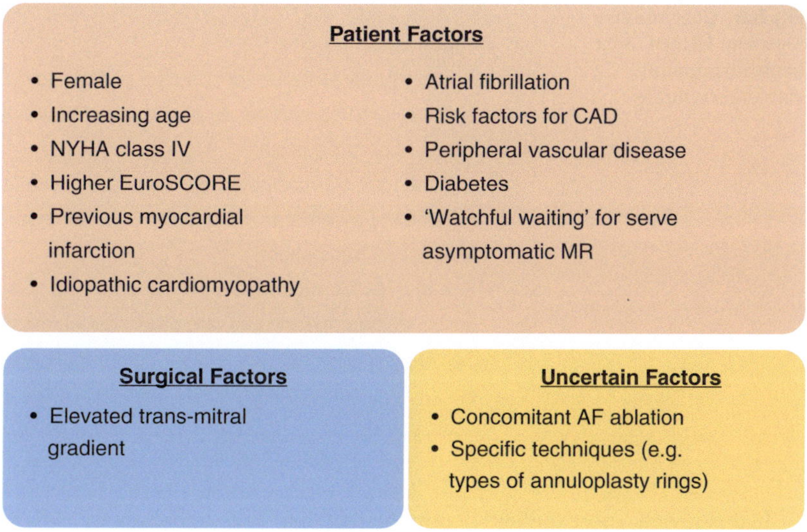

Patient Factors

- Female
- Increasing age
- NYHA class IV
- Higher EuroSCORE
- Previous myocardial infarction
- Idiopathic cardiomyopathy
- Atrial fibrillation
- Risk factors for CAD
- Peripheral vascular disease
- Diabetes
- 'Watchful waiting' for serve asymptomatic MR

Surgical Factors

- Elevated trans-mitral gradient

Uncertain Factors

- Concomitant AF ablation
- Specific techniques (e.g. types of annuloplasty rings)

It is promising that most studies confirm that HRQoL improves significantly post-intervention. It is further important to note that the level of post-interventional HRQoL in the patient population is comparable to healthy age-matched populations, including both the elderly and high-risk populations.

Study Limitations

While most studies provided a breakdown of aetiology leading to MV pathology, majority of studies unfortunately did not analyse baseline or HRQoL improvements according to aetiology. Of the 29 studies, many were of observational design with only two (6.9%) having randomisation included in their study design. The absence of randomisation resulted in considerable differences between baseline characteristics of patient cohorts—the typical MV patient presents with multiple chronic co-morbidities and various sequelae from MV disease. Furthermore, HRQoL instruments used and follow-up periods were significantly different between studies, making it difficult to compare outcomes between patients, interventions, and studies.

Whilst the MitraClip was the first of its kind which was designed specifically for a high-risk population, there has been a lack of studies reporting HRQoL after the use of other devices. Of the 29 studies currently available in the literature, nine (31.0%) were on devices other than the MitraClip. Additionally, twelve of these studies (60.0%) reported significant involvement of Abbott Vascular, with authors disclosing links to the company [8, 11, 12, 15, 16, 20, 22, 25, 26] or direct funding [7, 10, 21]. This, while not conclusive, might suggest institutional bias, with increased emphasis on this device due to increased funding. Studies might also fail to report poor outcomes due to conflicts of interest.

Suggestions for Further Research

It is recognised that patients value HRQoL more than clinical variables which are of more interest to clinicians and academics. HRQoL should become an essential tool to evaluate patient-centred benefits in the assessment of established as well as novel transcatheter MV devices. While most studies included in this review used the SF-36 in the assessment of patients' HRQoL, there is no consensus as to which instrument is best in determining HRQoL in this unique patient population undergoing transcatheter MV interventions and whether a separate disease-specific instrument is required altogether.

Chapter Conclusions:
- Transcatheter MV interventions are performed on heterogenous populations
- Innovative percutaneous designs are increasing the populations in which intervention is possible
- HRQoL after transcatheter mitral valve interventions is generally acceptable
- HRQoL improvements are maintained even in high-risk populations (including elderly and frail patients)
- Future trials should measure HRQoL at specific timepoints to allow determination of early and late predictors of impaired HRQoL
- Focusing on HRQoL outcomes in future trials will be required to allow for design of a disease/intervention specific HRQoL instrument

Fig. 8.2 Conclusions regarding HRQoL after transcatheter mitral valve interventions

In this review, most studies support the fact that transcatheter MV interventions have a significant impact on both physical and mental functioning and this impact is maintained even in elderly and high surgical risk patients. The measurement of physical functioning should be improved further, especially with the improvement of technology in accelerometers and activity monitors. Further research should include activity monitors to monitor physical activity before and after intervention, providing concrete data to reinforce HRQoL conclusions. Wrist-worn accelerometers or even smartphone applications that exploit built-in accelerometers are increasingly available, and these should be incorporated in future studies [39, 40].

Quantifiable predictors of HRQoL changes must also be identified in future research. For example, physiological biomarkers [41] may allow more innovative analysis, correlating magnitude of improvement to changes in these markers. Radiological measures (e.g. leaflet stress from MRI and coaptation depth/degree of left ventricular remodeling from echocardiography) were not analysed in any of the studies and should be used as future markers of functional outcome.

Conclusion

Transcatheter MV interventions are performed on heterogenous populations, with both young and old patients, presenting with a wide range of co-morbidities. This study confirms that HRQoL benefits of transcatheter MV interventions is generally acceptable, with certain populations showing better HRQoL when compared to age- and/or gender-matched normal populations. This improvement is maintained even in high surgical risk, elderly, and frail patients, with innovative percutaneous designs limiting the invasiveness of these interventions (Fig. 8.2). However, there are limitations in the current literature. Future randomised studies would benefit from baseline and follow-up HRQoL measurements at specific time points—this is suggested to be done pre-operatively and at 1-month, 1-year and 5-years post-operatively, enabling the determining of early and late predictors of impaired HRQoL. A common HRQoL instrument should be established, or indeed designed, for disease-specific use in transcatheter MV intervention studies. This would further support detailed comparison between devices. Use of newer technologies such as physical activity monitors, physiological biomarkers and radiological markers (e.g. leaflet stress from MRI and echocardiography) should be used as innovative markers of functional outcome.

References

1. Black N. Patient reported outcome measures could help transform healthcare. BMJ. 2013;346:f167.
2. Department of Health, Guidance on the routine collection of Patient Reported Outcome Measures (PROMs). 2010.
3. American College of Cardiology/American Heart Association Task Force on Practice Guidelines,

Society of Cardiovascular Anesthesiologists, Society for Cardiovascular Angiography and Interventions, Society of Thoracic Surgeons, Bonow RO, Carabello BA, et al. ACC/AHA 2006 guidelines for the management of patients with valvular heart disease: a report of the American College of Cardiology/American Heart Association Task Force on Practice Guidelines (writing committee to revise the 1998 Guidelines for the Management of Patients With Valvular Heart Disease): developed in collaboration with the Society of Cardiovascular Anesthesiologists: endorsed by the Society for Cardiovascular Angiography and Interventions and the Society of Thoracic Surgeons. Circulation. 2006;114(5):e84–231.

4. Bonow RO, Carabello BA, Chatterjee K, de Leon AC, Faxon DP, Freed MD, et al. 2008 Focused update incorporated into the ACC/AHA 2006 guidelines for the management of patients with valvular heart disease: a report of the American College of Cardiology/American Heart Association Task Force on Practice Guidelines (Writing Committee to Revise the 1998 Guidelines for the Management of Patients With Valvular Heart Disease): endorsed by the Society of Cardiovascular Anesthesiologists, Society for Cardiovascular Angiography and Interventions, and Society of Thoracic Surgeons. Circulation. 2008;118(15):e523–661.
5. Vahanian A, Alfieri O, Andreotti F, Antunes MJ, Barón-Esquivias G, Baumgartner H, et al. Guidelines on the management of valvular heart disease (version 2012): the Joint Task Force on the Management of Valvular Heart Disease of the European Society of Cardiology (ESC) and the European Association for Cardio-Thoracic Surgery (EACTS). Eur J Cardio-Thorac Surg. 2012;42(4):S1–44.
6. Tan MK, Jarral OA, Thong EH, Kidher E, Uppal R, Punjabi PP, et al. Quality of life after mitral valve intervention. Interact Cardiovasc Thorac Surg. 2017;24(2):265–72.
7. Arnold SV, Chinnakondepalli KM, Spertus JA, Magnuson EA, Baron SJ, Kar S, et al. Health status after transcatheter mitral-valve repair in heart failure and secondary mitral regurgitation: COAPT trial. J Am Coll Cardiol. 2019;73(17):2123–32.
8. Buzzatti N, Maisano F, Latib A, Taramasso M, Denti P, La Canna G, et al. Comparison of outcomes of percutaneous MitraClip versus surgical repair or replacement for degenerative mitral regurgitation in octogenarians. Am J Cardiol. 2015;115(4):487–92.
9. Edelman JJB, Dias P, Passage J, Yamen E. Percutaneous mitral valve repair in a high-risk Australian series. Heart Lung Circ. 2014;23(6):520–6.
10. Feldman T, Foster E, Glower DD, Kar S, Rinaldi MJ, Fail PS, et al. Percutaneous repair or surgery for mitral regurgitation. N Engl J Med. 2011;364(15):1395–406.
11. Franzen O, van der Heyden J, Baldus S, Schlüter M, Schillinger W, Butter C, et al. MitraClip® therapy in patients with end-stage systolic heart failure. Eur J Heart Fail. 2011;13(5):569–76.
12. Glower DD, Kar S, Trento A, Lim DS, Bajwa T, Quesada R, et al. Percutaneous mitral valve repair for mitral regurgitation in high-risk patients: results of the EVEREST II study. J Am Coll Cardiol. 2014;64(2):172–81.
13. Hellhammer K, Balzer J, Zeus T, Rammos C, Niebel S, Kubatz L, et al. Percutaneous mitral valve repair using the MitraClip® system in patients with anemia. Int J Cardiol. 2015;184:399–404.
14. Krawczyk-Ożóg A, Siudak Z, Sorysz D, Hołda MK, Płotek A, Dziewierz A, et al. Comparison of clinical and echocardiographic outcomes and quality of life in patients with severe mitral regurgitation treated by MitraClip implantation or treated conservatively. Postępy W Kardiologii Interwencyjnej. Adv Interv Cardiol. 2018;14(3):291.
15. Lim DS, Reynolds MR, Feldman T, Kar S, Herrmann HC, Wang A, et al. Improved functional status and quality of life in prohibitive surgical risk patients with degenerative mitral regurgitation after transcatheter mitral valve repair. J Am Coll Cardiol. 2014;64(2):182–92.
16. Maisano F, Franzen O, Baldus S, Schäfer U, Hausleiter J, Butter C, et al. Percutaneous mitral valve interventions in the real world: early and 1-year results from the ACCESS-EU, a prospective, multicenter, nonrandomized post-approval study of the MitraClip therapy in Europe. J Am Coll Cardiol. 2013;62(12):1052–61.
17. Metze C, Matzik A-S, Scherner M, Körber MI, Michels G, Baldus S, et al. Impact of frailty on outcomes in patients undergoing percutaneous mitral valve repair. JACC Cardiovasc Interv. 2017;10(19):1920–9.
18. Neuss M, Schau T, Schoepp M, Seifert M, Hölschermann F, Meyhöfer J, et al. Patient selection criteria and midterm clinical outcome for MitraClip therapy in patients with severe mitral regurgitation and severe congestive heart failure. Eur J Heart Fail. 2013;15(7):786–95.
19. Reichenspurner H, Schillinger W, Baldus S, Hausleiter J, Butter C, Schäefer U, et al. Clinical outcomes through 12 months in patients with degenerative mitral regurgitation treated with the MitraClip® device in the ACCESS-EUrope Phase I trial. Eur J Cardiothorac Surg. 2013;44(4):e280–8.
20. Rudolph V, Knap M, Franzen O, Schlüter M, de Vries T, Conradi L, et al. Echocardiographic and clinical outcomes of MitraClip therapy in patients not amenable to surgery. J Am Coll Cardiol. 2011;58(21):2190–5.
21. Rudolph V, Huntgeburth M, von Bardeleben RS, Boekstegers P, Lubos E, Schillinger W, et al. Clinical outcome of critically ill, not fully recompensated, patients undergoing MitraClip therapy. Eur J Heart Fail. 2014;16(11):1223–9.
22. Taramasso M, Maisano F, Denti P, Latib A, La Canna G, Colombo A, et al. Percutaneous edge-to-edge repair in high-risk and elderly patients with degenerative mitral regurgitation: midterm outcomes in a single-center experience. J Thorac Cardiovasc Surg. 2014;148(6):2743–50.

23. Terhoeven V, Nikendei C, Cranz A, Weisbrod M, Geis N, Raake PW, et al. Effects of MitraClip on cognitive and psychological function in heart failure patients: the sicker the better. Eur J Med Res. 2019;24(1):14.
24. Ussia GP, Cammalleri V, Sarkar K, Scandura S, Immè S, Pistritto AM, et al. Quality of life following percutaneous mitral valve repair with the MitraClip System. Int J Cardiol. 2012;155(2):194–200.
25. Van den Branden BJ, Swaans MJ, Post MC, Rensing BJ, Eefting FD, Jaarsma W, et al. Percutaneous edge-to-edge mitral valve repair in high-surgical-risk patients: do we hit the target? JACC Cardiovasc Interv. 2012;5(1):105–11.
26. Whitlow PL, Feldman T, Pedersen WR, Lim DS, Kipperman R, Smalling R, et al. Acute and 12-month results with catheter-based mitral valve leaflet repair: the EVEREST II (Endovascular Valve Edge-to-Edge Repair) High Risk Study. J Am Coll Cardiol. 2012;59(2):130–9.
27. Messika-Zeitoun D, Nickenig G, Latib A, Kuck K-H, Baldus S, Schueler R, et al. Transcatheter mitral valve repair for functional mitral regurgitation using the Cardioband system: 1 year outcomes. Eur Heart J. 2019;40(5):466–72.
28. Nickenig G, Hammerstingl C, Schueler R, Topilsky Y, Grayburn PA, Vahanian A, et al. Transcatheter mitral annuloplasty in chronic functional mitral regurgitation: 6-month results with the Cardioband percutaneous mitral repair system. JACC Cardiovasc Interv. 2016;9(19):2039–47.
29. Schofer J, Siminiak T, Haude M, Herrman JP, Vainer J, Wu JC, et al. Percutaneous mitral annuloplasty for functional mitral regurgitation: results of the CARILLON Mitral Annuloplasty Device European Union Study. Circulation. 2009;120(4):326–33.
30. Siminiak T, Wu JC, Haude M, Hoppe UC, Sadowski J, Lipiecki J, et al. Treatment of functional mitral regurgitation by percutaneous annuloplasty: results of the TITAN Trial. Eur J Heart Fail. 2012;14(8):931–8.
31. Wołoszyn M, Jerzykowska O, Kałmucki P, Link R, Firek L, Kuzemczak M, et al. Functional assessment of patients after percutaneous mitral valvuloplasty with Carillon™ device: a preliminary report. Kardiol Pol. 2011;69(3):228–33.
32. Arnold SV, Li Z, Vemulapalli S, Baron SJ, Mack MJ, Kosinski AS, et al. Association of transcatheter mitral valve repair with quality of life outcomes at 30 days and 1 year: analysis of the transcatheter valve therapy registry. JAMA Cardiol. 2018;3(12):1151–9.
33. Lim DS, Kar S, Spargias K, Kipperman RM, O'Neill WW, Ng MK, et al. Transcatheter valve repair for patients with mitral regurgitation: 30-day results of the CLASP study. JACC Cardiovasc Interv. 2019;12(14):1369–78.
34. MacHaalany J, Bilodeau L, Hoffmann R, Sack S, Sievert H, Kautzner J, et al. Treatment of functional mitral valve regurgitation with the permanent percutaneous transvenous mitral annuloplasty system: results of the multicenter international Percutaneous Transvenous Mitral Annuloplasty System to Reduce Mitral Valve Regurgitation in Patients with Heart Failure trial. Am Heart J. 2013;165(5):761–9.
35. Sorajja P, Moat N, Badhwar V, Walters D, Paone G, Bethea B, et al. Initial feasibility study of a new transcatheter mitral prosthesis: the first 100 patients. J Am Coll Cardiol. 2019;73(11):1250–60.
36. Nkomo VT, Gardin JM, Skelton TN, Gottdiener JS, Scott CG, Enriquez-Sarano M. Burden of valvular heart diseases: a population-based study. Lancet. 2006;368(9540):1005–11.
37. Taramasso M, Cioni M, Giacomini A, Michev I, Godino C, Montorfano M, et al. Emerging approaches of transcatheter valve repair/insertion. Cardiol Res Pract. 2010;2010:540749.
38. Preston-Maher GL, Torii R, Burriesci G. A technical review of minimally invasive mitral valve replacements. Cardiovasc Eng Technol. 2015;6(2):174–84.
39. Jarral OA, Kidher E, Patel VM, Nguyen B, Pepper J, Athanasiou T. Quality of life after intervention on the thoracic aorta. Eur J Cardiothorac Surg. 2016;49(2):369–89.
40. Tan MKH, Wong JKL, Bakrania K, Abdullahi Y, Harling L, Casula R, et al. Can activity monitors predict outcomes in patients with heart failure? A systematic review. Eur Heart J. 2019;5(1):11–21.
41. Bergler-Klein J, Gyöngyösi M, Maurer G. The role of biomarkers in valvular heart disease: focus on natriuretic peptides. Can J Cardiol. 2014;30(9):1027–34.

Percutaneous Interventions in Adult Congenital Heart Disease

9

Ana Barradas-Pires, Andrew Constantine, and Konstantinos Dimopoulos

Introduction

The emergence of a population of adults with congenital heart disease with reduced quality of life.

The field of adult congenital heart disease (ACHD) serves an emerging group of patients, who have benefitted greatly from improvements in surgical and percutaneous techniques. Prior to the 1970, half of the children with congenital heart disease (CHD) did not survive to adulthood. Current management results in over 90% of patients born with CHD reaching adulthood and, in Europe alone, this has translated into an ACHD population of over two million, and growing [1, 2].

A. Barradas-Pires
Adult Congenital Heart Centre and Centre for Pulmonary Hypertension, Cardiology Department, Royal Brompton Hospital, Guy's and St Thomas' NHS Foundation Trust, London, UK

Autonomous University of Barcelona, Barcelona, Spain

School of Public Health, Imperial College London, London, UK

A. Constantine · K. Dimopoulos (✉)
Adult Congenital Heart Centre and Centre for Pulmonary Hypertension, Cardiology Department, Royal Brompton Hospital, Guy's and St Thomas' NHS Foundation Trust, London, UK

Biomedical Research Unit, National Heart & Lung Institute, Imperial College London, London, UK

ACHD encompasses a wide spectrum of conditions of different severities. The prevalence of CHD has increased over time, but there has been a disproportionate increase in the proportion of patients with CHD of moderate or severe anatomic complexity, often with associated genetic syndromes and residual haemodynamic lesions even after successful repair [3]. Patients with repaired tetralogy of Fallot, for example, often present with pulmonary regurgitation, which requires further surgery. Depending on the underlying condition, ACHD patients are at risk of developing cardiac arrhythmias, heart failure, pulmonary hypertension and other extra-cardiac disease, such as kidney, liver and musculoskeletal abnormalities [4, 5]. As they age, ACHD patients are not spared from age-related acquired conditions, such as coronary atherosclerosis, cerebrovascular disease and dementia [6]. In recent years, ever more patients with extremely complex anatomy (e.g., hypoplastic left heart syndrome), survive to teenage and adult life and pose major challenges to paediatric and ACHD physicians. New structural and arrhythmic targets require novel transcatheter and surgical techniques to prevent and treat complications, thus, ensuring a good quality of life for these patients.

Despite CHD being a relatively rare cardiovascular condition within the wider cardiology population, the ACHD population is expanding rapidly and requires life-long highly specialised and multidisciplinary care. This comes at a sig-

T. Athanasiou et al. (eds.), *Patient Reported Outcomes and Quality of Life in Cardiovascular Interventions*,
https://doi.org/10.1007/978-3-031-09815-4_9

nificant cost to healthcare systems, both in terms of budget allocation and resource utilisation; such costs are likely to increase in the future, in parallel to the size and complexity of this population [7]. Our efforts and resources should be targeted towards achieving meaningful outcomes for our patients, in terms of morbidity, mortality and quality of life and care.

Quality of Care in Adults with Congenital Heart Disease

Healthcare quality indicators are typically developed based on the recommendations provided by international clinical guidelines, which use scientific evidence and expert opinion to inform standards of care. In ACHD, there is limited evidence and most guideline recommendations are based on expert consensus [8]. Indeed, CHD is a rare and heterogeneous condition, hence large randomised control trials are not feasible [9]. The development of robust quality indicators in ACHD is limited by the quality of the available evidence, which derives mostly from single-centre retrospective cohort studies and few small, randomised trials. The absence of established, disease-specific quality standards makes it challenging for individual ACHD centres and healthcare providers to measure and compare their outcomes in terms of efficiency, cost and user satisfaction.

In cardiovascular trials, classical or "hard" clinical endpoints such as all-cause and cardiovascular mortality, sudden cardiac death, transplantation and reoperation have been used to assess the efficacy of healthcare interventions and are considered acceptable surrogates of the quality of care. More recently, quality of health care measures have been broadened to incorporate patients' preferences and satisfaction levels, with the intent to deliver care in line with user needs and priorities. Indeed, the purely clinical outcomes listed above fail to capture patients' views and perceptions about their own health and care, and may not always match the priorities of the patient, e.g. how a procedure impacts on one's physical ability or mental health [10].

As a result of this unmet need, instruments to analyse patient-reported outcomes, or patient-reported outcome measures (PROMs), have been developed. PROMs are usually assessed by questionnaires, which might query general domains (such as patients' general wellbeing, quality of life [QoL], etc) or be focused on more disease-specific characteristics. It is worth mentioning that, although most PROMS studies use tools to assess specifically health-related quality of life (HRQoL) domains, QoL is a much broader concept, and incorporates unrelated healthcare dimensions such as social and familiar well-being.

Questionnaires assessing quality of life (mainly HRQoL) had their popularity increasing over time within general cardiology. The CHD field was also quick to embracing such instruments: the first article on QoL in adolescents with CHD was published in 1974 [11], and since then more than two hundred articles have been published on HRQoL and QoL in CHD patients up to 2019 [12, 13], even though knowledge gaps still persist.

Why use Quality of Life Indicators in Adults with Congenital Heart Disease?

ACHD field is well-suited for using PROMs and QoL measures in clinical care. It is a chronic, lifelong condition with frequent long-term complications and need for reinterventions. Many patients are reaching adulthood after multiple surgeries and other procedures, with the knowledge that they will require lifelong specialist follow-up. Exercise intolerance is also common in this population and influences the choices they make in life regarding sports, occupation and even family planning. The multiple challenges these patients face throughout their lives can impact on their individual perception of health, though little is known about the mechanisms and long-term implications of this perception.

The mantra of QoL research, that "living well is as important to most people as living longer", is especially true for CHD patients of all ages, who often have a worse QoL than control subjects [14]. For example, Matsuda et al. reported that at least 30% of children assessed one year after cardiac surgery described significant chronic pain, which considerably impaired their perceived health status [15]. Understanding the potential trade-off between conventional clinical endpoints versus QoL outcomes in ACHD would help model future research and help put patient priorities at the centre of future studies.

Challenges in Quality of Life Research in Adults with Congenital Heart Disease

In the last four decades, the ACHD community has conducted multiple studies involving QoL and PROMs in a variety of settings, but results are not consistent across the literature and are not extensive to all types of CHD [13]. Factors that contribute to these discrepancies are described below.

Firstly, a major challenge has been the lack of a uniform definition of QoL, which can be a broad and ambiguous concept. Moon and colleagues defined QoL as "the degree of overall life satisfaction that is positively or negatively influenced by an individual's perception of certain aspects of life that are important to them, including matters both related and unrelated to health" [16]. It is accepted that QoL is a multidimensional construct that goes beyond a health-care-related ideal, and incorporates non-medical domains such as family, social and work-related variables [16]. In ACHD, determinants of QoL would encompass domains such as demography (age, sex, nationality, education level, marital and employment status), family environment, support structure, physical status and spirituality (Fig. 9.1) [13, 14, 17]. Psychological factors, such as personality type, feelings of loneliness and the presence of depression or anxiety, also play an important role in perceived health status. More recently, the idea of the "sense of coherence" (SOC) was recognised as an important psychological tool for wellbeing. SOC is a measure of psychological resilience and is described as a life orientation or "personal way of thinking, being and acting, with an inner trust, which leads people to identify, benefit, use and re-use the resources at their disposal" [18, 19]. SOC questionnaire scores correlate well with the perceived health-related QoL in ACHD patients, even to a greater degree than exercise capacity [20]. ACHD patients often have a strong SOC, seeing the world as more predictable, manageable and meaningful than controls, perhaps as a result of the early onset of disease (typically diagnosed in childhood). This greater SOC enables the development of coping mechanisms against adversities and may be one reason why, in some studies, ACHD patients report a better QoL than healthy counterparts [20, 21].

Secondly, conceptual and methodological limitations in QoL research also account for some of the differences in the results of various CHD studies. Moon et al. appraised more than 70 articles focused on QoL in children and adults with CHD and found that the majority had significant methodological and conceptual problems [16]. Drawing conclusions from such studies is problematic. One of the first systematic reviews of QoL in ACHD, published in 2013, compiled data from more than 30 articles that used a wide spectrum of methodologies (varying definitions of QoL, use of matched controls, etc.) and at least 10 distinct QoL tools [22]. Most studies concluded that the CHD population experience a reduced physical function, but similar psychological and social functions to the general population. Overall, QoL in CHD was "worse, similar or even better" compared to matched controls, depending on the study analysed [14]. This is unhelpful in directing resources and aiding decision-making for healthcare professionals looking after these patients. The relation between CHD complexity and QoL is also inconsistent. In one meta-analysis of 33 studies and 4100 patients, data on the 36-item Short Form survey questionnaire (SF-36) pointed towards an inverse relationship of CHD complexity to physical function and general health perception [23]. This finding was not confirmed in a more recent synthesis of the literature, with no significant difference in QoL in young adult CHD patients when com-

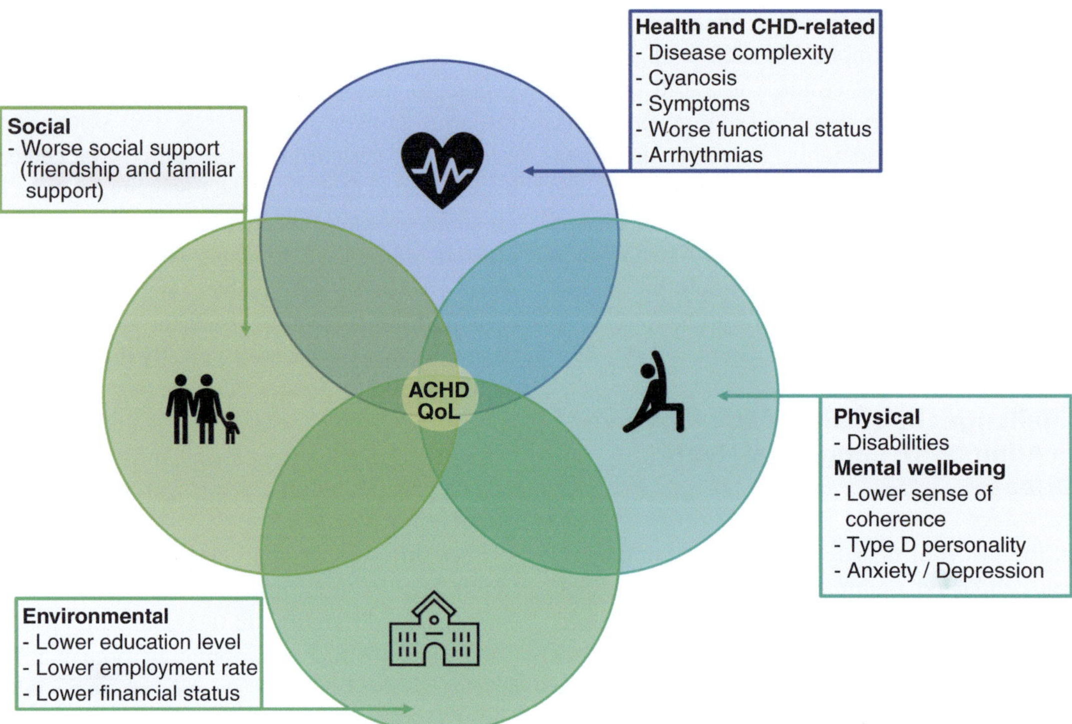

Fig. 9.1 Venn diagram representing the dimensions (in bold) and predictors of poor quality of life (QoL) in adult congenital heart disease (ACHD). (Adapted from [14, 25])

pared with age-matched controls, even after adjusting by disease complexity [24].

Thirdly, the multiplicity and heterogeneity of instruments used to assess QoL in CHD may also contribute to disparities in the results. At least 40 separate measures and variables have been used to assess QoL in CHD across the literature, including some older, more crude variables, such as the New York Heart Association (NYHA) functional class, 6-minute walk test and even simple symptoms description [16].

Finally, the lifelong nature of ACHD poses an additional major challenge to the assessment of QoL. Patients are usually followed from birth or early childhood, through adolescence, to adulthood. QoL measures and PROMs need to capture the changes in QoL after important treatment landmarks, such as surgery or interventional procedures, but also across different stages of their lives. The definition of QoL should, therefore, retain a dynamic component. Moon and colleagues exemplified this by showing that friendship is a core component of QoL in adolescents and young adults, but family and health become more important with age [25]. Therefore, a good QoL tool should capture the evolving nature of a patient's priorities.

Quality of Life Assessment Tools in ACHD

The most frequently used QoL assessment tools in ACHD are **generic** health-related QoL instruments, such as the SF-36 and the EuroQol five-dimensional (EQ-5D) health questionnaires. The SF-36 was designed to assess health status across different clinical conditions and make comparisons with the general population, and the EQ-5D to create comparable health index scores based on the responses obtained on five main health dimensions. In ACHD patients, these tools can be too simplistic to capture the full range of QoL domains that may be relevant to ACHD patients of different ages with different anatomies and previous palliative or corrective surgery. More **disease-specific tools** are also available, such as the Netherlands Organisation for Applied Scientific Research Academic Medical Centre (TNO-AZL) adult quality of life questionnaire (TAAQOL). The TAAQOL started as a generic Dutch health questionnaire and was further developed to focus on cardiac diseases, especially in the CHD field (CHD-TAAQOL) [26]. This tool aims to identify impairment in different health components (motor and social functioning, sleep, pain, etc) and to capture, if present, the psychological effect of those limitations. It also assesses the changes in QoL after surgical and interventional procedures. Finally, the most comprehensive and holistic assessment tools involve **open or semi-structured interviews** to capture information in a wide variety of domains [25]. Although open interviews can potentially uncover important topics for patients that might have been excluded from more structured questionnaires, the comparison of these results across individuals and different populations is often very challenging.

The potential utility and pitfalls of each one of these QoL instruments in the setting of ACHD interventional procedures are discussed later in this chapter.

Methods

QoL Tools in ACHD Interventions: Review of Existing Literature

In order to review the relation between QoL and percutaneous interventions in ACHD, we conducted a scoping review of the literature in the following electronic databases: PubMed online libraries, Google Scholar, and ClinicalTrials.gov (search date 1st February 2020). Furthermore, we manually examined reference lists from all selected articles and reviews to identify additional studies. Non-English language papers, for which an English translation was not available, were excluded.

As authors often use the terms 'quality of life', 'health status', 'functional status', 'HRQoL' and 'well-being' interchangeably, all studies using these terms were included. Nevertheless, we excluded all publications in which QoL was solely assessed using the NYHA functional class.

Results

Summary of Interventions

PROMs, mainly as HRQoL measures, have been used in the assessment of three types of percutaneous procedure:

- Percutaneous pulmonary valve implantation (PPVI)
- Percutaneous atrial septal defect (ASD) closure
- Percutaneous patent foramen ovale (PFO) closure

A description of the results obtained are described in the Table 9.1.

Percutaneous Pulmonary Valve Implantation

Three studies on QoL after percutaneous pulmonary valve implantation were identified. In a prospective, single-centre study of patients receiving PPVI with Melody (n = 56) or Sapien (n = 3) valves, Muller and colleagues found that almost all 8 domains assessed in the SF-36 questionnaire improved at 6 months following the procedure, accompanied by a significant improvement in peak oxygen uptake on cardiopulmonary exercise testing [27]. The authors found the QoL improvement was disproportionately higher than the change in peak oxygen uptake, which the authors suggested could have been due to a favourable perception of the minimally invasive intervention when compared to their previous experience of open-heart surgery.

Hager et al. measured QoL both at 6 months and 5 years after PPVI using the EQ-5D QoL utility index and a visual analogue scale (VAS) [28]. Improvement in utility scores and VAS were

Table 9.1 Studies using quality of life and patient reported outcome measures to assess the effectiveness of percutaneous procedures in adult congenital heart disease (ACHD)

	References	Study design	*N* (int. / control)	Age	Sex (% female)	Follow-up (months)	Instrument(s) used	Matching variables	Key findings
PPVI	Andresen et al. 2014	Case series, cross-sectional	10/–	17 [7–30]	30	3–6	Semi-structured interview	–	Patients happy with percutaneous procedures. Resuming normal life quickly after procedure was greatly valued
	Muller et al.2014	Case series, longitudinal	53/–	23 [17–30]	29	0, 6	SF-36	–	General improvement in most SF-36 domains, particularly in physical domains
	Hager et al. 2018	Case series, longitudinal	63/–	22 ± 11	33	0, 6, 60	EQ-5D, VAS	–	Utility indexes and VAS significantly improved at 6 months and 5 years after intervention
Percutaneous ASD closure	Cohen et al. 2010	Non-randomized, control study, cross-sectional	27/27	69 ± 6	63	12–84	TAAQOL	Age, sex	Patients reported high/very high levels of QoL after intervention. Significantly better QoL reported by the controls
	Hanninen et al. 2011	Retrospective chart review and prospective questionnaire, cross-sectional	54/–	69 [60–86]	72	28	SF-36	Age-adjusted Canadian reference group	All SF-36 domains similar to age-matched controls after procedure
	Mangiafico et al. 2013	Case series, longitudinal	30/–	49 ± 17	53	1, 6, 12	MCQ (patient symptoms)	–	Great improvement in symptoms after procedure, particularly in patients >40 years
	Komar et al. 2014	Case series, longitudinal	75/–	65 ± 16	60	0, 12	SF-36	–	All SF-36 domains improved significantly after the procedure
	Eren et a. 2015	Case series, cross-sectional	69/69	40 ± 14	74	18	SF-36	Age, sex, economic status, education level, marital and employment status	All SF-36 domains similar to age-matched controls after procedure

Percutaneous PFO closure (post-stroke)	Cohen et al. 2010	Non-randomized, control study, cross-sectional	89/60	54 ± 12	58	Not specified	TAAQOL	Age	Participants reported high quality of life after procedure, with no significant differences with the control group
	Evola et al. 2013	Case series, longitudinal	34/–	46 ± 10	59	0, 6	SF-36	–	All SF-36 domains improved significantly after the procedure
	Mirzada et al. 2018	Case series, cross-sectional	208/136/208 (ref.)	51 ± 12	37	36–156	SF-36	Age- and gender-matched Swedish reference group	All SF-36 domains similar to age-matched controls after procedure. Non-closure PFO group had significantly lower scores than the closure group and the matched controls

ASD, atrial septal defect; MCQ, multiple choice questions; PFO, patent foramen ovale; PPVI, percutaneous pulmonary valve implantation; VAS, visual analogue scale

reported on both periods. The improvement in the utility indexes was related to the severity of right ventricular obstruction in those receiving PPVI for pulmonary stenosis. Nevertheless, improvement in pulmonary regurgitation after the procedure was not related to QoL improvement.

Through semi-structured interviews of patients and their next-of-kin at 3–6 months following PPVI, Andresen et al. were able to garner the priorities of patients undergoing this procedure. Those interviewed emphasised the importance of regaining independence and taking control of daily life following the intervention [29]. Compared to previous surgical management, patients reported the physical burden of the procedure as being "minimal", and the next-of-kin highlighted the importance of a timely return to normal life following the procedure.

Percutaneous Atrial Septal Defect Closure

Most studies assessing QoL after percutaneous ASD closure have focused on patients over 60 years of age. Cohen et al. reported that almost 80% of patients had a "good" or "very good" quality of life after ASD closure [30]. Nevertheless, when compared to age-matched controls, their QoL was still significantly lower. QoL in these patients was associated with depression and anxiety scores, but not with functional class. In a Canadian study that included older adults following both surgical and percutaneous ASD repair, patients achieved similar scores on SF-36 QoL questionnaires to age-matched controls [31], associated with an improvement in functional class. Komar et al. corroborated these results in a longitudinal study, assessing older adults at 12 months following percutaneous ASD closure [32]. Patients reported a significant improvement in all the SF-36 domains along with a significant improvement in exercise capacity.

In younger patients who underwent ASD closure, QoL scores after the procedure in the SF-36 were similar to the general population [33]. An Italian group described similar results, although the authors did not use a specific QoL instrument and chose to assess QoL based on functional class, physical capacity and symptoms [34].

Patient Foramen Ovale Closure (Post-Stroke)

A patent foramen ovale (PFO) is a common condition, affecting around one quarter of the general population [35]. It is not considered a congenital heart defect, but is often managed by CHD specialists, especially in rare cases when a PFO allows paradoxical emboli causing (otherwise cryptogenic) strokes in younger patients. A meta-analysis of observational studies has shown a stronger association of PFO with cryptogenic stroke in patients <55 years compared to older patients, particularly when atrial septal aneurysms are present [36]. PFO closure following a cerebrovascular event is often performed by CHD interventionalists, who have experience in the percutaneous closure of other intra-cardiac communications.

Cohen and colleagues were the first authors to study the QoL implications of PFO closure, using the TAAQOL instrument [37]. Participants were divided into 2 age-groups and their responses were compared to age-matched controls. After PFO closure, the reported QoL was high in both age groups, with no difference to the matched controls. Optimism, estimated with a life orientation test (LOT-R), was higher in patients than in the control group. Older age and financial status were correlated to anxiety, depression and worse QoL. These three domains were highly interrelated, and negatively associated to optimism.

Evola et al. reported a significant improvement in QoL, measured using the SF-36 questionnaire, at 6 months after PFO closure [38]. This was largely attributed to an improvement in migraine symptoms. In a long term follow-up study, 3–12 years after PFO closure, Mirzada et al. reported a sustained improvement in QoL over time after the procedure [39]. Importantly, patients after PFO closure reported similar QoL metrics to a group of matched healthy adults, which was not the case for the non-closure group who described significant impairment in their physical, vitality, and general health domains.

Discussion

QoL After Percutaneous Procedures in ACHD

Surgical closure of atrial septal defects of pulmonary valve implantation have been the gold-standard in the ACHD field for the last 50 years. Nevertheless, percutaneous procedures have gained notoriety in the last three decades. In terms of QoL, longitudinal CHD studies reported a consistent improvement in different HRQoL domains after percutaneous intervention. These results contrast with a few studies of HRQoL after surgical intervention, where QoL was described as impaired compared to the general population [40–42]. These difference seems more pronounced for motor domains in patients with complex anatomies [43]. In more simple procedures, such as ASD closure, a small study comparing HRQoL after percutaneous versus surgical procedures showed that, although both groups improved their QoL, the patients in the percutaneous intervention group reported better scores in some SF-46 dimensions than their surgical counterparts [44]. Shorter admissions and speedy recovery time can explain some of the differences reported, as the amount of physically disability after surgery is seen as a core determinant of poor health status. Patients especially mention the ability to resume their usual daily activities quickly as one of the main positive experiences of percutaneous interventions compared to their previous surgical experience. Nevertheless, it is important to remember that patients undergoing surgery are more likely to have more complex CHD, which, together with comorbidities and CHD-related complications, might also influence their self-perceived QoL.

The Utility of Different Quality of Life Tools in the Setting of Percutaneous Procedures in Adult Congenital Heart Disease

Overall, studies assessing HRQoL around percutaneous procedures in ACHD patients have used 3 main instruments: SF-36, EQ-5D and TAAQOL. Each tool aims to assess a different set of domains (Fig. 9.2). The QoL instrument most frequently used in percutaneous interventions in ACHD was the SF-36 questionnaire, which is a generic assessment tool and also the most frequently used PROM in clinical trials worldwide [45]. It assesses health status using 36 items focused on 8 "health perception" domains: physical functioning, social functioning, role limitations due to physical problems, role limitations due to emotional problems, mental health, vitality, pain, and general health perceptions. It has been used in a variety of populations and clinical scenarios, including ACHD [43]. Therefore, it is a good choice for enabling comparisons between clinical groups or with healthy controls. Nevertheless, extrapolating general QoL from the results of the SF-36 questionnaires requires caution, as this tool tends to link general health perceptions with "health-related disability", when we know that patients with disabilities might still feel overall "healthy" [2]. Another common pitfall in the use of the SF-36 is reporting a total score based on all 8 dimensions. Each questionnaire domains should be reported separately, and the overall score that is often calculated using different algorithms is not standardised and has conceptual and methodological drawbacks [46, 47].

Another generic instrument used to assess QoL in ACHD patients after a pulmonary valve implantation was the EQ-5D. This HRQoL tool has been used for over 30 years [48]. It is simpler than the SF-36 and developed to standardise the value of QoL associated with health. The EQ-5D instrument asks subjects to describe their health status in 5 specific domains (mobility, self-care, main activity, pain/discomfort and anxiety/depression) and then requests an evaluation of

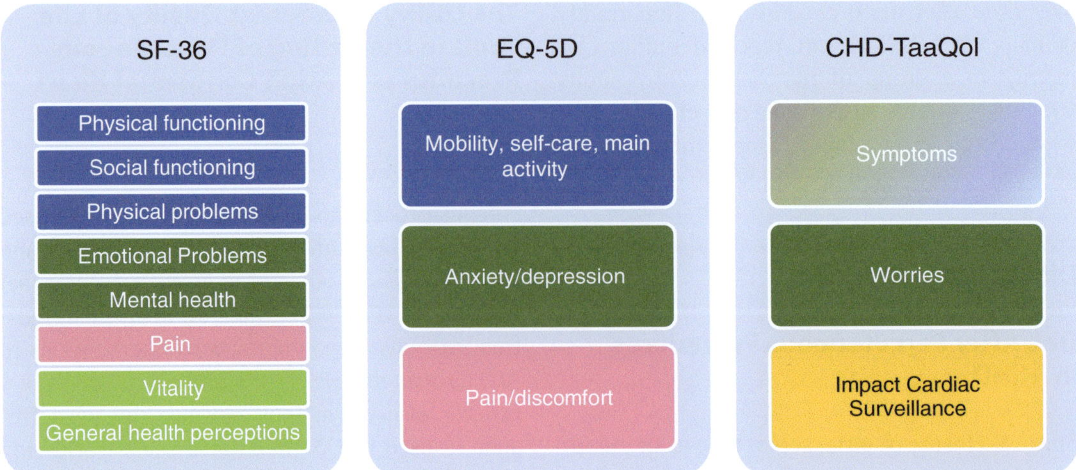

Fig. 9.2 Comparison of the domains included by the different tools used to investigate changes in quality of life (QoL) after percutaneous interventions in adult congenital heart disease (ACHD)

their "overall health status" using a Visual Analogue Scale (VAS). These components can be incorporated into one single index, facilitating comparison across different settings. As with the SF-36, however, this tool does not capture social or environmental domains, which are of interest in the ACHD population.

The third instrument used was the Netherlands Organisation for Applied Scientific Research Academic Medical Centre (TNO-AZL) adult quality of life questionnaire (TAAQOL). The TAAQOL was developed by Bruils et al. in 2001 as a generic HRQoL instrument [49, 50] and then adapted to the congenital cardiac setting by Kamphuis in 2004 under the name CHD-TAAQOL [26]. Since then, variations of this questionnaire have been validated in children, adolescents and adults with CHD. The TAAQOL tool has been used in 2 studies in this review, assessing patients following ASD and PFO closure [30, 37]. This tool focuses on three main domains: symptoms, worries, and the impact of cardiac surveillance on QoL. The final score ranges from 1 to 12 and, contrary to previous tools, higher scores describe a worse HRQoL. This tool is original for 2 reasons: firstly, it is designed to capture the perceptions and emotional reactions to illness; secondly, it aims to assesse the changes in a patient's QoL after surgery or other intervention. Both are particularly relevant to ACHD patients.

Overall, the instruments used to assess QoL after percutaneous interventions rely on PROMs that are often generic, simplistic and focused on health-related domains, therefore, interpretations on overall QoL should be avoided. Most of these tools also lack the sensitivity required to detect changes in QoL over time or around an intervention. New tools designed for the ACHD population are needed to better detect and report such changes, but these will need to be tested and validated against established measures. When reporting PROMs, statements should be limited to the dimensions directly assessed by the instruments used. Sweeping statements, such as that "QoL of patients with ACHD improves" after a given procedure, based only on the results of a single questionnaire, fail to recognise QoL as a broad, multidimensional concept and should be discouraged.

Comparison of PROMs with Other Established Health Outcomes

An association between functional class and QoL has previously been documented in ACHD patients, including those with cyanotic CHD or following a surgical procedure [42, 44]. Nevertheless, most studies assessing QoL in ACHD patients following percutaneous procedures failed to demonstrate a definitive link between QoL and more traditional outcome indicators, such as peak oxygen uptake, functional class or survival [51].

The association between QoL indicators and mortality was not addressed in any of the studies on percutaneous procedures in ACHD. In other settings, such as in patients with pulmonary arterial hypertension associated with CHD, negative changes in QoL measured by SF-36 questionnaires were identified as a mortality predictor, along with functional class, 6-min walk distance or BNP levels [52]. Favoccia et al. found that QoL measured by Emphasis-10 questionnaires in patients with pulmonary hypertension, including those with pulmonary arterial hypertension associated with CHD, was an independent predictor of mortality in addition to functional class or age [53]. In congenital patients with cyanosis or Eisenmenger syndrome, iron replacement therapy was also associated with an improvement in QoL [54].

This literature review has highlighted the significant heterogeneity in terms of methodology and population between studies measuring PROMs, including QoL, which is a significant barrier when attempting to compare or pool data (Table 9.2). Even within specific ACHD cohorts of patients undergoing the same procedure, study designs were heterogeneous, for example: longitudinal (such as pre- and post-procedural changes in QoL) versus cross-sectional; different control groups (local community versus general population or standardised QoL indices), etc. A wide range of QoL instruments were also used, from generic versus disease-specific, and directed questionnaires versus open-interview structures.

Table 9.2 Sources of heterogeneity encountered when measuring patient reported outcomes (PROMs) and quality of life (QoL) in adult congenital heart disease (ACHD) patients undergoing percutaneous interventions

Domain	Sources of heterogeneity
ACHD patients	Wide age range Anatomy and congenital heart disease complexity Pre-procedural symptoms
Procedure being assessed	First procedure, repeated or combined
Outcome measure	Choice of patient-reported outcome Definition of QoL
Scope, heterogeneity and applicability of QoL instruments/PROMs	Format of instrument (short questionnaire vs. semi-structured interview) QoL domains assessed Applicability to the ACHD population Reporting of results
Heterogeneity of study design	Longitudinal vs. cross-sectional Use and choice of control group

In order to expand and improve the use of HRQoL tools in daily practice worldwide, clinical guidelines and consensus statements should include QoL domains as desirable endpoints in cardiovascular studies and encourage its use in combination with more classical outcomes. This has been done for interventional procedures such as transcatheter aortic valve implantation (TAVI) and coronary interventions, where academic research consortiums have included QoL endpoints and provided guidance about tools and their interpretation [55, 56]. In the case of ACHD catheter interventions, to the best of our knowledge, no such guidance is yet available.

Concluding Remarks

QoL tools should be used more often in ACHD research and clinical practice and should complement functional status, imaging data and objective measures of exercise capacity (Fig. 9.3). PROMs associate with an intervention should be interpreted in a broader context, taking into account the patients' characteristics and all the factors that may influence their perception regarding the procedure's benefits and drawbacks (including age, CHD complexity and the presence of anxiety or depression).

Patient preference is fundamental in the management choices we make. The published ACHD QoL literature lacks standardisation in concepts and methodology, making it very difficult to compile and interpret outcomes. Standardisation is crucial in order to speak the same language and be able to compare information between different centres, diseases, ages etc. Moreover, particularly in the ACHD field where patients are followed throughout different stages of their lives, an effort to shift from health-related quality of life instruments to more comprehensive tools should be

Conclusions

1) Quality of life (QoL) tools should be used in clinical practice as complement to functional status, imaging data and objective measures of exercise capacity.

2) QoL in Adult Congenital Heart Disease (ACHD) extends beyond health-related dimensions, and its assessment should incorporate social, environmental, and physical and mental characteristics.

3) Patient-reported outcome measures in ACHD research should be able to capture the changes in QoL after important treatment landmarks, such as surgery or interventional procedures, but also across different stages of patients' lives. The definition of QoL should, therefore, retain a dynamic component.

4) Standardisation of QoL tools in research is key to compile and interpret outcomes from different studies.

5) Studies in health related QoL in ACHD suggest an improvement in some QoL domains after catheter interventions. Predictors of poor QoL after percutaneous interventions are scarce in ACHD research. Nevertheless, some studies have identified low educational or financial status, presence of symptoms and coexistence of depression / anxiety as poor predictors of QoL after procedures.

Fig. 9.3 Highlighted conclusions

made, so other significant QoL domains can be adequality captured and analysed in research, and then incorporated in our daily practice.

References

1. Khairy P, Ionescu-Ittu R, Mackie AS, Abrahamowicz M, Pilote L, Marelli AJ. Changing Mortality in Congenital Heart Disease. J Am Coll Cardiol. 2010;56:1149–57. https://doi.org/10.1016/j.jacc.2010.03.085.
2. Stout KK, Daniels CJ, Aboulhosn JA, Biykem B, Broberg CS, Colman JM, et al. AHA/ACC Guideline for the Management of Adults With Congenital Heart Disease: A Report of the American College of Cardiology/American Heart Association Task Force on Clinical Practice Guidelines. Circulation. 2018;2019(139):e698–800. https://doi.org/10.1161/CIR.0000000000000603.
3. Marelli AJ, Mackie AS, Ionescu-Ittu R, Rahme E, Pilote L. Congenital heart disease in the general population: changing prevalence and age distribution. Circulation. 2007;115:163–72. https://doi.org/10.1161/CIRCULATIONAHA.106.627224.
4. Neidenbach RC, Lummert E, Vigl M, Zachoval R, Fischereder M, Engelhardt A, et al. Non-cardiac comorbidities in adults with inherited and congenital heart disease: report from a single center experience of more than 800 consecutive patients. Cardiovasc Diagn Ther. 2018;8:423–31. https://doi.org/10.21037/cdt.2018.03.11.
5. Verheugt CL, Uiterwaal CSPM, van der Velde ET, Meijboom FJ, Pieper PG, van Dijk APJ, et al. Mortality in adult congenital heart disease. Eur Heart J. 2010;31:1220–9. https://doi.org/10.1093/eurheartj/ehq032.
6. Baumgartner H. Geriatric congenital heart disease: a new challenge in the care of adults with congenital heart disease? Eur Heart J. 2014;35:683–5. https://doi.org/10.1093/eurheartj/eht358.
7. Briston DA, Bradley EA, Sabanayagam A, Zaidi AN. Health Care Costs for Adults With Congenital Heart Disease in the United States 2002 to 2012. Am J Cardiol. 2016;118:590–6. https://doi.org/10.1016/j.amjcard.2016.05.056.
8. Fanaroff AC, Califf RM, Windecker S, Smith SC Jr, Lopes RD. Levels of Evidence Supporting American College of Cardiology/American Heart Association and European Society of Cardiology Guidelines, 2008–2018. JAMA. 2019;321:1069–80. https://doi.org/10.1001/jama.2019.1122.
9. Gurvitz M, Marelli A, Mangione-Smith R, Jenkins K. Building Quality Indicators to Improve Care for Adults With Congenital Heart Disease. J Am Coll Cardiol. 2013;62:2244. https://doi.org/10.1016/j.jacc.2013.07.099.
10. Øvretveit J, Zubkoff L, Nelson EC, Frampton S, Knudsen JL, Zimlichman E. Using patient-reported outcome measurement to improve patient care. Int J Qual Health Care. 2017;29:874–9. https://doi.org/10.1093/intqhc/mzx108.
11. Ferencz C. The Quality of Life the Adolescent Cardiac Patient. Postgrad Med. 1974;56:67–74. https://doi.org/10.1080/00325481.1974.11713904.
12. Bratt E-L, Moons P. Forty years of quality-of-life research in congenital heart disease: Temporal trends in conceptual and methodological rigor. Int J Cardiol. 2015;195:1–6. https://doi.org/10.1016/j.ijcard.2015.05.070.
13. Moons P, Luyckx K. Quality-of-life research in adult patients with congenital heart disease: current status and the way forward. Acta Paediatr. 2019;108:1765–72. https://doi.org/10.1111/apa.14876.
14. Apers S, Luyckx K, Moons P. Quality of Life in Adult Congenital Heart Disease: What Do We Already

Know and What Do We Still Need To Know? Curr Cardiol Rep. 2013;15:407. https://doi.org/10.1007/s11886-013-0407-x.
15. Matsuda M, Takemura H, Yamashita A, Matsuoka Y, Sawa T, Amaya F. Post-surgical chronic pain and quality of life in children operated for congenital heart disease. Acta Anaesthesiol Scand. 2019;63:745–50. https://doi.org/10.1111/aas.13346.
16. Moons P, Van Deyk K, Budts W, De Geest S. Caliber of Quality-of-Life Assessments in Congenital Heart Disease: A Plea for More Conceptual and Methodological Rigor. Arch Pediatr Adolesc Med. 2004;158:1062. https://doi.org/10.1001/archpedi.158.11.1062.
17. Apers S, Kovacs AH, Luyckx K, Thomet C, Budts W, Enomoto J, et al. Quality of Life of Adults With Congenital Heart Disease in 15 Countries. J Am Coll Cardiol. 2016;67:2237–45. https://doi.org/10.1016/j.jacc.2016.03.477.
18. Antonovsky A. Unraveling the mystery of health: How people manage stress and stay well. San Francisco, CA, US: Jossey-Bass; 1987.
19. Eriksson M, Lindström B. Antonovsky's sense of coherence scale and the relation with health: a systematic review. J Epidemiol Community Health. 2006;60:376–81. https://doi.org/10.1136/jech.2005.041616.
20. Müller J, Hess J, Hager A. Sense of coherence, rather than exercise capacity, is the stronger predictor to obtain health-related quality of life in adults with congenital heart disease. Eur J Prev Cardiol. 2014;21:949–55. https://doi.org/10.1177/2047487313481753.
21. Apers S, Moons P, Goossens E, Luyckx K, Gewillig M, Bogaerts K, et al. Sense of coherence and perceived physical health explain the better quality of life in adolescents with congenital heart disease. Eur J Cardiovasc Nurs. 2013;12:475–83. https://doi.org/10.1177/1474515113477955.
22. Fteropoulli T, Stygall J, Cullen S, Deanfield J, Newman SP. Quality of life of adult congenital heart disease patients: a systematic review of the literature. Cardiol Young. 2013;23:473–85. https://doi.org/10.1017/S1047951112002351.
23. Kahr PC, Radke RM, Orwat S, Baumgartner H, Diller G-P. Analysis of associations between congenital heart defect complexity and health-related quality of life using a meta-analytic strategy. Int J Cardiol. 2015;199:197–203. https://doi.org/10.1016/j.ijcard.2015.07.045.
24. Schrøder M, Boisen KA, Reimers J, Teilmann G, Brok J. Quality of life in adolescents and young adults with CHD is not reduced: a systematic review and meta-analysis. Cardiol Young. 2016;26:415–25. https://doi.org/10.1017/S104795111500181X.
25. Moons P, Van Deyk K, Marquet K, Raes E, De Bleser L, Budts W, et al. Individual quality of life in adults with congenital heart disease: a paradigm shift. Eur Heart J. 2005;26:298–307. https://doi.org/10.1093/eurheartj/ehi054.
26. Kamphuis M, Zwinderman KH, Vogels T, Vliegen HW, Kamphuis RP, Ottenkamp J, et al. A cardiac-specific health-related quality of life module for young adults with congenital heart disease: Development and validation. Qual Life Res. 2004;13:735–45. https://doi.org/10.1023/B:QURE.0000021690.84029.a3.
27. Müller J, Engelhardt A, Fratz S, Eicken A, Ewert P, Hager A. Improved exercise performance and quality of life after percutaneous pulmonary valve implantation. Int J Cardiol. 2014;173:388–92. https://doi.org/10.1016/j.ijcard.2014.03.002.
28. Hager A, Schubert S, Ewert P, Søndergaard L, Witsenburg M, Guccione P, et al. Five-year results from a prospective multicentre study of percutaneous pulmonary valve implantation demonstrate sustained removal of significant pulmonary regurgitation, improved right ventricular outflow tract obstruction and improved quality of life. EuroIntervention. 2017;12:1715–23. https://doi.org/10.4244/EIJ-D-16-00443.
29. Andresen B, Andersen MH, Lindberg H, Døhlen G, Fosse E. Perceived health after percutaneous pulmonary valve implantation: in-depth interviews of patients and next-of-kin. BMJ Open. 2014;4:e005102. https://doi.org/10.1136/bmjopen-2014-005102.
30. Cohen M, Daniela M, Yalonetsky S, Gagin R, Lorber A. Psychological functioning and health-related quality of life (HRQoL) in older patients following percutaneous closure of the secundum atrial septal defect (ASD). Arch Gerontol Geriatr. 2010;50:e5–8. https://doi.org/10.1016/j.archger.2009.04.003.
31. Hanninen M, Kmet A, Taylor DA, Ross DB, Rebeyka I, Muhll IFV. Atrial Septal Defect Closure in the Elderly Is Associated With Excellent Quality of Life, Functional Improvement, and Ventricular Remodelling. Can J Cardiol. 2011;27:698–704. https://doi.org/10.1016/j.cjca.2011.04.003.
32. Komar M, Przewlocki T, Olszowska M, Sobien B, Podolec P. The benefit of atrial septal defect closure in elderly patients*. Clin Interv Aging. 2014;9:1101–7. https://doi.org/10.2147/CIA.S62313.
33. Eren N, Kırdök AH, Kılıçaslan B, Kocabaş U, Düzel B, Berilgen R, et al. Quality of life of patients with atrial septal defect following percutaneous closure. Cardiol Young. 2015;25:42–6. https://doi.org/10.1017/S1047951113001479.
34. Mangiafico S, Monte IP, Tropea L, Lavanco V, Deste W, Tamburino C. Long-Term Results after Percutaneous Closure of Atrial Septal Defect: Cardiac Remodeling and Quality of Life. J Cardiovasc Echogr. 2013;23:53–9. https://doi.org/10.4103/2211-4122.123028.
35. Meissner I, Khandheria BK, Heit JA, Petty GW, Sheps SG, Schwartz GL, et al. Patent Foramen Ovale: Innocent or Guilty? J Am Coll Cardiol. 2006;47:440–5. https://doi.org/10.1016/j.jacc.2005.10.044.
36. Alsheikh-Ali AA, Thaler DE, Kent DM. Patent Foramen Ovale in Cryptogenic Stroke: Incidental or Pathogenic? Stroke. 2009;40:2349–55. https://doi.org/10.1161/STROKEAHA.109.547828.

37. Cohen M, Daniela M, Lorber A. Patent foramen ovale closure in post-CVA/TIA patients: psychological distress, quality of life and optimism: Patent foramen ovale closure and distress. Int J Clin Pract. 2009;64:182–7. https://doi.org/10.1111/j.1742-1241.2009.02251.x.
38. Evola S, Kauroo BAW, Trovato RL, Alioto L, D'Amico G, Fonte G, et al. The percutaneous closure of patent foramen ovale (PFO): Impact on the quality of life. Int J Cardiol. 2013;168:1622–3. https://doi.org/10.1016/j.ijcard.2013.01.015.
39. Mirzada N, Ladenvall P, Hansson P-O, Eriksson P, Taft C, Dellborg M. Quality of life after percutaneous closure of patent foramen ovale in patients after cryptogenic stroke compared to a normative sample. Int J Cardiol. 2018;257:46–9. https://doi.org/10.1016/j.ijcard.2018.01.120.
40. Landolt MA, Valsangiacomo Buechel ER, Latal B. Health-Related Quality of Life in Children and Adolescents after Open-Heart Surgery. J Pediatr. 2008;152:349–55. https://doi.org/10.1016/j.jpeds.2007.07.010.
41. Ladak LA, Hasan BS, Gullick J, Gallagher R. Health-related quality of life in congenital heart disease surgery in children and young adults: a systematic review and meta-analysis. Arch Dis Child. 2019;104:340–7. https://doi.org/10.1136/archdischild-2017-313653.
42. Pragt H, Pieper PG, van Slooten YJ, Freling HG, van Dijk APJ, Sieswerda GTJ, et al. Quality of Life Among Patients With Congenital Heart Disease After Valve Replacement. Semin Thorac Cardiovasc Surg. 2019;31:549–58. https://doi.org/10.1053/j.semtcvs.2019.02.002.
43. Kamphuis M. Health related quality of life and health status in adult survivors with previously operated complex congenital heart disease. Heart. 2002;87:356–62. https://doi.org/10.1136/heart.87.4.356.
44. Sun K-P, Xu N, Huang S-T, Chen L-W, Cao H, Chen Q. Comparison of Short-Term Quality of Life between Percutaneous Device Closure and Surgical Repair via Median Sternotomy for Atrial Septal Defect in Adult Patients. J Investig Surg. 2020:1–8. https://doi.org/10.1080/08941939.2020.1793037.
45. Scoggins JF, Patrick DL. The use of patient-reported outcomes instruments in registered clinical trials: Evidence from ClinicalTrials.gov. Contemp Clin Trials. 2009;30:289–92. https://doi.org/10.1016/j.cct.2009.02.005.
46. Lins L, Carvalho FM. SF-36 total score as a single measure of health-related quality of life: Scoping review. SAGE Open Med. 2016;4:2050312116671725. https://doi.org/10.1177/2050312116671725.
47. Hays RD, Hahn H, Marshall G. Use of the SF-36 and other health-related quality of life measures to assess persons with disabilities. Arch Phys Med Rehabil. 2002;83:S4–9. https://doi.org/10.1053/apmr.2002.36837.
48. EQ-5D n.d.. https://euroqol.org/. Accessed February 23, 2020.
49. Bruil J, Fekkes M, Vogels T, Verrips E. The validity and reliability of the TAAQOL: a health-related quality of life instrument comprising health-status weighted by the impact of health problems on well being. Qual Life Res. 2011:257.
50. Fekkes M, Kamphuis RP, Ottenkamp J, Verrips E, Vogels T, Kamphuis M, et al. Health-related quality of life in young adults with minor congenital heart disease. Psychol Health. 2001;16:239–50. https://doi.org/10.1080/08870440108405502.
51. Boukovala M, Müller J, Ewert P, Hager A. Effects of congenital heart disease treatment on quality of life. Am J Cardiol. 2019;123:1163–8. https://doi.org/10.1016/j.amjcard.2018.12.048.
52. Blok IM, van Riel ACMJ, Schuuring MJ, Duffels MG, Vis JC, van Dijk APJ, et al. Decrease in quality of life predicts mortality in adult patients with pulmonary arterial hypertension due to congenital heart disease. Neth Heart J. 2015;23:278–84. https://doi.org/10.1007/s12471-015-0666-9.
53. Favoccia C, Kempny A, Yorke J, Armstrong I, Price LC, McCabe C, et al. EmPHasis-10 score for the assessment of quality of life in various types of pulmonary hypertension and its relation to outcome. Eur J Prev Cardiol. 2019;26:1338–40. https://doi.org/10.1177/2047487318819161.
54. Tay ELW, Peset A, Papaphylactou M, Inuzuka R, Alonso-Gonzalez R, Giannakoulas G, et al. Replacement therapy for iron deficiency improves exercise capacity and quality of life in patients with cyanotic congenital heart disease and/or the Eisenmenger syndrome. Int J Cardiol. 2011;151:307–12. https://doi.org/10.1016/j.ijcard.2010.05.066.
55. Garcia-Garcia HM, McFadden EP, Farb A, Mehran R, Stone GW, Spertus J, et al. Standardized End Point Definitions for Coronary Intervention Trials: The Academic Research Consortium-2 Consensus Document. Circulation. 2018;137:2635–50. https://doi.org/10.1161/CIRCULATIONAHA.117.029289.
56. Généreux P, Piazza N, Alu MC, Nazif T, Hahn RT, Pibarot P, et al. Valve Academic Research Consortium 3: updated endpoint definitions for aortic valve clinical research. Eur Heart J. 2021;42:1825–57. https://doi.org/10.1093/eurheartj/ehaa799.

10 The Impact of Valve Surgery on the Health-Related Quality of Life of Elderly Patients: Systematic Review

Yusuf S. Abdullahi, Sanjay Chaubey, Roberto Casula, and Thanos Athanasiou

Aim: To investigate the impact of valvular heart surgery on the quality of life of elderly patients and highlight the predictors of poor quality of life post-operatively.

Introduction

The world health organisation (WHO) defines Quality of Life as "individual's perception of their position in life in the context of the culture and value systems in which they live and in relation to their goals, expectations, standards and concerns" [1].

One of the measures of quality of life (QOL) is the Health Related Quality of Life (HRQOL). Interest in HRQOL has significantly increased over the last decade amongst healthcare benefactors. Similarly, patient reported outcomes are also seen as an effective approach to measure QOL.

Furthermore, demographic trends show an undeniable increase in the average population age, particularly the 'very old' age group is growing at an unprecedented rate – a prominent phenomenon perhaps best seen in Europe [2]. Understandably, as the general population becomes older, age-related disease such as coronary artery disease and valvular heart disease become increasingly prevalent [3]. To address these problems, the field of cardiothoracic surgery has evolved in ways that see increasingly more complex operations carried out in a plethora of innovative ways to address the needs of an older population.

Some argue that a bygone golden era of cardiothoracic surgery has now been over-run by advances in interventional cardiology such as percutaneous coronary stents displacing coronary artery bypass grafts (CABG) as the new norm. Additionally, newer technologies such as transcatheter aortic and mitral valve replacements are on the rise, being utilized in an increasingly larger number of patients. While these options may provide an alternative to cardiac surgery, newer surgical techniques coupled with technological advances have demonstrated superior results for many patients groups [4].

To ascertain the benefits of undergoing cardiac surgery, many studies have been published on perioperative mortality and morbidity.

Y. S. Abdullahi (✉) · R. Casula · T. Athanasiou
Department of Cardiothoracic Surgery, Imperial College Healthcare NHS Trust, Hammersmith Hospital, London, UK

Department of Surgery and Cancer, Imperial College London, London, UK
e-mail: y.abdullahi14@imperial.ac.uk; Roberto.Casula@nhs.net; t.athanasiou@imperial.ac.uk

S. Chaubey
Department of Cardiothoracic Surgery, Imperial College Healthcare NHS Trust, Hammersmith Hospital, London, UK
e-mail: s.chaubey@nhs.net

T. Athanasiou et al. (eds.), *Patient Reported Outcomes and Quality of Life in Cardiovascular Interventions*,
https://doi.org/10.1007/978-3-031-09815-4_10

Typically, these figures compare surgical intervention to conservative treatment or catheter-based intervention. Statistics on valvular haemodynamic, blood loss and ICU stay are typically lauded when decisions are made whether to operate on patients or not [5]. However, while it must be acknowledged that these outcomes are indeed important, there is an increasing body of interest, particularly in older patient groups that advocates the incompleteness of these measures alone when assessing appropriateness of surgical intervention. Instead, some authors advocate a holistic approach to choosing guiding intervention—that is to say, the likely improvement of QOL [6].

Quality of life is a term which generally encompasses the well-being of individuals, observing life satisfaction, and multiple domains including but not limited to physical wellbeing [7]. Multiple scales exist to measure and quantify well-being, perhaps one of the most commonly used is the Short Form-36 (SF36) which measures well-being (as its name suggests) on a 36 item, 5-point Likert scale short form survey [8]. This survey is also unique in that it has been translated to multiple languages such as German and Arabic [9] to capture data from a variety of population groups. Once all items have been completed, scoring is sub-classified under one of eight domains [8].

From the research already conducted in QOL within a cardiothoracic context, there has been evidence that QOL is generally improve post-operatively compared to baseline levels [10]. Similarly, a large percentage – two-third of octogenarians were able to live independently one year following cardiac surgery [11]. However, in saying this, a paucity of data remains in certain areas—for example, when assessing QOL following valvular surgery in elderly populations.

Based on the above, it becomes evident that measuring and quantifying QOL for patients undergoing valvular heart surgery is of the utmost importance. As such, this paper will attempt to focus primarily on how QOL is affected by these operations. Furthermore, given the relevance of an aging population in the field of cardiac surgery—this chapter will have a focus on this age group.

Method

This systematic review study benefits from the protocol developed based on the preferred Reporting Items for Systematic Review and Meta-Analyses (PRISMA) [12].

Data Sources and Search

Data was sourced from EMBASE, CINAHL, MEDLINE, Cochrane, PubMed and other web based science electronic database for the period from 1980 to 2020. The following search terms were used to retrieve potential published articles for inclusion: ('Old', 'Frail', 'Elderly') AND "(Quality of life, HRQOL, PRO, QoL) AND (`Well-being, Physical health, Health status,) AND ('Risk', 'Risk score', 'Risk stratification', 'outcome',). AND (Mini, minimal invasive, minimally) AND (AVR, MVR, MVr, TVR, Transcatheter, Valve surgery, Cardiac surgery)". Other relevant articles were manually added and referenced.

Study Inclusion Criteria

The author independently retrieved potential articles using the aforementioned search terms. Cross-sectional or prospective studies evaluating the relationship between quality of life and elderly patients undergoing cardiac surgery were sourced. Abstract was reviewed and screened for inclusion. Selection criteria included (i) studies defining frailty and QoL as a multidimensional tool (ii) studies based on a patient population undergoing either cardiac or valve surgery; (iii) studies offering post cardiac surgery outcome data of elderly patients in relation to quality of

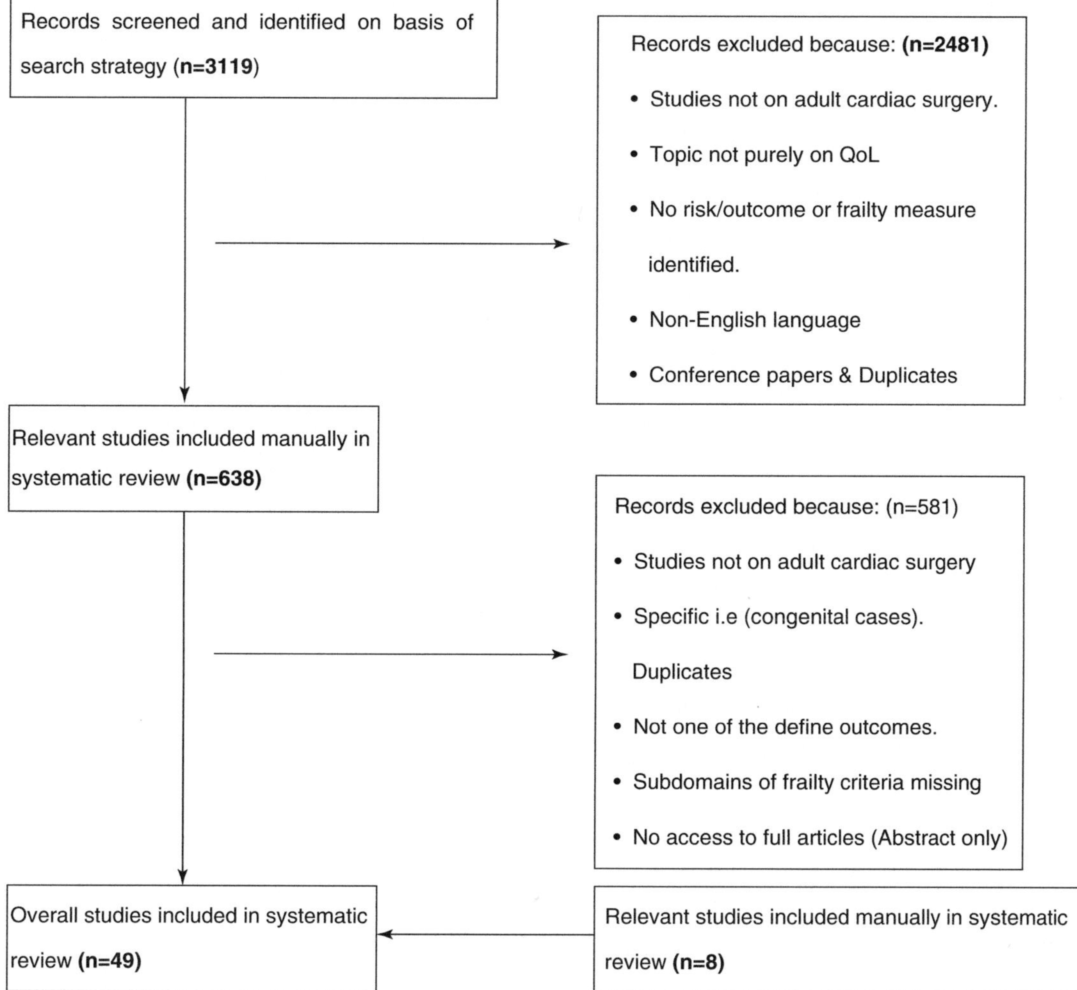

Fig. 10.1 Flow diagram of valve QoL study selection

life; (iv) articles written in English. Excluded studies were review articles, dissertations, and conference papers (Fig. 10.1).

Evaluation of Quality and Risk of Bias

Quality assessment of each study was performed by attributing a quality assessment score using a modified Newcastle–Ottawa scale [13]. The scale was modified to include all 17 EuroSCORE II cardiac risk factors as well as baseline physical, social and mental health function for comparability. The scoring criteria are shown in Table 10.1.

Results

Our literature search yielded 3119 studies, of which 49 articles with a patient population of 13,529 fulfilled our inclusion criteria (Fig. 10.1). A total of eighteen different quality of life measurement tools were applied in almost all of the articles individually with the exception of some studies that combined one or more tools (Tables 10.2, 10.3, 10.4). Most studies utilised SF-36 to assess and measure quality of life. Patient aged ranged from 34 to 85 years and included studies sample size ranged from 34 to 1833. The procedures undergone by these patients varied in terms

Table 10.1 Newcastle scoring system

Criteria for quality assessment. Modified Newcastle–Ottawa scoring criteria
Quality checklist
Selection
1. Assignment for treatment – any criteria reported? (If yes, 1-star)
2. How representative was the reference group in relation to the general population for aortic / mitral surgery (If yes, 1 star, no star if the patients were selected or selection of group was not described)
3. How representative was the comparison group in relation to the general population for aortic/mitral surgery? (If drawn from the same community as the reference group, 1-star, no star if drawn from a different source or selection of group was not described.
Comparability
Comparability variables: (1) age; (2) gender; (3) renal function; (4) extracardiac arteriopathy; (5) poor mobility; (6) previous cardiac surgery; (7) chronic lung disease; (8) active endocarditis; (9) critical preoperative state; (10) IDDM; (11) NYHA; (12) CCS IV; (13) LV function; (14) recent MI; (15) pulmonary hypertension; (16) urgency; (17) combined; (18) physical function score; (19) mental function score; (20) social function score
4. Groups comparable for 1, 2, 3, 4, 5, 6, 7, 8, 9 (If yes, 1-star was assigned for each of these. No star was assigned if the groups differed
5. Groups comparable for 10, 11, 12, 13, 14, 15, 16, 17(If yes, 1-star was assigned for each of these. No star was assigned if the two groups differed). 6. Groups comparable for 18, 19, 20 (If yes, 1-star assigned for each of these. No star was assigned if the groups differed)
Outcome assessment
6. Clearly defined outcome of interest (If yes, 1-star).
7. Follow-up (1-star if described)
IDDM = insulin dependent diabetes mellitus; MIVS = minimally invasive valve surgery; NYHA = New York Heart Association; ST = standard sternotomy. Comparability includes all the EuroSCORE II risk-factors

of incision method and operation type; open sternotomy was noted as the preferred choice over minimal access. All studies had a follow-up period ranged from 3 months to 8.4 years (Tables 10.2, 10.3, 10.4).

Most of the studies reported outcomes including in-hospital mortality, composite outcome and prolonged length of stay along with quality of life, however, studies failed to report on common endpoints which limited formal meta-analysis for these outcomes thereby limiting our interpretation of the best predictive value or score for quality of life tool to accurately measure valve surgery consequences on frail elderly patients.

Discussion

The growing elderly population worldwide places demands on health care providers and policy makers to formulate strategies in improving and maintaining quality of life during the extended years of life. Valvular surgery is increasingly becoming a common procedure in the elderly group. While the aforementioned demand for these procedures is driving the increase, improvements in surgical skills and advances in prosthesis models make these procedures safe and feasible.

This review aims to answer the question around whether improvements in QoL can be observed post valve related cardiac surgery and more specifically—highlight predictors of poor QoL post-operatively. To answer this question, one must first acknowledge that due to the nature of cardiac surgery—there are some inherent risks. These risks are well documented and can be both short and long term [14]. These risks are compounded in elderly patient who have a greater set of co-morbidities often placing them in the 'high risk' category [15]. Because of this – much focus is directed towards traditional markers of operative success. However, an increasing body of evidence informs us that elderly patients value regaining their independence and ability to enjoy improved quality of life post-operatively over and above the traditional markers of operative success [16].

Frailty Factor

Phenotype is often used a measure of frailty to aid clinicians in decision making on appropriate intervention for patients. Kojima et al. (2016) applied 36-item Short Form Health Survey instrument and demonstrated that patients rated as frail

Table 10.2 Multi-design studies on Aortic valve surgery and QoL

Author, year, Reference	Type of cardiac valve procedure	Study type	No. of patients at baseline	Age of patients	Follow-up duration (mean)	QoL Instruments	Conclusion	Physical component improved	Quality score
Detter, 2002 [32]	AVR: Minimally invasive ($n = 70$) vs. conventional replacement ($n = 70$)	Retrospective cohort	140	Mean 64.3 years Range 34–83 years	34 months (minimally invasive) 33.1 months (conventional)	SF-36	No significant differences in QoL between the groups at the end of the follow-up	N/A-No comparison with pre or norms	7
Aicher, 2001 [41]	AVR; repair ($n = 86$), mechanical replacement ($n = 41$), pulmonary autograft ($n = 39$)	Cross sectional study	166	40 ± 6 (repair) 46 ± 7 (mechanical replacement) 46 ± 7 (pulmonary autograft)	3–7 years	SF-36	Aortic valve repair and pulmonary autograft lead to less long term alteration from normal	N/A-No comparison with pre or norms	6
Grady, 2011 [24]	coronary artery bypass grafting, 136; aortic valve repair or replacement, 96; mitral valve repair or replacement, 92; Maze procedures, 46	Single-site prospective, longitudinal observational study	370	61.5 ± 11.9 years old	3 years	SF-36	Health-related quality of life improves early after operations and remains constant long-term independent of procedure	N/A-No comparison with pre or norms	5

(continued)

Table 10.2 (continued)

Author, year, Reference	Type of cardiac valve procedure	Study type	No. of patients at baseline	Age of patients	Follow-up duration (mean)	QoL Instruments	Conclusion	Physical component improved	Quality score
Goldsmith, 2001 [22]	Mitral Valve replacement (*n* = 21), Mitral Valve repair (*n* = 40)	Prospective cohort	61	65.9 ± 12.6 (MV repair) 65.6 ± 8.4 (MV replacement)	3 Months	SF-36	Significant improvement in QOL following mitral valve surgery, especially in repair. Impaired LV function/high end-systolic dimensions less likely to show improvement in QOL	Significant change in follow up from pre-op in QOL for almost all parameters in repair group, improvement in some parameters for replacement group	6
Notzold, 2001 [42]	Aortic Valve replacement; autograft (*n* = 40), mechanical (*n* = 40)	Retrospective cohort	80	57.58 ± 10.27 (Ross procedure) 59.18 ± 10.39 (mechanical)	2.21 ± 1.29 years (Ross procedure) 1.86 ± 0.69 years (mechanical)	SF-36 FPI-R EBF-24 SVF-66	Patients with pulmonary autograft have greater benefits in QOL compared to mechanical valve substitutes	N/A-No comparison with pre or norms	4
Zhao, 2007 [31]	Mitral valve repair (*n* = 163), mitral valve replacement (*n* = 104)	Multi-centre Prospective cohort	267	58.1 ± 12.2 (repair) 61.6 ± 12.9 (replacement)	12 months	SF-36	After mitral valve surgery, especially mitral valve repair, there is a significant improvement in NYHF class and health status	Scores for PCS were depressed at 1 month for both groups, but they showed marked improvements at 3 and 12 months after surgery for both groups (P .0001).	8

Aboud, 2009 [18]	Aortic valve replacement, mechanical (n = 83) vs bioprosthetic (n = 53)	Retrospective cohort	136	74 (52–87) (mechanical prosthesis) 64 (44–81) (Bioprosthetic)	21.4 ± 4.6 months	SF-36	Physical function scores were significantly better in patients with a mechanical prosthesis. Mental health indices were identical in both groups. Younger patients with mechanical valves and older patients with biological valves had significantly better item scores	Physical functioning index was significantly better in patients with mechanical prosthesis	2
Van Geldorp, 2012 [19]	Conservative management (n = 84) vs. aortic valve replacement [42] for aortic stenosis ** 22 patients crossed over from conservative to surgical	Multi-centre prospective cohort study	132	73.2 ± 10.9 (Conservative) 67.8 ± 12.2 (AVR)	18 months	SF-36v2TM	s Aortic valve replacement improves physical quality of life, general health and vitality in patients with symptomatic severe aortic stenosis	Physical functioning, improved significantly 1 year after aortic valve replacement. In conservatively treated patients physical quality of life deteriorated over time	5

(continued)

Table 10.2 (continued)

Author, year, Reference	Type of cardiac valve procedure	Study type	No. of patients at baseline	Age of patients	Follow-up duration (mean)	QoL Instruments	Conclusion	Physical component improved	Quality score
Tseng, 1997 [43]	Isolated AVR ($n = 247$)	Retrospective cohort study	247	76.2 ± 4.8 years	4.1 ± 3.1 years	SF-36	Patients undergoing AVR scored better than those who were 75 and older who did not (age adjusted norm), however, quality of life was similar between AVR group and those 65–74 who did not undergo AvR (age adjusted norm)	In areas of physical function, patients who underwent AVR scored better than did patients in the 75 years of age and older group and comparably with patients in the 65–74 year age group (age adjusted norm)	1
Casali, 2008 [37]	Aortic valve replacement with 17 mm St Jude Medical regent mechanical prosthesis ($n = 36$)	Retrospective cohort study	36	66.9 ± 12.1	4.1 ± 1.8	SF-36	Scores obtained in 7 of the 8 domains of the test were significantly higher than preoperative values	Post-operative physical function was improved compared to pre-operative physical functioning	2
Machaalany, 2013 [44]	Patients implantated with PTMA device ($n = 30$)	Muti-center prospective cohort study	43	72 ± 11	5.8 ± 3 months	Minnesota Living with Heart Failure Questionnaire EQ-5D questionnaires	Overall, PTMA had mild impact on MR reduction, left ventricular remodeling, QOL, and exercise capacity	N/A-No comparison with pre or norms	2

Markou, 2011 [25]	Isolated AVR ($n = 200$) vs. AVR + CABG ($n = 215$)	Retrospective cohort study	415	71.7 ± 7.3 (55–88)	1 year (only 239 patients)	EQ-5D	Postoperatively, all patients Experienced significantly better health-related QOL. However, the patients undergoing combined surgery experienced more benefit from their operation	N/A-No comparison with pre or norms	9
Vicchio, 2012 [26]	Isolated AVR ($n = 406$) vs. AVR + CABG ($n = 112$)	Retrospective cohort study	520	74.2 ± 3.6 years 74.3 ± 3.6 (AVR) 74 ± 3.3 in (AVR + CABG)	4.2 ± 3.3 years	SF-36	The scores obtained in the SF-36 test were similar in the two groups and significantly higher than those of the general population matched for country, age and sex ($p < 0.001$ in all domains)	Physical functioning score was higher in both groups compared to the elderly Italian population	8
Whitlow, 2011 [38]	Underwent MitraClip procedure ($n = 78$)	Prospective cohort study	78	77	1 year	SF36	The MitraClip device reduced MR in a majority of patients deemed at high risk of surgery, resulting in improvement in clinical symptoms and quality of life	The physical component of SF36 improved from 31.6 ± 9.1 to 36.5 ± 10.6	10

(continued)

Table 10.2 (continued)

Author, year, Reference	Type of cardiac valve procedure	Study type	No. of patients at baseline	Age of patients	Follow-up duration (mean)	QoL Instruments	Conclusion	Physical component improved	Quality score
Ussia, 2012 [39]	Mitral valve repair with the MitraClip (*n* = 39)	Prospective cohort	39	72 ± 11	6 months	SF12 (v2)	early marked improvement in functional status and physical and mental health in patients underwent percutaneous mitral valve repair with the MitraClip System	At 6 month follow up point, a drastic improvement in PCS was observed (PCS 35.44 vs 44.67, P < 0.0001)	2
Maliwa, 2003 [40]	Underwent mechanical AVR (*n* = 312)	Retrospective cohort	312	41 ± 12	30 ± 1.8 years	SF36 EuroQol (EQ-5D)	At long term follow-up (mean 30 years) of patients who had mAVR. QoL was relatively high	Physical functioning QOL subscale was lower than that of other populations e.g. Dutch population	2
Sedrakyan, 2003 [18]	Aortic Valve replacement (*n* = 72) Mitral Valve repair (*n* = 72)	Prospective cohort	148*220 initally sampled, but only 148 had complete data	66.5 ± 14.4	18 Months	SF36	Age does not appear to limit the QOL benefits of surgery	Physical functioning improved significantly for all age groups	9
Florath, 2005 [28]	Bioprosthetic AVR (*n* = 247) Mechanical AVR (*n* = 145)	Retrospective cohort	392	Bioprosthetic: 76 ± 5 Mechanical: 71 ± 4	3 to 66 months	Nottingham health profile	Elderly people receiving stentless bioprostheses benefit emotionally because of the avoidance of coumarin	Physical functioning comparable to general German population, females in the study scored higher	9

Jokinen, 2007 [36]	MV Repair: ($n = 85$) MV Replacement: ($n = 99$)	Prospective cohort	184	MV Repair: 62.2 ± 9.2 MV Replacement: 61.3 ± 9.4	7.3 ± 1.4	Nottingham Health Profile	Survival is longer after MV repair than after MV replacement. The quality of life of not differ from each other	Physical activity was statistically significantly worse in the MV replacement and repair groups than in the reference population	8
Lam, 2004 [20]	Aortic Valve replacement in >80 years age ($n = 58$)	Prospective Cohort	58	83.7 ± 3.4	35.3 ± 25.3	SF36	Despite higher operative risk and greater morbidity, QOL indicators in patients ≥80 years were equivalent to or better than their counterparts	N/A-No comparison with pre or norms	1
Zacek, 2016 [29]	Aortic valve-sparing procedure, age < 50 ($n = 36$) Aortic valve-sparing procedure, age > 50 ($n = 52$) Ross procedure ($n = 22$) Mechanical aortic valve replacement ($n = 29$)	Cross sectional study	139	Aortic valve-sparing procedure, age < 50 36.3 ± 6.1 Aortic valve-sparing procedure, age > 50 59.2 ± 7.7 Ross procedure 37.8 ± 11.9 Mechanical aortic valve replacement 39.7 ± 7.3	Median 26.9 months	SF36	Postoperative quality of life is influenced by the type of aortic valve procedure and is negatively linked with mechanical prosthesis implantation and long-term anticoagulation	Younger valve repair patients and Ross patients scored significantly better than the patients after mechanical valve replacement in all four physical subscales	7

(continued)

Table 10.2 (continued)

Author, year, Reference	Type of cardiac valve procedure	Study type	No. of patients at baseline	Age of patients	Follow-up duration (mean)	QoL Instruments	Conclusion	Physical component improved	Quality score
Maisano, 2009 [23]	Isolated mitral valve surgery ($n = 225$) sub study (Combination aortic/mitral valve surgery) (n = 208)	Retrospective Cohort	225	77 ± 3.2 years	2.8 ± 1.2 years	Minnesota Living with Heart Failure (MLHF) questionnaire	Quality of life following mitral valve surgery is suboptimal in more than half of elderly patients. MLHF score at follow-up is mostly related to preoperative conditions. Type of surgery does not influence MLHF score, however, quality of life is worse in patients with recurrent/ residual MR following repair		2
Folkmann, 2010 [11]	AvR with CABG ($n = 80$) AvR without CABG ($n = 74$)	Retrospective Cohort	154	82.9 ± 2.5	1 year	Seattle Angina Questionnaire	Surgery in the aortic valve without CABG is associated with a good outcome. The improvement in QoL after one year supports the decision to operate on patients older than 80 years of age	Assessment of QoL revealed a substantial improvement of physical fitness in all 126 patients (who survived to be followed up at 1 year)	1

Klomp, 2016 [34]	Age < 80 $N = 597$ Age > 80 $N = 163$	Prospective single-canter cohort study	762	Age < 80 71 (66–75) Age > 80 82 (81–83)	1 year	SF-36	Surgical aortic valve replacement in octogenarians could be performed with very low mortality, and with a relevant and significant increase of the quality of life towards normal values	PCS increased from baseline for both group at 1 year follow up	8
Vicchio, 2007 [30]	Bioprosthetic AVR $N = 62$ Mechanical AVR $N = 98$	Retrospective cohort	160	Bioprosthetic group: 82.9 ± 2.7 Mechanical group: 81.8 ± 1.8	3.4 ± 2.8	SF-36	Long-term survival after AVR in selected octogenarians was similar to that of the general elderly population. The device type exerted no influence on QOL	N/A-No comparison with pre or norms	11
Aoyagi, 2010 [35]			60	82.3 ± 1.9	3.4 ± 3.1 years		Some 97.6% of late survivors reported that their activity level was equal to or better than the preoperative level	N/A-No comparison with pre or norms	2
Oliveira, 2011 [33]	>75 year old patients that underwent AVR ($n = 114$)	Retrospective cohort	114	78.5 ± 2.5 years	47.2 ± 23.4 months		At follow-up, most achieved improvement of QoL and remained autonomous		2

Table 10.3 RCT trial studying Aortic valve surgery and QoL

Author, year, Ref	Intervention	Study type	No. of patients at baseline	Follow-up duration (mean)	HRQOL Instruments	Conclusion	Physical component improved	Quality score
PARTNER1A – surgically operable at high risk (Mack et al. 2015) [45]	TAVI vs SAVR	RCT	TAVI ($n = 348$) SAVR ($n = 351$)	5 year	SF-12, EQ-5D, KCCQ	Greater improvement on both physical and mental scores in TAVI group at 1 month. No difference at 1 year	TAVI better over the first year	14
US CoreValve Trial- surgically operable at high risk (Deeb et al. 2016) [46]	TAVI vs. SVAR	RCT	TAVI ($n = 394$) SAVR ($n = 401$)	5 years	SF-12, KCCQ	Greater improvement on both physical and mental scores in TAVI group at 1 month. At 6 months statistically significant difference in mental score. No difference at 1 year	TAVI better over the first year	13
SURTAVI Trial-surgically operable at intermediate risk (Reardon et al. 2017) [47]	TAVI vs. SAVR	RCT	TAVI ($n = 864$) SAVR ($n = 796$)	2 years	KCCQ	The QoL was assessed using the KCCQ and they have shown a significant improvement for both TAVI and sAVR at 24 months of follow-up	Both showed similar improvement in QoL	14
PARTNER 2–surgically operable at intermediate risk (Baron et al. 2017) [48]	TAVI vs. SAVR	RCT	TAVI ($n = 950$) SAVR ($n = 883$)	2 years	SF-36, EQ-5D, KCCQ	Both TAVI and sAVR were associated with significant improvements in both disease-specific (16–22 points in the KCCQ-OS scale) and generic health status (3.9–5.1 points in the SF-36 physical scale). There were no significant differences between TAVI and sAVR in any health status measures at 1- or 2-year follow-up	Comparable improvement in QoL	14
PARTNER 3–surgically operable at low risk (Mack et al. 2019) [49]	TAVI vs. SAVR	RCT	TAVI ($n = 496$) SAVR ($n = 454$)	1 year	KCCQ, NYHA class, 6 min walk test	TAVI patient showed the more rapid improvement in all QoL metrics	TAVI better over the first year	13

EVOLUT trial– surgically operable at low risk (Popma et al. 2019) [50]	TAVI vs. SAVR	RCT	TAVI ($n = 725$) SAVR ($n = 678$)	1 year	KCCQ	TAVI was non-inferior to sAVR for the composite end point of death or disabling stroke at 24 months In relation to QoL analysis, assessed using the KCCQ, both TAVI and surgery offered similar functional improvement at 12 months, with better early, 30-day recovery observed in the TAVI group	TAVI and surgery similar over first year	14
Aris et al. 1999 [51]	Limited vs Full sternotomy	RCT	Limited ($n = 20$) Full ($n = 20$)		**Primary outcomes:** cross-clamp and pump times, time to extubation, chest drainage (24 h), number of blood transfusions, ICU stay, total postoperative length of stay **Secondary outcomes:** pain scores (daily) and cosmetic evaluation (discharge)	Pain scores similar Lung function better	NA	11
Bonacchi et al. 2002 [52]	Limited vs Full sternotomy	RCT	Limited ($n = 40$) Full ($n = 40$)	Peri operative assessment	**Outcomes:** in-hospital death, re-exploration for bleeding, mean mediastinal drainage or bleeding >800 mL, blood transfusion, atrial fibrillation, atelectasis, respiratory insufficiency, sternal wound infection, sternal instability, mechanical ventilation time, oxygen requirements (pre- and post extubation), pain scores (1 and 12 h), analgesia requirements, ICU stay, hospital stay, spirometry (5 days and 1 to 2 months)	Pain scores reduced Blood loss reduced ITU and total length of stay reduced Less post-op ventilation	NA	12

(continued)

Table 10.3 (continued)

Author, year, Ref	Intervention	Study type	No. of patients at baseline	Follow-up duration (mean)	HRQOL Instruments	Conclusion	Physical component improved	Quality score
Borger 2015 [53]	Limited vs. Full sternotomy	RCT	Limited ($n = 46$) Full ($n = 48$)	Peri operative assessment	**Primary outcomes:** cross-clamp and CPB time **Secondary outcomes:** haemodynamic performance, quality of life (EQ-5D), NYHA class **Safety outcomes:** cardiac reoperation, thromboembolism, renal failure, paravalvular leak, permanent pacemaker insertion, resternotomy, major bleeding events, endocarditis, myocardial infarction, deep sternal wound infection, cerebrovascular accident, respiratory failure	QoL scores similar	NA	14
Calderon et al. 2009 [54]	Limited vs. Full sternotomy	RCT	Limited ($n = 38$) Full ($n = 39$)	Peri operative assessment	**Primary outcomes:** respiratory parameters **Secondary outcomes:** bleeding, transfusion, pain status **Other reported outcomes:** intraoperative and postoperative blood loss, transfusion rates, CPB and cross-clamp times, operation time, mechanical ventilation time, ICU stay, hospital stay, systemic inflammatory response syndrome, re-exploration for bleeding, death, spirometry (1, 2, and 7 days), pain scores, cardiac output studies	Pain scores similar Blood loss less	NA	12

Dogan et al. 2003 [55]	Limited vs. Full sternotomy	RCT	Limited ($n = 20$) Full ($n = 20$)	Peri operative assessment	**Primary outcomes:** operative time, CPB and cross-clamp time, postoperative ventilation, 24-h chest tube drainage, ICU stay, hospital stay **Secondary outcomes:** spirometry (postoperative day 6 or 7), pain scores (days 2 to 3 and 6 to 7), neuropsychological and biochemical tests	ITU length of stay less Pain scores similar Blood loss less	NA	12
Machler et al. 1999 [56]	Limited vs. Full sternotomy	RCT	Limited ($n = 60$) Full ($n = 60$)	Peri operative assessment	**reported outcomes:** cross-clamp time, CPB time, operation time, postoperative ejection fraction, duration of ventilation, chest tube drainage at 24 h, reoperation requirements, pericardial effusions, conversion to full sternotomy, arrhythmias, strokes, wound infection, sternal instability, sternal pain	Reduced AF	NA	13
Moustafa et al. 2007 [57]	Limited vs Full sternotomy	RCT	Limited (n = 30) Full (n = 30)	Peri operative assessment	**Reported outcomes:** pulmonary function tests (1 week and 1 month post), length of incision, operating time, CPB time, ventilation time, chest drainage at 24 hours, blood transfusions, ICU stay, total hospital stay, participant survey of cosmetic effect, analgesia use	ITU and total length of stay less Blood loss less Lung function better Less post-op ventilation	NA	13
Nair et al. 2018 [58]	Limited vs. Full sternotomy	RCT	Limited ($n = 118$) Full ($n = 104$)	Hospital stay		No difference in hospital stay		9

Table 10.4 Trials and others studying mitral valve surgery and QoL

Author, year, Reference	Intervention	Study type	No. of patients at baseline	Follow-up duration (mean)	HRQOL Instruments	Conclusion	Physical component improved	Quality score
Aker et al. 2014 [59]	MVr vs. MVR (ischaemic)	RCT	MVr $N = 126$ MVR $N = 125$	12 months	SF-12, MLHF	No significant difference was seen	Similar improvement	14
Ay et al. 2013 [60]	MVr vs. MVR	Prospective	MVr $N = 32$ MVR $N = 24$	6 months	SF-36	QoL may be better in MVr	AF, female gender, MVR affected physical component negatively	10
Immer et al. 2003 [61]	MVr vs. MVR	Retrospective	MVr $N = 53$ MVR $N = 62$	37 months	SF-36	MVr had better scores in physical health, role function, general health	Mid-term result scores where similar	11
Jokinen et al. 2007 [36]	MVr vs. MVR	Prospective	MVr $N = 85$ MVR $N = 99$	7 years	NHP	QoL similar between MVr and MVR	Mobility scores lower than general population	8
Maisano et al. 2009 [23]	MVr/MVR (elderly)	Retrospective	$N = 225$	2 years	MLHF	MVr/MVR and choice of prosthesis did not predict MLHF scores	MLHF scores related to pre-operative conditions	2
Sedrakyan et al. 2006 [18]	MVr vs. MVR	Prospective	MVr $N = 45$ MVR $N = 25$	18 months	SF-36	More improvement in both physical and mental component in MVr	MVr showed more improvement	9
Zhao et al. 2007 [31]	MVr vs. MVR	Prospective	MVr $N = 163$ MVR $N = 104$	12 months	NYHA, SF-36	NHYA more improved after MVr MVr showed more in mental component improvement	Physical improvement similar	8
Suri et al. 2007 [62]	MVr (sternotomy vs. robotic assisted)	Prospective	Sternotomy $N = 72$ Robotic $N = 69$	24 months	DASI, SF-12	Robotic was associated with slightly improved scores in first year	QoL scores better after robotic approach	11
Goldsmith et al. 2001 [22]	MVr or MVR	Retrospective	MVr $N = 40$ MVR $N = 21$	3 months	SF-36	MVr showed better improvement in QoL Impaired LV function showed no improvement in QoL	MVr shows improvement in QoL however this is unlikely with LV impairment	8
Hansen et al. 2010 [63]	MVr	Retrospective	$N = 663$	4.1 year	NYHA, SF-36	QoL was comparable across aetiology of MR. QoL determined by females and LV function	QoL determined by co-morbidities	12

Heikkinen et al. 2005 [64]	MVr	Retrospective	$N = 130$ (FU = 109)		RAND-36	Health survey variables of study group were similar to age and gender adjusted general population	Patient after MVr have similar QoL to general population	12
Mesana et al. 2013 [65]	MVr (complete ring vs. partial band)	Retrospective	Band $N = 65$ Ring $N = 42$	4.3 years	SF-36, 6 min walk	Lower scores for patient following ring	Complete ring may have worse QoL	11
van Leeuwen et al. 2013 [66]	MVr (asymptomatic)	Retrospective	$N = 46$	8.4 years	NYHA, SF-36	QoL (SF-36) assessment showed comparable physical and mental components as compared to age and gender matched population	MVr in asymptomatic patients resulted in excellent QoL	12
Timek et al. 2014 [67]	MVr (ischaemic)	Retrospective	$N = 86$ (FU = 49)	50 months	NYHA SF36 (compared to general population)	No significant difference was seen in individual or composite (mental or physical) scores	MVr with Geoform ring established similar well being matched general population	12

or intermediate frail according to the Phenotype Frailty score have been shown to correlate to have lower physical and mental quality of life scores [17] but a numerous body of evidence challenges this conclusion.

Studies presented age alone should not be a precluding factor of worsening QoL post-surgery [5, 18, 19]. In fact, Sedrakyan et al. (2003) show that not only is age not correlated with QoL post-surgery, but that benefits reaped from valvular surgery seem to be prominent regardless of age. Additionally, Lam and Hendry [20] found that in octogenarians undergoing aortic valve replacement, quality of life post-operatively was equivalent to, or better than their counterparts.

HRQOL Outcome: PCS vs. MCS

A significant improvement in QoL following valve surgery was overwhelmingly reported regardless of the different QoL tools used, even for the studies that pre-selected baseline characteristics, or grouped patients into cohorts of middle and advanced age. Similarly articles that compared their study to country specific age matched population norms noted overall improvement in quality of life. However, majority of the articles 25 reported improvement in PCS and general health compared to 8 articles for marked improvement in MCS. Four studies reported MCS did not improve while Van Geldorp and Tseng added MCS score was lower than population norms and didn't benefit from surgery concurring with the study by Maliwa and colleagues.

Given that the overwhelming majority of literature indicated QoL is generally improved by surgical intervention, this study aimed to assess predictors of poor quality of life post valvular surgery.

Predictors of Quality of Life

Assessing predictors of QoL was a difficult task as data on the subject matter is extremely limited; in fact, more than half of the studies didn't evaluated any predictors of QoL post-surgery. The predictors identified in the studies are briefly discussed below and summarised in Fig. 10.2.

Female Gender

Goldsmith et al. (2001) reported female gender as an independent predictor of lower QoL following an open Mitral valve repair or replacement. This was previously reported in a large study of 741 patients that also included concomitant procedure with (212 MVP and MVR patients) by Flameng and colleagues [21]. The decline in general health for female gender in the first 3 months post-surgery is not yet well known.

Mitral Regurgitation

Studies [22, 23] investigated the impact of mitral regurgitation/residual following MR on the QoL. They noted non-significant improvement in QoL 3 months post-surgery when compared to baseline data in both open MV repair and replacement, with patients presenting etiology of mitral regurgitation (MR) with end systolic dimensions of more than 45 mm disadvantaged. Conversely patients with functional MR had improved their QoL post-surgery compared to those presenting degenerative MR in minimal invasive based MV repair.

Coronary Artery Disease

Four studies [11, 24–26] focused on the impact of coronary artery disease on the quality of life of patients undergoing aortic valve replacement. Studies reported previous myocardial infarction (MI) was predictive of rapid improvement in the physical component of QoL shortly after cardiac surgery. They however indicated non-significant mental health component improvement regardless of patient's history of coronary artery disease, acute MI, previous PCI intervention or repeat CABG surgery. Interestingly one study

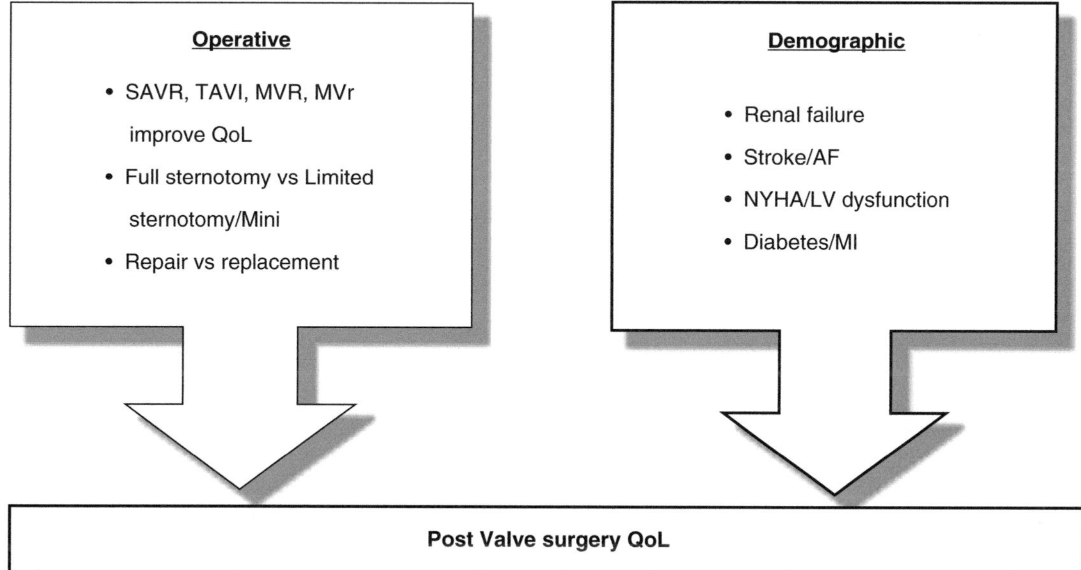

Fig. 10.2 Factors affecting HRQOL post valve surgery

reported that concomitant CABG and AVR is associated with poor QoL, precipitating higher mortality rates compared to sole AVR, however, on regression analysis—CABG alone was not significantly responsible for this increase [26]. This was further challenged by Markou and colleagues who reported in their prospective study of 215 concomitant (CABG+AVR) and 200 isolated valve that patients undergoing combined surgery exhibited greater benefit from their surgery than their counterpart.

Ejection Fraction, NYHA and LV function

Three studies pre-selected ejection fraction, LV function and NHYA class to evaluate any improvement in QoL post-surgery. Work by Goldsmith et al. (2001) revealed significant improvement in QoL following mitral valve repair but noted impaired LV function or end-systolic dimension is less likely to aid improvement in QoL. Likewise he presented higher NYHA functional score being independent predictor of low improvement in QoL and general health status post mitral valve surgery. Conversely Zhao et al. [27] reported significant improvement in NYHA class and health status for mitral repair patients.

Other Determinants of Quality of Life

Type of Prosthesis

Prosthesis type was reported as another important indicator of QoL post-operatively. Some studies have pointed out that even though surgery improves QoL, certain prosthesis result in better gains than others. One example is the research done by Florath et al. (2005) who have concluded that elderly patients receiving a stentless bioprosthetic aortic valve had a greater gain in the emotional QoL component due to the avoidance of warfarin [28]. This point was further supported by Zacek et al. [29] who stated QoL post-operatively is influenced by the specific type of aortic valve and greater quality of life and freedom is preserved by procedures that avoid life-long anticoagulation.

On the other hand Vicchio et al. [30] found that while survival in selected octogenarians was similar to the general elderly population, quality of life was not influence by the type of aortic valve used—that is to say, there was no difference in quality of life between patients with bioprosthetic or mechanical valves.

Type of Surgery

QoL following mitral valve surgery has been a closely followed topic. Much of the literature suggests that patients undergoing mitral repair experiencing a greater QoL improvement whereas mitral valve replacement yield inferior QoL gains [31]. Interestingly, Jokinen et al. (2007) assert that their research indicated quality-of life post-operatively was not significantly different between mitral valve replacement or repair, whereas survival was longer after mitral valve replacement as compared to repair. Furthermore, when compared to an age- and sex-matched population, scores around energy and mobility were lower. Juxtaposed to this, Maisano et al. [23] found that quality of life following mitral valve surgery is suboptimal in almost half of all elderly patients, particularly those with residual mitral regurgitation.

Transcatheter aortic valve implantation (TAVI) has been used for over a decade as a less invasive option for those who cannot undergo SAVR due to high risk of surgical complications. Following continuous advancements in TAVI technology with the aim of reducing complications, the use of TAVI has been extended to patients for whom SAVR is considered suitable but poses a high risk and also intermediate and lower risk patient populations, including younger patients with fewer comorbidities [45].

The all-cause mortality up to 5 years of follow-up did not differ significantly between TAVI and SAVR in patients surgically operable at a high risk, but favoured TAVI over medical therapy in patients surgically inoperable. Although TAVI was non-inferior to SAVR inpatients surgically operable at a high risk, shorter term benefits were observed for those patients undergoing TAVI regarding QoL, NYHA classification, overall incidence and severity of prosthesis-patient mismatch and lower incidence of acute kidney injury [45–47].

QoL after MVr and MVR improves. Improvement in QoL after surgery was seen in elderly group, asymptomatic and ischaemic mitral regurgitation patient. Though not conclusive, MVr showed more improvement in QoL especially over the first year. The use of robotic or mini mitral approach also confers benefits to post operative QoL [59–61, 64].

Incision Factor

The impact of full sternotomy on patient's post-operative quality of life and the perceived benefit of minimally invasive approach were investigated by Detter and colleagues [32] in their study of 140 patients that were separated equally to their respective cohort (minimal vs. conventional) group, and with a mean age 64.3 years and 34 months follow-up.

Interestingly they presented the absence of any significant difference between the two groups in any of the 8 domains of the quality of life tool used (SF 36). Furthermore, they reported patient's satisfaction and scar judgement after the operation was not influence by the incision style. None the less their study has few limitations and to begin with their postop follow-up was not done at 3 months or at 12 months, hence they haven't reported early mobilisation or the stability of the sternum at any given point. Similarly, their post-op complication list didn't not account for surgical site infection on which case if considered and reported it may have influence the patient's satisfaction and quality of life results [32].

There was uncertainty on mortality or extracorporeal support times with upper hemisternotomy for aortic valve replacement compared to full median sternotomy. The evidence to support a reduction in total hospital length of stay or intensive care stay was low in quality. There was also uncertainty of any difference in the rates of other, secondary outcome measures or adverse events (blood loss, deep sternal wound infection, pain scores, QoL(SF-36), post-op AF, re-exploration) with minimally invasive limited sternotomy approaches to aortic valve replacement [54–58, 68].

Limitation

In conducting this review, multiple limitations must be acknowledged. While some of the studies reviewed were prospective in nature, many were retrospective (see table of studies above). Similarly, many studies were single centre, which can affect the generalisability of results. Quality analysis demonstrated some of the most common flaws in the studies – namely patient selection, which must be acknowledge is largely due to ethical and technical consideration rather than poor selection.

We were specifically interested in identifying predictors of poor QoL gains post-operatively, and given the paucity of data around the subject, this was particularly difficult. In all of the literature identified, only few studies directly broached this topic. This provides a bottleneck in terms of validating the findings of these articles as well as limiting the scope of other potential factors which can negatively affect QoL post-operatively.

Conclusion

Increases in average population age across developed countries means there is a greater prevalence of valvular heart disease. Elderly patients can safely undergo valvular surgery with excellent post-operative outcomes. While mortality and morbidity are both important measures of operative success, it is imperative that a quality of life measure be included when evaluating the success of valvular surgery in elderly patients. Our literature review identified that quality of life gains post-operatively for elderly patients undergoing valvular heart surgery are both evident and significant when compared to pre-operative state. In saying that, we identified certain factors which can be correlated to limited QoL improvement—these included prosthetic type, valve dimensions, renal failure, AF, LV dysfunction, gender, NYHA score and replacement as compared to repair in mitral valve surgery (Fig. 10.3).

Conclusion

- Variety of tools to measure QoL make Comparing across studies difficult
- Risk factors like diabetes, LV function, Gender, renal failure negatively impact post -op QoL
- Limited upper sternotomy may benefit in regards to secondary endpoints
- TAVI approach helps QoL in the first year
- QoL similar to between TAVI and SVAR by I year
- QoL improve after MVR but possibly more after MVr
- Mini Mitral approach allows for better QoL over the first 12 months

Fig. 10.3 Conclusions

References

1. WHO. Study protocol for the World Health Organization project to develop a Quality of Life assessment instrument (WHOQOL). Qual Life Res. 1993;2(2):153–9.
2. Shephard RJ. Limits to the measurement of habitual physical activity by questionnaires. Br J Sports Med. 2003;37(3):197–206.
3. Odden MC, et al. The impact of the aging population on coronary heart disease in the United States. Am J Med. 2011;124(9):827–33 e5.
4. Iribarne A, et al. The golden age of minimally invasive cardiothoracic surgery: current and future perspectives. Futur Cardiol. 2011;7(3):333–46.
5. Sedrakyan A, et al. Age does not limit quality of life improvement in cardiac valve surgery. J Am Coll Cardiol. 2003;42(7):1208–14.
6. Tully PJ. Quality-of-Life Measures for Cardiac Surgery Practice and Research: A Review and Primer. J Extra Corpor Technol. 2013;45(1):8–15.
7. Kim D. Correlation between physical function, cognitive function, and health-related quality of life in elderly persons. J Phys Ther Sci. 2016;28(6):1844–8.
8. Ware JE Jr, Sherbourne CD. The MOS 36-item short-form health survey (SF-36). I. Conceptual framework and item selection. Med Care. 1992;30(6):473–83.
9. Wagner AK, et al. Cross-cultural comparisons of the content of SF-36 translations across 10 countries: results from the IQOLA Project. International Quality of Life Assessment. J Clin Epidemiol. 1998;51(11):925–32.
10. Shan L, et al. A systematic review on the quality of life benefits after aortic valve replacement in the elderly. J Thorac Cardiovasc Surg. 2013;145(5):1173–89.

11. Folkmann S, et al. Quality-of-life in octogenarians one year after aortic valve replacement with or without coronary artery bypass surgery. Interact Cardiovasc Thorac Surg. 2010;11(6):750–3.
12. Moher D, Liberati A, Tetzlaff J. Preferred reporting items for systematic reviews and meta-analyses: the PRISMA statement. PLoS Med. 2009;6(7):e1000097.
13. Wells, G., Shea, B., O'Connell, D., Peterson, J., Welch, V., Losos, M. and Tugwell, P. The Newcastle-Ottawa Scale (NOS) for assessing the quality of non-randomised studies in meta-analyses. 2014; Available from: http://www.ohri.ca/programs/clinical_epidemiology/oxford.asp
14. Nicolini F, et al. The Evolution of Cardiovascular Surgery in Elderly Patient: A Review of Current Options and Outcomes. Biomed Res Int. 2014;2014:10.
15. Wang W, et al. Association between older age and outcome after cardiac surgery: a population-based cohort study. J Cardiothorac Surg. 2014;9(1):177.
16. Cleveland JC Jr. Frailty, Aging, and Cardiac Surgery Outcomes: The Stopwatch Tells the Story *. J Am Coll Cardiol. 2010;56(20):1677–8.
17. Kojima G, et al. Association between frailty and quality of life among community-dwelling older people: a systematic review and meta-analysis. J Epidemiol Community Health. 2016;70(7):716–21.
18. Aboud A, et al. Quality of life after mechanical vs. biological aortic valve replacement. Asian Cardiovasc Thorac Ann. 2009;17(1):35–8.
19. van Geldorp MWA, et al. The effect of aortic valve replacement on quality of life in symptomatic patients with severe aortic stenosis. Neth Hear J. 2013;21(1):28–35.
20. Lam BK, Hendry PJ. Patients over 80 years: quality of life after aortic valve replacement. Age Ageing. 2004;33(3):307–9.
21. Flameng WJ, et al. Determinants of early and late results of combined valve operations and coronary artery bypass grafting. Ann Thorac Surg. 1996;61(2):621–8.
22. Goldsmith IR, Lip GY, Patel RL. A prospective study of changes in patients' quality of life after aortic valve replacement. J Heart Valve Dis. 2001;10(3):346–53.
23. Maisano F, et al. Quality of Life of elderly patients following valve surgery for chronic organic mitral regurgitation. Eur J Cardiothorac Surg. 2009;36(2):261–6.
24. Grady KL, Lee R, Subacius H. Improvements in health-related quality of life before and after isolated cardiac operations. Ann Thorac Surg. 2011;91:777–83.
25. Markou ALP, de Jager MJ, Noyez L. The impact of coronary artery disease on the quality of life of patients undergoing aortic valve replacement. Interact Cardiovasc Thorac Surg. 2011;13(2):128–32.
26. Vicchio M, et al. Coronary artery bypass grafting associated to aortic valve replacement in the elderly: survival and quality of life. J Cardiothorac Surg. 2012;7:13.
27. Yusuf S, et al. Effect of coronary artery bypass graft surgery on survival: overview of 10-year results from randomised trials by the Coronary Artery Bypass Graft Surgery Trialists Collaboration. Lancet. 1994;344(8922):563–70.
28. Florath I, et al. Mid term outcome and quality of life after aortic valve replacement in elderly people: mechanical versus stentless biological valves. Heart. 2005;91(8):1023–9.
29. Zacek P, et al. Quality of life after aortic valve repair is similar to Ross patients and superior to mechanical valve replacement: a cross-sectional study. BMC Cardiovasc Disord. 2016;16:63.
30. Vicchio M, et al. Tissue Versus Mechanical Prostheses: Quality of Life in Octogenarians. Ann Thorac Surg. 2007;85(4):1290–5.
31. Zhao L, et al. Comparison of recovery after mitral valve repair and replacement. J Thorac Cardiovasc Surg. 2007;133(5):1257–63.
32. Detter C, et al. Midterm results and quality of life after minimally invasive vs. conventional aortic valve replacement. Thorac Cardiovasc Surg. 2002;50(6):337–41.
33. Oliveira SM, et al. Long-Term Survival, Autonomy, and Quality of Life of Elderly Patients Undergoing Aortic Valve Replacement. J Card Surg. 2012;27(1):20–3.
34. Jansen Klomp WW, et al. Survival and quality of life after surgical aortic valve replacement in octogenarians. J Cardiothorac Surg. 2016;11(1):38.
35. Aoyagi S, et al. Heart valve surgery in octogenarians: operative and long-term results. Heart Vessel. 2010;25(6):522–8.
36. Jokinen JJ, et al. Mitral valve replacement versus repair: propensity-adjusted survival and quality-of-life analysis. Ann Thorac Surg. 2007;84(2):451–8.
37. Casali G, et al. Della Echocardiographic follow-up after implanting 17-mm Regent mechanical prostheses. Asian Cardiovasc Thorac Ann. 2008;16:208–11.
38. Whitlow PL, et al. Acute and 12-month results with catheter-based mitral valve leaflet repair: the EVEREST II (Endovascular Valve Edge-to-Edge Repair) High Risk Study. J Am Coll Cardiol. 2012;59(2):130–9.
39. Ussia GP, et al. Quality of life following percutaneous mitral valve repair with the MitraClip System. Int J Cardiol. 2012;155(2):194–200.
40. Maliwa MA, et al. Quality of Life and NYHA Class 30 Years after Mechanical Aortic Valve Replacement. Cardiovasc Surg. 2003;11(5):381–7.
41. Aicher D, et al. Quality of life after aortic valve surgery: replacement versus reconstruction. J Thorac Cardiovasc Surg. 2011;142(2):e19–24.
42. Notzold A, et al. Quality of life in aortic valve replacement: pulmonary autografts versus mechanical prostheses. J Am Coll Cardiol. 2001;37(7):1963–6.
43. Tseng EE, et al. Aortic valve replacement in the elderly. Risk factors and long-term results. Ann Surg. 1997;225(6):793–802; discussion 802–4
44. Machaalany J, et al. Treatment of functional mitral valve regurgitation with the permanent percutaneous transvenous mitral annuloplasty system: results of the multicenter international Percutaneous Transvenous

Mitral Annuloplasty System to Reduce Mitral Valve Regurgitation in Patients with Heart Failure trial. Am Heart J. 2013;165(5):761–9.
45. Mack MJ, Leon MB, Smith CR, Miller DC, Moses JW, Tuzcu EM, et al. 5-year outcomes of transcatheter aortic valve replacement or surgical aortic valve replacement for high surgical risk patients with aortic stenosis (PARTNER 1): a randomised controlled trial. Lancet. 2015;385:2477–84. https://doi.org/10.1016/S0140-6736(15)60308-7.
46. Deeb GM, Reardon MJ, Chetcuti S, Patel HJ, Grossman PM, Yakubov SJ, et al. 3-Year Outcomes in High-Risk Patients Who Underwent Surgical or Transcatheter Aortic Valve Replacement. J Am Coll Cardiol. 2016;67:2565–74. https://doi.org/10.1016/j.jacc.2016.03.506.
47. Reardon MJ, Van Mieghem NM, Popma JJ, Kleiman NS, Sondergaard L, Mumtaz M, et al. Surgical or transcatheter aortic-valve replacement inintermediate-risk patients. N Engl J Med. 2017;376:1321–31.
48. Baron SJ, Arnold SV, Wang K, Magnuson EA, Chinnakondepali K, Makkar R, et al. for the PARTNER 2 Investigators. Health status benefits of transcathetervs surgical aortic valve replacement in patients with severe aorticstenosis at intermediate surgical risk: results from the PARTNER 2randomized clinical trial. JAMA Cardiol. 2017;2:837–45.
49. Mack MJ, Leon MB, Thourani VH, Makkar R, Kodali SK, Russo M, et al. Transcatheter aortic-valve replacement with a balloon-expandable valvein low-risk patients. N Engl J Med. 2019;380:1695–705.
50. Popma JJ, Deeb GM, Yakubov SJ, Mumtaz M, Gada H, O'Hair D, et al. Evolut Low Risk Trial Investigators. Transcatheter aortic-valve replacementwith a self-expanding valve in low-risk patients. N Engl J Med. 2019;380:1706–15.
51. Aris A, Camara ML, Montiel J, Delgado LJ, Galan J, Litvan H. Ministernotomy versus median sternotomy for aortic valve replacement: a prospective, randomized study. Ann Thorac Surg. 1999;67:1583–7.
52. Bonacchi M, PriPi E, Giunti G, Frati G, Sani G. Does ministernotomy improve postoperative outcome in aortic valve operation? A prospective randomized study. Ann Thorac Surg. 2002;73:460–5.
53. Borger MA, Moustafine V, Conradi L, Knosalla C, Richter M, Merk DR, et al. A randomized multicenter trial of minimally invasive rapid deployment versus conventional full sternotomy aortic valve replacement. Ann Thorac Surg. 2015;99:17–25.
54. Calderon J, Richebe P, Guibaud JP, CoiJic A, Branchard O, Asselineau J, et al. Prospective randomized study of early pulmonary evaluation of patients scheduled for aortic valve surgery performed by ministernotomy or total median sternotomy. J Cardiothorac Vasc Anesth. 2009;23:795–801.
55. Dogan S, Dzemali O, Wimmer-Greinecker G, Derra P, Doss M, Khan MF, et al. Minimally invasive versus conventional aortic valve replacement: a prospective randomized trial. J Heart Valve Dis. 2003;12:76–80.
56. Mächler HE, Bergmann P, Anelli-Monti M, Dacar D, Rehak P, Knez I, et al. Minimally invasive versus conventional aortic valve operations: a prospective study in 120 patients. Ann Thorac Surg. 1999;67:1001–5.
57. Moustafa MA, Abdelsamad AA, Zakaria G, Omarah MM. Minimal vs median sternotomy for aortic valve replacement. Asian Cardiovasc Thorac Ann. 2007;15:472–5.
58. Nair SK, Sudarshan CD, Thorpe BS, Singh J, Pillay T, Catarino P, Valchanov K, Codispoti M, Dunning J, Abu-Omar Y, Moorjani N, Matthews C, Freeman CJ, Fox-Rushby JA, Sharples LD. Mini-Stern Trial: A randomized trial comparing mini-sternotomy to full median sternotomy for aortic valve replacement. J Thorac Cardiovasc Surg. 2018;156(6):2124–2132.e31. https://doi.org/10.1016/j.jtcvs.2018.05.057. Epub 2018 Jun 4
59. Acker MA, Parides MK, Perrault LP, Moskowitz AJ, Gelijns AC, Voisine P, et al. Mitral-valve repair versus replacement for severe ischemic mitral regurgitation. N Engl J Med. 2014;370:23–32.
60. Ay Y, Kara I, Aydin C, Ay NK, Inan B, Basel H, et al. Comparison of the health related quality of life of patients following mitral valve surgical procedures in the 6-months follow-up: a prospective study. Ann Thorac Cardiovasc Surg. 2013;19:113–9.
61. Immer FE, Donati O, Wyss T, Immer-Bansi AS, Schmidli J, Berdat PA, et al. Quality of life after mitral valve surgery: differences between reconstruction and replacement. J Heart Valve Dis. 2003;12:162–8.
62. Suri RM, Antiel RM, Burkhart HM, Huebner M, Li Z, Eton DT, et al. Quality of life after early mitral valve repair using conventional and robotic approaches. Ann Thorac Surg. 2012;93:761–9.
63. Hansen L, Winkel S, Kuhr J, Bader R, Bleese N, Riess FC. Factors influencing survival and postoperative quality of life after mitral valve reconstruction. Eur J Cardiothorac Surg. 2010;37:635–44.
64. Heikkinen J, Biancari F, Satta J, Salmela E, Juvonen T, Lepojarvi M. Quality of life after mitral valve repair. J Heart Valve Dis. 2005;14:722–6.
65. Mesana TG, Lam BK, Chan V, Chen K, Ruel M, Chan K. Clinical evaluation of functional mitral stenosis after mitral valve repair for degenerative disease: potential affect on surgical strategy. J Thorac Cardiovasc Surg. 2013;146:1418–23; discussion 23–5
66. van Leeuwen WJ, Head SJ, de Groot-de Laat LE, Geleijnse ML, Bogers AJ, Van Herwerden LA, et al. Single-centre experience with mitral valve repair in asymptomatic patients with severe mitral valve regurgitation. Interact Cardiovasc Thorac Surg. 2013;16:731–7.
67. Timek TA, Hooker RL, Collingwood R, Davis AT, Alguire CT, Willekes CL, et al. Five-year real world outcomes of GeoForm ring implantation in patients with ischemic mitral regurgitation. J Thorac Cardiovasc Surg. 2014;148:1951–6.
68. Hauptman PJ, Rector TS, Wentworth D, Kubo S. Quality of life in advanced heart failure: role of mitral regurgitation. Am Heart J. 2006;151:213–8.

Quality of Life After Mitral Valve and Tricuspid Valve Surgery

11

Nicola Di Bari, Marco Moscarelli, Giuseppe Nasso, and Giuseppe Speziale

Quality of Life After Mitral Valve Surgery

Introduction

Recent years have seen a rising interest in measuring quality of life (QoL) as an outcome of cardiac surgery for mitral valve repair/replacement rather than focusing solely on postoperative morbidity and mortality. Consistent with available guidelines [1], the current clinical trend is to treat severe degenerative mitral disease surgically in the early phase when patients are still asymptomatic. Earlier treatment makes preserving patient QoL a high priority and an important benchmark for procedural success.

Alongside a focus on postoperative QoL, cardiac centers are increasingly opting for minimally invasive surgical approaches as a way to minimize surgical risk. Recent strides forward in surgical technique have made fully endoscopic mitral valve repair/replacement a safe, common procedure that produces similar outcomes to the sternotomy approach in terms of morbidity and mortality. To this end, it is imperative to examine QoL as an additional important outcome of minimally invasive and percutaneous procedures, as has been recently done for traditional surgical approaches.

Methods for Assessing the Quality of Life

Several instruments are used to measure QoL after cardiac surgery. Generic tools (i.e., non-disease specific tools) include the Short-Form (SF) 36 [2], RAND SF-36 [3], SF-12 [4], Linear Analogue Scale Assessment [4], 6-Domain Australian QoL Index [5], Nottingham Health Profile Questionnaire [6], Patient Component of the Global Assessment [7], and the EuroQoL-5D [8]. Disease-specific tools include the Minnesota Living with Heart Failure Questionnaire (MLHFQ) [9], Kansas City Cardiomyopathy Questionnaire (KCCQ) [7], and Duke Activity Status index (DASI) [10]. These instruments can be used individually or in combination to assess QoL as an outcome of cardiac surgery.

The most widely used assessment among studies reported in the literature is the SF-36. Advantages of the SF-36 questionnaire include its brevity (on average, the survey takes no longer than 10 min to complete) and precision (validity and reproducibility). The 36 questions of the

N. Di Bari (✉)
Division of Cardiac Surgery, Department of Emergency and Organ Transplant, Policlinico Hospital, University of Bari, Bari, Italy

M. Moscarelli · G. Nasso · G. Speziale
Department of Cardiovascular Surgery, GVM Care & Research Anthea Hospital, Bari, Italy
e-mail: m.moscarelli@imperial.ac.uk; gnasso@libero.it; gspeziale@gvmnet.it

T. Athanasiou et al. (eds.), *Patient Reported Outcomes and Quality of Life in Cardiovascular Interventions*,
https://doi.org/10.1007/978-3-031-09815-4_11

SF-36 are subdivided into 8 different scales and 2 indices that summarize physical and mental health. A higher score indicates better self-perceived health. With regard to disease-specific scales, the KCCQ is most widely used and is structured in 23 items representing 6 dimensions, with higher scores indicating better QoL.

Negative Predictors of Quality of Life

In most studies, variables that negatively influence QoL after mitral valve surgery are female sex, older age, and higher New York Heart Association (NYHA) class [11, 12]. Other factors such as coronary heart disease (and associated risk factors) and previous myocardial infarction also negatively impact QoL in this context (Fig. 11.1).

In one study, Ay et al. [2] reported that preoperative atrial fibrillation, oral anticoagulation, peripheral vascular disease, and female sex negatively influenced mental score. Similarly, Maisano et al. [13] identified preoperative atrial fibrillation, diabetes mellitus, high creatinine level, Euroscore, degree of mitral insufficiency (MI), and pulmonary artery pressure as negative predictors after mitral valve surgery.

Quality of Life in Relation to Prosthesis Type and Surgical Approach

Biological Versus Mechanical Heart Valve Replacement

In a study conducted by Molero Junior et al. [14], QoL was assessed using the SF-36 in 36 patients (16 men, mean age 51 years) who underwent mitral valve replacement surgery. The authors found that prosthesis type did not influence postoperative QoL after an average follow-up period of 32.5 months. In contrast, a recent study of 150 patients by Huang et al. [15] found that mechanical mitral valve replacement with the ATS valve (ATS Medical, Inc., Minneapolis, Minn) was associated with better QoL at discharge (determined using the Chinese version of the SF-36) compared to replacement with the Sorin and St. Jude Medical (SJM) valves, although this difference gradually decreased at 3 and 12 months of follow-up. Another study by the same group [16] compared postoperative QoL after replacement with the Star GK (85 patients) and SJM (87 patients) and found no significant difference between groups.

Predictors of Impaired HRQOL after mitral valve intervention	
Patient factors	**Surgical factors**
Higher NYHA Class	Replacement instead of repair
Female	Elevated trans-mitral gradient
Increasing age	Residual mitral regurgitation
Previous myocardial infarction	Use of mechanical instead of bioprosthetic valves
Atrial fibrillation	
Higher EuroSCORE	
Risk factors for CAD	
Peripheral vascular disease	
Diabetes	

Predictors of impared health-related quality of life (HRQOL) improvement.

Fig. 11.1 Predictors of Impaired HRQOL after mitral valve intervention.

Conventional Mitral Valve Intervention (Surgical Repair or Replacement) Via Median Sternotomy

Several studies have reported the use of single assessment tools in patients undergoing conventional mitral repair or replacement surgery with median sternotomy. In general, patients exhibit improvements in QoL during the postoperative period with scores similar to or even higher than the normal population, especially for the physical component [6, 17, 18]. Some studies illustrate this effect to be larger in patients undergoing repair rather than replacement [9, 19]. On the other hand, a prospective randomized study identified no significant difference in postoperative QoL after repair versus replacement, even in patients with moderate or severe MI at follow-up [10].

Hansen et al. [11] found that QoL improved in all patients (n = 663) undergoing conventional valve repair surgery regardless of etiology. Moreover, patients treated for mitral degeneration showed a higher physical well-being score than a population sample matched for age and gender. Patients with idiopathic dilated cardiomyopathy had the worst QoL scores at follow-up, especially if they were women, despite higher comorbidities among men.

Conventional Mitral Valve Interventions (Surgical Repair or Replacement) versus Minimally Invasive Approach

In two studies comparing patients undergoing conventional versus minimally invasive mitral valve surgery, QoL (assessed using the SF-12 and SF-36, respectively) was superior in patients undergoing minimally invasive surgery at short-term follow-up, but there was no difference during long-term follow-up [20, 21]. Similarly, Suri et al. [20] identified a benefit of robotic surgery to conventional surgery during the first year of follow-up, but observed no significant difference at 12 or 24 months. Nasso et al. [21] conducted a randomized controlled trial in 160 patients with Barlow's disease and found that patients undergoing minimally invasive mitral surgery had better physical activity and general well-being at 6 months, but there was no benefit in terms of SF-36 score at 1 year. Two other studies similarly detected no difference in QoL outcomes after conventional versus minimally invasive procedures beyond the immediate postoperative period [4, 22]. These studies do however confirm the non-superiority of minimally invasive surgery to conventional surgery for postoperative QoL, supporting the adoption of minimally invasive surgery as the gold standard for mitral repair/replacement at many cardiac surgery centers.

A recent study by Zhao et al. [23] compared QoL measured with the SF-12 at 30 days and 6 months after mitral valve replacement with a robotic (da Vinci) versus conventional approach (47 patients in each group). In this study, QoL was initially better in the robotic group, but this difference diminished at 6 months. However, the robotic approach is less invasive, favors quick postoperative recovery, and has higher patient satisfaction.

Another study retrospectively compared the effect of fully endoscopic versus conventional mitral surgery on QoL in a population of 163 patients using the Chinese version of the Medical Outcome Study (MOS) SF-36. At 3 months follow-up, the authors noted a significant group difference in bodily pain and mental pain scores in favor of the minimally invasive group. In conclusion, compared to median sternotomy, endoscopic surgery has a noninferior therapeutic effect and improves QoL with a better cosmetic effect and lower pain [5].

MitraClip Implantation

Edge-to-edge percutaneous mitral repair significantly reduces mitral regurgitation with a low complication rate in patients with severe MI who are not eligible for conventional surgery. Many studies in the literature have reported a significant improvement in QoL among patients receiving a MitraClip implant [24–26]. In a study by Agata Krawczyk-Ożóg et al. [27], the MitraClip was compared to conventional conservative treatment in 33 patients with severe mitral regurgitation on a functional basis, as the efficacy and benefit of this procedure is not yet fully established. Compared to conservative treatment, MitraClip implantation improved the clinical condition of patients measured as significant decrease in NYHA class; reduced the extent of regurgitation, effective regurgitant orifice area of the vena contracta, regurgitation volume, and end diastolic left ventricular diameter; and improved QoL measured on the EQ-5D-3L and SF-12v2 at a mean follow-up of 8.0 ± 2.3 months. Other studies have reported no significant difference between the MitraClip implant and conventional surgery in this context [28, 29].

In a cohort study used by the Society of Thoracic Surgeons/American College of Cardiology Transcatheter Valve Therapy registry, Arnold et al. [7] analyzed data from patients with severe MI treated between 2013 and 2017 at 217 US hospitals and measured changes in disease-specific health status (KCCQ-Overall Summary [OS] score; range 0-100 points, with higher scores indicating better health status) at 30 days and 1 year after the procedure. Risk factors associated with 30-day KCCQ-OS were also evaluated. KCCQ data were available from 81.2% of patients at baseline, 69.3% of survivors at 30 days, and 47.4% of survivors at 1 year. Among 4226 patients who underwent transcatheter mitral valve repair, KCCQ-OS increased from 41.9 before the procedure to 66.7 at 30 days and scores remained stable to 1 year post-procedure. In the multivariable analysis, atrial fibrillation, permanent pacemaker, severe lung disease, home oxygen, in-hospital renal failure, and lower KCCQ-OS scores at baseline were independently associated with lower 30-day KCCQ-OS scores. In estimates calculated with inverse probability weighting, 54.2% of patients were alive and well at 1-year follow-up, 23.0% had died, 21.9% had persistently poor health status (KCCQ-OS <60 points), 5.5% had a health status decline from baseline, and 4.6% had both poor health status and health status decline.

Other Percutaneous Mitral Valve Interventions

With regard to other percutaenous interventions, studies have demonstrated improvements in QoL after implantation with the Carillon Mitral Countou System [8, 30].

The Viacor percutaneous transvenous mitral annuloplasty device was used in one study, but the trial was terminated prematurely due to perioperative complications and no observable improvement [31].

A study by Barth et al. [32] examined QoL at 5 months after treatment with the PASCAL device in 31 patients: 63% had functional MI, 29% had degenerative disease, and 9.7% had mixed etiology. Eighty-seven percent of the cohort completed follow-up including the KCCQ and EuroQoL5D. The authors detected postoperative QoL improvements of 31 and 9 points, respectively, supporting safety and efficacy of the device. Another work by Lim et al. [33] used the same QoL measures and identified improvements of 17 and 10 points, respectively, in 62 patients at 30 days after PASCAL device implantation.

Finally, a study by Okoh et al. [34] evaluated QoL in 15 patients undergoing transcatheter valve-in-valve implantation for previous biological valve degeneration using the Sapien XT, Sapien, or Sapien S3 and reported QoL improvement in 10 out of 11 patients evaluated at 30 days follow-up.

Quality of Life After Tricuspid Valve Surgery

Severe tricuspid insufficiency is relatively common and higher severity is associated with higher morbidity and mortality. Treatments for isolated forms are limited. For most patients, both medical therapy and conventional surgery can be effective; however, transcatheter repair surgery has become a treatment of choice and produces significant improvements in QoL and mortality. Davidson et al. [35] reported outcomes of first-time treatment with the Cardioband device in US cohort of 30 patients and found that 75% of patients were NYHA class I or II and showed a KCCQ score improvement of 16 points at 30 days follow-up. Another study by Nickenig et al. [36] demonstrated an increase in follow-up KCCQ score of 14 points after the same procedure.

Guillem Muntanè-Carol et al. [37] described an initial experience with the FORMA device for transcatheter tricuspid repair in high-risk patients. Patients showed significant improvements in both heart disease symptoms and QoL. Positive results were also obtained with the TrialignTM device, which represents a new percutaneous tricuspid annuloplasty technique for functional insufficiency [38]. The edge-to-edge transcatheter technique has also been shown to be safe and effective for reducing tricuspid insufficiency and improves QoL by 16% [39].

Although there is considerable clinical experience with transcatheter repair in the literature, repair is not possible or may not optimally reduce the severity of tricuspid regurgitation in a large number of patients. A large coaptation gap (>6–8 mm) and non-central regurgitant jets are associated with poor procedural success. Moreover, the presence of calcification and immobile or severely retracted leaflets (especially the septal leaflet) with extensive tenting distances are also negative predictors of outcome after repair. Transcatheter replacement is the preferred treatment option in cases of moderate or severe tricuspid regurgitation after repair. Valves currently in use include orthotopic types (Cardiovalve, Evoque, Lux-Valve, Navigate, TriSol, Intrepid, TriCares) and heterotopic types (Sapien XT, TricValve, Tricento), both of which appear to positively influence QoL [40].

References

1. Baumgartner H, Falk V, Bax JJ, Bonis MD, Hamm C, Holm PJ, et al. 2017 ESC/EACTS Guidelines for the management of valvular heart disease. Eur Heart J. 2017;38:2739–91.
2. Ay Y, Kara I, Aydin C, Ay NK, Inan B, Basel H, et al. Comparison of the health related quality of life of patients following mitral valve surgical procedures in the 6-months follow-up: a prospective study. Ann Thorac Cardiovasc Surg. 2013;19:113–9.
3. Heikkinen J, Biancari F, Satta J, et al. Quality of life after mitral valve repair. J Heart Valve Dis. 2005;14:722–6.
4. Walther T, Falk V, Metz S, Diegeler A, Battellini R, Autschbach R, et al. Pain and quality of life after minimally invasive versus conventional cardiac surgery. Ann Thorac Surg. 1999;67:1643–7.
5. Huang L, Chen D, Chen L, et al. Health-related quality of life following minimally invasive totally endoscopic mitral valve surgery. J Cardiothorac Surg. 2020;15:194.
6. Mesana TG, Lam BK, Chan V, Chen K, Ruel M, Chan K. Clinical evaluation of functional mitral stenosis after mitral valve repair for degenerative disease: potential affect on surgical strategy. J Thorac Cardiovasc Surg. 2013;146:1418–23.
7. Arnold SV, Li Z, Vemulapalli S, Baron SJ, et al. Association of Transcatheter Mitral Valve Repair with quality of life outcomes at 30 days and 1 year. Analysis of the Transcatheter Valve Therapy Registry. JAMA Cardiol. 2018;3(12):1151–9.
8. Siminiak T, Wu JC, Haude M, Hoppe UC, et al. Treatment of functional mitral regurgitation by percutaneous annuloplasty:results of the TITAN Trial. Eur J Heart Fail. 2012;14:931–8.
9. Immer FE, Donati O, Wyss T, Immer-Bansi AS, Schmidli J, Berdat PA, et al. Quality of life after mitral valve surgery: differences between reconstruction and replacement. J Heart Valve Dis. 2003;12:162–8.
10. Acker MA, Parides MK, Perrault LP, Moskowitz AJ, Gelijns AC, Voisine P, et al. Mitral-valve repair versus replacement for severe ischemic mitral regurgitation. N Engl J Med. 2014;370:23–32.
11. Goldsmith I, Lip GY, Patel RL. A prospective study of changes in the quality of life of patients following mitral valve repair and replacement. Eur J Cardiothorac Surg. 2001;20:949–55.
12. Hansen L, Winkel S, Kuhr J, Bader R, Bleese N, Riess FC. Factors influencing survival and postoperative quality of life after mitral valve reconstruction. Eur J Cardiothorac Surg. 2010;37:635–44.
13. Maisano F, Franzen O, Baldus S, Schafer U, Hausleiter J, Butter C, et al. Percutaneous mitral valve interventions in the real world: early and 1-year results from the ACCESS-EU, a prospective, multicenter, nonrandomized post-approval study of the MitraClip therapy in Europe. J Am Coll Cardiol. 2013;62:1052–61.
14. Junior MJC, Raimundo RD, Tonon do Amaral JA, de Abreu LC, Breda JR. Bioprosthesis versus mechanical valve heart prosthesis: assessment of quality of life. Int J Cardiovasc Sci. 2020;33(1):36–42.
15. Huang JS, Sun KP, Xu N, Chen Q, Chen LW, Kuo YR. Effect of the sounds of different mechanical mitral valves on quality of life at different follow-up times: a single-center study. Ann Thorac Cardiovasc Surg. 2020;26(4):209–15.
16. Huang JS, Xu N, Sun KP, Hong ZN, Chen LW, Kuo YR, Chen Q. Comparison of quality of life in patients who underwent mechanical mitral valve replacement: star GK vs SJM. J Cardiothorac Surg. 2020;15:2.

17. Goldsmith I, Lip GY, Kaukuntla H, Patel RL. Hospital morbidity and mortality and changes in quality of life following mitral valve surgey in the elderly. J Heart Valve Dis. 1999;8:702–7.
18. Grady KL, Lee R, Subacius H, Malaisrie SC, McGee EC Jr, Kruse J, et al. Improvements in health-related quality of life before and after isolated cardiac operations. Ann Thorac Surg. 2011;91:777–83.
19. Jokinen JJ, Hippelainen MJ, Pitkanen OA, et al. Mitral valve replacement versus repair:propensity-adjusted survival and quality-of-life analysis. Ann Thorac Surg. 2007;84:451–8.
20. Suri RM, Antiel RM, Burkhart HM, Huebner M, Li Z, Eton DT, et al. Quality of life after early mitral valve repair using conventional and robotic approaches. Ann Thorac Surg. 2012;93:761–9.
21. Nasso G, Bonifazi R, Romano V, Bartolomucci F, Rosano G, Massari F, et al. Three-year results of repaired Barlow mitral valves via right minithoracotomy versus median sternotomy in a randomized trial. Cardiology. 2014;128:97–105.
22. Bayer-Topilsky T, Suri RM, Topilsky Y, Marmor YN, Trenerry MR, Antiel RM, et al. Psychoemotional and quality of life response to mitral operations in patients with mitral regurgitation: a prospective study. Ann Thorac Surg. 2015;99:847–54.
23. Zhao H, Zhang H, Yang M, Xiao C, Wang Y, Gao C, Wanf R. Comparison of quality of life and long-term outcomes following mitral valve replacement through robotically assisted versus median sternotomy approach. Nan Fang Yi Ke Da Xue Xue Bao. 2020;40(11):1557–63.
24. Edelman JJ, Dias P, Passage J, Yamen E. Percutaneous mitral valve repair in a high-risk Australian series. Heart Lung Circ. 2014;23:520–6.
25. Franzen O, van der Heyden J, Baldus S, et al. MitraClip(R) therapy in patients with end-stage systolic heart failure. Eur J Heart Fail. 2011;13:569–76.
26. Neuss M, Schau T, Schoepp M, Seifert M, et al. Patient selection criteria and midterm clinical outcome for MitraClip therapy in patients with severe mitral regurgitation and severe congestive heart failure. Eur J Heart Fail. 2013;15:786–95.
27. Ozog AK, Siudak Z, Sorysz D, Holda M, Plotek A, et al. Comparison of clinical and echocardiographic outcomes and quality of life in patients with severe mitral regurgitation treated by MitraClip implantation or treated conservatively. Postepy Kardiol Interwencyjnej. 2018;14(3):291–8.
28. Buzzatti N, Maisano F, Latib A, Taramasso M, et al. Comparison of outcomes of percutaneous MitraClip versus surgical repair or replacement for degenerative mitral regurgitation in octogenarians. Am J Cardiol. 2015;115:487–92.
29. Rudolph V, Knap M, Franzen O, Schluter M, et al. Echocardiograohic and clinical outcomes of MitraClip therapy in patients not amenable to surgery. J Am Coll Cardiol. 2011;58:2190–5.
30. Schofer J, Siminiak T, Haude M, Herman JP, et al. Percutaneous mitral annuloplasty for functional mitral regurgitation: results of the CARILLON Mitral Annuloplasty Device European Union Study. Circulation. 2009;120:326–33.
31. Machaalany J, Bilodeau L, Hoffmann R, Sack S, et al. Treatment of functional mitral valve regurgitation with the permanent percutaneous transvenous mitral annuloplasty system: results of the multicenter international Percutaneous Transvenous Mitral Annuloplasty System to Reduce Mitral Valve Regurgitation in Patients with Heart Failure trial. Am Heart J. 2013;165:761–9.
32. Barth S, Hautmann MB, Arvaniti E, Kikec J, Kerber S, Zacher M, et al. Mid-term hemodynamic and functional results after transcatheter mitral valve leaflet repair with the new PASCAL device. Clin Res Cardiol. 2021;110(5):628–39.
33. Lim DS, Kar S, Spargias K, Kipperman RM, O'Neill WW, Ng MKC, et al. Transcatheter Valve Repair for Patients With Mitral Regurgitation: 30-Day Results of the CLASP Study. JACC Cardiovasc Interv. 2019;12(14):1369–78.
34. Okoh AK, Shah A, Kang N, Almaz B, Resnick J, Ghaffar A, Chen C, Haik B, Cohen M, Russo MJ. Outcomes After Transcatheter Mitral Valve-in-Valve Replacement in Patients With Degenerated Bioprosthesis: A Single-Center Experience. J Invasive Cardiol. 2020;32(2):49–54.
35. Davidson CJ, Lim DS, Smith RL, Kodali SK, Kipperman RM, Eleid MF, Reisman M, Whisenant B, Puthumana J, Abramson S, Fowler D, Grayburn P, Hahn RT, Koulogiannis K, Pislaru SV, Zwink T, Minder M, Dahou A, Deo SH, Vandrangi P, Deuschl F, Feldman TE, Gray WA, Investigators CTREFS. Early Feasibility Study of Cardioband Tricuspid System for Functional Tricuspid Regurgitation: 30-Day Outcomes. JACC Cardiovasc Interv. 2021;14(1):41–50.
36. Ickenig G, Weber M, Schüler R, Hausleiter J, Nabauer M, von Bardeleben RS, et al. Tricuspid valve repair with the Cardioband system: two-year outcomes of the multicentre, prospective TRI-REPAIR study. EuroIntervention. 2021;16(15):e1264–71.
37. Muntané-Carol G, Del Val D, Bédard E, Philippon F, Rodés-Cabau J. Transcatheter innovations in tricuspid regurgitation: FORMA device. Prog Cardiovasc Dis. 2019;62(6):496–9.
38. Besler C, Meduri CU, Lurz P. Transcatheter Treatment of Functional Tricuspid Regurgitation Using the Trialign Device. Interv Cardiol. 2018;13(1):8–13.
39. Orban M, Besler C, Braun D, Nabauer M, Zimmer M, Orban M, Noack T, Mehilli J, Hagl C, Seeburger J, Borger M, Linke A, Thiele H, Massberg S, Ender J, Lurz P, Hausleiter J. Six-month outcome after transcatheter edge-to-edge repair of severe tricuspid regurgitation in patients with heart failure. Eur J Heart Fail. 2018;20(6):1055–62.
40. Goldberg YH, Ho E, Chau M, Latib A. Update on Transcatheter Tricuspid Valve Replacement Therapies. Front Cardiovasc Med. 2021;15(8):619558. https://doi.org/10.3389/fcvm.2021.619558.

Quality of Life and Patient Reported Outcomes in Paediatric Cardiac Surgery Patients

12

Robyn Lotto, Amer Harky, and Attilio Lotto

Introduction

This chapter provides an overview of the literature examining patient related outcome measures following paediatric cardiac surgery. The findings are divided into five sections reflecting five dimensions of patient reported outcomes, namely: quality of life or more specifically health related quality of life, functional status, symptoms and symptom burden, patient experience and health behaviours.

R. Lotto
Faculty of Health, Liverpool John Moores University, Liverpool, England

Liverpool Centre for Cardiovascular Science, Liverpool, England
e-mail: r.r.lotto@ljmu.ac.uk

A. Harky
Department of Cardiothoracic Surgery, Liverpool Heart and Chest Hospital, Liverpool, England

Department of Integrative Biology, Faculty of Health and Sciences, University of Liverpool, Liverpool, England

Liverpool Centre for Cardiovascular Science, Liverpool, England

A. Lotto (✉)
Faculty of Health, Liverpool John Moores University, Liverpool, England

Liverpool Centre for Cardiovascular Science, Liverpool, England

Department of Cardiac Surgery, Alder Hey Children's, NHS Foundation Trust, Liverpool, England
e-mail: Attilio.Lotto@alderhey.nhs.uk

Background

Congenital heart disease (CHD) is the most frequently occurring congenital anomaly, affecting around 0.8% of live births [1]. It is a heterogeneous group of cardiac anomalies ranging from innocent malformation to severe anomalies carrying significant risk of neonatal death if not recognized and managed appropriately [2, 3]. Annually, around 5500 operations are performed in the United Kingdom [4]. These may be classed as either corrective or palliative. Whilst corrective surgery has traditionally been viewed as curative, palliative correction is directed to improving functional capacity, often requiring several operations or interventions during the patient's lifetime.

Following the introduction of the cardiopulmonary bypass machine in the early 1950s, cardiac surgery quickly developed as a speciality [5]. Nonetheless, developments in CHD surgery lagged behind, with the majority of complex surgical cases treated with palliative procedures, and few options for definitive surgery. As a result, many patients require multiple surgeries, often associated with high morbidity, and poor quality of life (QoL) [6]. The last two decades have witnessed a significant reduction in both mortality and morbidity following CHD surgery, most noticeable in the treatment of complex, previously incurable conditions [7]. This has ultimately led to an increased life expectancy for the

T. Athanasiou et al. (eds.), *Patient Reported Outcomes and Quality of Life in Cardiovascular Interventions*,
https://doi.org/10.1007/978-3-031-09815-4_12

majority of patients; with most now surviving into adulthood [8].

The impact of a chronic disease, on a developing child and their family, is complex, and combined with underline pathology management can have a significant effect on their QoL and their ability to psychologically adjust [9, 10]. As mortality decreases, the need for a better understanding of the long-term impact of QoL and other patient reported outcomes in patients following CHD diagnosis has increased (Table 12.1) [11].

Table 12.1 Summary of key systematic reviews in quality of life in cardiac patients

Study	Focus of the study	Summary of key findings
Parents and families		
Tesson et al. [12] 11 studies included, involving nine interventions.	Review of psychological interventions for children, adolescents and adults with CHD and their family's efficacy-wise. Four interventions involved adolescents and adults, five involved parents.	Patient focus interventions allowed for alleviation of anxiety and worry maternal mental health wise and better coping and family functioning.
Gregory et al. [13] 33 cross sectional or cohort studies included	Review of how parental QoL may be affected with children diagnosed with CHD.	The main factors which affected parental QoL included: severity of illness, age at which child was diagnosed, perceived levels of support and financial resources available.
Golfenshtein et al. [14] 66 observational studies included	Parental stress and experience of raising children with CHD, pediatric cancer, and ASD.	Future research and assessment of parenting stress should account for the illness course and family needs should be addressed.
Vo et al. [15] 15 studies included Narrative synthesis presented	Systematic review of the literature available on the psychosocial impact of 22q11 deletion syndrome.	Study found that a lot of complex and conflicting emotions were experienced by family members of those with 22q11 deletion syndrome.
Childhood		
Clancy et al. [16] 28 studies included	Psychosocial outcomes of infants and young children with CHD who had cardiac surgery early in life.	The study found a high prevalence of low severity emotional and behavioural dysregulation. Comorbidity was shown to increase impairment, with evident externalisation. The study encouraged assessment and monitoring of behaviour and social development to enable early detection and intervention.
Drakouli et al. [17] 32 studies included	Assessing the QoL in children and adolescents with CHD.	QoL is determined by factors such as parental support, economic support, physical ability, and overall mental health.
Huisenga et al. [18] 185 studies included	Developmental outcomes from infancy to adolescence with children with CHD who underwent surgery.	Children with complex CHD can beat increased risk of poorer developmental outcomes. Single-ventricle CHD has worse outcomes than two-ventricle CHDs. There is no constant association between preoperative factors and patient outcomes.
Lane et al. [19] Cochrane review. No papers included	Psychological interventions in children with CHD with depression.	Depression can exacerbate the physical impact of CHD. There has been no efficacy proven in non-pharmacological treatments.

Table 12.1 (continued)

Study	Focus of the study	Summary of key findings
Adolescents and adulthood		
Journiac et al. [20] 32 studies included	Psychosocial outcomes and experiences of young adult cardiac patients (18–55 years old).	In comparison to the general population, young adult cardiac patients demonstrated worse health behaviour profiles. Women were shown to have increased levels of depression, stress and distress and overall a lower QoL.
Kahr et al. [21] Systematic review and meta analysis. 234 studies included with a total of 47,471 patients included in analysis	QoL in CHD patients (Mean age 24, with 84% of studies adult participants only)	QoL is impaired in moderate or complex CHD.
Schrøder et al. [22] Systematic review and meta analysis. 18 studies included with 1986 patients included in analysis	QoL in adolescents and young adults.	Social functioning was found to be comparable, or better compared with controls. In some subdomains, patients appeared to have reduced QoL. Overall, adolescents and young adults do not have reduced QoL.
Xu et al. [23] Meta analysis of nine RCTs	Post-op effects of exercise training on QoL, biomarkers, exercise capacity and vascular function in CHD.	NT-proBNP levels were lower in individuals who engaged in exercise training. Exercise interventions were also shown to increase the score in QoL from the score prior to intervention.
Fteropoulli et al. [24] 31 studies included	Relationship between disease severity and QoL in adult patients with CHD.	The QoL of adult congenital heart disease patients can be compromised in physical disease.

Patient Reported Outcomes (PROs) and Patient Reported Outcome Measures (PROMs)

PROMS are tools used to measure outcomes that matter to patients; reflecting patients' or caregivers' perspective of the impact of the condition on their lives, including how illness is experienced [25]. An example could be 'can I climb my stairs?', rather than 'has my cardiac output improved?' The completion and compilation of PROMS by patients plays an important role in patient assessment, assisting clinical decision-making, and tracking patient progress. There is growing evidence to support the use of PROMS to improve care processes and outcomes in part through supporting communication between clinicians and patients [26] as well as improve patient engagement and satisfaction with care [27]. PROs can be characterised into five dimensions namely: functional status; symptoms and symptom burden; patient experience; health behaviours; and quality of life or more specifically health related quality of life [28]. Figure 12.1 Despite the growing interest in PROMs, at the time of writing, no PROM for congenital heart disease in children [29], and one newly validated PROM for the adult congenital heart disease (ACHD) population [30] has been identified. Tools identified in the literature are presented in Table 12.2.

Quality of Life

Quality of life is a multidimensional concept and focusses on the self-perceptions of an individual's current state of mind [31]. It consists of a combination of objective and subjective indicators within a broad range of life domains, including physical, psychological, social and

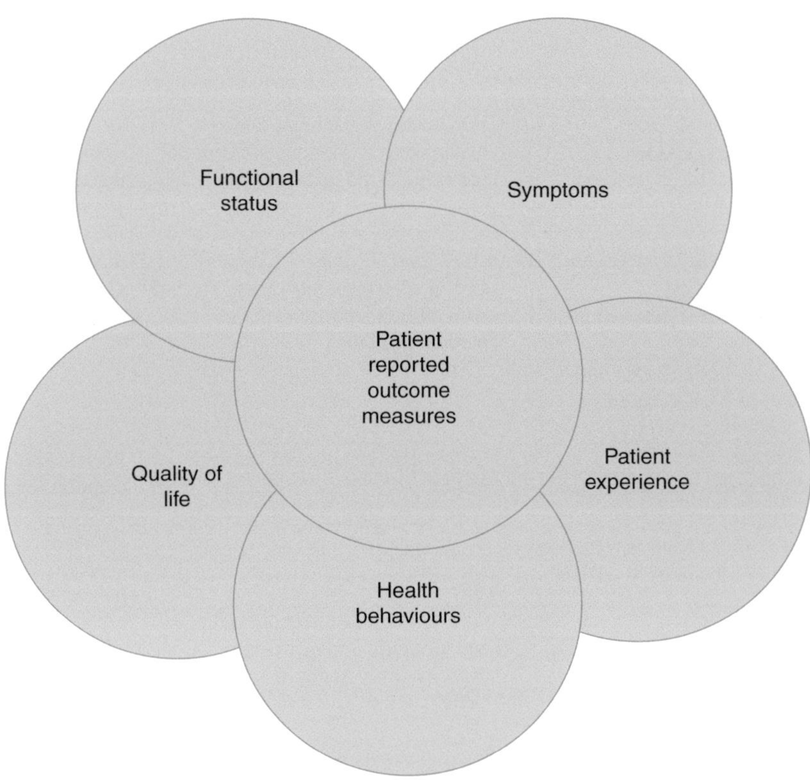

Fig. 12.1 Patient reported outcomes

Table 12.2 Summary table of different assessment tools of quality of life

Tool	Description	Comments
TNO-AZL Adult's Health Related Quality of Life (TAAQOL)	This survey is consisting of several questionnaires to enable a systematic and reliable description of Health-Related Quality of Life of people of 16 years and older. This is defined as a person's health status, weighted by the emotional response of the person to his/her health status problems	Parents usually fill this out, however the child version can be filled out by the children who are able to express the reported questionnaire
Sickness Impact Profile (SIP)	A particular type of health assessment using behaviourally-based measure of health status in terms of the impact of the disease on physical and emotional functioning and it has two main domains: physical and psychosocial. It is usually used to assess a person's perception of their health status with respect to their disease impact.	It is a general form and not specific to CHD.
World Health Organization Quality of Life-Bref (WHOQOL-Bref)	A WHO defined quality of life assessment tool using four key domains (1) Physical health, (2) Psychological, (3) Social relationships and (4) Environment	General quality of life assessment and not specific to CHD.
Subjective Quality of Life (SQoL)	This is usually used to refer to a person's own assessment of self-well-being and satisfaction with life. It is a multidimensional concept involving various life domains using self-appraisal techniques.	Usually directed toward adults and not specific for CHD.
Linear Analogue Scale (LAS)	This is a self-assessment technique whereby a numeric lines with anchoring descriptions are placed and the patients is asked to mark their state on specific symptom on a scale level of 100 mm lines.	General assessment tool and not specific for CHD patients.

Table 12.2 (continued)

Tool	Description	Comments
Schedule for the Evaluation of Individual Quality of Life-Direct Weighting (SEIQoL-DW)	This assessment is an interview-based tool for the assessment of quality of life. This can be used for a variety of patient groups; however, its use is mostly limited to illnesses which impair cognitive functioning or motivational state.	General adults but can be used for children that can express or understand the form of the interview.
Congenital Heart Disease-TNO-AZL Adult's Quality of Life (CHD-TAAQOL)	This is a similar tool of TAAQOL but devoted to patients with congenital heart disease with the domains being focused mostly on the CHD related outcomes. Including questions related to Symptoms, the Impact cardiac surveillance and Worries domains.	This is a CHD specific questionnaire of TAAQOL.
PedsQL 3.0 Cardiac Module PedsQL 4.0 Generic Core Scales CHQ (Child Health Questionnaire)	A special, paediatric model used to measure the HRQOL in children who have health issues. This module has five scales related to symptoms, perceived physical appearance, treatment anxiety, cognitive problems, and communication.	Specific for paediatric age group, parents are used as proxy and children aged 8–18
TACQOL (Child Quality of Life)	This is mainly derived from the HRQoL with focused conceptualization of assessing the health of children aged 6–15 years using their parents as a proxy. This includes the assessment of feasibility and psychometric performance.	Specific for children but not CHD.
KINDL-R (health related quality of life for children and adolescents)	A German designed generic tool to assess quality of life in children and adolescent. It mostly involves psychometric testing in that age group.	Specific for children but not for CHD.
SF-36 and SF-36 (36-Item Short Form Health Survey) PedsQL	It is a similar form of PedsQL but derived from 36-Item Short Form Health Survey questionnaire (SF-36) and focuses on eight scales: physical functioning (PF), role physical (RP), bodily pain (BP), general health (GH), vitality (VT), social functioning (SF), role emotional (RE), and mental health (MH).	Specific for paediatric age group but not for CHD.
CBCL—internal/ external and total behaviour problems	This is a popular method, questionnaire that is currently used to assess the child's behavioural and emotional problems. CBCL is now called *Achenbach System of Empirically Based Assessment.*	This is mediated through the parents as proxy and not specific for CHD patients.
The Vineland Adaptive Behavior Scales (VABS—social)	A special assessment tool used to assess the adaptability of children with specific diseases such as Autism Spectrum Disorders (ASD) without intellectual disabilities.	A disease specific assessment tool for paediatric age group but not specific for CHD patients.
TAPQoL	A particular tool for pre-school children to assess their quality of life and see the impact of diseases and treatments on children's life. It consists of 43 items to measure	This is for paediatric age group but not specific for CHD cohort.
KIDSCREEN	This tool is used for children between the age of 8–18 years old to subjectively assess their health and well-beings. It was developed as a self-reporting system for healthy and chronically ill children. It has three models of KIDSCREEN-52, -27 and -10.	This tool is filled out by the children and can be used in different formats of -52, -27 or -10, depending on assessment level and components.
Manual for the child behavior checklist and revised child behavior profile	This is a specially designed questionnaire to understand the behaviour and behaviour profile of the children using different items to perform such assessments.	The test focuses mostly on behaviour pattern and profile of the child and how this affects the daily life.
Quality of life Child Health Questionnaire, parent form (CHQ-PF)	Generic questionnaire that is developed to assess the health-related quality of life in children between ages of 5–12 years old.	This assessment consists of 14 domains and it is filled out using the parents as proxy

(continued)

Table 12.2 (continued)

Tool	Description	Comments
Child Health Questionnaire, child form (CHQ-CF)	A designated child health questionnaire form which consists of 87-generic item related to paediatric health-related quality of life.	The questionnaire is usually conducted with different domains and scales to assess the health-related quality of life of the child.
Inventory for the Assessment of the Quality of life in Children and Adolescents (IQLC)	This assessment in consisting of nine items including subjective quality of life: school, family, other children, loneliness, health, humour/nerves, total quality of life, and, in addition to stress from illness and stress from therapy.	This assessment is generally for paediatric group of patients and used to measure many domains in the cohort
25-item Healthcare Needs Scale for Youth with Congenital Heart Disease—CHEN	A devoted tool for assessing quality of life for patients with congenital heart disease. This questionnaire is consisting of 25 items.	This questionnaire is targeting CHD patients and is mainly aimed at adolescence patients.
Health Behaviour Scale for CHD	This is a comprehensive tool that is measuring health compromising behaviors in children with congenital heart disease. This scale is consisted of 15 domains that has wide range of activities recorded.	The scale is specific for CHD patients and can be a useful tool to predict possible issues with quality of life of patients with CHD.
Bayley Scales of Infant Development	A comprehensive tool that is used to examine all the aspects of a child's development through five key developmental domains of cognition, language, social-emotional, motor and adaptive behaviour.	This is usually done by using the parent as a proxy, the target age cohort is 1–42 months old.
Baecke questionnaire	This tool is mainly used to assess the physical activity of patient in relation to quality of life.	The questionnaire is not specific for CHD patients but rather overall paediatric patients
Leuven Knowledge Questionnaire for CHD (LKQCHD).	This is a special tool that is used to test the level of patient's own knowledge of CHD. It is consisting of four main domains: (1) the disease and its treatment; (2) the prevention of complications; (3) physical activities; and (4) reproductive issues.	The study is filled out by the patients directly, however parents can be used as proxy if needed.
Consultation and relational Empathy (CARE) Measure	This study focuses on patients experience when they encounter health care service provision and how this affects them afterwards	This assessment is not specific for CHD but rather overall population of patients to assess the interpersonal quality of healthcare encounters mainly in primary care
Patient Perception of Patient-Centeredness (PPPC)	It measures the perception of the patient of patient-centered care during the last clinical visit. This tool has 14 items using a 4-point Likert scale from completely to not at all, and no subscales.	A generic tool used mostly in primary care without specialization to CHD patients.

environmental factors, as well as incorporating individual values [32]. Translating this concept into empirical terms is not simple, and even less so when examining the concept within the paediatric population [33]. Children's perceptions and values are likely to differ from those of adults, but will also change as they move from childhood to adolescents and early adulthood [34]. In addition, the importance of contextual variables, such as family and peer support systems cannot be underestimated [35].

There are an increasing number of systematic reviews comparing QoL of CHD patients to healthy peers or siblings. These are presented in Table 12.2, and findings summarised in Fig. 12.2. CHD patients are heterogeneous in their presenta-

	Parents and Family	***Childhood***	***Adolescence and young adulthood***
Physical	Timing of diagnosis	Comorbidities	Disease severity
	Complexity of the anomaly	Physical ability/ reduced exercise tolerance	Reduced exercise tolerance
Psychological	Parental stress	Depression	Depression, stress and distress
		Poor body image	Poor body image
Social	Poor parental support		
	Social isolation		Social isolation
Environmental	Low income		
	High deprivation		
	Low parental education levels		Low educational attainment

Fig. 12.2 Predictors of poor quality of life

tion, with evidence highly conflicting. Findings from studies examining factors such as the complexity of the underline anomaly, and the number of surgical interventions on QoL have come to differing conclusions [18, 23]. One recent study demonstrated a lower QoL in those with complex CHD compared with peers with moderate and simple cases [36]. However, another study reported impaired QoL in moderate and complex CHD patients only with no difference in simple CHD cases [21]. Other studies have demonstrated no difference in QoL between all cohorts of CHD patients when compared to their control peers [22]. However, others suggest that QoL is higher in girls with CHD during childhood, and boys and girls during adolescence, with severity of disease not shown to affect the overall outcomes [37].

Findings appear more consistent and nuanced across the limited evidence examining specific domains of QoL. A study by [11] focusing on QoL within the physical and psychosocial domains, reported impaired physical QoL during young adulthood, but no deficit in the mental and psychological domains. This was exacerbated when associated with a lower physical exercise tolerance, female gender, reduced social support and lower educational level predictors of reduced overall QoL.

A number of reviews have compared QoL of specific subgroups of the CHD population, to peers. In a review by Dahan-Oliel et al. [38], disease complexity was associated with a poorer HRQoL. However, this became particularly noticeable in the cohort of patients born preterm, as well as those with additional impairments. This difference remained the case for adolescents and young adults.

Social determinants such as parental unemployed as a result of the child's needs or families who experienced financial difficulties have also been associated with lower QoL, compared to of control groups [39].

Few studies have compared QoL of children with CHD to that of children with other chronic conditions. Again, findings are contradictory, with one study reporting that children with CHD after surgery experience a better proxy-reported QoL than other children with chronic disease [40] while the opposite was found in another study [41].

Parents and Caregiver Prospective

Children with CHD, especially those with complex underline pathologies, may need several operations, and often associated with prolonged hospital stays. This can have significant effect on the parental life, with parents suffering psychological, emotional and financial difficulties, in some instances resulting in post-traumatic stress disorder (PTSD) [42–44]. A recent study showed that up to 22% of the parents have persistent psychological issues when they have a child with CHD, regardless of the complexity of the disease [45]. Therefore, maintaining the well-being of the parents can be significant contributing factor in promoting the long-term wellbeing and QoL of the child [46].

Timing of the diagnosis may also influence the impact on the family. Developments in antenatal testing and diagnosis has meant that many parents will have engaged with the clinical team prior to birth. This provides time to prepare both psychologically and physically for the arrival of a neonate who will require medical intervention. Regular counselling and an understanding of the pathology and the requirement for intervention can enables parents to prepare for the birth, and any immediate requirements for intervention [47]. Ongoing counselling, parents and peer support, and external support can be of great help to reduce the burden on the parents [48]. The provision of comprehensive information packs, group support, or individual sessions detailing the care needs of a child with CHD throughout their lifetime is therefore essential. Parental perception of QoL peri-operatively may also have an effect on their children's QoL perception [49]. If parental mental health is affected by their children's condition, it may in turn lead to poor engagement in ensuring that their children develop according to their milestones, segregation from others, as well as reduced social opportunities.

Whilst the psychological impact on parents is considerable, there is evidence to suggest it reduces over time (Bevilacqua et al. 2013; [44]). Nonetheless, such parental stress can have negative implications on the life of the child if not addressed, with some parents becoming defensive and overprotective of the child, resulting in barriers to interaction between the child and other children in the same family or at school [50]. Siblings add to the complexity of the family dynamics [47], affecting not only the relationship between parent and child, but between parents, with over 40% of parents reporting strains on their relationships as a result of caring for a child with CHD [51]. By maximizing children's developmental stages, long term poor QoL outcomes may be prevented [52].

Functional Status

Functional status refers to the ability of a patient to perform age specific activities of daily life [53]. Within the context of CHD, neurodevelopmental disability is the most common complication for survivors of surgery for congenital heart disease (CHD) [54], with the impact reflective of their functional status.

A limited number of prospective studies are reported in a systematic review addressing neurodevelopmental outcomes in young CHD patients. The included studies consistently revealed cognitive and motor delay in children after cardiac surgery during early infancy [55]. These findings were reflected in a subsequent large-scale international study involving over 1700 participants [56]. Primary outcome measures included were Psychomotor Development Index (PDI), and Mental Development Index (MDI). Findings suggested that early neurodevelopmental outcomes have improved modestly over time, but only after adjustment for innate patient risk factors. Lower birth weight and genetic or extracardiac anomalies were associated with reduced PDI and MDI. Risk factors for lower PDI also included white race, and for MDI, male gender and lower maternal education.

In addition, age, supplemental tube feeding, longer cardiopulmonary bypass time, and shorter time since last hospitalization have been reported as significant predictors of developmental outcomes [57]. Lower performance on intelligence and alertness assessment have also been reported, which may contribute to difficulties in daily life and school [58].

Heterogeneity in assessment methods, small sample sizes, and substantial heterogeneity in the group with CHD are likely to limit the interpretation and go some way to explain the different findings reported. The neurodevelopmental outcomes of infants with single-ventricle CHD is generally reported to be inferior to those with two-ventricle CHD Similarly, those with complex CHD are at increased risk of impaired developmental outcome [18].

Whilst literature around long term impact is generally lacking, there is some evidence to suggest that children with two-ventricle CHD gradually grow out of their initial developmental impairment [18]. However, these are often still pertinent as the child commences school, with a range of developmental difficulties often present at school entry which enhance the risk of learning challenges and subsequent decreased social participation [59].

Symptom and Symptom Burden

Symptoms are defined as "the subjective evidence of disease or physical disturbance observed by a patient" [60]. The negative nature of symptoms is implicit, as is the requirement for the symptoms to be observed and experienced by the patient and can only be known through patient reporting. Symptom burden captures the combination of both symptom severity and impact experienced with a specific disease or treatment [61]. The most commonly described symptoms in children with CHD are anorexia, difficulty in activities, palpitations, shortness of breath, weakness, and fatigue [62]. Symptoms such as chest pain, fatigue, and breathlessness, have been described as living "at war with" and "against the body" ([63], p. 246). These symptoms impact on physical and educational development, with many experiencing concentration and memory difficulties at school [64, 65] This is exacerbated by hospital appointments and procedures that resulted in missed school and academic assessments [66]. The impact of symptom burden is clearly reflected within the patient experience discussed below.

Patient Experience

Over the past two decades, patient satisfaction and experience have become a key dimension of patient-centered care [67]. They have been used as measures to reflect quality, inform patient choice, and drive change [68, 69]. Measurement of this concept is complex and relates to perceived needs, expectations as well as experience of care [70] Literature relating to patient experience of paediatric congenital cardiac surgery patients is extremely limited. Of the papers available, the focus is predominantly on parental perceptions, with some literature around adolescents and young adulthood, in particular the transition period.

Becoming a parent of a child with CHD can be traumatic, with the need to manage a chronic condition, interspersed with acute medical crises [71]. Parents have to manage the long term implications of a CHD but also aspects of life-threatening treatments such as surgery followed by high-technology intensive care [72]. Research examining the lived experience of parents suggests they encounter intense and fluctuating emotions [73], with increased levels of distress leading up to surgery [74].

Parents, but particularly mothers, are at risk of psychological distress, presenting with symptoms of anxiety, depression, hopelessness, as well as posttraumatic stress symptoms [43, 75]. This may subsequently influence the mother's responsiveness to her child [76]. Long term, most parents successfully adapt, but approximately 40% report a need for psychosocial care [76], with around 30% of parents of children with critical CHD presenting with posttraumatic stress (PTS) symptoms [43]. In addition, parents face numerous additional physical, financial, and practical challenges [76], requiring the whole family to undergo a stressful adjustment process [77]. Parents describe financial costs as broader than monetary terms, including family burden and emotional burdens [78]. Disease complexity, as well as parental socioeconomic status appear to be linked to higher levels of financial cost, and associated emotional and family burden [78]. The difficulties experienced by parents following the birth of a child with CHD are widely documented. However, the degree of burden reported varies considerably. These inconsistency may again reflect different approaches to how and what to measure [79]. Indeed, reliance on quantitative measures is drawn into question, where qualitative approaches have been shown to provide a 'more complete' picture [80].

A small, predominantly qualitative literature base was identified examining childhood experiences. This included a recent narrative synthesis, drawing the studies together [66] The findings highlight the difficulties encountered by children, and is presented across six themes: disrupting normality; powerlessness in deteriorating health; enduring medical ordeals; warring with the body; hampering potential; and establishing one's own pace. These themes highlight the vulnerability of the children as they oscillation between health and illness, burdened by physical symptoms, and traumatised by invasive interventions, whilst coping with treatment failure and preoccupation with mortality.

Many of these themes are reflected in the literature exploring the experiences of adolescents, particularly in relation to transition to adult services, Qualitative literature discusses the 'ambivalence' experienced by adolescents in relation to daily life and encounters with the health care system [81]. Similar themes run through much of the literature, describing the needs of adolescents to strike a balance between being different and not being different; being sick and being healthy; revealing or hiding their congenital heart disease, and therefore living with a hidden handicap [81–84]. Despite this, adolescents stressed the importance of "seeing possibilities instead of restrictions" [85].

Health Behaviours

Data derived from health behaviour PROMs may serve several important clinical purposes. They enable clinicians to monitor risk behaviours and intervene early, but also identifies areas for implementing (and subsequent evaluation of) risk reduction and health promotion interventions [28].

CHD is a chronic condition requiring lifelong follow-up, and as such, patients are at increased risk of a number of health concerns, such as cardiac related morbidities including coronary artery disease and heart failure, as well as endocarditis, stroke, and pregnancy complications [86]. In order to optimise long-term outcomes, health-promoting behaviours are recommended [87]. However, few studies have examined health behaviours in young people with CHD [88–92].

Those available have reported increased levels of 'risky behaviour' including frequent poor oral health care practices [88], relatively high rates of substance use [90, 92], and low levels of physical activity, particularly as patients age [89].

Physical activity (PA) is an important part of normal childhood development, promoting healthy growth and improving the child's general fitness [93]. Even children who have undergone a Fontan procedure may obtain beneficial effects from PA participation and exercise interventions, with improvements in their cardiovascular fitness and quality of life [94–96]. However, children with CHD (regardless of the severity of their condition) show lower PA levels and a higher proportion of sedentary time compared to their peers [97], something that worsens with age and that especially affects girls, those with siblings, younger children, and those from areas of higher deprivation [97]. Maternal anxiety and depression negatively impacts the self-efficacy of these children with CHD, with consequential negative impact on their activity level [98]. Different barriers to participation, such as social stigma and parental overprotection, make engaging this group of children and adolescents in physical activities more complex [94], and currently no consensus on what constitutes optimal PA levels in this population has been reached. However, as with other chronic diseases, it is likely that physical activity programmes require tailoring to individual needs and abilities and are likely to change over the life-course.

Tools and Measures

QOL has been increasingly studied amongst the CHD population, with notable heterogeneity of QOL scores [17, 99] Any QoL measures should conform to scientific standards, and should be reliable and valid, reflecting quality. In addition, they should reflect, or be combined to reflect, the multiple domains associated with QoL. There is some debate over the validity of adult based tools when examining the QoL in a paediatric population, with specific paediatric tools perceived as preferable [9]. Rationale includes the potential failure of adult measures to explore specific aspects of QoL that are important to a child, but also the accessibility of adult based measures that impose considerable response burden for children, in terms of length, reading skills and response scale [9]. Nonetheless, there is evidence to suggest that children are able to self-report of their QoL from as early as 5 years of age [100] Calls to improve the rigour and methodological approach to assessing QoL in the CHD population have been made, with many of the studies assessed deemed to be of a poor quality or exhibiting methodological flaws [101, 102].

Whilst there is some debate within the wider literature around the validity of parental proxy measures [103, 104], evidence from cardiac based studies, supports the use of these tools, with patients and parents broadly in agreement on the impact of congenital heart disease on the QoL of children and adolescents [105].

A number of tools for measuring QoL and health related QoL (HRQoL) were identified within the literature. The majority of measures employed are generic QoL, reliant on parents to complete on behalf of the child. Only one CHD specific measure was identified, which could be completed by older children or adolescents [106]. The heterogeneity of the tools applied makes inter-study comparisons difficult. However, all the measure include some form of measure of a physical, mental and social component. Despite this, the lack of validated CHD specific measures is likely to impact on our understanding of the QoL of this population [39].

Tools employed are presented in Table 12.2.

Summary and Conclusion

Overall, evidence remains extremely variable, with conflicting findings when examining the risk factors associated with QoL and PROs in children with CHD. Few studies examine the same risk factors, and heterogeneity of sample populations make comparisons difficult. This is compounded by the use of a number of different tools, most of which are not validated specifically within the CHD population. Quality of papers has been criticized previously, further obscuring our understanding.

Highlighted Conclusions

- CHD is the most common congenital anomaly
- The reduction in mortality associated with CHD has resulted in renewed efforts to better understand patient reported outcomes (PROMS) including Quality of Life
- Important to consider the wider domains of (PROMS) including functional status, symptoms and symptom burden, patient experience and health behaviours, alongside QoL to inform practice.
- Evidence reporting QoL within the CHD population is poor, with heterogeneity of participants and tools making comparisons difficult

Future Research

- Development and validation of age-appropriate tools to assess PROMS including QoL within the CHD population
- Exploring practicalities in parents and patients involvements in developing PROMS
- Age specific studies examining specific PROMS and QoL indicators

References

1. Bouma BJ, Mulder BJ. Changing landscape of congenital heart disease. Circ Res. 2017;120:908–22.
2. Lopes LM, Tartar M, Bailey S, Kowlessar T. Prenatal diagnosis of cardiac malposition's and situs anomalies. Perin Cardiol. 2020:154.
3. Marantz P, Sáenz Tejeira MM, Peña G, Segovia A, Fustiñana C. Fetal and neonatal mortality in patients with isolated congenital heart diseases and heart conditions associated with extracardiac abnormalities. Perin Cardiol. 2013;111(5):418–22.
4. Nicor NIFCOR. National congenital heart disease audit report. 2017. https://www.nicor.org.uk/wp-content/uploads/2018/08/09729-ucl-congenital-report-2013-16-updates-july-2018-v1.pdf. Accessed 10 Nov 2018.
5. Cohn Lawrence H. Fifty years of open-heart surgery. Circulation. 2003;107:2168–70.
6. Martin GR, Jonas RA. Surgery for congenital heart disease: improvements in outcomes. Am J Perinatol. 2018;35:557–60.
7. Spector LG, Menk JS, Knight JH, Mccracken C, Thomas AS, Vinocur JM, Oster ME, St Louis JD, Moller JH, Kochilas L. Trends in long-term mortality after congenital heart surgery. J Am Coll Cardiol. 2018;71:2434–46.
8. Ottaviani G, Buja LM. Update on congenital heart disease and sudden infant/perinatal death: from history to future trends. J Clin Pathol. 2017;70(7):555–62.
9. Eiser C, Morse R. A review of measures of quality of life for children with chronic illness. Arch Dis Child. 2001;84:205–11.
10. Silva GVD, Moraes DEB, Konstantyner T, Leite HP. [Social support and quality of life of families with children with congenital heart disease]. Cien Saude Colet. 2020;25:3153–62.
11. Rometsch S, Greutmann M, Latal B, et al. Predictors of quality of life in young adults with congenital heart disease. Eur Heart J Qual Care Clin Outcomes. 2019;5(2):161–8.
12. Tesson S, Butow PN, Sholler GF, Sharpe L, Kovacs AH, Kasparian NA. Psychological interventions for people affected by childhood-onset heart disease: a systematic review. Health Psychol. 2019;38:151.
13. Gregory MRB, Prouhet PM, Russell CL, Pfannenstiel BR. Quality of life for parents of children with congenital heart defect: a systematic review. J Cardiovasc Nurs. 2018;33:363–71.
14. Golfenshtein N, Srulovici E, Medoff-Cooper B. Investigating parenting stress across pediatric

health conditions-a systematic review. Comprehens Child Adolesc Nurs. 2016;39:41–79.
15. Vo OK, Mcneill A, Vogt KS. The psychosocial impact of 22q11 deletion syndrome on patients and families: a systematic review. Am J Med Genet A. 2018;176:2215–25.
16. Clancy T, Jordan B, De Weerth C, Muscara F. Early emotional, behavioural and social development of infants and young children with congenital heart disease: a systematic review. J Clin Psychol Med Settings. 2020;27:686–703.
17. Drakouli M, Petsios K, Giannakopoulou M, Patiraki E, Voutoufianaki I, Matziou V. Determinants of quality of life in children and adolescents with CHD: a systematic review. Cardiol Young. 2015;25:1027.
18. Huisenga D, La Bastide-Van Gemert S, Van Bergen A, Sweeney J, Hadders-Algra M. Developmental outcomes after early surgery for complex congenital heart disease: a systematic review and meta-analysis. Dev Med Child Neurol. 2020;63:29.
19. Lane DA, Millane TA, Lip GY. Psychological interventions for depression in adolescent and adult congenital heart disease. Cochrane Database Syst Rev. 2013;10:CD004372.
20. Journiac J, Vioulac C, Jacob A, Escarnot C, Untas A. What do we know about young adult cardiac patients' experience? A systematic review. Front Psychol. 2020;11:1119.
21. Kahr PC, Radke RM, Orwat S, Baumgartner H, Diller G-P. Analysis of associations between congenital heart defect complexity and health-related quality of life using a meta-analytic strategy. Int J Cardiol. 2015;199:197–203.
22. Schrøder M, Boisen KA, Reimers J, Teilmann G, Brok J. Quality of life in adolescents and young adults with CHD is not reduced: a systematic review and meta-analysis. Cardiol Young. 2016;26:415–25.
23. Xu C, Su X, Ma S, Shu Y, Zhang Y, Hu Y, Mo X. Effects of exercise training in postoperative patients with congenital heart disease: a systematic review and meta-analysis of randomized controlled trials. J Am Heart Assoc. 2020;9:E013516.
24. Fteropoulli T, Stygall J, Cullen S, Deanfield J, Newman SP. Quality of life of adult congenital heart disease patients: a systematic review of the literature. Cardiol Young. 2013;23:473–85.
25. Makrinioti H, Bush A, Griffiths C. What are patient-reported outcomes and why they are important: improving studies of preschool wheeze. Arch Dis Childh Educ Pract. 2020;105:185–8.
26. Nelson E, Eftimovska E, Lind C, Hager A, Wasson J, Lindblad S. Patient reported outcome measures in practice. BMJ. 2015;350:G7818.
27. Field J, Holmes MM, Newell D. Proms data: can it be used to make decisions for individual patients? a narrative review. Pat Relat Outc Measur. 2019;10:233.
28. Cella D, Hahn EA, Jensen SE, Butt Z, Nowinski CJ, Rothrock N, Lohr KN. Patient-reported outcomes in performance measurement. Research Triangle Park, NC: RTI Press; 2015.
29. Algurén B, Coenen M, Malm D, Fridlund B, Mårtensson J, Årestedt K. A scoping review and mapping exercise comparing the content of patient-reported outcome measures (proms) across heart disease-specific scales. J Pat Rep Outc. 2020;4:7.
30. Cedars AM, Ko JM, John AS, Vittengl J, Stefanescu-Schmidt AC, Jarrett RB, Kutty S, Spertus JA. Development of a novel adult congenital heart disease–specific patient-reported outcome metric. J Am Heart Assoc. 2020;9:E015730.
31. Bonomi AE, Patrick DL, Bushnell DM, Martin M. Validation of the United States' version of the world health organization quality of life (WHOQOL) instrument. J Clin Epidemiol. 2000;53(1):1–12.
32. Koot H, Wallander J. Quality of life in child and adolescent illness: concepts, methods and findings. London: Routledge; 2014.
33. Matza LS, Swensen AR, Flood EM, Secnik K, Leidy NK. Assessment of health-related quality of life in children: a review of conceptual, methodological, and regulatory issues. Value Health. 2004;7:79–92.
34. Bullinger M, Schmidt S, Petersen C, Group D. Assessing quality of life of children with chronic health conditions and disabilities: a European approach. Int J Rehabil Res. 2002;25:197–206.
35. Thiyagarajan A, Bagavandas M, Kosalram K. Assessing the role of family well-being on the quality of life of Indian children with thalassemia. BMC Pediatr. 2019;19:1–6.
36. Ladak LA, Hasan BS, Gullick J, Awais K, Abdullah A, Gallagher R. Health-related quality of life in surgical children and adolescents with congenital heart disease compared with their age-matched healthy sibling: a cross-sectional study from a lower middle-income country, Pakistan. Arch Dis Child. 2019;104(5):419–25.
37. Reiner B, Oberhoffer R, Ewert P, Müller J. Quality of life in young people with congenital heart disease is better than expected. Arch Dis Child. 2019;104(2):124–8.
38. Dahan-Oliel N, Majnemer A, Mazer B. Quality of life of adolescents and young adults born at high risk. Phys Occup Ther Pediatr. 2011;31(4):362–89.
39. Latal B, Helfricht S, Fischer JE, Bauersfeld U, Landolt MA. Psychological adjustment and quality of life in children and adolescents following open-heart

surgery for congenital heart disease: a systematic review. BMC Pediatr. 2009;9:6.
40. Mussatto K, Tweddell J. Quality of life following surgery for congenital cardiac malformations in neonates and infants. Cardiol Young. 2005;15:174.
41. Dunbar-Masterson C, Wypij D, Bellinger DC, Rappaport LA, Baker AL, Jonas RA, Newburger JW. General health status of children with d-transposition of the great arteries after the arterial switch operation. Circulation. 2001;104:I-138-I-142.
42. Bevilacqua F, Palatta S, Mirante N, et al. Birth of a child with congenital heart disease: emotional reactions of mothers and fathers according to time of diagnosis. J Matern Fetal Neonatal Med. 2013;26(12):1249–53.
43. Woolf-King SE, Arnold E, Weiss S, Teitel D. "There's no acknowledgement of what this does to people": a qualitative exploration of mental health among parents of children with critical congenital heart defects. J Clin Nurs. 2018;27:2785.
44. Helfricht S, Latal B, Fischer JE, Tomaske M, Landolt MA. Surgery-related posttraumatic stress disorder in parents of children undergoing cardiopulmonary bypass surgery: a prospective cohort study. Pediatr Crit Care Med. 2008;9(2):217–23.
45. Lawoko S, Soares JJ. Distress and hopelessness among parents of children with congenital heart disease, parents of children with other diseases, and parents of healthy children. Pediatr Crit Care Med. 2002;52(4):193–208.
46. Kasparian NA, Kan JM, Sood E, Wray J, Pincus HA, Newburger JW. Mental health care for parents of babies with congenital heart disease during intensive care unit admission: Systematic review and statement of best practice. Early human development. 2019;139:104837.
47. Biber S, Andonian C, Beckmann J, et al. Current research status on the psychological situation of parents of children with congenital heart disease. Cardiovasc Diagn Ther. 2019;9(Suppl 2): S369–S376.
48. Ruggiero KM, Hickey PA, Leger RR, Vessey JA, Hayman LL. Parental perceptions of diseaseseverity and health-related quality of life in school-age children with congenital heart disease. J Spec Pediatr Nurs. 2018;23(1).
49. Nousi D, Christou A. Factors affecting the quality of life in children with congenital heart disease. Health Sci J. 2010;4:94.
50. Soulvie MA, Desai PP, White CP, Sullivan BN. Psychological distress experienced by parents of young children with congenital heart defects: A comprehensive review of literature. Journal of Social Service Research. 2012;38(4):484–502.
51. Kolaitis GA, Meentken MG, Utens E. Mental health problems in parents of children with congenital heart disease. Front Pediatr. 2017;5:102.
52. Ringle ML, Wernovsky G. Functional, quality of life, and neurodevelopmental outcomes after congenital cardiac surgery. Semin Perinatol. 2016;40(8):556–70. https://doi.org/10.1053/j.semperi.2016.09.008. PMID: 27989374.
53. Cohen ME, Marino RJ. The tools of disability outcomes research functional status measures. Arch Phys Med Rehabil. 2000;81:S21–9.
54. Cassidy AR, Ilardi D, Bowen SR, Hampton LE, Heinrich KP, Loman MM, Sanz JH, Wolfe KR. Congenital heart disease: a primer for the pediatric neuropsychologist. Child Neuropsychol. 2018;24:859–902.
55. Snookes SH, Gunn JK, Eldridge BJ, Donath SM, Hunt RW, Galea MP, Shekerdemian L. A systematic review of motor and cognitive outcomes after early surgery for congenital heart disease. Pediatrics. 2010;125:E818–27.
56. Gaynor JW, Stopp C, Wypij D, Andropoulos DB, Atallah J, Atz AM, Beca J, Donofrio MT, Duncan K, Ghanayem NS, Goldberg CS, Hövels-Gürich H, Ichida F, Jacobs JP, Justo R, Latal B, Li JS, Mahle WT, Mcquillen PS, Menon SC, Pemberton VL, Pike NA, Pizarro C, Shekerdemian LS, Synnes A, Williams I, Bellinger DC, Newburger JW, For The International Cardiac Collaborative On Neurodevelopment, I. Neurodevelopmental outcomes after cardiac surgery in infancy. Pediatrics. 2015;135:816–25.
57. Mussatto KA, Hoffmann RG, Hoffman GM, Tweddell JS, Bear L, Cao Y, Brosig C. Risk and prevalence of developmental delay in young children with congenital heart disease. Pediatrics. 2014;133:E570–7.
58. Sterken C, Lemiere J, Vanhorebeek I, Van Den Berghe G, Mesotten D. Neurocognition after paediatric heart surgery: a systematic review and meta-analysis. Open Heart. 2015;2:e000255.
59. Majnemer A, Limperopoulos C, Shevell M, Rohlicek C, Rosenblatt B, Tchervenkov C. Developmental and functional outcomes at school entry in children with congenital heart defects. J Pediatr. 2008;153:55–60. e1.
60. Merriam-Webster's Collegiate Dictionary (10th ed.). (1999). Merriam-Webster Incorporated.
61. Cleeland CS. Symptom burden: multiple symptoms and their impact as patient-reported outcomes. J Natl Cancer Inst Monogr. 2007:16–21.
62. Bektas İ, Kır M, Yıldız K, Genç Z, Bektas M, Ünal N. Symptom frequency in children with congenital heart disease and parental care burden in predicting the quality of life of parents in Turkey. J Pediatr Nurs. 2020;53:E211–6.
63. Gantt LT. Growing up heartsick: the experiences of young women with congenital heart disease. Health Care Women Int. 1992;13:241–8.
64. Birks Y, Sloper P, Lewin R, Parsons J. Exploring health-related experiences of children and young people with congenital heart disease. Health Expect. 2007;10:16–29.
65. Cornett L, Simms J. At the 'heart' of the matter: an exploration of the psychological impact of living with congenital heart disease in adulthood. J Health Psychol. 2014;19:393–406.

66. Chong LS, Fitzgerald DA, Craig JC, Manera KE, Hanson CS, Celermajer D, Ayer J, Kasparian NA, Tong A. Children's experiences of congenital heart disease: a systematic review of qualitative studies. Eur J Pediatr. 2018;177:319–36.
67. Lapin BR, Honomichl RD, Thompson NR, Rose S, Sugano D, Udeh B, Katzan IL. Association between patient experience with patient-reported outcome measurements and overall satisfaction with care in neurology. Value Health. 2019;22:555–63.
68. Coulter A. Patient feedback for quality improvement in general practice. Br Med J. 2016;352:e913.
69. Van Velthoven MH, Atherton H, Powell J. A cross sectional survey of the UK public to understand use of online ratings and reviews of health services. Patient Educ Couns. 2018;101:1690–6.
70. Williams B. Patient satisfaction: a valid concept? Soc Sci Med. 1994;38:509–16.
71. Sjostrom-Strand A, Terp K. Parents' experiences of having a baby with a congenital heart defect and the child's heart surgery. Comprehens Child Adolesc Nurs. 2017;42:1–14.
72. Franich Ray C, Bright MA, Anderson V, Northam E, Cochrane A, Menahem S, Jordan B. Trauma reactions in mothers and fathers after their infant's cardiac surgery. J Pediatr Psychol. 2013;38:494–505.
73. Mcmahon E, Chang Y-S. From surviving to thriving-parental experiences of hospitalised infants with congenital heart disease undergoing cardiac surgery: a qualitative synthesis. J Pediatr Nurs. 2020;51:32–41.
74. Wray J, Sensky T. Psychological functioning in parents of children undergoing elective cardiac surgery. Cardiol Young. 2004;14:131–9.
75. Lotto R, Jones I, Seaton SE, Dhannapuneni R, Guerrero R, Lotto A. Congenital cardiac surgery and parental perception of risk: a quantitative analysis. World J Pediatr Congenit Heart Surg. 2019;10:669–77.
76. Kolaitis GA, Meentken MG, Utens EM. Mental health problems in parents of children with congenital heart disease. Front Pediatr. 2017;5:102.
77. Lan S-F, Mu P-F, Hsieh K-S. Maternal experiences making a decision about heart surgery for their young children with congenital heart disease. J Clin Nurs. 2007;16:2323–30.
78. Connor JA, Kline NE, Mott S, Harris SK, Jenkins KJ. The meaning of cost for families of children with congenital heart disease. J Pediatr Health Care. 2010;24:318–25.
79. Wei H, Roscigno CI, Hanson CC, Swanson KM. Families of children with congenital heart disease: a literature review. Heart Lung. 2015;44: 494–511.
80. Utens EM, Versluis-Den Bieman HJ, Verhulst FC, Witsenburg M, Bogers AJ, Hess J. Psychological distress and styles of coping in parents of children awaiting elective cardiac surgery. Cardiol Young. 2000;10:239–44.
81. Berghammer M, Dellborg M, Ekman I. Young adults experiences of living with congenital heart disease. Int J Cardiol. 2006;110:340–7.
82. Berghammer MC, Brink E, Rydberg AM, Dellborg M, Ekman I. Committed to life: adolescents' and young adults' experiences of living with Fontan circulation. Congenit Heart Dis. 2015;10:403–12.
83. Chiang YT, Chen CW, Su WJ, Wang JK, Lu CW, Li YF, Moons P. Between invisible defects and visible impact: the life experiences of adolescents and young adults with congenital heart disease. J Adv Nurs. 2015;71:599–608.
84. Lee S, Kim S, Choi JY. Coping and resilience of adolescents with congenital heart disease. J Cardiovasc Nurs. 2014;29:340–6.
85. Mcmurray R, Kendall L, Parsons J, Quirk J, Veldtman G, Lewin R, Sloper P. A life less ordinary: growing up and coping with congenital heart disease. Coron Health Care. 2001;5:51–7.
86. Jackson JL, Tierney K, Daniels CJ, Vannatta K. Disease knowledge, perceived risk, and health behavior engagement among adolescents and adults with congenital heart disease. Heart Lung. 2015;44:39–44.
87. Janssens A, Goossens E, Luyckx K, Budts W, Gewillig M, Moons P, Investigators I-D. Exploring the relationship between disease-related knowledge and health risk behaviours in young people with congenital heart disease. Eur J Cardiovasc Nurs. 2016;15: 231–40.
88. Chen C-W, Chen Y-C, Chen M-Y, Wang J-K, Su W-J, Wang H-L. Health-promoting behavior of adolescents with congenital heart disease. J Adolesc Health. 2007;41:602–9.
89. Lunt D, Briffa T, Briffa NK, Ramsay J. Physical activity levels of adolescents with congenital heart disease. Austr J Physiother. 2003;49:43–50.
90. Massin MM, Hövels-Gürich H, Seghaye M-C. Atherosclerosis lifestyle risk factors in children with congenital heart disease. Eur J Cardiovasc Prev Rehabil. 2007;14:349–51.
91. Reid GJ, Webb GD, Mccrindle BW, Irvine MJ, Siu SC. Health behaviors among adolescents and young adults with congenital heart disease. Congenit Heart Dis. 2008;3:16–25.
92. Uzark K, Vonbargen-Mazza P, Messiter E. Health education needs of adolescents with congenital heart disease. J Pediatr Health Care. 1989;3:137–43.
93. Malina RM. Physical activity and fitness: pathways from childhood to adulthood. Am J Hum Biol. 2001;13:162–72.
94. Moola F, Mccrindle BW, Longmuir PE. Physical activity participation in youth with surgically corrected congenital heart disease: devising guidelines so johnny can participate. Paediatr Child Health. 2009;14:167–70.
95. Takken T, Hulzebos H, Blank A, Tacken M, Helders P, Strengers J. Exercise prescription for patients with a Fontan circulation: current evidence and future directions. Neth Hear J. 2007a;15:142–7.
96. Takken T, Tacken MH, Blank AC, Hulzebos EH, Strengers JL, Helders PJ. Exercise limita-

tion in patients with Fontan circulation: a review. J Cardiovasc Med. 2007b;8:775–81.
97. Voss C, Duncombe SL, Dean PH, De Souza AM, Harris KC. Physical activity and sedentary behavior in children with congenital heart disease. J Am Heart Assoc. 2017;6:E004665.
98. Dulfer K, Duppen N, Van Dijk AP, Kuipers IM, Van Domburg RT, Verhulst FC, Van Der Ende J, Helbing WA, Utens EM. Parental mental health moderates the efficacy of exercise training on health-related quality of life in adolescents with congenital heart disease. Pediatr Cardiol. 2015;36:33–40.
99. Ernst MM, Marino BS, Cassedy A, Piazza-Waggoner C, Franklin RC, Brown K, Wray J. Biopsychosocial predictors of quality of life outcomes in pediatric congenital heart disease. Pediatr Cardiol. 2018;39:79–88.
100. Sluys KP, Lannge M, Iselius L, Eriksson LE. Six years beyond pediatric trauma: child and parental ratings of children's health-related quality of life in relation to parental mental health. Qual Life Res. 2015;24:2689–99.
101. Bratt EL, Moons P. Forty years of quality-of-life research in congenital heart disease: temporal trends in conceptual and methodological rigor. Int J Cardiol. 2015;195:1–6.
102. Moons P, Van Deyk K, Budts W, De Geest S. Caliber of quality-of-life assessments in congenital heart disease: a plea for more conceptual and methodological rigor. Arch Pediatr Adolesc Med. 2004;158:1062–9.
103. Cohen ML, Tulsky DS, Boulton AJ, Kisala PA, Bertisch H, Yeates KO, Zonfrillo MR, Durbin DR, Jaffe KM, Temkin N. Reliability and construct validity of the Tbi-Qol communication short form as a parent-proxy report instrument for children with traumatic brain injury. J Speech Lang Hear Res. 2019;62:84–92.
104. Fayed N, Avery L, Davis AM, Streiner DL, Ferro M, Rosenbaum P, Cunningham C, Lach L, Boyle M, Ronen GM. Parent proxy discrepancy groups of quality of life in childhood epilepsy. Value Health. 2019;22:822–8.
105. Marino BS, Tomlinson RS, Drotar D, Claybon ES, Aguirre A, Ittenbach R, Welkom JS, Helfaer MA, Wernovsky G, Shea JA. Quality-of-life concerns differ among patients, parents, and medical providers in children and adolescents with congenital and acquired heart disease. Pediatrics. 2009;123:E708–15.
106. Kamphuis M, Zwinderman K, Vogels T, et al. A cardiac-specific health-related quality of life module for young adults with congenital heart disease: development and validation. Quality of Life Research. 2004;13(4):735–45.

13 Percutaneous Coronary Intervention

Adam Hartley and Sukhjinder Nijjer

Introduction

Percutaneous Coronary Intervention (PCI), the catheter-based implantation of intra-coronary arterial stents of various types, has evolved rapidly since its inception as balloon angioplasty in 1974 [1]. Whilst initially performed electively in patients with angina pectoris, it is now most frequently performed in patients admitted into hospitals with acute coronary syndromes (ACS). Importantly, when performed acutely for rupture of atherosclerotic plaque, it has proven prognostic benefit in those suffering ST-segment elevation myocardial infarction (STEMI), as well as in non-ST elevation myocardial infarction (NSTEMI) [2]. Advancing techniques have meant more complex coronary disease can be treated without a significant increase in procedure associated morbidity and mortality rates [3].

In the elective setting, PCI is typically performed to relieve angiographically-narrow, flow-limiting epicardial coronary stenoses, in the belief that improved blood flow will reduce patient symptoms. While some have hoped to find prognostic benefit here, there have been no contemporary studies that demonstrate any reduction in risk of ischaemic cardiovascular events or mortality over and above optimised modern medical therapy [4, 5]. There are specific subsets that may still have prognostic advantage. Revascularisation of the left main stem (the initial branch of the left coronary artery that supplies ~80% of blood to the left ventricle in left-dominant coronary circulation [6]) may provide prognostic benefit. This patient subgroup is typically excluded from these trials and is commonly treated with coronary artery bypass grafting (CABG) surgery when patient factors allow. Meta-analysis has also suggested that selected patients with chronic total occlusions (CTO)s, defined as total obstruction of a coronary artery lasting for at least 3 months, appear to have prognostic advantage when successfully treated by PCI [7]. However, this specific intervention carries greater procedural risks and is still largely performed for relief of clinical angina pectoris rather than for prognosis.

Given that PCI in the setting of stable coronary artery disease (CAD) is performed primarily for symptomatic reasons, quantification of health-related quality of life (HRQOL) are essential. Utilisation of patient reported outcome measures (PROMs) goes hand-in-hand with a greater patient-centred focus and cost efficiency that is emphasised in modern healthcare. Additionally,

A. Hartley
National Heart and Lung Institute, Imperial College London, London, UK

Imperial College Healthcare NHS Trust, London, UK
e-mail: adam.hartley12@imperial.ac.uk

S. Nijjer (✉)
National Heart and Lung Institute, Imperial College London, London, UK
e-mail: s.nijjer@imperial.ac.uk

T. Athanasiou et al. (eds.), *Patient Reported Outcomes and Quality of Life in Cardiovascular Interventions*,
https://doi.org/10.1007/978-3-031-09815-4_13

the use of PROMs has the ability to improve the overall quality of healthcare delivered [8].

This systematic review aims to provide an up-to-date analysis of all published literature examining HRQOL outcome measures in patients undergoing PCI in any setting. This permits the assessment of the real benefits of PCI as reported by patients, whilst also identifying recommendations for clinical practice and future research.

Materials and Methods

Search Strategy

This study was performed according to the 'Preferred Reporting Items for Systematic reviews and Meta-Analyses' guidelines for studies that evaluate healthcare interventions [9]. A systematic search of EMBASE and MEDLINE databases was performed using the search terms 'quality of life' AND ('percutaneous coronary intervention' or 'PCI') up until January 2020. Further suitable articles for inclusion were identified from hand-searching of selected papers.

Inclusion and Exclusion Criteria

All articles were included that detailed patient reported quality of life outcome instrument scores in relation to PCI and a comparison group. Papers reporting PCI outcome measures but without a contemporaneous control group were excluded. In some instances, the comparison was a conventional control group undergoing medical therapy or placebo procedure, whilst in other studies PCI was compared to other techniques, for example CABG. In addition, the PCI group had to be definable (i.e. PCI could not be a component of a composite 'invasive revascularisation' approach), and outcome measures had to be reported at both baseline pre-intervention and at a minimum of one post-procedural timepoint. Papers were further restricted to research articles published in English.

Outcomes of Interest and Data Extraction

Studies were analysed independently by two reviewers (A.H. and S.N.). Conflicts between reviewers were resolved through face-to-face discussion. Data extraction for each study included the following: author; publication year; geographical areas of participant inclusion; study design; purpose and setting of study; age; sex; number of study participants in both the PCI and comparator groups; duration of follow up and proportion that completed follow up; HRQOL instrument(s) used and scores at relevant timepoints (ideally 3-, 6-, 12-months and 3- and 5-years). If studies included both an interventional and non-interventional PCI comparator, the non-interventional comparator was chosen for assessment. In some studies PCI outcomes were split into different subsets for comparison, e.g. by age group; when possible these subgroups were combined to form a whole PCI cohort for analysis. In studies that utilised HRQOL instruments comprising various domains, the summary score was assessed if this was reported. The proportion of participants followed up at the latest timepoint was taken as the follow up percentage when there were multiple follow up episodes.

Quality Scoring

Included studies were assessed for quality of methodology and data reporting. Observational studies were assessed using the Newcastle-Ottawa Scale, which attributes stars based on three domains (participant selection, group comparability and outcome assessment) [10]. A score of five or less represents a high likelihood of bias, out of a maximum of nine points [11]. The quality of randomised studies was assessed using the Jadad score, a five-point scale assessing randomisation, blinding and withdrawals or dropout. A score of less than three suggests poor quality [12].

Results

Selected Studies

The literature search identified 3516 records and a further five records were added after reference review of selected papers. After duplicates were removed and the search was restricted to English language only, 2597 records were included for further assessment. 2341 articles were then excluded during screening, leaving 256 full-text articles to be evaluated. Following study exclusion based on article-level analysis, 25 studies were included in the review [13–37]. Data from these studies were extracted and displayed in Tables 13.1, 13.2, 13.3, and 13.4. The search strategy is displayed in Fig. 13.1.

Study Objectives, Design and Population

The 25 included papers covered a wide time period, with the earliest published in 1990, and the latest in 2019. In total, there were 16,482 patients enrolled across all studies. The mean age of included participants was 64.3 (± standard deviation 3.5) years and were 24.7% female, although one study did not report sex [36] and one further study did not report any patient demographics [37]. Follow up was carried out for a median of 12 months (interquartile range (IQR) 6, 12). The studies were evenly split between randomised and non-randomised—13 (52%) were randomised controlled trials, whilst 12 (48%) were non-randomised observational studies.

The studies covered a wide geographical distribution, with six (24%) from North America, nine (36%) from Europe, three (12%) from both North America and Europe, four (16%) from Asia and three (12%) enrolled patients from three or more continents. 11 (44%) of studies reported 100% patient follow up at the latest timepoint, with five of these being observational studies. Seven (28%) studies reported follow up of between 80% and 99.9%, whilst four (16%) reported 60–79.9% participants completed follow up. Three (12%) studies did not report the number of participants that completed follow up.

The clinical setting that PCI was performed varied across the included studies. 11 studies included patients with CAD but did not specify further [17, 19–22, 26, 30, 32, 35–37]. Six studies included patients with stable CAD [14, 18, 28, 31, 33, 34]. Five studies were performed in the setting of ACS, of which two were in NSTEMI [13, 25], one was in STEMI [23], whilst two did not specify further [27, 29]. Three studies were performed for CTOs [15, 16, 24].

Quality of Included Studies

The studies varied in quality and risk of bias according to the assessment tools, although overall, were of a high standard. Of the randomised studies, 11/13 (84.6%) [13, 15–19, 23, 26, 30, 34, 36] were assessed as being high quality with Jadad scores of three or more. The median score for randomised studies was three (IQR 3, 4). 12/12 (100%) of the non-randomised studies scored six or more on the Newcastle-Ottawa Scale, and were therefore considered high quality with a low risk of bias. The median score for non-randomised studies was eight (IQR 8, 8).

Health-Related Quality of Life Measures Used

Various HRQOL assessment instruments were utilised across the studies, amounting to a total of 13 separate tools used. The average number of tools used per study was one (IQR 1, 2). The most widely used of these was a disease-specific tool, the Seattle Angina Questionnaire (SAQ), which is a patient-completed questionnaire consisting of five domains (angina frequency, physical limitation, quality of life, angina stability and treatment satisfaction) relevant to CAD [38]. This instrument was used in 12 (48%) studies [16–21, 24–26, 31, 34, 35], of which only one

Table 13.1 Patient related outcome measures in studies focusing on percutaneous coronary intervention for stable coronary artery disease

Study	Study intent	Study design	Quality score RCT	Quality score observational	Age	Sex (% female)	Other relevant demographics (race, employment, obesity, diabetes, physical activity, smoking, alcohol, no leisure physical activity)	No. of patients	Follow-up (months)	Instrument(s)		Control	Data spread	Pre-op control (PCS)	Pre-op control (PCS) standard deviation	Pre-op intervention (PCI)	Pre-op intervention (PCI) standard deviation	1 month control (PCS)	1 month control (PCS) standard deviation	1 month intervention (PCI)	1 month intervention (PCI) standard deviation	6 month control (PCS)	6 month control (PCS) standard deviation	6 month intervention (PCI)	6 month intervention (PCI) standard deviation	12 month control (PCS)	12 month control (PCS) standard deviation	12 month intervention (PCI)	12 month intervention (PCI) standard deviation	3 year control (PCS)	3 year control (PCS) standard deviation	3 year intervention (PCI)	3 year intervention (PCI) standard deviation	5 year control (PCS)	5 year control (PCS) standard deviation	5 year intervention (PCI)	5 year intervention (PCI) standard deviation
Nishi et al. 2018	FAME 1&2: quality of life outcomes in patients treated with PCI for significant lesions by FFR vs MT for non-significant lesions by FFR	Observational		8	64 (10)	PCI—146 (20.4%), Reference—67 (36.2%)	Stable CAD	428 (243 lowest FFR subgroup, 185 reference)	12 months	EQ-5D		MT	SD	0.821	0.153	0.807	0.167	0.817	0.188	0.891	0.148	X	X	X	X	0.814	0.198	0.876	0.158	X	X	X	X	X	X	X	X
Al-Lamee et al. 2017	ORBITA: sham-controlled trial of PCI in stable CAD	RCT	5		66.0 (9.0)	54 (27%)	Stable CAD	200	6 weeks	SAQ	Physical limitation	MT	SD	69.1	24.7	71.3	22.5	74.1*	24.7*	78.6*	24*	X	X	X	X	X	X	X	X	X	X	X	X	X	X	X	X
										SAQ	Angina frequency	MT	SD	60	25.1	63.2	20.4	67.7*	22.1*	74.4*	21.4*	X	X	X	X	X	X	X	X	X	X	X	X	X	X	X	X
										SAQ	Angina stability	MT	SD	68.5	24.3	64.7	25.5	63.5*	25.6*	60.5*	23.7*	X	X	X	X	X	X	X	X	X	X	X	X	X	X	X	X
Al-Lamee et al. 2017	ORBITA: sham-controlled trial of PCI in stable CAD	RCT	5		66.0 (9.0)	54 (27%)	Stable CAD	200	6 weeks	EQ-5D		MT	SD	0.79	0.22	0.8	0.21	0.82*	0.2*	0.83*	0.21*	X	X	X	X	X	X	X	X	X	X	X	X	X	X	X	X
Wijeysundera et al. 2014	APPROACH registry: quality of life outcomes in patients with CTOs with MT vs PCI vs CABG	Observational		8	66.4 (10.7)	67 (17.3%)	Stable non-CTO	387	12 months	EQ-5D		MT vs non-CTO	SD	0.76	0.15	0.82	0.14	X	X	X	X	X	X	X	X	0.86	0.15	0.88	0.13	X	X	X	X	X	X	X	X
Wijeysundera et al. 2014	APPROACH registry: quality of life outcomes in patients with CTOs with MT vs PCI vs CABG	Observational		8	66.4 (10.7)	67 (17.3%)	Stable non-CTO	387	12 months	SAQ	Physical limitation	MT vs PCI-non-CTO	SD	69.4	25.2	68.9	22.3	X	X	X	X	X	X	X	X	71.5	23.3	75.2	25.7	X	X	X	X	X	X	X	X
										SAQ	Angina frequency	MT vs PCI-non-CTO	SD	85.8	19.2	78.5	24.7	X	X	X	X	X	X	X	X	84	22.8	90.3	17.3	X	X	X	X	X	X	X	X
										SAQ	Angina stability	MT vs PCI-non-CTO	SD	61.8	27.9	64.7	32.7	X	X	X	X	X	X	X	X	67.9	26.5	69.5	27	X	X	X	X	X	X	X	X
										SAQ	Disease perception	MT vs PCI-non-CTO	SD	65.7	24.6	55.6	26.4	X	X	X	X	X	X	X	X	71.4	21.8	73.8	22.7	X	X	X	X	X	X	X	X
										SAQ	Treatment satisfaction	MT vs PCI-non-CTO	SD	87.2	16.3	87.5	14.8	X	X	X	X	X	X	X	X	88.1	16.9	89.6	15	X	X	X	X	X	X	X	X
Loponen et al. 2009	Quality of life outcomes following PCI vs CABG in stable CAD	Observational		8	PCI—64.5 (10.2), CABG—66.1 (8.8)	121 (25.8%)	Stable CAD	469	6 months	15D		CABG	SD	0.83	0.09	0.83	0.1	X	X	X	X	0.86	0.11	0.85	0.11	X	X	X	X	X	X	X	X	X	X	X	X
Weintraub et al. 2008	COURAGE: quality of life outcomes following PCI vs MT in stable CAD	RCT	1		62 (10)	340 (14.9%)	Stable CAD	2287	36 months	SAQ	Physical limitation	MT	SD	66	25	66	25	70	24	73	24	72	24	77	23	73	24	75	24	74	24	74	24	X	X	X	X
										SAQ	Angina stability	MT	SD	53	32	54	33	73	28	81	26	73	28	76	28	70	28	74	27	70	28	72	28	X	X	X	X
										SAQ	Angina frequency	MT	SD	69	26	68	26	76	24	82	23	83	22	87	20	84	21	87	19	88	18	89	18	X	X	X	X
										SAQ	Treatment satisfaction	MT	SD	86	16	88	15	88	15	92	12	90	14	92	13	90	14	92	12	92	11	92	12	X	X	X	X
										SAQ	Quality of life	MT	SD	51	25	51	25	62	24	68	24	70	23	75	22	73	22	76	21	77	20	79	20	X	X	X	X
Weintraub et al. 2008	COURAGE: quality of life outcomes following PCI vs MT in stable CAD	RCT	1		62 (10)	340 (14.9%)	Stable CAD	2287	36 months	SF-36	Physical functioning	MT	SD	59	27	58	27	61	27	65	27	66	26	68	27	66	28	69	27	64	28	66	29	X	X	X	X
										SF-36	Role limitation—physical	MT	SD	37	42	38	41	46	43	47	42	57	43	62	42	61	42	64	42	60	42	66	42	X	X	X	X
										SF-36	Role limitation—emotional	MT	SD	56	43	57	43	62	42	62	42	68	41	70	41	70	40	73	38	68	42	71	40	X	X	X	X
										SF-36	Energy/fatigue	MT	SD	47	23	47	24	48	24	53	23	53	23	56	23	54	24	56	23	52	24	56	23	X	X	X	X
										SF-36	Emotional wellbeing	MT	SD	71	20	71	20	73	19	74	19	75	19	75	19	75	20	75	19	74	20	75	19	X	X	X	X
										SF-36	Social functioning	MT	SD	70	27	71	27	75	26	75	25	79	26	81	24	80	25	81	25	79	26	80	26	X	X	X	X
										SF-36	Pain	MT	SD	62	26	61	26	66	25	68	26	70	26	71	26	70	27	72	25	68	27	70	27	X	X	X	X
										SF-36	General health	MT	SD	55	20	57	20	55	20	61	20	58	21	61	21	58	21	61	21	57	22	60	22	X	X	X	X
Benzer et al. 2003	Quality of life outcomes with PCI vs CABG vs MT in stable CAD	Observational		8	64.5 (10.3)	43 (33.3%)	Stable CAD	130	12 months	MacNew	Global scale	MT	SD	4.9	1.3	5	1.3	X	X	X	X	X	X	X	X	5.2	NR	5.6	NR	X	X	X	X	X	X	X	X
Zhang et al. 2003	SoS: quality of life outcomes with PCI vs CABG in stable CAD	RCT	4		61.4	207 (21%)	Stable CAD	988	12 months	SAQ	Physical limitation	CABG	SD	54.3	22	56.6	22.6	X	X	X	X	76.5	21.2	73.6	22.4	76.6	20.7	75.2	21.3	X	X	X	X	X	X	X	X
										SAQ	Angina frequency	CABG	SD	53.8	28	55.8	27.9	X	X	X	X	89.7	17.8	83.8	23.1	89.6	18.2	86.9	19.8	X	X	X	X	X	X	X	X
										SAQ	Treatment satisfaction	CABG	SD	86.2	15	86.7	14.4	X	X	X	X	90.1	16.3	89.2	15.1	90	16	91.2	13.1	X	X	X	X	X	X	X	X
										SAQ	Quality of life	CABG	SD	37	20.5	39.5	20	X	X	X	X	69.1	21.4	65.4	24.5	71.5	21.4	69.8	23	X	X	X	X	X	X	X	X

MT medical therapy; *CTO* chronic total occlusion; *CABG* coronary artery bypass grafting; *PCI* percutaneous coronary intervention; *CAD* coronary artery disease; *SD* standard deviation; *RCT* randomised controlled trial; *NR* not reported; *IQR* interquartile range

* 6 weeks

Table 13.2 Patient related outcome measures in studies focusing on percutaneous coronary intervention for acute coronary syndromes

Study	Study intent	Study design	Quality score RCT	Quality score observational	Age	Sex (% female)	Other relevant demographics (race, employment, obesity, diabetes, physical activity, smoking, alcohol, no leisure physical activity)	No. of patients	Follow-up (months)	Instrument(s)		Control	Data spread	Pre-op control (PCS)	Pre-op control (PCS) standard deviation	Pre-op intervention (PCI)	Pre-op intervention (PCI) standard deviation	1 month control (PCS)	1 month control (PCS) standard deviation	1 month intervention (PCI)	1 month intervention (PCI) standard deviation	6 month control (PCS)	6 month control (PCS) standard deviation	6 month intervention (PCI)	6 month intervention (PCI) standard deviation	12 month control (PCS)	12 month control (PCS) standard deviation	12 month intervention (PCI)	12 month intervention (PCI) standard deviation	3 year control (PCS)	3 year control (PCS) standard deviation	3 year intervention (PCI)	3 year intervention (PCI) standard deviation	5 year control (PCS)	5 year control (PCS) standard deviation	5 year intervention (PCI)	5 year intervention (PCI) standard deviation
Lee et al. 2019	CABG-ACS: PCI vs MT in NSTEMI with prior CABG	RCT	5		71 (9)	17 (28%)	ACS (NSTEMI)	60	12 months	EQ-5D		MT	IQR	0.863	(0.596–0.924)	0.602	(0.360–0.881)	X	X	X	X	0.89	(0.67–0.95)	0.67	(0.34–0.94)	0.83	(0.72–0.95)	0.72	(0.56–0.94)	X	X	X	X	X	X	X	X
Bohmer et al. 2014	NORDISTEMI substudy: quality of life outcomes of early invasive therapy vs conservative therapy in STEMI after thrombolysis	RCT	3		PCI—60(9), CT—59 (10)	57 (23.0%)	ACS (STEMI)	248	12 months	SF-6D		MT	SD	0.77	0.14	0.79	15	0.71	0.13	0.7*	0.12	0.8*	0.14*	0.8*	0.13*	0.78	0.15	0.78	0.15	X	X	X	X	X	X	X	X
										15D		MT	SD	0.91	0.09	0.91	0.09	0.88	0.1	0.8*	0.08	0.9	0.09	0.91	0.09	0.9	0.1	0.91	0.09	X	X	X	X	X	X	X	X
Yang et al. 2014	Quality of life outcomes in PCI vs CABG in NSTEMI	Observational		8	PCI—67.6 (12), CABG—67.1 (9)	306 (30.2%)	ACS (NSTEMI)	1012	6 months	SAQ	Angina frequency	CABG	SD	61	17	58	18	X	X	X	X	93	9	79	14	X	X	X	X	X	X	X	X	X	X	X	X
										SAQ	Treatment satisfaction	CABG	SD	70	12	72	17	X	X	X	X	80	9	76	13	X	X	X	X	X	X	X	X	X	X	X	X
										SAQ	Quality of life	CABG	SD	48	14	40	23	X	X	X	X	56	11	43	17	X	X	X	X	X	X	X	X	X	X	X	X
Li et al. 2012	Quality of life outcomes in ACS with PCI vs MT	Observational		8	PCI— 64.1 (11), MT—73 (11)	157 (34.8%)	ACS	451	6 months	SF-36	Physical component	MT	SD	29	15	32	15	X	X	X	X	35	15	42	13	X	X	X	X	X	X	X	X	X	X	X	X
										SF-36	Mental component	MT	SD	53	14	51	12	X	X	X	X	54	11	53	10	X	X	X	X	X	X	X	X	X	X	X	X
Mark et al. 2009	OAT: quality of life outcomes in persistent occlusion of the infarct-related artery beyond 72 hours with PCI vs MT	RCT	2		59.2 (11.1)	206 (21.7%)	ACS	951	24 months	Duke Activity Status Index		MT	SD	37.3	19.6	36.3	19.7	X	X	X	X	X	X	X	X	37	20	36	20.1	X	X	X	X	X	X	X	X
Mark et al. 2009	OAT: quality of life outcomes in persistent occlusion of the infarct-related artery beyond 72 hours with PCI vs MT	RCT	2		59.2 (11.1)	206 (21.7%)	ACS	951	24 months	Rand Short-Form 36 Mental Health Inventory 5		MT	SD	74.7	18.6	72.6	19.3	X	X	X	X	X	X	X	X	77.4	18.5	77	18.9	X	X	X	X	X	X	X	X

MT medical therapy; *CTO* chronic total occlusion; *CABG* coronary artery bypass grafting; *PCI* percutaneous coronary intervention; *CAD* coronary artery disease; *SD* standard deviation; *RCT* randomised controlled trial; *NR* not reported; *IQR* interquartile range

* 7 months

Table 13.3 Patient related outcome measures in studies focusing on percutaneous coronary intervention for chronic total occlusions

Study	Study intent	Study design	Quality score RCT	Quality score observational	Age	Sex (% female)	Other relevant demographics (race, employment, obesity, diabetes, physical activity, smoking, alcohol, no leisure physical activity)	No. of patients	Follow-up (months)	Instrument(s)		Control	Data spread	Pre-op control (PCS)	Pre-op control (PCS) standard deviation	Pre-op intervention (PCI)	Pre-op intervention (PCI) standard deviation	1 month control (PCS)	1 month control (PCS) standard deviation	1 month intervention (PCI)	1 month intervention (PCI) standard deviation	6 month control (PCS)	6 month control (PCS) standard deviation	6 month intervention (PCI)	6 month intervention (PCI) standard deviation	12 month control (PCS)	12 month control (PCS) standard deviation	12 month intervention (PCI)	12 month intervention (PCI) standard deviation	3 year control (PCS)	3 year control (PCS) standard deviation	3 year intervention (PCI)	3 year intervention (PCI) standard deviation	5 year control (PCS)	5 year control (PCS) standard deviation	5 year intervention (PCI)	5 year intervention (PCI) standard deviation
Obedinskiy et al. 2018	IMPACTOR-CTO: PCI vs MT for RCA CTO CAD	RCT	3		56.6 (8.1)	12 (16.7%)	CTO	72	12 months	SF-36	Physical functioning	MT	IQR	40	(30–45)	40	(23–45)	41*	(31–45)*	45*	(45–75)*	X	X	X	X	40	(30–45)	45	(45–70)	X	X	X	X	X	X	X	X
										SF-36	Role—physical functioning	MT	IQR	25	(0–75)	25	(0–50)	25*	(25–75)*	75*	(50–75)*	X	X	X	X	25	(25–50)	75	(50–75)	X	X	X	X	X	X	X	X
										SF-36	Bodily pain	MT	IQR	41	(22–51)	41	(22–41)	40*	(40–51)*	62*	(41–62)*	X	X	X	X	41	(32–51)	51	(41–62)	X	X	X	X	X	X	X	X
										SF-36	General health	MT	IQR	40	(25–50)	25	(20–45)	45*	(20–50)*	50*	(35–57)*	X	X	X	X	40	(20–50)	50	(45–55)	X	X	X	X	X	X	X	X
										SF-36	Vitality	MT	IQR	33	(25–45)	30	(20–38)	35*	(25–45)*	45*	(35–50)*	X	X	X	X	33	(25–40)	45	(40–50)	X	X	X	X	X	X	X	X
										SF-36	Social functioning	MT	IQR	50	(25–63)	50	(25–54)	50*	(38–75)*	75*	(50–75)*	X	X	X	X	50	(37–63)	63	(50–75)	X	X	X	X	X	X	X	X
										SF-36	Role—emotional	MT	IQR	38	(36–69)	36	(33–67)	40*	(34–68)*	100*	(67–100)*	X	X	X	X	67	(33–67)	100	(66–100)	X	X	X	X	X	X	X	X
										SF-36	Mental health	MT	IQR	40	(32–52)	40	(30–46)	40*	(32–52)*	52*	(44–62)*	X	X	X	X	40	(32–48)	52	(48–60)	X	X	X	X	X	X	X	X
Werner et al. 2018	EUROCTO: PCI vs MT for CTO CAD	RCT	3		65 (9.7)	63 (16%)	CTO	396 (259 PCI, 137 MT)	12 months	SAQ	Angina frequency	MT	SD	80.6	24.2	77.2	23.8	X	X	X	X	X	X	X	X	87.6	18.7	91.8	16.3	X	X	X	X	X	X	X	X
										SAQ	Physical limitation	MT	SD	71.2	24.7	67.1	24.9	X	X	X	X	X	X	X	X	76.6	22.9	80.2	22.4	X	X	X	X	X	X	X	X
										SAQ	Quality of life	MT	SD	59.8	26.2	55.3	24.9	X	X	X	X	X	X	X	X	71.8	25.5	76.6	23	X	X	X	X	X	X	X	X
										SAQ	Angina stability	MT	SD	53.4	23.4	52	22.7	X	X	X	X	X	X	X	X	56.2	20.2	57.7	19.6	X	X	X	X	X	X	X	X
										SAQ	Treatment satisfaction	MT	SD	88.2	13.7	84.1	17.6	X	X	X	X	X	X	X	X	89.2	13.9	90	15.3	X	X	X	X	X	X	X	X
Wijeysundera et al. 2014	APPROACH registry: quality of life outcomes in patients with CTOs with MT vs PCI vs CABG	Observational		8	66.4 (10.7)	67 (17.3%)	CTO	387	12 months	EQ-5D		CABG vs PCI-CTO	SD	0.76	0.15	0.82	0.16	X	X	X	X	X	X	X	X	0.9	0.14	0.89	0.15	X	X	X	X	X	X	X	X
Wijeysundera et al. 2014	APPROACH registry: quality of life outcomes in patients with CTOs with MT vs PCI vs CABG	Observational		8	66.4 (10.7)	67 (17.3%)	CTO	387	12 months	SAQ	Physical limitation	CABG vs PCI-CTO	SD	64.1	24	72.2	25.9	X	X	X	X	X	X	X	X	84.7	18.8	85.5	19.7	X	X	X	X	X	X	X	X
										SAQ	Angina frequency	CABG vs PCI-CTO	SD	78.3	23.2	77.6	22.7	X	X	X	X	X	X	X	X	94.9	12.7	90.6	14.7	X	X	X	X	X	X	X	X
										SAQ	Angina stability	CABG vs PCI-CTO	SD	55.1	29.7	67.4	29.7	X	X	X	X	X	X	X	X	76.1	25.9	80.1	25.2	X	X	X	X	X	X	X	X
										SAQ	Disease perception	CABG vs PCI-CTO	SD	50.8	27.7	53.3	26.5	X	X	X	X	X	X	X	X	81	20	78.9	21.4	X	X	X	X	X	X	X	X
										SAQ	Treatment satisfaction	CABG vs PCI-CTO	SD	88.2	15.5	84.3	19.2	X	X	X	X	X	X	X	X	92.3	18.8	91.1	15.2	X	X	X	X	X	X	X	X

MT medical therapy; *CTO* chronic total occlusion; *CABG* coronary artery bypass grafting; *PCI* percutaneous coronary intervention; *CAD* coronary artery disease; *SD* standard deviation; *RCT* randomised controlled trial; *NR* not reported; *IQR* interquartile range

* 2 months

Table 13.4 Patient related outcome measures in studies focusing on percutaneous coronary intervention for undifferentiated coronary artery disease

Study	Study intent	Study design	Quality score RCT	Quality score observational	Age	Sex (% female)	Other relevant demographics (race, employment, obesity, diabetes, physical activity, smoking, alcohol, no leisure physical activity)	No. of patients	Follow-up (months)	Instrument(s)		Control	Data spread	Pre-op control (PCS)	Pre-op control (PCS) standard deviation	Pre-op intervention (PCI)	Pre-op intervention (PCI) standard deviation	1 month control (PCS)	1 month control (PCS) standard deviation	1 month intervention (PCI)	1 month intervention (PCI) standard deviation	6 month control (PCS)	6 month control (PCS) standard deviation	6 month intervention (PCI)	6 month intervention (PCI) standard deviation	12 month control (PCS)	12 month control (PCS) standard deviation	12 month intervention (PCI)	12 month intervention (PCI) standard deviation	3 year control (PCS)	3 year control (PCS) standard deviation	3 year intervention (PCI)	3 year intervention (PCI) standard deviation	5 year control (PCS)	5 year control (PCS) standard deviation	5 year intervention (PCI)	5 year intervention (PCI) standard deviation
Abdallah et al. 2017	SYNTAX: quality of life outcomes in PCI vs CABG	RCT	4		PCI—65.2(9.7), CABG—64.8 (9.9)	385 (21.4%)	CAD	1800	60 months	SF-36	Physical component	CABG	SD	40.4	10.2	40.4	10	38.8	NR	46.6	NR	47.1	NR	47.6	NR	X	X	X	X	X	X	X	X	46	NR	45.8	NR
										SF-36	Mental component	CABG	SD	45.2	12	45.2	12.4	45.7	NR	48.8	NR	48.9	NR	49.4	NR	X	X	X	X	X	X	X	X	50.7	NR	49.3	NR
Abdallah et al. 2017	SYNTAX: quality of life outcomes in PCI vs CABG	RCT	4		PCI—65.2(9.7), CABG—64.8 (9.9)	385 (21.4%)	CAD	1800	60 months	SAQ	Angina frequency	CABG	SD	69.5	26.7	69.6	25.8	89.2	NR	90.5	NR	93.6	NR	91.2	NR	X	X	X	X	X	X	X	X	95.3	NR	92.8	NR
										SAQ	Physical limitation	CABG	SD	65.3	25	65.1	24.7	66.4	NR	78.3	NR	79.5	NR	80.9	NR	X	X	X	X	X	X	X	X	77.6	NR	75.5	NR
										SAQ	Quality of life	CABG	SD	44.8	22.8	45.6	23	66.2	NR	71.3	NR	76.8	NR	74.7	NR	X	X	X	X	X	X	X	X	81.6	NR	79	NR
										SAQ	Treatment satisfaction	CABG	SD	85.6	16	86.7	15.9	89.3	NR	90.3	NR	91	NR	92.2	NR	X	X	X	X	X	X	X	X	90.7	NR	91.7	NR
Baron et al. 2017	EXCEL: quality of life outcomes in PCI vs CABG in patients with LMS CAD	RCT	4		PCI—66.0 (9.6), CABG—65.8 (9.5)	402 (22.5%)	CAD	1788	24 months	SAQ	Angina frequency	CABG	SD	69.2	24.5	70.2	24.9	91.8	NR	93.1	NR	X	X	X	X	95	NR	94.1	NR	95.7	NR	95.8	NR	X	X	X	X
										SAQ	Physical limitation	CABG	SD	66.1	25	65.2	25	69	NR	84.5	NR	X	X	X	X	83.4	NR	83.7	NR	83	NR	84.2	NR	X	X	X	X
										SAQ	Quality of life	CABG	SD	47.7	23.8	48.4	23.8	51.2	NR	53	NR	X	X	X	X	51.6	NR	53.2	NR	51.5	NR	52	NR	X	X	X	X
										SAQ	Treatment satisfaction	CABG	SD	89.6	14.4	90	14.2	114.5	NR	118.2	NR	X	X	X	X	124.6	NR	121.9	NR	125.2	NR	124.9	NR	X	X	X	X
Baron et al. 2017	EXCEL: quality of life outcomes in PCI vs CABG	RCT	4		PCI—66.0 (9.6), CABG—65.8 (9.5)	402 (22.5%)	CAD	1788	24 months	PHQ-8		CABG	SD	5.6	5.4	5.8	5.4	5.5	NR	5.4	NR	X	X	X	X	5.3	NR	5.4	NR	5.2	NR	5.4	NR	X	X	X	X
Baron et al. 2017	EXCEL: quality of life outcomes in PCI vs CABG	RCT	4		PCI—66.0 (9.6), CABG—65.8 (9.5)	402 (22.5%)	CAD	1788	24 months	SF-12	Physical component	CABG	SD	38.2	11	38.5	10.8	37	NR	45.4	NR	X	X	X	X	46.6	NR	45.6	NR	45.7	NR	45.9	NR	X	X	X	X
										SF-12	Mental component	CABG	SD	49.8	11.1	49.3	11.1	52.1	NR	53	NR	X	X	X	X	52.5	NR	53	NR	52.4	NR	53.3	NR	X	X	X	X
Baron et al. 2017	EXCEL: quality of life outcomes in PCI vs CABG	RCT	4		PCI—66.0 (9.6), CABG—65.8 (9.5)	402 (22.5%)	CAD	1788	24 months	EQ-5D		CABG	SD	0.791	0.183	0.789	0.187	0.807	NR	0.886	NR	X	X	X	X	0.88	NR	0.869	NR	0.876	NR	0.876	NR	X	X	X	X
McGrath et al. 2017	APPROACH registry: PCI vs CABG in diabetic patients with multi-vessel disease requiring revascularisation	Observational		8	PCI—65 (9.6), CABG—66.1 (8.6)	402 (22.5%)	CAD	1319	60 months	SAQ	Physical limitation	CABG	95% CI	64.9	(61.9–68.0)	74.2	(71.9–76.5)	X	X	X	X	X	X	X	X	81.5	(79.9–83.2)	80.8	(78.9–82.2)	79.8	(77.9–81.7)	78.9	(77.1–80.7)	77.3	(75.1–79.5)	78.1	(75.8–80.4)
										SAQ	Angina stability	CABG	95% CI	64.7	(60.8–68.6)	78.6	(76.0–81.2)	X	X	X	X	X	X	X	X	81.2	(79.1–83.3)	75.8	(73.8–77.8)	80.6	(78.3–82.8)	76.3	(74.2–78.5)	77.8	(75.4–80.2)	75.6	(73.0–78.1)
										SAQ	Angina frequency	CABG	95% CI	78.8	(75.4–82.3)	84.9	(82.9–86.9)	X	X	X	X	X	X	X	X	92.9	(91.7–94.2)	91	(88.8–91.4)	93.3	(92.0–94.6)	92	(90.6–93.3)	93.5	(92.2–94.9)	91.6	(90.0–93.2)
										SAQ	Treatment satisfaction	CABG	95% CI	86.4	(84.2–88.6)	89.2	(87.8–90.5)	X	X	X	X	X	X	X	X	93.2	(92.3–94.2)	90.5	(89.4–91.6)	93	(91.9–94.1)	91.8	(90.7–92.9)	93.8	(92.7–94.8)	92.4	(91.1–93.6)
										SAQ	Quality of life	CABG	95% CI	58	(54.5–61.5)	69.5	(67.3–71.7)	X	X	X	X	X	X	X	X	82.5	(81.0–84.0)	77.4	(75.9–79.0)	83.3	(81.7–84.5)	81.2	(79.7–83.3)	84.2	(82.5–85.9)	81.8	(80.1–83.6)
Fakhrzad et al. 2016	Quality of life outcomes with PCI vs CABG	Observational		6	PCI—58.7 (11.2), CABG—60.2 (12.5)	147 (37.2%)	CAD	395	6 months	SAQ		CABG	SD	56.3	12.7	60	13.3	X	X	X	X	71.8	13.1	70.5	14.6	X	X	X	X	X	X	X	X	X	X	X	X
Fakhrzad et al. 2016	Quality of life outcomes with PCI vs CABG	Observational		6	PCI—58.7 (11.2), CABG—60.2 (12.5)	147 (37.2%)	CAD	395	6 months	SF-36		CABG	SD	59.5	21.2	59.2	20.5	X	X	X	X	67.8	18.7	63.8	18.3	X	X	X	X	X	X	X	X	X	X	X	X
Zajac et al. 2016	PCI of native vessels/ grafts vs MT in patients with prior CABG	Observational		8	70.4 (8.7)	16 (20.6%)	CAD	78	12 months	EQ-5D		MT vs PCI of native vessel	SD	0.66	0.08	0.65	0.06	X	X	X	X	X	X	X	X	0.67	0.7	0.72	0.05	X	X	X	X	X	X	X	X
										EQ-5D		MT vs PCI of grafts	SD	0.66	0.08	0.66	0.04	X	X	X	X	X	X	X	X	0.67	0.7	0.7	0.06	X	X	X	X	X	X	X	X
Abdallah et al. 2013	FREEDOM: quality of life outcomes in diabetic patients and multivessel CAD with PCI vs CABG	RCT	3		PCI—63.2 (8.9), CABG—63.0 (9.2)	535 (28%)	CAD	1880	60 months	SAQ	Angina frequency	CABG	95% CI	70.9	(69.3–72.5)	71.4	(69.8–73.0)	93.3	(92.3–94.3)	93.7	(92.8–94.5)	95.8	(95.0–96.6)	94.2	(93.2–95.1)	95.8	(94.9–96.6)	95.1	(94.2–95.9)	95.7	(94.8–96.7)	95.1	(94.1–96.1)	94	(91.9–96.1)	95.4	(93.6–97.1)
										SAQ	Physical limitation	CABG	95% CI	67.3	(65.7–68.9)	69.9	(68.4–71.4)	74.4	(72.4–76.4)	86.5	(85.2–87.8)	88.1	(86.9–89.3)	88.2	(87.0–89.4)	87	(85.7–88.4)	85.6	(84.2–86.9)	87.8	(86.2–89.4)	85.4	(83.7–87.1)	85.2	(82.2–88.2)	85.2	(82.4–88.1)
										SAQ	Quality of life	CABG	95% CI	47.8	(46.1–49.4)	49.2	(47.5–50.8)	74.9	(73.5–76.4)	77.6	(76.4–78.9)	80.4	(79.1–81.7)	79	(77.7–80.3)	80.7	(79.3–82.0)	78.8	(77.5–80.2)	82.2	(80.7–83.7)	80.8	(79.3–82.3)	83.3	(80.9–85.8)	79.5	(77.0–82.1)
Thiele et al. 2009	MIDCAB Versus DES in Proximal LAD Lesions: PCI vs minimally invasive CABG for LAD CAD	RCT	4		66	39 (30%)	CAD	130	12 months	SF-36	Physical functioning	CABG	SD	17.1	4.5	17.1	4.1	X	X	X	X	X	X	X	X	19.8	4	19.3	4	X	X	X	X	X	X	X	X
										SF-36	Role—physical functioning	CABG	SD	13.3	3.9	12.2	4.8	X	X	X	X	X	X	X	X	14.2	4.1	14.4	3.9	X	X	X	X	X	X	X	X
										SF-36	Bodily pain	CABG	SD	6.9	2.5	7.2	2.6	X	X	X	X	X	X	X	X	9.3	2.4	9.6	2.5	X	X	X	X	X	X	X	X
										SF-36	General health	CABG	SD	16.2	3.4	15.7	3.3	X	X	X	X	X	X	X	X	17.6	3.2	17.3	3.5	X	X	X	X	X	X	X	X
										SF-36	Vitality	CABG	SD	12	2.8	11.8	3.3	X	X	X	X	X	X	X	X	13.2	3.2	12.9	3.3	X	X	X	X	X	X	X	X
										SF-36	Social functioning	CABG	SD	7.7	1.9	8	2.1	X	X	X	X	X	X	X	X	8.6	1.7	8.6	1.6	X	X	X	X	X	X	X	X
										SF-36	Role—emotional	CABG	SD	10.5	3.2	10.4	4	X	X	X	X	X	X	X	X	11.5	3.1	11.5	2.9	X	X	X	X	X	X	X	X

(continued)

Table 13.4 (continued)

Study	Study intent	Study design	Quality score RCT	Quality score observational	Age	Sex (% female)	Other relevant demographics (race, employment, obesity, diabetes, physical activity, smoking, alcohol, no leisure physical activity)	No. of patients	Follow-up (months)	Instrument(s)		Control	Data spread	Pre-op control (PCS)	Pre-op control (PCS) standard deviation	Pre-op intervention (PCI)	Pre-op intervention (PCI) standard deviation	1 month control (PCS)	1 month control (PCS) standard deviation	1 month intervention (PCI)	1 month intervention (PCI) standard deviation	6 month control (PCS)	6 month control (PCS) standard deviation	6 month intervention (PCI)	6 month intervention (PCI) standard deviation	12 month control (PCS)	12 month control (PCS) standard deviation	12 month intervention (PCI)	12 month intervention (PCI) standard deviation	3 year control (PCS)	3 year control (PCS) standard deviation	3 year intervention (PCI)	3 year intervention (PCI) standard deviation	5 year control (PCS)	5 year control (PCS) standard deviation	5 year intervention (PCI)	5 year intervention (PCI) standard deviation
										SF-36	Mental health	CABG	SD	17.7	3.4	17.8	4	X	X	X	X	X	X	X	X	18.7	3.7	18.7	3.3	X	X	X	X	X	X	X	X
Thiele et al. 2009	MIDCAB Versus DES in Proximal LAD Lesions: PCI vs minimally invasive CABG for LAD CAD	RCT	4		66	39 (30%)	CAD	130	12 months	MacNew		CABG	SD	4.8	1	4.9	1	X	X	X	X	X	X	X	X	5.5	1	5.5	0.9	X	X	X	X	X	X	X	X
Hofer et al. 2006	Quality of life outcomes with PCI vs CABG vs MT	Observational		8	PCI—61.5 (11.2), MT 62.8 (9.1)	45 (28.8%)	CAD	156	3 months	SF-36	Physical component	MT	SD	40.14	10.31	39.28	8.27	42.02	11.08	42.98	10.2	X	X	X	X	X	X	X	X	X	X	X	X	X	X	X	X
										SF-36	Mental component	MT	SD	47.38	9.91	46.75	10.32	47.13	11.25	49.13	10.08	X	X	X	X	X	X	X	X	X	X	X	X	X	X	X	X
Hofer et al. 2006	Quality of life outcomes with PCI vs CABG vs MT	Observational		8	PCI—61.5 (11.2), MT 62.8 (9.1)	45 (28.8%)	CAD	156	3 months	MacNew	Global scale	MT	SD	4.89	1.01	4.93	0.97	5.12	1.16	5.4	0.93	X	X	X	X	X	X	X	X	X	X	X	X	X	X	X	X
Hofer et al. 2006	Quality of life outcomes with PCI vs CABG vs MT	Observational		8	PCI—61.5 (11.2), MT 62.8 (9.1)	45 (28.8%)	CAD	156	3 months	HADS	Anxiety	MT	SD	6.52	3.62	6.55	3.67	6.04	4.12	5.61	3.25	X	X	X	X	X	X	X	X	X	X	X	X	X	X	X	X
										HADS	Depression	MT	SD	4.88	3.38	5.06	3.86	5.27	4.25	4.27	3.52	X	X	X	X	X	X	X	X	X	X	X	X	X	X	X	X
Borkon et al. 2002	Quality of life outcomes with PCI vs CABG	Observational		8	PCI—64 (13), CABG—67 (10.9)	157 (33%)	CAD	475	12 months	SAQ	Angina frequency	CABG	SD	65.7	1.7	60	1.8	84.2	1.9	81	1.9	90	1.9	83.1	1.9	93.2	2	87.7	1.9	X	X	X	X	X	X	X	X
										SAQ	Physical limitation	CABG	SD	64.6	1.7	67.6	1.6	52	2.4	65.1	2.4	78.6	2.4	72	2.4	83.6	2.4	76.7	2.4	X	X	X	X	X	X	X	X
										SAQ	Quality of life	CABG	SD	53.6	1.5	50.7	1.4	65	2.3	70.4	2.3	83.4	2.3	77.3	2.2	87.6	2.3	80.9	2.2	X	X	X	X	X	X	X	X
Strauss et al. 1995	ACME: quality of life outcomes with PCI vs MT with stable single vessel CAD	RCT	3		PCI—62, MT—63	NR	CAD	212	6 months	QoL score (from the Psychological General Well-being Index and the McMaster Health Index Questionnaire)		MT	SD	96	18.6	96.7	20.1	X	X	X	X	98	NR	104.1	NR	X	X	X	X	X	X	X	X	X	X	X	X
Allen et al. 1990	Quality of life outcomes with PCI vs CABG	Observational		8	NR	NR	CAD	170	12 months	Functional Status Questionnaire	Physical activity	CABG	SD	59	25	75	26	X	X	X	X	X	X	X	X	91	14	92	18	X	X	X	X	X	X	X	X
											Social activity	CABG	SD	76	35	89	24	X	X	X	X	X	X	X	X	99	5	95	17	X	X	X	X	X	X	X	X
											Work performance	CABG	SD	81	24	79	23	X	X	X	X	X	X	X	X	93	11	89	17	X	X	X	X	X	X	X	X
											Mental Health	CABG	SD	61	23	67	19	X	X	X	X	X	X	X	X	82	14	77	17	X	X	X	X	X	X	X	X
											Quality of interaction	CABG	SD	77	16	80	13	X	X	X	X	X	X	X	X	84	13	80	13	X	X	X	X	X	X	X	X

MT medical therapy; *CTO* chronic total occlusion; *CABG* coronary artery bypass grafting; *PCI* percutaneous coronary intervention; *CAD* coronary artery disease; *SD* standard deviation; *RCT* randomised controlled trial; *NR* not reported; *IQR* interquartile range

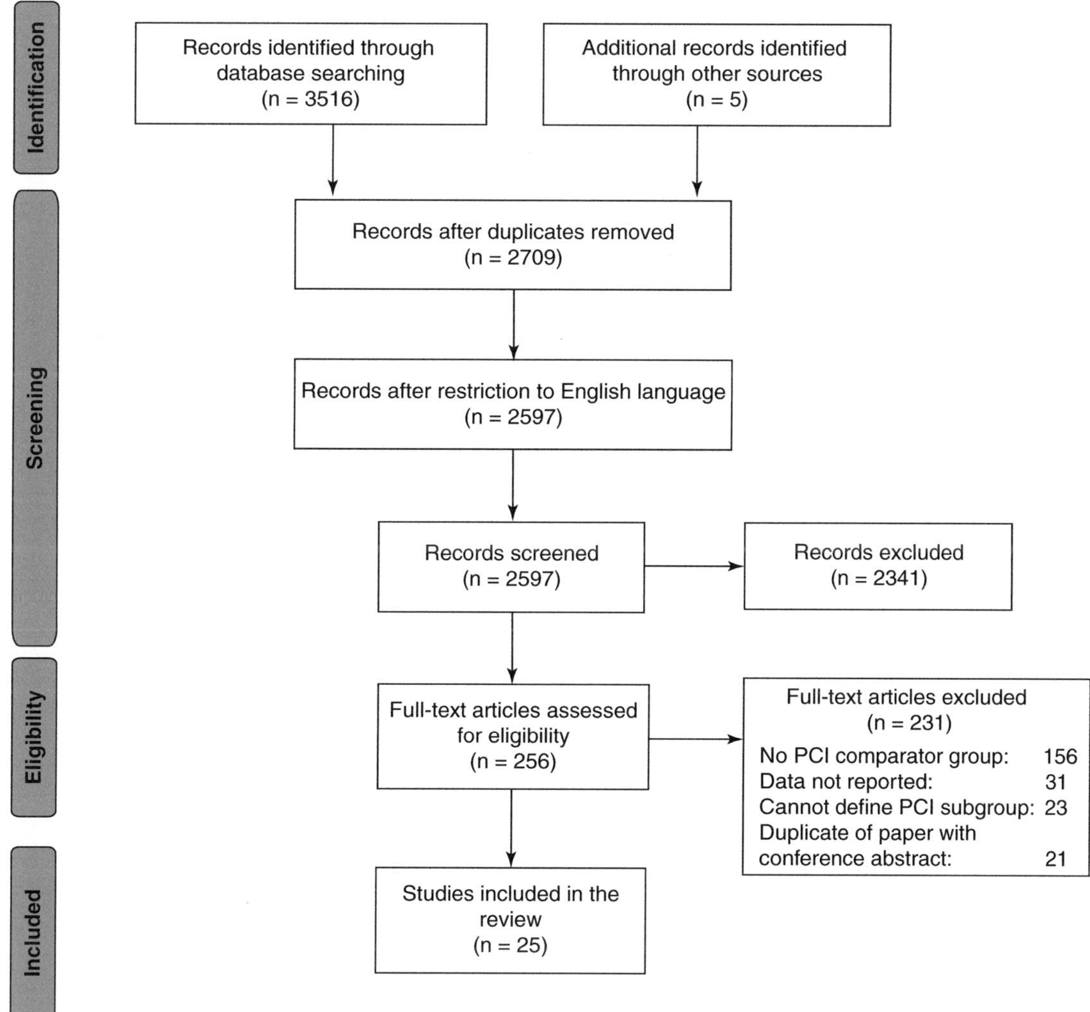

Fig. 13.1 PRISMA flow diagram

was performed in the setting of ACS [25]. However only four of these studies reported all five of the SAQ domains [16, 20, 24, 31] and one study reported one SAQ score only [21]. Other utilised disease-specific instruments include the MacNew Heart Disease HRQOL instrument [30, 32, 33] and the Duke Activity Status Index [29]; both of which were designed for cardiovascular disease [39, 40]. The PHQ-8 (eight-item Patient Health Questionnaire depression scale) [41] was reported in one study [19], whilst the HADS (Hospital Anxiety and Depression Scale) [42] was also reported in one study [32]. Two studies [19, 26] reported the Rose Dyspnoea Scale [43], however this measure was not included in the final analysis due to the reporting of binary responses to four questions, and therefore being less quantifiable.

Generic HRQOL status instruments provide a comprehensive assessment of health status, permitting their use across a variety of treatments or conditions at different time points, but with the trade-off of less sensitivity for detecting temporal change than disease-specific instruments. The most commonly used generic HRQOL instrument was the SF-36 [15, 17, 21, 27, 30–32, 44]. Other generic tools used included the SF-36 Mental Health Inventory 5 (SF-36 MHI 5) [45] (a subscale of the broader SF-36) [29], and the Short Form 12 (SF-12, [46] an abridged version of the SF-36) [19]. One study combined two instruments (the Psychological General Well-being Index [47] and the McMaster Health Index Questionnaire [48]) to generate an overall quality of life score [36]. The earliest study that was performed prior to the widespread use of other well-validated HRQOL instruments utilised the Functional Status Questionnaire [37, 49].

Preference-based HRQOL instruments were also reported, which focus primarily on health-related outcomes to an intervention. The EuroQOL-5D (EQ-5D) [50] is one such widely used measure which comprises two sections: the first is a health state description which has five dimensions (mobility, self-care, usual activities, pain/discomfort and anxiety/depression) and the second is a health state evaluation which is provided by the EuroQOL-Visual Analogue Scale (EQ-VAS) [51]. The EQ-5D was utilised in six studies [13, 14, 18, 19, 22, 24]. Other preference-based HRQOL instruments used include the 15-D [23, 28, 52] and the Short Form 6D (SF-6D, a subclassification of the SF-36 and SF-12 for economic evaluation) [23, 53].

PCI in Stable Coronary Artery Disease

PCI was performed in the setting of stable CAD in seven studies (Table 13.1). All studies were well-matched at baseline for HRQOL scores. Of these, three studies utilised the SAQ tool and demonstrated an early post-procedure improvement in the angina frequency domain with PCI versus medical therapy [18, 20, 31]. One study compared PCI to CABG in this setting and identified significant improvements across most SAQ domains for both groups from baseline, with no significant differences between revascularisation modalities [34]. A combined analysis of the FAME 1 and 2 studies found PCI to have superior improvements in EQ-5D score that persisted out to 1 year versus medical therapy [14], but this was not replicated in the smaller, but blinded ORBITA study [18]. There were no other significant differences identified with the other HRQOL scores.

PCI in Acute Coronary Syndromes

Five studies investigated differences in HRQOL scores in patients undergoing urgent revascularisation for ACS (Table 13.2). Four studies compared PCI to medical therapy. It is difficult to draw major inferences from the data in this cohort owing to the variety of HRQOL measures used. Moreover, follow up was relatively short, with no studies extending beyond 12 months. Only one study compared PCI to CABG, reporting greater improvements in SAQ score with cardiothoracic surgery across all domains [25]. Of the studies comparing PCI to medical therapy, most revealed no substantial differences. There was also no difference demonstrated in SF-6D or 15D scores in patients post-thrombolysis for STEMI randomised to either early PCI or medical therapy [23].

PCI in Chronic Total Occlusions

Only three studies assessed PCI for CTOs (Table 13.3). These studies were performed more recently than other procedural indications, with the earliest study published in 2014 [24]. Two studies utilised the SAQ tool. The IMPACTOR-CTO trial reported large HRQOL improvements with CTO-PCI of the right coronary artery versus medical therapy [15], with similar findings reported in the EURO-CTO trial, which undertook CTO-PCI of unselected coronary arteries [16]. However, an observational study comparing CTO-PCI to CABG found PCI to be inferior when compared to change from reference SAQ scores (although the CABG group had significantly lower scores at baseline, suggesting some case selection bias) [24].

PCI in Undifferentiated Coronary Artery Disease

A total of 11 studies comprised patients with CAD that was not defined further, and thus could include PCI performed in stable or unstable settings (Table 13.4). These studies were generally older, or involved patients with less common CAD subtypes, for example left main stem disease [17, 19], patients with prior CABG [22] or diabetic patients with multi-vessel CAD [20]. The majority (6/11, 55%) utilised the SAQ and only three (27%) had a non-interventional comparator [22, 32, 36]. In general, baseline HRQOL scores were well-matched between PCI and comparator groups, with the exception of lower scores for patients undergoing CABG in some observational studies [20, 37]. In the studies reporting SAQ scores, initial improvements were found in the PCI versus CABG groups in the physical limitation and quality of life domains at 1 month [17, 19, 26, 35]. However, this discrepancy levelled out by 6 months. At 5 years, the SAQ scores were generally even across all domains, except for perhaps a trend towards improved angina stability with CABG. Other studies comparing HRQOL following PCI or CABG also generally demonstrated improved PCI scores early post-procedure in the physical domains of SF-36 and EQ-5D, which again equalised by 6 months [17, 19, 30].

Discussion

This systematic review represents over 16,000 patients undergoing PCI in a variety of clinical settings over a 30-year period with PROMs reported in PCI and comparator groups. 92% of the studies were assessed as being of high quality and a low risk of bias. Throughout this analysis there has been a notable increase in HRQOL measure reporting, as evidenced by 15 of the studies being published in the last 10 years (as opposed to ten studies in the preceding 20 years). Indeed, some of the included papers were published as stand-alone quality of life sub-studies as prespecified secondary endpoints of large studies, further demonstrating the growing weight of PROMs in PCI. Although many HRQOL measures were reported across the included studies, the SAQ was utilised widely and appears to be predominating. Figure 13.2 highlights key patient and procedural factors that predict poor quality of life outcomes with PCI.

As discussed above, the importance of symptomatic improvement in PCI for stable CAD and

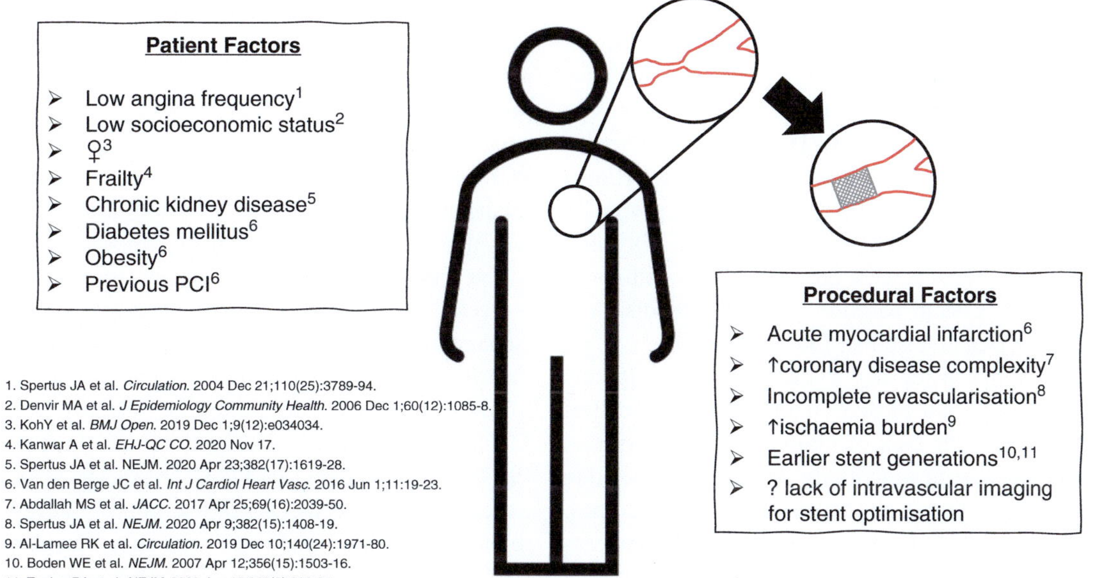

Fig. 13.2 Predictors of poor quality of life outcomes with PCI

CTOs is paramount, and quantifiable HRQOL outcome measures are increasingly viewed with significance. It is with great interest therefore that we report a potential observed improvement in symptoms with PCI in stable CAD and CTO-PCI versus medical therapy. However, this benefit was often limited to a few domains of the HRQOL tools. In order to justify PCI in this setting, with its associated cost and safety implications, the symptomatic gain needs to be significant. Thus, it is important to note that PCI was comparable to the more invasive and expensive CABG surgery in many settings. However, the initial PROM gains seen in PCI versus CABG cohorts are likely related to the much more prolonged and intensive post-operative recovery of cardiothoracic surgery.

The International Study of Comparative Health Effectiveness with Medical and Invasive Approaches (ISCHEMIA) trial, a large multicentre study of 5179 patients with moderate or severe ischemia who were randomised to either an initial invasive strategy (angiography and revascularisation when feasible), in addition to medical therapy, or to an initial conservative strategy of medical therapy alone, reported in 2020. This critical trial demonstrated no effect of revascularisation (74% PCI, 26% CABG) on ischaemic cardiovascular events or all-cause mortality over a median of 3.2 years [4]. The quality of life substudy of ISCHEMIA confirmed the findings of this systematic review, reporting a modest increase in HRQOL outcomes with an invasive versus a conservative strategy. Of note, HRQOL benefits were greater in those with more severe angina at baseline (35% of patients were angina-free at baseline) [54].

When considering so-called 'soft' endpoints in clinical trials (unlike 'hard' endpoints such as mortality), the lack of blinding of the physician and participant potentially results in knowledge of the treatment allocation affecting outcomes. Of course, blinding the patient to an interventional procedure is difficult to achieve; this is in comparison to giving a similar-looking placebo drug in a pharmaceutical trial. The absence of blinding in trials reporting PROMs may mean that if the patient 'believes' that the treatment they are receiving (be it PCI or CABG) is going to be more effective than the medical therapy they have already been taking (typically unsuccessfully, as failure of anti-anginal medical therapy is an indication for revascularisation), then the interventional arm may receive better HRQOL scores. This is as relevant in PCI versus medical therapy as it is to PCI versus CABG, where patient awareness to treatment allocation has the potential to affect the overall outcome. Blinding for CABG is especially challenging, as it would be unethical to perform a sternotomy without performing revascularisation. Moreover, after CABG, patients have a constant reminder of their operation with a scar and lifestyle modifications necessary for sternal healing. In contrast, after PCI, there may be no visible mark of the procedure.

In an attempt to remove these issues, meticulous patient blinding was performed in the landmark ORBITA trial [18]. This was the first study to explore the use of a placebo procedure in PCI; patients with severe single vessel disease were randomised to either traditional PCI or sham-procedure. Patients were sedated and underwent an invasive procedure, but in those randomised to placebo, pressure wire assessment was performed as per protocol, but no PCI was performed. As reported here, the ORBITA trial demonstrated no substantial HRQOL improvement between the PCI and sham procedure arms when maximal medical therapy was delivered to both arms. This was also true for other markers of symptoms such as exercise time, albeit with follow up only to 6 weeks. Conversely, more objective markers of ischaemia such as stress echocardiography were clearly improved by PCI. Thus, the overall impact of presence/absence of blinding on PROMs with PCI requires further investigation—the lack of PROM improvement in ORBITA raises some uncertainty over results in other randomised trials reported in this analysis, and their modest HRQOL improvements.

There are other potential sources of confounding in the use of PROMs with PCI. For example, procedural factors may significantly affect results. These include site of access for the procedure (radial versus femoral), use of sedation (which is not commonplace practice), length and complexity of the procedure as well as the presence of any procedural complications, which can all affect patient satisfaction and therefore PROM measures. The acute success of the procedure is also a contributing factor. As PCI has near instant feedback on angiographic markers of technical success, this can contribute to PROMs. For example, in patients who are told that the procedure was *less* successful, PROMs are likely to be adversely affected regardless of actual patient symptoms. Other potential obstacles include the reason for PCI being undertaken—e.g. if a patient is undergoing a repeat procedure for stent failure or in-stent restenosis, this will negatively affect their perceived HRQOL gains. In contrast, an emergency procedure for ACS in which PCI can immediately alleviate the associated chest discomfort may positively inflate the perceived benefits. Alternatively, as many patients do not experience angina prior to an ACS, and ACS-related chest pain may be short lived if successfully treated, long term HRQOL benefits may be under-reported in PROMs.

A further issue is that many patients do not like taking medications long term and in countries where medication costs are high—this can alter patient behaviours and preferences. PCI routinely predicates the use of dual antiplatelet agents for 6 months or more; in addition, multiple anti-anginals and statins will be started which may alter patient perception of the treatment. While procedural-related factors are more likely to influence outcomes closer to the time of procedure, longer term follow up may demonstrate different results as patient preferences change. Longer-term follow up may also help to reduce the potential confounding, and moreover will give a fairer representation of the long-lasting effects of the intervention. Although lack of blinding is an issue with randomised trials, there are other major sources of potential bias in observational studies, including selection bias, indication bias and significant confounding variables.

Study Limitations

Interpretation of this systematic review must be tempered with understanding of the limitations of the data synthesis and studies themselves. Inclusion was restricted to studies reporting raw baseline HRQOL outcome measures and at least one further timepoint. This significantly adds weight to the analysis, but does result in the exclusion of a large number of studies. In addition, not all studies reported spread of data ranges for all outcomes, limiting subsequent quantitative analysis. As above, there are inherent biases in PROM data, which also include reporter level bias, observer bias if interviews are used and self-selection bias if surveys are used for follow up.

Other limitations of this systematic review include the wide time span of included studies with significantly evolving technology and techniques, which may restrict the generalisability of results to present day practice. Early studies did not utilise stents but relied upon balloon angioplasty alone, which is recognised to have poor longer-term outcomes, specifically requiring repeat procedures. Secondly, each of the studies have varying patient characteristics and comorbidities which can affect PROMs. Thirdly, with the observational studies in particular, baseline HRQOL scores were not always well-matched, and lastly, studies were included with either active (CABG) and passive (medical therapy) comparators, further limiting global evaluation.

Suggestions for Future Research

PROMs in PCI have a growing importance which is set to continue. In order to maximise the potential of future research in this area it is important that investigators focus on a select few HRQOL tools to ensure optimal generalisability with previous and forthcoming studies. To this end, the SAQ appears to be gaining increasing use, which should be encouraged. Further studies investigating HRQOL outcomes with PCI, especially in the setting of stable CAD or CTOs where appropriate, ideally in comparison to optimal medical therapy, should be endorsed and will help iden-

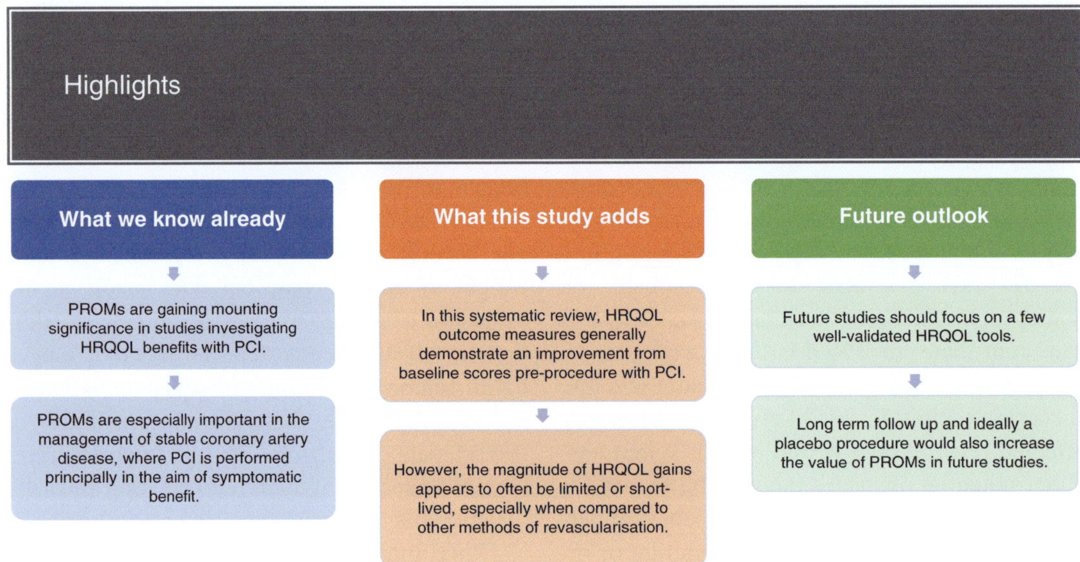

Fig. 13.3 Study highlights

tify the true symptomatic benefit of elective PCI. In addition, there is now consensus in the cardiology community on what constitutes a myocardial infarction [55] and major adverse bleeding [56] for reporting in clinical trials of PCI. However, no such consensus exists for quality of life outcomes. Thus, there is a real need for the formulation of an expert working group, aiming to clarify issues and standardise practice on HRQOL reporting following PCI.

Separately, given that PROMs are 'soft' endpoints that can be affected by patient knowledge of treatment allocation, serious consideration should be given to the use of placebo procedures, or some other method of patient blinding, in future RCTs. Where this is not possible, or in the case of observational studies, long term follow up should be supported.

Conclusions

PROMs are increasingly fashionable and gaining mounting significance in studies investigating potential HRQOL benefits with PCI. This is the case most pertinently in elective PCI procedures, predominantly carried out for symptomatic gains, where quantifiable improvements are both important and necessary. In this study HRQOL outcome measures with PCI generally demonstrate an improvement from baseline scores pre-procedure. However, the magnitude of these gains appears to be limited, and in some instances, relatively short-lived when compared to other methods of revascularisation or medical therapy. Future studies should focus on a few well-validated HRQOL tools, provide long term follow up and ideally use a placebo procedure. Figure 13.3 highlights the key findings of this analysis.

Funding A.H. is funded by a Wellcome Trust Clinical Research Fellowship.

Conflict of Interest None declared.

References

1. Grüntzig A, Hopff H. [Percutaneous recanalization after chronic arterial occlusion with a new dilator-catheter (modification of the Dotter technique) (author's transl)]. Dtsch Med Wochenschr. 1974;99(49):2502–10, 11.
2. Chacko L, James PH, Rajkumar C, Nowbar AN, Kane C, Mahdi D, et al. Effects of percutaneous coronary intervention on death and myocardial infarction strati-

fied by stable and unstable coronary artery disease: a meta-analysis of randomized controlled trials. Circ Cardiovasc Qual Outc. 2020;13(2):e006363.

3. Tavakol M, Ashraf S, Brener SJ. Risks and complications of coronary angiography: a comprehensive review. Global J Health Sci. 2012;4(1):65–93.
4. Maron DJ, Hochman JS, Reynolds HR, Bangalore S, O'Brien SM, Boden WE, et al. Initial invasive or conservative strategy for stable coronary disease. N Engl J Med. 2020;382(15):1395–407.
5. Boden WE, O'Rourke RA, Teo KK, Hartigan PM, Maron DJ, Kostuk WJ, et al. Optimal medical therapy with or without PCI for stable coronary disease. N Engl J Med. 2007;356(15):1503–16.
6. Leaman DM, Brower RW, Meester GT, Serruys P, van den Brand M. Coronary artery atherosclerosis: severity of the disease, severity of angina pectoris and compromised left ventricular function. Circulation. 1981;63(2):285–99.
7. Christakopoulos GE, Christopoulos G, Carlino M, Jeroudi OM, Roesle M, Rangan BV, et al. Meta-analysis of clinical outcomes of patients who underwent percutaneous coronary interventions for chronic total occlusions. Am J Cardiol. 2015;115(10):1367–75.
8. Black N. Patient reported outcome measures could help transform healthcare. BMJ. 2013;346:f167.
9. Liberati A, Altman DG, Tetzlaff J, Mulrow C, Gotzsche PC, Ioannidis JP, et al. The PRISMA statement for reporting systematic reviews and meta-analyses of studies that evaluate healthcare interventions: explanation and elaboration. BMJ. 2009;339:b2700.
10. Stang A. Critical evaluation of the Newcastle-Ottawa scale for the assessment of the quality of nonrandomized studies in meta-analyses. Eur J Epidemiol. 2010;25(9):603–5.
11. Luchini C, Stubbs B, Solmi M, Veronese N. Assessing the quality of studies in meta-analyses: advantages and limitations of the Newcastle Ottawa Scale. World J Meta Anal. 2017;5(4):80–4.
12. Jadad AR, Moore RA, Carroll D, Jenkinson C, Reynolds DJ, Gavaghan DJ, et al. Assessing the quality of reports of randomized clinical trials: is blinding necessary? Control Clin Trials. 1996;17(1):1–12.
13. Lee MMY, Petrie MC, Rocchiccioli P, Simpson J, Jackson CE, Corcoran DS, et al. Invasive versus medical management in patients with prior coronary artery bypass surgery with a non-ST segment elevation acute coronary syndrome. Circ Cardiovasc Interv. 2019;12(8):e007830.
14. Nishi T, Piroth Z, De Bruyne B, Jagic N, Mobius-Winkler S, Kobayashi Y, et al. Fractional flow reserve and quality-of-life improvement after percutaneous coronary intervention in patients with stable coronary artery disease. Circulation. 2018;138(17):1797–804.
15. Obedinskiy AA, Kretov EI, Boukhris M, Kurbatov VP, Osiev AG, Ibn Elhadj Z, et al. The IMPACTOR-CTO trial. JACC Cardiovasc Interv. 2018;11(13):1309–11.
16. Werner GS, Martin-Yuste V, Hildick-Smith D, Boudou N, Sianos G, Gelev V, et al. A randomized multicentre trial to compare revascularization with optimal medical therapy for the treatment of chronic total coronary occlusions. Eur Heart J. 2018;39(26):2484–93.
17. Abdallah MS, Wang K, Magnuson EA, Osnabrugge RL, Kappetein AP, Morice MC, et al. Quality of life after surgery or DES in patients with 3-vessel or left main disease. J Am Coll Cardiol. 2017;69(16):2039–50.
18. Al-Lamee R, Thompson D, Dehbi HM, Sen S, Tang K, Davies J, et al. Percutaneous coronary intervention in stable angina (ORBITA): a double-blind, randomised controlled trial. Lancet. 2018;391(10115):31–40.
19. Baron SJ, Chinnakondepalli K, Magnuson EA, Kandzari DE, Puskas JD, Ben-Yehuda O, et al. Quality-of-life after everolimus-eluting stents or bypass surgery for left-main disease: results from the EXCEL trial. J Am Coll Cardiol. 2017;70(25):3113–22.
20. McGrath BM, Norris CM, Hardwicke-Brown E, Welsh RC, Bainey KR. Quality of life following coronary artery bypass graft surgery vs. percutaneous coronary intervention in diabetics with multivessel disease: a five-year registry study. Eur Heart J Qual Care Clin Outc. 2017;3(3):216–23.
21. Fakhrzad NGR, Barouni M, Kojuri J, Jahani Y. Examining the health-related quality of life after coronary artery bypass grafting and percutaneous coronary intervention in Iran via SF-36 and SAQ. Int Cardiovasc Res J. 2016;1(10):123–8.
22. Zajac P, Zycinski P, Qawoq H, Jankowski L, Peruga J, Wcislo T, et al. Outcomes of percutaneous coronary intervention in patients after previous coronary artery bypass surgery. Kardiol Pol. 2016;74(4):322–30.
23. Bohmer E, Kristiansen IS, Arnesen H, Halvorsen S. Health-related quality of life after myocardial infarction, does choice of method make a difference? Scand Cardiovasc J. 2014;48(4):216–22.
24. Wijeysundera HC, Norris C, Fefer P, Galbraith PD, Knudtson ML, Wolff R, et al. Relationship between initial treatment strategy and quality of life in patients with coronary chronic total occlusions. EuroIntervention. 2014;9(10):1165–72.
25. Yang LX, Zhou YJ, Wang ZJ, Li YP, Chai M. Impact of invasive treatment strategy on health-related quality of life six months after non-ST-elevation acute coronary syndrome. J Geriatr Cardiol. 2014;11(3):206–11.
26. Abdallah MS, Wang K, Magnuson EA, Spertus JA, Farkouh ME, Fuster V, et al. Quality of life after PCI vs CABG among patients with diabetes and multivessel coronary artery disease: a randomized clinical trial. JAMA. 2013;310(15):1581–90.
27. Li R, Yan BP, Dong M, Zhang Q, Yip GW, Chan CP, et al. Quality of life after percutaneous coronary intervention in the elderly with acute coronary syndrome. Int J Cardiol. 2012;155(1):90–6.
28. Loponen P, Luther M, Korpilahti K, Wistbacka JO, Huhtala H, Laurikka J, et al. HRQoL after coronary artery bypass grafting and percutaneous coronary intervention for stable angina. Scand Cardiovasc J. 2009;43(2):94–9.

29. Mark DB, Pan W, Clapp-Channing NE, Anstrom KJ, Ross JR, Fox RS, et al. Quality of life after late invasive therapy for occluded arteries. N Engl J Med. 2009;360(8):774–83.
30. Thiele H, Neumann-Schniedewind P, Jacobs S, Boudriot E, Walther T, Mohr FW, et al. Randomized comparison of minimally invasive direct coronary artery bypass surgery versus sirolimus-eluting stenting in isolated proximal left anterior descending coronary artery stenosis. J Am Coll Cardiol. 2009;53(25):2324–31.
31. Weintraub WS, Spertus JA, Kolm P, Maron DJ, Zhang Z, Jurkovitz C, et al. Effect of PCI on quality of life in patients with stable coronary disease. N Engl J Med. 2008;359(7):677–87.
32. Hofer S, Doering S, Rumpold G, Oldridge N, Benzer W. Determinants of health-related quality of life in patients with coronary artery disease. Eur J Cardiovasc Prev Rehabil. 2006;13(3):398–406.
33. Benzer W, Hofer S, Oldridge NB. Health-related quality of life in patients with coronary artery disease after different treatments for angina in routine clinical practice. Herz. 2003;28(5):421–8.
34. Zhang Z, Mahoney EM, Stables RH, Booth J, Nugara F, Spertus JA, et al. Disease-specific health status after stent-assisted percutaneous coronary intervention and coronary artery bypass surgery: one-year results from the Stent or Surgery trial. Circulation. 2003;108(14):1694–700.
35. Borkon AM, Muehlebach GF, House J, Marso SP, Spertus JA. A comparison of the recovery of health status after percutaneous coronary intervention and coronary artery bypass. Ann Thorac Surg. 2002;74(5):1526–30; discussion 30.
36. Strauss WE, Fortin T, Hartigan P, Folland ED, Parisi AF. A comparison of quality of life scores in patients with angina pectoris after angioplasty compared with after medical therapy. Outcomes of a randomized clinical trial. Veterans Affairs Study of Angioplasty Compared to Medical Therapy Investigators. Circulation. 1995;92(7):1710–9.
37. Allen JK, Fitzgerald ST, Swank RT, Becker DM. Functional status after coronary artery bypass grafting and percutaneous transluminal coronary angioplasty. Am J Cardiol. 1990;66(12):921–5.
38. Spertus JA, Winder JA, Dewhurst TA, Deyo RA, Prodzinski J, McDonell M, et al. Development and evaluation of the Seattle Angina Questionnaire: a new functional status measure for coronary artery disease. J Am Coll Cardiol. 1995;25(2):333–41.
39. Höfer S, Lim L, Guyatt G, Oldridge N. The MacNew heart disease health-related quality of life instrument: a summary. Health Qual Life Outcomes. 2004;2:3.
40. Hlatky MA, Boineau RE, Higginbotham MB, Lee KL, Mark DB, Califf RM, et al. A brief self-administered questionnaire to determine functional capacity (The Duke Activity Status Index). Am J Cardiol. 1989;64(10):651.
41. Kroenke K, Strine TW, Spitzer RL, Williams JB, Berry JT, Mokdad A. The PHQ-8 as a measure of current depression in the general population. J Affect Disord. 2009;114(1–3):163.
42. Snaith RP. The hospital anxiety and depression scale. Health Qual Life Outcomes. 2003;1(1):1–4.
43. Rose GA, Blackburn H. Cardiovascular survey methods. Monograph series. Geneva: World Health Organization; 1968. p. 56.
44. Ware JE, Sherbourne C. The MOS 36-item Short-Form Health Survey (SF-36). I. Conceptual framework and item selection. Med Care. 1992;30(6):473.
45. Berwick DM, Murphy JM, Goldman PA, Ware JE, Barsky AJ, Weinstein M. Performance of a five-item mental health screening test. Med Care. 1991;29(2):169.
46. Ware J, Kosinski M, Keller S. A 12-Item Short-Form Health Survey: construction of scales and preliminary tests of reliability and validity. Med Care. 1996;34(3):220.
47. Dupuy HJ. PGWBI - psychological general well-being index. New York, NY: Le Jacq Publishing; 1984.
48. Chambers LW, Macdonald LA, Tugwell P, Buchanan WW, Kraag G. The McMaster health index questionnaire as a measure of quality of life for patients with rheumatoid disease. J Rheumatol. 1982;9(5):780.
49. Jette AM, Davies AR, Cleary PD, Calkins DR, Rubenstein LV, Fink A, et al. The functional status questionnaire: reliability and validity when used in primary care. J Gen Intern Med. 1986;1(3):143.
50. EuroQol-Group. EuroQol--a new facility for the measurement of health-related quality of life. Health Policy. 1990;16(3):199.
51. Feng Y, Parkin D, Devlin NJ. Assessing the performance of the EQ-VAS in the NHS PROMs programme. Qual Life Res. 2014;23:977–89.
52. Sintonen H. The 15D instrument of health-related quality of life: properties and applications. Ann Med. 2001;33(5):328.
53. Brazier J, Usherwood T, Harper R, Thomas K. Deriving a preference-based single index from the UK SF-36 health survey. J Clin Epidemiol. 1998;51(11):1115.
54. Spertus JA, Jones PG, Maron DJ, O'Brien SM, Reynolds HR, Rosenberg Y, et al. Health-status outcomes with invasive or conservative care in coronary disease. N Engl J Med. 2020;382(15):1408–19.
55. Thygesen K, Alpert JS, Jaffe AS, Chaitman BR, Bax JJ, Morrow DA, et al. Fourth universal definition of myocardial infarction. Circulation. 2018;138(20):e618–e51.
56. Mehran R, Rao SV, Bhatt DL, Gibson CM, Caixeta A, Eikelboom J, et al. Standardized bleeding definitions for cardiovascular clinical trials: a consensus report from the Bleeding Academic Research Consortium. Circulation. 2011;123(23):2736–47.

Quality of Life and Patient Reported Outcome Measures Following Carotid Artery Intervention

14

Leonard L. Shan, Akshat Saxena, and Alun H. Davies

Abbreviations

ACAS	Asymptomatic carotid atherosclerosis study
ACST	The asymptomatic carotid surgery trial
CREST	Carotid revascularisation endarterectomy versus stenting trial
ECST	European carotid surgery trial
NASCET	The North American symptomatic carotid endarterectomy trial
SAPPHIRE	Stenting and angioplasty with protection in patients at high risk for endarterectomy trial

L. L. Shan (✉)
St. Vincent's Hospital Melbourne, Melbourne, VIC, Australia

Department of Surgery, The University of Melbourne, Melbourne, VIC, Australia
e-mail: leonard.shan@unimelb.edu.au

A. Saxena
Department of Cardiothoracic Surgery and Transplantation, Fiona Stanley Hospital, Murdoch, WA, Australia

A. H. Davies
Charing Cross, London, UK

St. Mary's Hospital, London, UK

Vascular Surgery, Department of Surgery and Cancer, Imperial College London, London, UK
e-mail: a.h.davies@imperial.ac.uk

Introduction

Stroke and transient ischemic attacks are a serious public health problem which commonly causes persistent disability and poor quality of life (QOL) [1–3]. A significant proportion of ischemic strokes (18–29%) are attributable to carotid artery disease [4, 5] and are preventable by revascularisation [6]. The benefit of carotid revascularisation by either carotid endarterectomy (CEA) or carotid stenting (CAS) has been well established previously. However, these focus on technical outcomes such as morbidity, mortality, and stroke prevention. Whilst these are important, they provide only one aspect of the intervention outcome.

From the early 1990s the concept of QOL and patient reported outcomes measures (PROMS) were identified as an important assessment of post-operative outcomes [7]. In particular, QOL after surgery is a patient-focussed assessment that complements traditional outcome measures such as post-operative stroke and death [8].

This chapter summarises the available literature on QOL and PROMS after carotid artery intervention. The current literature provides mainly QOL outcomes after CEA or CAS in atherosclerotic disease. This is therefore the focus of this chapter. Other indications and procedures are outside of the scope of this chapter.

T. Athanasiou et al. (eds.), *Patient Reported Outcomes and Quality of Life in Cardiovascular Interventions*,
https://doi.org/10.1007/978-3-031-09815-4_14

Current Interventions on the Carotid Artery

Carotid Endarterectomy

Several landmark trials have provided strong evidence for CEA in stroke prevention. The benefit is greatest in symptomatic carotid stenosis as outlined in the NASCET and ECST trials [9, 10]. The ACAS and ASCT trials demonstrated that CEA is also beneficial in carefully selected asymptomatic patients with few comorbidities, good life expectancy, and low institutional perioperative stroke and mortality rates [11–14]. The combined peri-procedural mortality and stroke rate after CEA is 3.2–6.7% in symptomatic patients [10, 15–18] and 2.9–3.1% in asymptomatic patients [13, 19–21]. However, many of these trials are now outdated with changes in treatment algorithms. In particular, preoperative digital subtraction angiography is no longer routine and perioperative medical therapy is much improved.

Carotid Stenting

Even though CEA is still the preferred method in most patients [17], the emergence of CAS has triggered key trials comparing CAS to CEA. CAS may be more appropriate for younger patients with favourable anatomy and symptomatic patients at high risk of complications from CEA [22]. The SAPPHIRE [23] and CREST [16] trials, and Carotid Stenting Trialist's Collaboration meta-analysis [15] showed CAS prevents strokes and is not inferior to CEA in highly selected circumstances. The recent European Society for Vascular Surgery guidelines indicate that CEA should be the first consideration in symptomatic patients with >50% carotid stenosis and average risk asymptomatic patients with >60% carotid stenosis and >5 years life expectancy [24].

Quality of Life Instruments and Proms in Carotid Intervention

Definition of Quality of Life and Patient Reported Outcome Measures

PROMS ask patients to assess elements of their own health, QOL, and functioning [25]. The aim is to understand the impact of a treatment and its recovery, allow comparison of different patients' outcomes with the same intervention [25]. QOL is the major element of PROMS and is defined as a patient's perception of health as assessed in multiple domains [26, 27]. The use of QOL instruments in carotid revascularisation have been previously described [28].

One of the important considerations in QOL assessment is the type of instrument used and the measurement time points and time frame within which these assessments will be made. Previous recommendations have been provided for core outcome sets and reporting in carotid intervention [29, 30]. However, these documents provide very little detail on QOL measurement. Until these are specified in detail for QOL outcomes, investigators will need to use clinical judgment on the most appropriate methods of assessment.

Commonly Used Quality of Life Instruments in Carotid Intervention

QOL can be assessed by study designed questionnaires, and disease-specific or generic instruments. These instruments assess an individual's physical, emotional and psychological health as well as social and functional status [26, 27].

Individual study designed questionnaires are constructed by study authors as arbitrary measures of QOL outcomes [31–33]. Disease-specific QOL instruments are validated QOL scoring systems that measure the effect of an illness or treatment on a specific condition [27]. Generic QOL instruments are validated QOL scoring systems that measure QOL in a broad range of health domains and allow comparisons with other conditions and reference populations [27]. Generic scoring systems used by studies in this review are Medical Outcomes Short Form 36 (SF-36) and 12 (SF-12) [34], Sickness Impact Profile (SIP) [35], Hospital Anxiety and Depression Scale (HAD) [36], Katz Index of Independence in Activities of Daily Living (ADL) [37], European Quality of Life EQ-5D Questionnaire (EQ-5D) [38], Multidimensional Index of Life Quality Questionnaire (MILQ) [39], and the World Health Organisation Quality of Life BREF (WHOQOL-BREF) [40]. These instruments are described in previous chapters.

Quality of Life and Patient Reported Outcomes

There have been numerous randomised trials and meta-analyses on CEA and CAS in various subgroups of patients [11–16, 41], but these have focussed on technical outcomes of the procedure. Recent reviews have highlighted the importance of QOL outcomes [28, 42, 43]. This chapter assesses the currently available evidence. To date QOL is the primary method of PROMS. Study characteristics and a brief quality appraisal is outlined in Table 14.1 and the QOL outcomes are summarised in Table 14.2. This section describes the key QOL findings.

Table 14.1 Study characteristics and quality appraisal

Original studies

Author Year	Patients	Study design	Patient demographics	Validated QOL instrument	QOL instruments used	Follow-up method reported	Response rate
Sirrka [31] 1992	84	R	Male: NR, Age: 66, Asymptomatic: 0%, Symptomatic: 100%, Level stenosis: "significant"	No	Study questionnaire	No	49%
Study objectives:			Long-term QOL and cognitive performance after CEA (CEA vs. non-operative group)				
Martin [32] 1998	200	R	*CEA* Male: 61%, Age: 65, Asymptomatic: 0%, Symptomatic: 100%, Level stenosis: >70% *Medical treatment* Male: 62%, Age: 66, Asymptomatic: 0%, Symptomatic: 100%, Level stenosis: <70%	Yes	SF-36	Yes	83%
Study objectives:			Short-term QOL after CEA (CEA vs. medical management in those inappropriate for CEA, CEA or medical therapy vs. general population)				
Vriens [44] 1998	86	P	Male: 78.6%, Age: 65 (44–82), Asymptomatic: 34%, Symptomatic: 66%, Level stenosis: NR	Yes	SIP	No	81.4%

(continued)

Table 14.1 (continued)

Original studies							
Author / **Year**	**Patients**	**Study design**	**Patient demographics**	**Validated QOL instrument**	**QOL instruments used**	**Follow-up method reported**	**Response rate**
Study objectives:			To investigate whether QOL improves after CEA (preoperative vs. postoperative)				
			Does haemodynamic improvement have an impact				
Dardik [45] 2001	50	P	Male: 78%, Age: 67.1 (49–83), Asymptomatic: 0%, Symptomatic: 100%, Level stenosis: >65%	Yes	SF-36	No	100%
Study objectives:			Short-term QOL after CEA (preoperative vs. postoperative, postoperative vs. general population)				
Middleton [46] 2001	238	R	*RPAH Hospital*	Yes	SF-36	Yes	90%
			Male: 72.8%, Age: 82.4% <75, Asymptomatic: 32%, Symptomatic: 68%, Level stenosis: NR				
			CRGH Hospital				
			Male: 66.4%, Age: 69.9% <75, Asymptomatic: 32%, Symptomatic: 68%, Level stenosis: NR				
Study objectives:			Mid-term QOL after CEA (CEA vs. general population)				
			Mortality rate and causes of death after CEA				
Lloyd [47] 2004	100	P	Male: 64%, Age: 69 (45–87), Asymptomatic: 13%, Symptomatic: 87%, Level stenosis: NR	Yes	SF-36, HAD, EQ-5D	Yes	92%
Study objectives:			Short-term QOL and cognitive function after CEA (preoperative vs. postoperative)				
Diethrich [48] 2005	397	P	*CEA*	Yes	MILQ	No	48%
			Male: 63%, Age: 71.4, Asymptomatic: 67%, Symptomatic: 33%, Level stenosis: 89% patients >75% stenosis				
CARESS Trial			*CAS*				
			Male: 60%, Age: 71.2, Asymptomatic: 69%, Symptomatic: 31%, Level stenosis: 94% patients >75% stenosis				

Table 14.1 (continued)

Original studies							
Author / **Year**	**Patients**	**Study design**	**Patient demographics**	**Validated QOL instrument**	**QOL instruments used**	**Follow-up method reported**	**Response rate**
Study objectives:			Short-term QOL after CEA and CAS (CEA vs. CAS)				
Abelha [49] 2008	63	P	Male: 76%, Age: 70 (44–84), Asymptomatic: 21%, Symptomatic: 79%, Level stenosis: all patients ≥65%	Yes	SF-36, ADL	Yes	76%
Study objectives:			Short-term QOL and independence with activities of daily living after CEA (preoperative vs. postoperative, postoperative vs. general population)				
Stolker [50] 2010 SAPHHIRE Trial	310	RCT	*CEA* Male: 68%, Age: 72, Asymptomatic: 72%, Symptomatic: 28%, Level stenosis: symptomatic >50%, asymptomatic >80% *CAS* Male: 68%, Age: 72, Asymptomatic: 70%, Symptomatic: 30%, Level stenosis: symptomatic >50%, asymptomatic >80%	Yes	SF-36, EQ-5D, LS	No	80%
Study objectives:			Short-term QOL after CEA compared to CAS (CEA vs. CAS, preoperative vs. postoperative)				
Attigah [51] 2011	102	P	Male: 68.6%, Age: 70 (42–86), Asymptomatic: 74.5%, Symptomatic: 25.5%, Level stenosis: >70%	Yes	HAD, EQ-5D	Yes	100%
Study objectives:			Short-term QOL and satisfaction after CEA (preoperative vs. postoperative)				
Cohen [52] 2011 CREST trial	2502	RCT	Male: 65%, Age: 69, Asymptomatic: 47%, Symptomatic: 53%, Level stenosis: >85% of patients >70% stenosis	Yes	SF-36, LS	Yes	85%
Study objectives:			Short-term QOL after CEA compared to CAS (CEA vs. CAS, preoperative vs. postoperative)				
Kazmierski [33] 2012	102	P	Male: 70.6%, Age: 65.8 (34–84), Asymptomatic: 0%, Symptomatic: 100%, Level stenosis: >50%	Yes	SIP, LS	No	100%

(continued)

Table 14.1 (continued)

Original studies							
Author **Year**	**Patients**	**Study design**	**Patient demographics**	**Validated QOL instrument**	**QOL instruments used**	**Follow-up method reported**	**Response rate**
Study objectives:			Short-term QOL after CEA (preoperative vs. postoperative)				
Hsu [53] 2014	61	P	Male: 83%, Age: 73.3, Asymptomatic: 71%, Symptomatic: 29%, Level stenosis: symptomatic >60%, asymptomatic >80%	Yes	SF-36, LS	No	66%
Study objectives:			QOL after CAS in patients with dizziness (preoperative vs. postoperative)				
Kazmierski [54] 2014	102	P	Male: 71%, Age: 65.8, Asymptomatic: 0%, Symptomatic: 100%, Level stenosis: >70%	Yes	mRS, LS	No	NR
Study objectives:			Short-term QOL, neurological status and disability after CEA (preoperative vs. postoperative)				
Yan [55] 2014	65	P	*CAS* Male: 56%, Age: 72.1, Asymptomatic: 0%, Symptomatic: 100%, Level stenosis: >70% *Medical treatment* Male: 48%, Age: 73.1, Asymptomatic: 0%, Symptomatic: 100%, Level stenosis: >70%	Yes	WHOQOL-BREF, HAM-D, HAM-A	Yes	NR
Study objectives:			Short-term QOL and cognition after CAS in elderly patients (preoperative vs. postoperative, CAS vs. medical treatment)				
Carta [56] 2015	46	P	*CEA* Male: 57%, Age: 71.6, Asymptomatic: 69%, Symptomatic: 31%, Level stenosis: symptomatic >50%, asymptomatic >70% *Medical treatment* Male: 80%, Age: 72.1, Asymptomatic: 64%, Symptomatic: 36%, Level stenosis: symptomatic >50%, asymptomatic >70%	Yes	SF-12	Yes	87%
Study objectives:			Short-term QOL, mood, cognition after CEA compared to medical treatment (preoperative vs. postoperative, CEA vs. medical treatment in those who refused surgery)				
Hye [57] 2015 CREST trial	53	RCT	Male: 62%, Age: 67, Asymptomatic: 43%, Symptomatic: 57%, Level stenosis: >85% of patients >70% stenosis	Yes	SF-36, LS	Yes	98%

Table 14.1 (continued)

Original studies							
Author **Year**	**Patients**	**Study design**	**Patient demographics**	**Validated QOL instrument**	**QOL instruments used**	**Follow-up method reported**	**Response rate**
Study objectives:			QOL after CEA in those who sustained cranial nerve injury				
Reviews							
Al-Damluji [42] 2013		Review	Total studies: 28, Studies on QOL: 2, Total patients in studies on QOL: 2812				
Study objectives:			Periprocedural safety and long-term efficacy of CEA compared to CAS				
Shan [28] 2015		Review	Total studies: 12, Studies on QOL: 12, Total patients in studies on QOL: 4224				
Study objectives:			QOL after CEA, QOL after CAS, QOL after CEA vs. CAS, QOL compared to reference populations				
Chabowski [43] 2017		Review	Total studies: NR, Studies on QOL: NR, Total patients in studies on QOL: NR				
Study objectives:			QOL in stroke survivors and after CEA				

ADL activities of daily living, *CaRESS* carotid revascularization using endarterectomy or stenting systems trial, *CAS* carotid artery stenting, *CEA* carotid endarterectomy, *CREST* carotid revascularization endarterectomy versus stenting trial, *HAD* hospital anxiety and depression scale, *QOL* quality of life, *MILQ* multidimensional index of life quality, *NA* not applicable, *NR* not recorded, *P* prospective, *R* retrospective, *RCT* randomized control trial, *SAPPHIRE* stenting and angioplasty with protection in patients at high risk for endarterectomy, *SF-36* medical outcomes survey short form 36 questions, *SIP* sickness impact profile, *LS* Likert scale, *EQ-5D* Euro-QOL 5 dimensions, *mRS* modified Rankin scale, *HAM-D* Hamilton depression rating scale, *HAM-A* Hamilton anxiety rating scale, *WHOQOL-BREF* World Health Organisation quality of life-BREF

Table 14.2 Quality of life results

Original studies				
Author **Year**	**Procedure**	**Follow-up time**	**Peri-operative mortality**	**Peri-operative stroke**
Sirrka [31] 1992	CEA	8–11 years	NR	NR
	Key findings:	QOL similar between CEA and non-operated groups at long-term follow-up		
		Non-operative patients who had a stroke had better physical condition than those who had CEA		
Martin [32] 1998	CEA	1 year	3%	1%
	Key findings:	SF-36 scores similar between CEA and medical therapy group at 1 year across all domains		
		Superior improvement in self-perceived general health and treatment success after CEA compared to medical therapy.		
		Similar levels of anxiety over future strokes or TIAs		
		CEA and medical groups both have worse physical health domains at 1 year compared to general population, but mental health domains are similar		
Vriens [44] 1998	CEA	3 months	0%	3%
	Key findings:	No significant change in QOL observed 3 months post-op based on SIP measurement		
		Significant QOL improvement after CEA limited to only patients with contralateral carotid occlusion.		

(continued)

Table 14.2 (continued)

Original studies				
Author **Year**	**Procedure**	**Follow-up time**	**Peri-operative mortality**	**Peri-operative stroke**
Dardik [45] 2001	CEA	3 months	0%	8%
	Key findings:	Perceived improved overall health after CEA		
		SF-36 scores in all domains similar at 3 months compared to baseline		
		Postoperative physical health similar to chronically ill general population		
		Postoperative mental health similar to healthy general population		
Middleton [46] 2001	CEA	NR	1.7%	NR
	Key findings:	At 1 year, majority of patients consider overall health to be similar to pre-op		
		SF-36 scores higher in CEA cohort than population norms for Australian >55 years old who had experienced a stroke, but not compared to general healthy population		
Lloyd [47] 2004	CEA	6 months	0%	NR
	Key findings:	CEA did not cause deterioration of QOL at 6 months		
		Significantly less anxiety after the operation based on HAD scale		
		Significant improvement in QOL according to EQ-5D scale		
CaRESS [48] 2005	CAS CEA	30 days, 1 year	0.0% CAS vs. 0.4% CEA	2.1% CAS vs. 3.6% CEA
	Key findings:	No significant differences between CEA and CAS groups in change of QOL and MILQ score		
		CAS experienced greater decline in QOL after intervention, but it was not statistically significant		
Abelha [49] 2008	CEA	6 months	0%	4.8%
	Key findings:	Improved subjective perception of QOL		
		Higher levels of dependency in activities of daily living		
		Worse SF-36 scores compared to general population		
Stolker [50] 2010 SAPPHIRE	CAS CEA	2 weeks, 1 month, 6 months, 12 months	NR	NR
	Key findings:	Physical health domains decline at 2 weeks after CEA, and return to baseline by 1 month		
		At 2 weeks, CAS patients had better scores in SF-36 physical scale compared to CEA		
		No significant difference in SF-36 scores at 1 month, 6 months, 12 months		
		Mental health scores similar at all time intervals		
		EQ-5D utility score similar		
		At 2 weeks CAS patients reported less difficulty eating, swallowing, difficulty driving and less neck pain. These differences resolved by the 1 month follow-up assessment		
Attigah [51] 2011	CEA	Baseline, 2 days	0%	0%
	Key findings:	Procedural satisfaction better in those who already have worse HADS scores		

Table 14.2 (continued)

Original studies				
Author **Year**	**Procedure**	**Follow-up time**	**Peri-operative mortality**	**Peri-operative stroke**
Cohen [52] 2011 CREST	CAS CEA	2 weeks, 1 month, 1 year	CAS 5.2% vs. CEA 4.5%	4.1% CAS vs. 2.3% CEA
	Key findings:	After CEA, physical and functional health domains of SF-36 worse at 2 weeks, but return to baseline or better by 12 months		
		After CEA, mental health domains of SF-36 continuously improve, including at 2 weeks		
		Better SF-36 scores for CAS at 2 weeks compared to CEA (SF-36, disease specific scales, pain scale), but not after 1 month, and are the same at 1 year		
		LS scores for pain and function similar for both CEA and CAS at 1 year		
		Postoperative stroke has negative impact on QOL, but not myocardial infarct or cranial nerve injury		
Kazmierski [33] 2012	CEA	1 year	NR	NR
	Key findings:	Mean QOL after surgery increased 1 year after surgery		
		Before surgery: "poor" (more than half). After surgery "good" (86%).		
Hsu [53] 2014	CAS	Baseline, 1 month, 6 months	0%	0%
	Key findings:	All SF-36 domains similar to baseline at 1 month after CAS		
		At 6 months, physical and general health domains better, less pain, emotional and social function better		
		Asymptomatic patients maintain preoperative QOL		
Kazmierski [54] 2014	CEA	Baseline, 1 year	NR	NR
	Key findings:	Majority of patients have significant functional improvement after CEA		
		Patient's life quality improved in 67% patients		
Yan [55] 2014	CAS	Baseline, 1 month, 3 months, 6 months, 12 months	0%	0%
	Key findings:	WHOQOL-BREF improved at 1 month, 3 months, 6 months, 12 months after CAS compared to baseline		
		HAM-D and HAM-A were better after CAS compared to medical therapy at all postoperative time points		
Carta [56] 2015	CEA	6–7 months	NR	NR
	Key findings:	SF-12 score similar between CEA and medical treatment groups		
		Positive trend towards better QOL outcomes after CEA, but 6 months not enough to demonstrate this		
		No significant difference between preoperative and postoperative scores		
Hye [57] 2015	CEA	Baseline, 2 weeks, 1 month, 12 months	NR	NR
	Key findings:	No difference in QOL between patients with and without cranial injury after CEA		
		LS showed cranial nerve injury had some negative impact on functional status		

(continued)

Table 14.2 (continued)

Original studies				
Author / **Year**	**Procedure**	**Follow-up time**	**Peri-operative mortality**	**Peri-operative stroke**
Reviews				
Al-Damluji [42] 2013	Key findings:	CAS patients have better QOL at 2 weeks postop compared to CEA patients, but no difference by 1 year		
Shan [28] 2015	Key findings:	CEA and CAS maintain preoperative QOL for at least 1 year Minimal differences between CEA and CAS		
Chabowski [43] 2017	Key findings:	Early postoperative QOL after CEA declines, but returns to baseline at 1 year 1 year QOL similar to chronically ill general population		

ADL activities of daily living, *BP* bodily pain, *CaRESS* carotid revascularization using endarterectomy or stenting systems trial, *CAS* carotid artery stenting, *CEA* carotid endarterectomy, *CREST* carotid revascularization endarterectomy versus stenting trial, *EQ-5D* European quality of life questionnaire EQ-5D, *GHP* general health perception, *QOL* quality of life, *ICU* intensive care unit, *MH* mental health, *MILQ* multidimensional index of life quality, *NA* not applicable, *NR* not recorded, *NS* not significant, *PF* physical function, *Post-op* post-operative, *Pre-op* pre-operative, *RE* role emotional/mental, *RP* role physical, *SAPPHIRE* stenting and angioplasty with protection in patients at high risk for endarterectomy, *SF* social functioning, *SF-36* medical outcomes survey short form 36 questions, *VAS* visual analogue scale, *VT* energy/vitality

Quality of Life After Carotid Endarterectomy (18 Studies) [28, 31–33, 42–52, 54, 56, 57]

The vast majority of QOL evidence pertains to CEA. Numerous studies demonstrate that patients maintain pre-operative QOL after CEA. The pattern of recovery varies across different domains in different studies. There is a temporary decline in QOL at 2 weeks to 1 month especially in physical health and functional domains. This is only transient and is consistent with the expected initial postoperative decline after open surgery. However, by 6 months to 1 year, all domains are at least as good as pre-operatively.

The preservation of mental health is important after carotid intervention, particularly in prophylactic procedures. Patients with carotid stenosis already have a baseline level of anxiety and poor perception of health related to overall poor cardiovascular health [47]. Studies included in this chapter show that unlike the physical health domains, mental health domains did not demonstrate the same pattern of initial decline after surgery. Instead, QOL appears to be maintained throughout.

A major limitation of these studies should be highlighted here. There remains only one study with QOL data beyond 12 months [31]. This study is one of the earliest studies on QOL after CEA and is therefore limited because modern operative techniques and validated QOL instruments haven't been used. While it is difficult to draw strong conclusions, these authors demonstrated that after 8–11 years' follow-up, QOL remained similar between the CEA and non-operative groups with relatively similar response rates. This suggests a positive long-term QOL outcome after CEA.

Quality of Life After Carotid Stenting (Seven Studies) [28, 42, 48, 50, 52, 53, 55]

Overall, QOL does not appear to deteriorate after CAS. Earlier studies show that although some health domains were temporarily worse, QOL at 1 year is similar to baseline. Contemporary studies suggest that CAS patients have similar QOL by 1 month and may actually experience an improvement in their physical and general health domains with better emotional and social function by 6 months. To date there is no data on QOL after CAS beyond 1 year.

Quality of Life After Endarterectomy Compared to Stenting (Five Studies) [28, 42, 48, 50, 52]

CAS may be superior to CEA in the early post-procedure period in physical health domains from as early as 2 weeks. However, these differences were not present at 1 year. A similar pattern is observed in functional performance with no difference in walking, eating and driving ability by 1 year. Mental health domains do not appear to be impacted by the type of procedure. Based on these results where QOL is similar, the choice between CEA and CAS is likely to be influenced by other factors.

Quality of Life Compared to Reference Populations (Seven Studies) [31, 32, 45, 46, 49, 55, 56]

Comparisons have been made between carotid intervention and medical treatment groups or the general population. It is clear that current data remains insufficient to be definitive. After CEA, there does not appear to a clear difference in QOL between intervention and medical treatment groups at follow-up of up to 1 year, especially in physical health domains. Treatment satisfaction remains high, but anxiety over future strokes or TIA may remain. These anxieties appear to be lesser after CAS at short follow-up. CEA patients have worse physical health compared to the general population, but mental health may be similar. The lack of benefit compared with medical treatment groups and the general population is largely due to the short term follow-up. Stroke prevention in carotid intervention is greater the longer the follow-up. Therefore, it is likely that there has not been enough time elapsed to identify a QOL benefit of intervention.

Cognitive Function

There has been a greater interest recently in cognitive outcomes after carotid intervention. A number of reviews and meta-analyses have been published on this subject, but definitive conclusions have not been reached due to significant heterogeneity. CEA may be associated with both preservation and improvement of cognitive function depending on the domain tested [58–61]. This includes memory, attention, mini mental state exams, and executive function. CAS may be associated with improved global cognition, memory, attention and psychomotor speed, although executive function and language may not change [62]. The difference between CEA and CAS remains unclear [61].

Utility of Quality of Life Tools

Importance of Quality of Life Assessment and PROMS

A recent review by the Australian Commission on Safety and Quality in Health Care has identified some key aspects of PROMS and QOL [25]. QOL and PROMS are used because patients are the best judges of the effect on their QOL and function. This allows a patient centered model of care and helps improve the quality and safety of various treatments. The effectiveness of different treatments can therefore be more accurately determined.

With carotid revascularisation, the inference previously has been that intervention prevents QOL deterioration due to stroke prevention. It is only recently that QOL outcomes have been formally reviewed [28, 42, 43], showing the positive outcome of carotid revascularisation on QOL and PROMS. There should be distinction between asymptomatic and symptomatic patients in order to use QOL in clinical practice.

QOL should not necessarily be expected to improve after revascularisation, particularly for previously asymptomatic patients who have prophylactic procedures. The outcome is positive if QOL is maintained after intervention because the intervention served to prevent a stroke. This is especially important in prophylactic procedures, especially if performed on asymptomatic patients who would otherwise not have had a detriment to their QOL as a result of the disease process. Similarly, because they were asymptomatic, they were unlikely to gain a great benefit from intervention other than in mental health domains.

In symptomatic patients who have had a stroke, there may be a significant deterioration in QOL before intervention. Subsequent revascularisation and resolution of symptoms in conjunction with rehabilitation may then improve QOL. The recovery in QOL will then likely be longer than in asymptomatic patients. There will also likely be positive effects on mobility indices, Rankin score, and mini mental state, but these are yet to be elucidated in studies. Existing QOL studies do not make a distinction between transient ischemic attacks and stroke as the indication for carotid revascularisation. By definition, patients with transient ischemic attacks don't have residual physical neurological deficits and therefore physical domains of QOL are much less impacted than a patient with stroke. Mobility and disability are also likely to be different. Fear of subsequent stroke is more likely to be a key feature in transient ischemic attacks, and this affects mental health domains much more.

With implementation of these guidelines, important and clinically relevant information would be obtained. This information provides improved patient-focused outcomes data which facilitates improved quality of care to patients and more accurate analysis of the effectiveness of an intervention. In addition, perhaps the greatest benefit will be its use in policy making, cost-effectiveness analysis, and ultimately resource allocation. For example, CEA has been shown to be cost effective even in asymptomatic patients less than 75 years of age if a threshold of £20,000 per quality of life year and background stroke rate of less than 1% per year is used [63]. The cost effectiveness of CAS compared to CEA is not so clear [64–66]. QOL and cognitive function have not yet been included in such cost-effectiveness analyses.

Need for Further Research

There are several key issues identified from previous QOL studies that should be addressed in future studies [28].

Firstly, and perhaps most importantly, there needs to be investigation into the long-term QOL outcomes after carotid intervention. The benefit of stroke prevention is likely to be greater the longer the follow-up. This is especially important in asymptomatic carotid intervention. Current QOL outcomes are largely limited to 1 year, but these outcomes would be more even more relevant if follow-up extended up to 5 years.

Secondly, there is a clear lack of evidence on the use of currently available QOL and PROM instruments after carotid revascularisation [67]. These disease-specific QOL instruments are useful measures of change in QOL specific to a treatment and disease process [27]. However, there are significant difficulties with developing such QOL instruments because there would need to be separation of symptomatic and asymptomatic patients, transient ischemic attack and stroke patients, as well as degree of stenosis. It may be better to apply the currently available neurological QOL instruments and mobility and disability indices in carotid intervention.

Thirdly, there needs to be a standardised set of results that are reported to facilitate objective assessment with meta-analyses. Ideally a standardised common instrument should be used by all studies. QOL data should be expressed as mean ± standard deviation and results given at pre-determined follow-up time points including baseline and final follow-up, rather than a range or median of variable follow-up time points.

Fourthly, there was a relatively low response rate in previously conducted studies. High response rates are compulsory to minimise bias.

Fifthly, the distinction between symptomatic and asymptomatic patients for both CEA and CAS is unclear. These are markedly different subgroups of patients in regard to baseline QOL, expected QOL gains, and importantly the patient's own expectations after intervention.

Finally, the effect of morbidity, frailty and disability as a variable for QOL outcomes is underappreciated. The burden of comorbidities is a risk factor for frailty, which in turn predisposes to disability [68]. This is because frailty causes decreased reserve and less ability to deal with adverse outcomes [68]. Comorbidities, frailty and disability are therefore separate entities. They are important because they are increasingly prevalent with an ageing population, who are increasingly offered intervention. There are also specific stent technologies, stent brands, and adjuncts to improve procedural success of CAS in specific anatomical set ups. However, the impact of these on QOL outcomes have not been investigated.

With implementation of these guidelines, important and clinically relevant information would be obtained. The logistical challenges faced will be in the design of an instrument which is simple and thorough enough for patients to participate in, as well as the data collection which needs to be consistent and accurate without significant loss to follow-up. The importance of this aspect of treatment is often underestimated as the traditional teaching heavily emphasises the importance of technical outcomes alone. This paradigm now needs to incorporate QOL outcomes as a complement to technical outcomes as a routine part of clinical practice.

Effect of Other Outcomes on Quality of Life and Proms

Predictors of QOL outcomes have been studied after CEA (Fig. 14.1) [43, 69]. Worse QOL is likely after severe stroke, older age, comorbidities, lack of proper treatment and rehabilitation, and poor socioeconomic factors [43]. Mental health domains of QOL after significantly affected by contralateral stenosis, dizziness improvement, and hoarseness [69]. This shows that although uncommon, vagus nerve injury should be avoided during CEA by meticulous dissection and avoidance of retractor injury.

The mortality, survival, morbidity and complications of CEA and CAS are well described in the literature. These are outside of the scope of this text. In order assess the relevance of QOL outcomes, it is more important to assess the reported morbidity and mortality in the studies that report QOL. Any patients who do not participate in QOL assessment or are lost to follow-up are more likely to have a worse QOL due to a greater burden of comorbidities and physical impairments [49, 50]. The difficulty in interpreting QOL assessments is compounded by the fact that post-operative stroke and death renders it unlikely that such patients will complete QOL questionnaires. According to previous guidelines, a response rate of >85% (loss to follow-up <15%) is considered ideal [70]. This rate is achieved in only eight studies in the literature [33, 45–47, 51, 52, 56, 57]. It is therefore possible that QOL outcomes are overestimated, at least in the shorter term. At the same time, the lack of adequate long-term follow-up may also underestimate the QOL benefit because the benefit of CEA for stroke prevention is more apparent the longer the follow-up duration. It is therefore important to assess the both the shorter and longer-term response rates to identify risk of bias in conjunction with the technical outcomes to put the QOL outcomes into perspective.

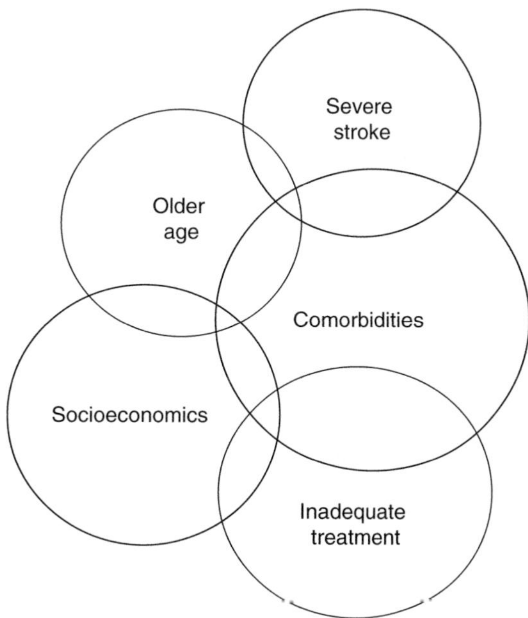

Fig. 14.1 Predictors of poor QOL

Statistical techniques to deal with missing data have been developed to resolve issues such as mentioned above. This includes multiple imputation which is a statistical method of dealing with missing data by combining the results of several different possible data sets [71]. There are particular biases that occur as a result of the missing data, depending on the reason why the data is missing. Multiple imputation may be helpful in both epidemiological studies and randomised controlled trials, but there are potential pitfalls that warrant input from a statistician [71, 72]. Future studies may benefit from incorporation of this technique.

Perioperative mortality and stroke was analysed in studies reporting QOL data. The perioperative mortality and stroke rate are CEA was 0.0–4.5% and 0–8.0%, respectively [32, 44–49, 51, 52], while after CAS it was 0.0–5.2% and 0–5.8%, respectively [48, 52, 53, 55]. Perioperative myocardial infarction was 0.8–6.6% in CEA and 0.0–1.9% in CAS [16, 23, 48, 50, 52]. The 1-year stroke rates for CEA and CAS were 7.7–9.8% and 5.5–5.8%, respectively [23, 48, 50]. These results are reflective of the studies included which were not designed to evaluate stroke and mortality rates, with few randomised controlled trials and high quality studies in this regard. While the results don't necessarily reflect that of currently accepted standards, they do provide an indication of how the QOL results from these studies can be interpreted. The mortality and stroke rates are in general higher, meaning QOL outcomes may be worse than if QOL data were derived from higher quality studies.

Few studies reported comprehensive morbidity data. Patients in included studies experienced fewer stroke symptoms after CEA compared to CAS [33]. Symptoms including headache, leg pain were similar in CEA and CAS after 1 year [52], although there may be more neck pain with CEA [50]. Cranial nerve palsies occurred in 0.3% and 4.7% of CAS and CEA patients respectively [52]. However, cranial nerve injury does not appear to cause a detriment to overall QOL [57]. The effect of perioperative morbidity and complications on QOL outcomes and PROMS remains unclear. Given the relatively low incidence of complications in experienced centres, it may not be possible to demonstrate a statistically significant impact. However, clinically it would be prudent to avoid complications and improve morbidity to avoid a negative impact on QOL.

Cognitive function is a relatively new area of interest in carotid intervention. The reason for cognitive impairment from carotid disease and intervention may relate to brain injury which occurs due to embolism, thrombosis or hyperperfusion/hypoperfusion [73]. Atheroembolism in particular is associated with worse short and long term cognitive function [74, 75]. There is also a theory that the greater embolization rate during CAS may account for a worse cognitive outcome, but this is not yet confirmed [61]. Cognitive outcomes following carotid revascularisation are important because these affect how a patient perceives their QOL and also how they report their QOL. Furthermore, if a patient has severe cognitive impairment, it may significantly limit their ability to accurately report on their own QOL. Further research is necessary to identify the impacts of cognitive function on PROMS in these patients.

Conclusion

Currently available studies show that CEA and CAS maintain pre-operative QOL for at least 1 year (Fig. 14.2). Long-term data is lacking and there is insufficient evidence to differentiate CEA and CAS. QOL and PROMS are a critical aspect of outcomes assessment in modern surgical practice. This is particularly pertinent to preventative procedures such as CEA and CAS. Significant limitations of the currently available literature are identified with the view that these be used as a guideline for future research. This information provides improved patient-focused outcomes data which facilitates improved quality of care to patients and more accurate analysis of the effectiveness of an intervention. In addition, perhaps the greatest benefit will be its use in policy making, cost-effectiveness analysis, and ultimately resource allocation.

Conclusions

1. QOL and PROMS are critical in contemporary outcomes assessment after carotid artery intervention.
2. CEA and CAS maintain pre-operative QOL for at least one year.
3. Long-term data is lacking and there is insufficient evidence to differentiate CEA and CAS.
4. Severe stroke, older age, comorbidities, lack of proper treatment and rehabilitation, and poor socioeconomic factors are predictors of poor QOL after CEA.
5. Future studies are needed to improve methods of QOL assessment and evaluate factors that affect QOL outcomes especially after CAS.

Fig. 14.2 Conclusions

References

1. Go AS, Mozaffarian D, Roger VL, Benjamin EJ, Berry JD, Blaha MJ, et al. Heart disease and stroke statistics--2014 update: a report from the American Heart Association. Circulation. 2014;129(3):e28–e292.
2. Sprigg N, Selby J, Fox L, Berge E, Whynes D, Bath PM. Very low quality of life after acute stroke: data from the Efficacy of Nitric Oxide in Stroke trial. Stroke. 2013;44(12):3458–62.
3. Luengo-Fernandez R, Gray AM, Bull L, Welch S, Cuthbertson F, Rothwell PM. Quality of life after TIA and stroke: ten-year results of the Oxford Vascular Study. Neurology. 2013;81(18):1588–95.
4. Zhu CZ, Norris JW. Role of carotid stenosis in ischemic stroke. Stroke. 1990;21(8):1131–4.
5. Petty GW, Brown RD Jr, Whisnant JP, Sicks JD, O'Fallon WM, Wiebers DO. Ischemic stroke subtypes: a population-based study of incidence and risk factors. Stroke. 1999;30(12):2513–6.
6. WHO. Surveillance in brief: update of noncommunicable diseases and mental health surveillance activities, vol. 5. Geneva: WHO; 2003. p. 1–5.
7. Adar R, Cohen E, Kreitler S. Carotid endarterectomy for symptom-free stenosis: the patient's point of view. Cardiovasc Surg. 1994;2(5):582–5.
8. Herrera FJ, Wong J, Chung F. A systematic review of postoperative recovery outcomes measurements after ambulatory surgery. Anesth Analg. 2007;105(1):63–9.
9. European Carotid Surgery Trialists' Collaborative Group. Randomised trial of endarterectomy for recently symptomatic carotid stenosis: final results of the MRC European Carotid Surgery Trial (ECST). Lancet. 1998;351(9113):1379–87.
10. Barnett HJ, Taylor DW, Eliasziw M, Fox AJ, Ferguson GG, Haynes RB, et al. Benefit of carotid endarterectomy in patients with symptomatic moderate or severe stenosis. North American Symptomatic Carotid Endarterectomy Trial Collaborators. N Engl J Med. 1998;339(20):1415–25.
11. Fisher M, Martin A, Cosgrove M, Norris JW. The NASCET-ACAS plaque project. North American symptomatic carotid endarterectomy trial. Asymptomatic carotid atherosclerosis study. Stroke. 1993;24(12 Suppl):I24–5; discussion I31–2.
12. Young B, Moore WS, Robertson JT, Toole JF, Ernst CB, Cohen SN, et al. An analysis of perioperative surgical mortality and morbidity in the asymptomatic carotid atherosclerosis study. ACAS Investigators. Asymptomatic Carotid Atherosclerosis Study. Stroke. 1996;27(12):2216–24.
13. Halliday A, Mansfield A, Marro J, Peto C, Peto R, Potter J, et al. Prevention of disabling and fatal strokes by successful carotid endarterectomy in patients without recent neurological symptoms: randomised controlled trial. Lancet. 2004;363(9420):1491–502.
14. Halliday A, Harrison M, Hayter E, Kong X, Mansfield A, Marro J, et al. 10-year stroke prevention after successful carotid endarterectomy for asymptomatic stenosis (ACST-1): a multicentre randomised trial. Lancet. 2010;376(9746):1074–84.
15. Bonati LH, Dobson J, Algra A, Branchereau A, Chatellier G, Fraedrich G, et al. Short-term outcome after stenting versus endarterectomy for symptomatic carotid stenosis: a preplanned meta-analysis of individual patient data. Lancet. 2010;376(9746):1062–73.
16. Brott TG, Hobson RW II, Howard G, Roubin GS, Clark WM, Brooks W, et al. Stenting versus endarterectomy for treatment of carotid-artery stenosis. N Engl J Med. 2010;363(1):11–23.
17. Ederle J, Dobson J, Featherstone RL, Bonati LH, van der Worp HB, de Borst GJ, et al. Carotid artery stenting compared with endarterectomy in patients with symptomatic carotid stenosis (International Carotid Stenting Study): an interim analysis of a randomised controlled trial. Lancet. 2010;375(9719):985–97.

18. Orrapin S, Rerkasem K. Carotid endarterectomy for symptomatic carotid stenosis. Cochrane Database Syst Rev. 2017;6:CD001081.
19. Chambers BR, Donnan GA. Carotid endarterectomy for asymptomatic carotid stenosis. Cochrane Database Syst Rev. 2005;4:CD001923.
20. Hobson RW II, Weiss DG, Fields WS, Goldstone J, Moore WS, Towne JB, et al. Efficacy of carotid endarterectomy for asymptomatic carotid stenosis. The Veterans Affairs Cooperative Study Group. N Engl J Med. 1993;328(4):221–7.
21. Walker MD, et al. Endarterectomy for asymptomatic carotid artery stenosis. Executive Committee for the asymptomatic carotid atherosclerosis study. JAMA. 1995;273(18):1421–8.
22. Grotta JC. Clinical practice. Carotid stenosis. N Engl J Med. 2013;369(12):1143–50.
23. Yadav JS, Wholey MH, Kuntz RE, Fayad P, Katzen BT, Mishkel GJ, et al. Protected carotid-artery stenting versus endarterectomy in high-risk patients. N Engl J Med. 2004;351(15):1493–501.
24. Naylor AR, Ricco JB, de Borst GJ, Debus S, de Haro J, Halliday A, et al. Editor's choice - management of atherosclerotic carotid and vertebral artery disease: 2017 clinical practice guidelines of the European society for vascular surgery (ESVS). Eur J Vasc Endovasc Surg. 2018;55(1):3–81.
25. Williams KSJ, Morris D, Grootemaat P, Thompson C. Patient-reported outcome measures: literature review. Sydney, NSW: Healthcare ACoSaQi; 2016.
26. Testa MA, Simonson DC. Assessment of quality-of-life outcomes. N Engl J Med. 1996;334(13):835–40.
27. Urbach DR. Measuring quality of life after surgery. Surg Innov. 2005;12(2):161–5.
28. Shan L, Shan J, Saxena A, Robinson D. Quality of life and functional status after carotid revascularisation: a systematic review and meta-analysis. Eur J Vasc Endovasc Surg. 2015;49(6):634–45.
29. Timaran CH, McKinsey JF, Schneider PA, Littooy F. Reporting standards for carotid interventions from the Society for Vascular Surgery. J Vasc Surg. 2011;53(6):1679–95.
30. Nedeltchev K, Pattynama PM, Biaminoo G, Diehm N, Jaff MR, Hopkins LN, et al. Standardized definitions and clinical endpoints in carotid artery and supra-aortic trunk revascularization trials. Catheter Cardiovasc Interv. 2010;76(3):333–44.
31. Sirkka A, Salenius JP, Portin R, Nummenmaa T. Quality of life and cognitive performance after carotid endarterectomy during long-term follow-up. Acta Neurol Scand. 1992;85(1):58–62.
32. Martin PJ, Fotopoulou M, Baker GA, Humphrey PR. Health-related quality of life after transient ischemic attack and minor stroke: is medical or surgical treatment influential? J Stroke Cerebrovasc Dis. 1998;7(1):70–5.
33. Kazmierski P, Kasielska A, Bogusiak K, Lysakowski M, Stelagowski M. Influence of internal carotid endarterectomy on patients' life quality. Polski Przeglad Chirurgiczny. 2012;84(1):17–22.
34. Ware JE Jr, Sherbourne CD. The MOS 36-item short-form health survey (SF-36). I. Conceptual framework and item selection. Med Care. 1992;30(6):473–83.
35. de Bruin AF, de Witte LP, Stevens F, Diederiks JP. Sickness impact profile: the state of the art of a generic functional status measure. Soc Sci Med. 1992;35(8):1003–14.
36. Lewis G, Wessely S. Comparison of the general health questionnaire and the hospital anxiety and depression scale. Br J Psychiatry. 1990;157:860–4.
37. Katz S, Downs TD, Cash HR, Grotz RC. Progress in development of the index of ADL. The Gerontologist. 1970;10(1):20–30.
38. EuroQol Group. EuroQol--a new facility for the measurement of health-related quality of life. Health Policy. 1990;16(3):199–208.
39. Avis NE, Smith KW, Hambleton RK, Feldman HA, Selwyn A, Jacobs A. Development of the multidimensional index of life quality. A quality of life measure for cardiovascular disease. Med Care. 1996;34(11):1102–20.
40. WHO. WHOQOL-BREF. Geneva: WHO; 1996. https://www.who.int/mental_health/publications/whoqol/en/.
41. Ederle J, Bonati LH, Dobson J, Featherstone RL, Gaines PA, Beard JD, et al. Endovascular treatment with angioplasty or stenting versus endarterectomy in patients with carotid artery stenosis in the Carotid and Vertebral Artery Transluminal Angioplasty Study (CAVATAS): long-term follow-up of a randomised trial. Lancet Neurol. 2009;8(10):898–907.
42. Al-Damluji MS, Nagpal S, Stilp E, Remetz M, Mena C. Carotid revascularization: a systematic review of the evidence. J Interv Cardiol. 2013;26(4):399–410.
43. Chabowski M, Grzebien A, Ziomek A, Dorobisz K, Lesniak M, Janczak D. Quality of life after carotid endarterectomy: a review of the literature. Acta Neurol Belg. 2017;117(4):829–35.
44. Vriens EM, Post MW, Jacobs HM, van Huffelen AC, Eikelboom BC. Changes in health-related quality of life after carotid endarterectomy. Eur J Vasc Endovasc Surg. 1998;16(5):395–400.
45. Dardik A, Minor J, Watson C, Hands LJ. Improved quality of life among patients with symptomatic carotid artery disease undergoing carotid endarterectomy. J Vasc Surg. 2001;33(2):329–33.
46. Middleton S, Donnelly N, Harris J, Lusby R, Ward J. Audit of long-term mortality and morbidity outcomes for carotid endarterectomy. Aust Health Rev. 2002;25(4):81–91.
47. Lloyd AJ, Hayes PD, London NJ, Bell PR, Naylor AR. Does carotid endarterectomy lead to a decline in cognitive function or health related quality of life? J Clin Exp Neuropsychol. 2004;26(6):817–25.
48. CaRESS Steering Committee. Carotid Revascularization Using Endarterectomy or Stenting Systems (CaRESS) phase I clinical trial: 1-year results. J Vasc Surg. 2005;42(2):213–9.
49. Abelha FJ, Quevedo S, Barros H. Quality of life after carotid endarterectomy. BMC Cardiovasc Disord. 2008;8:33.

50. Stolker JM, Mahoney EM, Safley DM, Pomposelli FB Jr, Yadav JS, Cohen DJ. Health-related quality of life following carotid stenting versus endarterectomy: results from the SAPPHIRE (Stenting and Angioplasty with Protection in Patients at HIgh Risk for Endarterectomy) trial. JACC Cardiovasc Interv. 2010;3(5):515–23.
51. Attigah N, Kutter J, Demirel S, Hakimi M, Hinz U, Motsch J, et al. Assessment of patients' satisfaction in carotid surgery under local anaesthesia by psychometrical testing--a prospective cohort study. Eur J Vasc Endovasc Surg. 2011;41(1):76–82.
52. Cohen DJ, Stolker JM, Wang K, Magnuson EA, Clark WM, Demaerschalk BM, et al. Health-related quality of life after carotid stenting versus carotid endarterectomy: results from CREST (Carotid Revascularization Endarterectomy Versus Stenting Trial). J Am Coll Cardiol. 2011;58(15):1557–65.
53. Hsu LC, Chang FC, Teng MM, Chern CM, Wong WJ. Impact of carotid stenting in dizzy patients with carotid stenosis. J Chin Med Assoc. 2014;77(8):403–8.
54. Kazmierski P, Stelagowski M, Kasielska-Trojan A, Bogusiak K, Glabinski A. Neurologic and functional long-term outcome after carotid endarterectomy. J Stroke Cerebrovasc Dis. 2014;23(4):686–93.
55. Yan Y, Yuan Y, Liang L, Chen T, Shen Y, Zhong C. Influence of carotid artery stenting on cognition of elderly patients with severe stenosis of the internal carotid artery. Med Sci Monit. 2014;20:1461–8.
56. Carta MG, Lecca ME, Saba L, Sanfilippo R, Pintus E, Cadoni M, et al. Patients with carotid atherosclerosis who underwent or did not undergo carotid endarterectomy: outcome on mood, cognition and quality of life. BMC Psychiatry. 2015;15:277.
57. Hye RJ, Mackey A, Hill MD, Voeks JH, Cohen DJ, Wang K, et al. Incidence, outcomes, and effect on quality of life of cranial nerve injury in the Carotid Revascularization Endarterectomy versus Stenting Trial. J Vasc Surg. 2015;61(5):1208–14.
58. Dempsey RJ, Jackson DC, Wilbrand SM, Mitchell CC, Berman SE, Johnson SC, et al. The preservation of cognition 1 year after carotid endarterectomy in patients with prior cognitive decline. Neurosurgery. 2018;82(3):322–8.
59. Wang Q, Zhou M, Zhou Y, Ji J, Raithel D, Qiao T. Effects of carotid endarterectomy on cerebral reperfusion and cognitive function in patients with high grade carotid stenosis: a perfusion weighted magnetic resonance imaging study. Eur J Vasc Endovasc Surg. 2015;50(1):5–12.
60. De Rango P, Caso V, Leys D, Paciaroni M, Lenti M, Cao P. The role of carotid artery stenting and carotid endarterectomy in cognitive performance: a systematic review. Stroke. 2008;39(11):3116–27.
61. Paraskevas KI, Lazaridis C, Andrews CM, Veith FJ, Giannoukas AD. Comparison of cognitive function after carotid artery stenting versus carotid endarterectomy. Eur J Vasc Endovasc Surg. 2014;47(3):221–31.
62. Antonopoulos CN, Kakisis JD, Sfyroeras GS, Moulakakis KG, Kallinis A, Giannakopoulos T, et al. The impact of carotid artery stenting on cognitive function in patients with extracranial carotid artery stenosis. Ann Vasc Surg. 2015;29(3):457–69.
63. Thapar A, Garcia Mochon L, Epstein D, Shalhoub J, Davies AH. Modelling the cost-effectiveness of carotid endarterectomy for asymptomatic stenosis. Br J Surg. 2013;100(2):231–9.
64. Sternbergh WC III, Crenshaw GD, Bazan HA, Smith TA. Carotid endarterectomy is more cost-effective than carotid artery stenting. J Vasc Surg. 2012;55(6):1623–8.
65. Vilain KR, Magnuson EA, Li H, Clark WM, Begg RJ, Sam AD II, et al. Costs and cost-effectiveness of carotid stenting versus endarterectomy for patients at standard surgical risk: results from the Carotid Revascularization Endarterectomy Versus Stenting Trial (CREST). Stroke. 2012;43(9):2408–16.
66. Featherstone RL, Dobson J, Ederle J, Doig D, Bonati LH, Morris S, et al. Carotid artery stenting compared with endarterectomy in patients with symptomatic carotid stenosis (International Carotid Stenting Study): a randomised controlled trial with cost-effectiveness analysis. Health Technol Assess. 2016;20(20):1–94.
67. Essat M, Aber A, Phillips P, Poku E, Woods HB, Howard A, et al. Patient-reported outcome measures in carotid artery revascularization: systematic review and psychometric analysis. Ann Vasc Surg. 2018;50:275–83.
68. Fried LP, Tangen CM, Walston J, Newman AB, Hirsch C, Gottdiener J, et al. Frailty in older adults: evidence for a phenotype. J Gerontol A Biol Sci Med Sci. 2001;56(3):M146–56.
69. Jiang Q, Lin T, Qu L. Predictors of health-related quality of life for mental health status in patients after carotid endarterectomy. World Neurosurg. 2019;126:e379–e84.
70. Wright RW, Brand RA, Dunn W, Spindler KP. How to write a systematic review. Clin Orthop Relat Res. 2007;455:23–9.
71. Sterne JA, White IR, Carlin JB, Spratt M, Royston P, Kenward MG, et al. Multiple imputation for missing data in epidemiological and clinical research: potential and pitfalls. BMJ. 2009;338:b2393.
72. Jakobsen JC, Gluud C, Wetterslev J, Winkel P. When and how should multiple imputation be used for handling missing data in randomised clinical trials - a practical guide with flowcharts. BMC Med Res Methodol. 2017;17(1):162.
73. Goldberg JB, Goodney PP, Kumbhani SR, Roth RM, Powell RJ, Likosky DS. Brain injury after carotid revascularization: outcomes, mechanisms, and opportunities for improvement. Ann Vasc Surg. 2011;25(2):270–86.
74. Zhou W, Baughman BD, Soman S, Wintermark M, Lazzeroni LC, Hitchner E, et al. Volume of subclinical embolic infarct correlates to long-term cognitive changes after carotid revascularization. J Vasc Surg. 2017;65(3):686–94.
75. Hitchner E, Baughman BD, Soman S, Long B, Rosen A, Zhou W. Microembolization is associated with transient cognitive decline in patients undergoing carotid interventions. J Vasc Surg. 2016;64(6):1719–25.

Quality of Life and Patient Reported Outcome Measures Following Percutaneous Aortic Intervention for Aortic Aneurysms and Dissection

15

Leonard L. Shan, Akshat Saxena, and Alun H. Davies

Abbreviations

ADSORB	Acute dissection: stent graft or best medical therapy
AJAX	Amsterdam acute aneurysm trial
DREAM	Dutch randomised endovascular aneurysm management
ECAR	Endovasculaire ou Chirurgie dans les Anevrysmes aorto-iliaques rompus
EVAR-1	United Kingdom endovascular aneurysm repair trial 1
EVAR-2	United Kingdom endovascular aneurysm repair trial 2
IMPROVE	Immediate management of patients with rupture: open versus endovascular repair
INSTEAD	Randomised comparison of strategies for type B aortic dissection: the investigation of stent graft in aortic dissection
INSTEAD XL	Randomised comparison of strategies for type B aortic dissection: the investigation of stent graft in aortic dissection with extended follow-up
OVER	Open versus endovascular repair veterans affairs cooperative study

L. L. Shan (✉)
St. Vincent's Hospital Melbourne,
Melbourne, VIC, Australia

Department of Surgery, The University of Melbourne,
Melbourne, VIC, Australia
e-mail: leonard.shan@unimelb.edu.au

A. Saxena
Department of Cardiothoracic Surgery and Transplantation, Fiona Stanley Hospital,
Murdoch, WA, Australia

A. H. Davies
Charing Cross, London, UK

St. Mary's Hospital, London, UK

Vascular Surgery, Department of Surgery and Cancer,
Imperial College London, London, UK
e-mail: a.h.davies@imperial.ac.uk

Introduction

Aortic aneurysms and dissection are important public health issues. Screening studies report a prevalence of abdominal aortic aneurysms (AAA) of 4–8%, with an annual incidence of new diagnoses at 0.4–0.67% in Western populations [1–5]. Unlike AAA where the diagnosis is increasingly being made during an investigation for another abdominal pathology, thoracic aortic pathology tends to be silent until the acute presentation. The prevalence of thoracic aortic aneurysms (TAA) is estimated at 0.16–0.34%, with an annual incidence of up to 0.016% [6]. Forty

T. Athanasiou et al. (eds.), *Patient Reported Outcomes and Quality of Life in Cardiovascular Interventions*,
https://doi.org/10.1007/978-3-031-09815-4_15

percent of TAA involves the descending thoracic or thoracoabdominal aorta [7]. The annual incidence of aortic dissection is difficult to measure, but is estimated at 5–30 per one million people [8]. Even though the overall incidence of thoracic aortic pathology is relatively low, there is a significant associated morbidity and mortality which is particularly poignant in the setting of rupture [1–6, 8, 9].

Endovascular intervention is often the preferred method of treatment for aortic pathologies in relation to aneurysms and dissection. Simple endovascular procedures include abdominal endovascular aneurysm repair (EVAR) and thoracic endovascular aneurysm repair (TEVAR). Complex endovascular procedures include fenestrated endovascular aneurysm repair (FEVAR), chimney endovascular aneurysm repair (CHEVAR), branched endovascular aneurysm repair (BEVAR), and custom made devices. Procedural outcomes for each of these are continually improving over time. The concept of quality of life (QOL) and patient reported outcomes measures (PROMS) has been introduced since the early 1990s as an important aspect of outcomes assessment [10], but it is only recently that these are being integrated into modern practice and management of aortic pathologies.

This chapter summarises the available literature on QOL and PROMS after percutaneous aortic intervention for aortic aneurysms and dissection. However, aortic interventions are a broad set of procedures that can be categorised according to anatomical site, pathology, indication for surgery, and type of surgery. It is therefore necessary to differentiate between these groups in order to accurately report on QOL and PROMS outcomes.

Currently, evidence exists for QOL and PROMS after endovascular intervention for; (a) standard EVAR for AAA, (b) standard TEVAR for TAA and type B aortic dissection (TBAD), and (c) thoracoabdominal aneurysms (TAAA). There is currently no published data on QOL or PROMS after (a) complex endovascular repair of AAA (FEVAR, CHEVAR, BEVAR, custom-made devices), (b) endovascular repair of abdominal aortic dissection, (c) endovascular repair of ascending aortic and aortic arch pathology (which still generally requires open surgery), and (d) complex endovascular interventions for TAA, TAAA, TBAD (FEVAR, BEVAR, custom-made devices). Hence, four key groups of patients are presented in this chapter: (a) standard EVAR for AAA, (b) standard TEVAR for TAA, (c) standard TEVAR for TBAD, and (d) endovascular repair of TAAA. These include both elective and emergency procedures.

Current Interventions on the Aorta

Abdominal Aorta

Abdominal Aortic Aneurysms

The endovascular treatment options for AAA include EVAR, FEVAR, BEVAR, CHEVAR, and custom-made devices. Evidence on QOL and PROMS are limited to standard EVAR and this forms the focus of this section. In contemporary practice, elective EVAR is often the preferred option in patients with suitable anatomy.

The outcomes and relative merits of EVAR and open AAA repair in the elective setting are well described in numerous trials and meta-analyses including EVAR-1, EVAR-2, OVER, and DREAM [11–18]. EVAR has a proven low perioperative morbidity and mortality which is the primary reason for it is use in AAA. The trade-off is a greater rate of secondary reintervention compared to open AAA repair. The survival benefit of EVAR is also generally thought to be lost after 2–3 years. A recent study suggests EVAR may actually have a worse long-term mortality compared to open AAA repair [19].

The ideal treatment for emergency cases is less clear. The IMPROVE, AJAX, and ECAR trials, as well as meta-analyses of these trials show no difference in early outcomes after EVAR compared to open AAA repair in the setting of rupture [20–24]. However, mid-term results from the IMPROVE trial suggest a survival advantage in EVAR patients [25].

Thoracic Aorta

Thoracic and Thoracoabdominal Aortic Aneurysms

The endovascular treatment options for TAA and TAAA include TEVAR, BEVAR, and custom-made devices. In contemporary practice, TEVAR is regarded as the preferred option in the majority of cases.

The preference for TEVAR over open repair for TAA and TAAA is based mainly on retrospective and observational studies coupled with anecdotal evidence and experience. Recent reviews and meta-analyses have supported this practice, demonstrating superior morbidity and mortality of TEVAR over traditional open repair techniques [26–28]. Evidence is still limited in regard to which method of repair is better for emergency cases, but TEVAR would still be preferred in most centres due to the much lesser invasiveness of TEVAR.

Type B Thoracic Aortic Dissection

This chapter focusses specifically on TBAD as these are amenable to TEVAR. When intervention is required for the ascending aorta or aortic arch, some element of open repair is still required. TBAD can be classed as acute, subacute and chronic. Medical management was the traditional treatment paradigm for uncomplicated acute and subacute TBAD, with operative intervention reserved for complicated TBAD (refractory pain and hypertension, malperfusion, rupture). Treatment for chronic TBAD largely relates to aneurysmal dilatation and prevention of long-term rupture risk. In contemporary practice, TEVAR is the preferred treatment option in a large proportion of acute and chronic TBAD, with selected cases requiring FEVAR, BEVAR or custom made devices.

Most patients with complicated acute and subacute TBAD will receive urgent treatment. In uncomplicated TBAD, the ADSORB, INSTEAD, and INSTEAD XL trials supported the use of TEVAR in the subacute setting in carefully selected patients to decrease long-term aneurysm related mortality [29–32]. Chronic TBAD is treated with similar techniques to TAA and TAAA as this is usually the primary indication for treatment. There is limited evidence on the best management of residual TBAD after repair of type A dissection.

Quality of Life Instruments and Proms in Aortic Intervention

Definition of Quality of Life and Patient Reported Outcome Measures

PROMS ask patients to assess elements of their own health, QOL, and functioning [33]. The aim is to understand the impact of a treatment and its recovery, allow comparison of different patients' outcomes with the same intervention [33]. QOL is the major element of PROMS and is defined as a patient's perception of health as assessed in multiple domains [34, 35]. QOL is also the most frequently used form of assessment and their use in aortic intervention has been previously described [36].

One of the important considerations in QOL assessment is the type of instrument used and the measurement time points and time frame within which these assessments will be made. There is currently no consensus on this. However, research is underway to help determine these with core outcome sets in AAA [37]. Until then, investigators will need to use clinical judgment on the most appropriate methods of assessment.

Commonly Used Quality of Life Instruments in Aortic Intervention

QOL can be assessed by study designed questionnaires, and disease-specific or generic instruments. These instruments assess an individual's physical, emotional and psychological health as well as social and functional status [34, 35].

Individual study designed questionnaires are constructed by study authors as arbitrary measures of QOL outcomes. Disease-specific QOL instruments are validated QOL scoring systems that measure the effect of an illness or treatment on a specific condition [35]. These include Aneurysm-Dependent QOL Questionnaire (AneurysmDQOL) [38], Aneurysm Symptom Rating Questionnaire (AneurysmSRQ) [38], and Aneurysm Treatment Satisfaction Questionnaire (Aneurysm TSQ) [38]. Generic QOL instruments are validated QOL scoring systems that measure holistic QOL in a broad range of domains and allow comparisons with other conditions and reference populations [35]. Generic scoring systems used by studies reviewed in this chapter are Medical Outcomes Short Form 36 (SF-36) and 12 (SF-12) and 8 (SF-8) [39], Hospital Anxiety and Depression Scale (HAD) [40], European Quality of Life EQ-5D VASC Vascular Questionnaire (EQ-5D VASC) [41], and Nottingham Health Profile (NHP) [42]. These instruments are described in earlier chapters.

Quality of Life and Patient Reported Outcomes

The aforementioned trials on the management of aortic aneurysms and dissection have focussed on technical outcomes after EVAR and TEVAR. However, recent reviews have highlighted the importance of QOL outcomes [23, 36, 43–47]. To date QOL has been the primary method of PROMS assessment. Study characteristics and a brief quality appraisal is outlined in Table 15.1. Detailed study information and QOL outcomes are shown in Table 15.2. This section describes the key QOL findings. Some of this information has been described in prior reviews [36, 43, 45].

Abdominal Aorta (29 Studies) [12, 16, 18, 25, 38, 48–68, 70–72]

The vast majority of studies focus on elective standard EVAR [12, 16, 18, 38, 48–64, 67, 68, 70, 72]. Broadly similar QOL outcomes have been reported across all the instruments used. There is an initial postoperative decline after EVAR. Most health domains return to baseline levels between 1 and 4 months. Between 6 months and 2 years, QOL is maintained at preoperative levels. Within this time period, it should be noted that mental health has a distinct benefit. A number of studies describe mental health domains to be superior to preoperative levels. This is an important aspect of treatment benefit that is likely attributed to the alleviation of fear of rupture. After 2 years, there was a gradual, but progressive age-related decline in all QOL domains up to 8 years.

Compared to open AAA repair, EVAR has a more rapid recovery in QOL. This is particularly pertinent to physical health domains and is consistent with the greater physical toll from open aortic surgery. However, this difference is resolved by 6 months and QOL remains similar up to 1 year. Functional status and participation in activities of daily living is also similar in both groups at 1 year. Patients perceive long-term surveillance and secondary reintervention be more difficult after EVAR whereas early physical recovery is the difficulty after open AAA. This is an important concept because surveillance will tend to affect mental health domains more. The longer the surveillance occurs, the more likely there will be a detriment to mental health. This is an important trade-off for the early benefits of EVAR. There is also some evidence that EVAR has worse QOL compared to open AAA repair.

Recently, three studies have reported QOL after emergency intervention [25, 65, 71]. Early QOL is similar or slightly better after EVAR compared to open AAA repair. However, the advantages of EVAR are lost after 3–4 years, with one study suggesting there is a better QOL after open AAA repair. This mirrors the longer term technical outcomes and durability advantage of open AAA repair.

The population is ageing with an ever increasing life expectancy. Aneurysmal disease of the aorta becomes more prevalent with increased age and the patients being treated for AAA will be increasingly elderly. This is an important subgroup because elderly patients have more comorbidities and are more likely to have EVAR over open AAA repair, yet they also have known increased anatomical challenges for EVAR compared to their younger counterparts. Outcomes

Table 15.1 Study characteristics and quality appraisal

Author / Year	Patients	Study design	Patient demographics	Validated QOL instrument	QOL instruments used	Follow-up method reported	Response rate
Original studies—abdominal aorta							
Lloyd [48]	EVAR	P	Male: NR, Age: 73, HTN: NR, DM: NR,	Yes	SF-36	Yes	78%
2000	n = 34		Smoking: NR, IHD: NR, CVA: NR, CKD: NR				
	OR		Elective: NR, Emergency: NR				
	n = 48		Aortic pathology: AAA				
Study objectives:			QOL and cognitive function after open AAA repair or EVAR (preoperative vs. postoperative, EVAR vs. open AAA repair)				
Malina [49]	EVAR	P	*EVAR*	Yes	NHP	Yes	95%
2000	n = 21		Male: 81%, Age: 74, HTN: 24%, DM: NR,				
	OR		Smoking: NR, IHD: 24%, CVA: NR, CKD: NR				
	n = 21		Elective: 100%, Emergency: 0%				
			Aortic pathology: AAA				
			Open AAA repair				
			Male: 76%, Age: 74, HTN: 52%, DM: NR				
			Smoking: NR, IHD: 24%, CVA: NR, CKD:				
			Elective: 100%, Emergency: 0%				
			Aortic pathology: AAA				
Study objectives:			QOL and functional status after open AAA repair or EVAR (preoperative vs. postoperative, EVAR vs. open AAA repair)				
Aquino [50]	EVAR	P	*EVAR*	Yes	SF-36	Yes	61%
2001	n = 25		Male: 93%, Age: 71, HTN: 84%, DM: 11.5%,				
	OR		Smoking: NR, IHD: 48%, CVA: NR, CKD: NR				
	n = 26		Elective: NR, Emergency: NR				
			Aortic pathology: AAA				
			Open AAA repair				
			Male: 73%, Age: 70, HTN: 80%, DM: 38%,				
			Smoking: NR, IHD: 42%, CVA: NR, CKD: NR				
			Elective: NR, Emergency: NR				
			Aortic pathology: AAA				

(continued)

Table 15.1 (continued)

Original studies—abdominal aorta							
Author **Year**	**Patients**	**Study design**	**Patient demographics**	**Validated QOL instrument**	**QOL instruments used**	**Follow-up method reported**	**Response rate**
Study objectives:			QOL and functional status after open AAA repair or EVAR (preoperative vs. postoperative, EVAR vs. open AAA repair)				
Arko [51]	EVAR	P	*EVAR*	Yes	Study questionnaire	Yes	39%
2003	n = 153		Male: 83%, Age: 74, HTN: 56%, DM: 36%,				
	OR		Smoking: NR, IHD: 79%, CVA: NR, CKD: 6%				
	n = 141		Elective: 100%, Emergency: 0%				
			Aortic pathology: AAA				
			Open AAA repair				
			Male: 86%, Age: 74, HTN: 61%, DM: 29%,				
			Smoking: NR, IHD: 76%, CVA: NR, CKD: 9%				
			Elective: 100%, Emergency: 0%				
			Aortic pathology: AAA				
Study objectives:			Compare periprocedural survival, and recovery times after EVAR and open AAA repair				
			Compare early (<6 months) and late (>6 months) functional outcomes after EVAR and open AAA repair (preoperative vs. postoperative, EVAR vs. open AAA repair)				
Lederle [52]	EVAR	P	*Immediate Open AAA repair*	Yes	SF-36	Yes	85%
2003	n = 567		Male: 99%, Age: 68, HTN: 57.8%, DM: 9.7%,				
	OR		Smoking: 41.4%, IHD: 43.6%, CVA: 12%, CKD: NR				
	n = 569		Elective: 100%, Emergency: 0%				
			Aortic pathology: AAA				
			Surveillance				
			Male: 99.6%, Age: 68, HTN: 54.9%, DM: 9.9%,				
			Smoking: 36.9%, IHD: 40.2%, CVA: 12.7%, CKD: NR				
			Elective: 100%, Emergency: 0%				
			Aortic pathology: AAA				

Study objectives:			Long-term QOL after open AAA repair or surveillance for sub-threshold AAA (preoperative vs. postoperative, surveillance vs. repair)				
Ballard [53]	EVAR	P	*EVAR*	Yes	SF-12	Yes	65%
2004	n = 22		Male: 90%, Age: 77, HTN: 62%, DM: 38%				
	OR		Smoking: NR, IHD: 81%, CVA: NR, CKD: 10%				
	n = 107		Elective: 100%, Emergency: 0%				
			Aortic pathology: AAA				
			Open AAA repair				
			Male: 76%, Age: 72, HTN: 81%, DM: 19%,				
			Smoking: NR%, IHD: 79%, CVA: NR, CKD: 18%				
			Elective: 100%, Emergency: 0%				
			Aortic pathology: AAA				
Study objectives:			QOL after EVAR and retroperitoneal open AAA repair (preoperative vs. postoperative, EVAR vs. open AAA repair)				
Lottman [54]	OR	P	*EVAR*	Yes	SF-36, EuroQOL	NR	91%
2004	n = 19		Male: 95%, Age: 69, HTN: NR, DM: NR,				
	EVAR		Smoking: NR, IHD: NR, CVA: NR, CKD: NR				
	n = 57		Elective: 100%, Emergency: 0%				
			Aortic pathology: AAA				
			Open AAA repair				
			Male: 64%, Age: 68, HTN: NR, DM: NR,				
			Smoking: NR, IHD: NR, CVA: NR, CKD: NR				
			Elective: 100%, Emergency: 0%				
			Aortic pathology: AAA				

(continued)

Table 15.1 (continued)

Original studies—abdominal aorta							
Author Year	**Patients**	**Study design**	**Patient demographics**	**Validated QOL instrument**	**QOL instruments used**	**Follow-up method reported**	**Response rate**
Study objectives:			Short-term QOL after EVAR compared to open AAA repair (preoperative vs. postoperative, EVAR vs. open AAA repair)				
Prinssen [55]	EVAR	P	*EVAR*	Yes	SF-36, EQ-5D VASC	Yes	73%
2004	n = 78		Male: 92%, Age: 70.5, HTN: 51%, DM: 6%,				
	OR		Smoking: 62%, IHD: 32%, CVA: NR, CKD: 8%				
	n = 75		Elective: 100%, Emergency: 0%				
			Aortic pathology: AAA				
			Open AAA repair				
			Male: 92%, Age: 69, HTN: 48%, DM: 5%,				
			Smoking: 31%, IHD: 44%, CVA: NR, CKD: 7%				
			Elective: 100%, Emergency: 0%				
			Aortic pathology: AAA				
Study objectives:			Short-term QOL after EVAR compared to open AAA repair (preoperative vs. postoperative, EVAR vs. open AAA repair)				
EVAR-2 [16]	EVAR	P	*EVAR*	Yes	EQ-5D VASC, SF-36	Yes	83%
2005	n = 166		Male: 85 %, Age: 76.8, HTN: NR, DM: 15%				
	Surveillance		Smoking: 17%, IHD: 65%, CVA: NR, CKD: NR				
	n = 172		Elective: 100%, Emergency: 0%				
			Aortic pathology: AAA				
			Surveillance				
			Male: 85%, Age: 76.0, HTN: NR, DM: 13%,				
			Smoking: 16%, IHD: 73%, CVA: NR, CKD: NR				
			Elective: 100%, Emergency: 0%				
			Aortic pathology: AAA				
Study objectives:			Does EVAR decrease risk of aneurysm related death and improve QOL compared to medical treatment in patients not fit for open AAA repair (preoperative vs. postoperative, EVAR vs. medical treatment)				

EVAR-1 [56]	EVAR	P	*EVAR*	Yes	SF-36, EQ-5D VASC	Yes	100%
2005	n = 543		Male: 91%, Age: 74.2, HTN: NR, DM: 9%,				
	OR		Smoking: 21%, IHD: 44%, CVA: NR, CKD: NR				
	n = 539		Elective: 100%, Emergency: 0%				
			Aortic pathology: AAA				
			Open AAA repair				
			Male: 91%, Age: 74.0, HTN: NR, DM: 12%,				
			Smoking: 22%, IHD: 43%, CVA: NR, CKD: NR				
			Elective: 100%, Emergency: 0%				
			Aortic pathology: AAA				
Study objectives:			Compare mortality, durability, QOL, costs for EVAR compared to open AAA repair (preoperative vs. postoperative, EVAR vs. open AAA repair)				
Soulez [57]	EVAR	P	*EVAR*	Yes	SF-36, Karnofsky	Yes	NR
2005	n = 20		Male: 95%, Age: 70.3, HTN: 40%, DM: 5%,				
	OR		Smoking: 25%, IHD: 65%, CVA: NR, CKD: 5%				
	n = 20		Elective: 100%, Emergency: 0%				
			Aortic pathology: AAA				
			Open AAA repair				
			Male: 100%, Age: 71.2, HTN: 50%, DM: 25%,				
			Smoking: 15%, IHD: 70%, CVA: NR, CKD: 25%				
			Elective: 100%, Emergency: 0%				
			Aortic pathology: AAA				
Study objectives:			Functional autonomy, QOL, pain, after EVAR compared to open AAA repair (preoperative vs. postoperative, EVAR vs. open AAA repair)				
Vogel [58]	EVAR	R	*EVAR*	Yes	SF-36	Yes	NR
2005	n = 92		Male: 87%, Age: 71.5, HTN: 72%, DM: 13%,				
	OR		Smoking: NR, IHD: 54%, CVA: NR, CKD: 8%				
	n = 126		Elective: 100%, Emergency: 0%				
			Aortic pathology: AAA				
			Open AAA repair				
			Male: 68%, Age: 70.8, HTN: 65%, DM: 11%,				
			Smoking: NR, IHD: 46%, CVA: NR, CKD: 6%				
			Elective: 100%, Emergency: 0%				
			Aortic pathology: AAA				

(continued)

Table 15.1 (continued)

Original studies—abdominal aorta							
Author **Year**	**Patients**	**Study design**	**Patient demographics**	**Validated QOL instrument**	**QOL instruments used**	**Follow-up method reported**	**Response rate**
Study objectives:			Factors that influence independence and functional health after EVAR or open AAA repair (EVAR vs. open AAA repair)				
Aljabri [59]	EVAR	P	*EVAR*	Yes	SF-36	Yes	NR
2006	n = 43		Male: 86.1%, Age: 76.1, HTN: 62.8%, DM: 11.6%,				
	OR		Smoking: NR, IHD: 67.4%, CVA: 13.9%, CKD: NR				
	n = 33		Elective: 100%, Emergency: 0%				
			Aortic pathology: AAA				
			Open AAA repair				
			Male: 75.8%, Age: 68.6, HTN: 57.6%, DM: 21.2%				
			Smoking: NR, IHD: 66.7%, CVA: 9.1%, CKD: 3%				
			Elective: 100%, Emergency: 0%				
			Aortic pathology: AAA				
Study objectives:			QOL after EVAR compared to open AAA repair (preoperative vs. postoperative, EVAR vs. open AAA repair)				
Dick [60]	EVAR	R	*EVAR*	Yes	SF-36	Yes	86.8%
2008	n = 68		Male: 94.1%, Age: 71.7, HTN: 54.4%, DM: 8.8%				
	OR		Smoking: 44.1%, IHD: 41.2%, CVA: NR, CKD: NR				
	n = 244		Elective: 100%, Emergency: 0%				
	EOR		Aortic pathology:				
	n = 89		*Open AAA repair*				
			Male: 83.2%, Age: 66.4, HTN: 45.5%, DM: 14.3%				
			Smoking: 38.5%, IHD: 41.2%, CVA: NR, CKD: NR				
			Elective: 100%, Emergency: 0%				
			Aortic pathology: AAA				
			Emergency Open AAA repair.				
			Male: 92.1%, Age: 70.6, HTN: 58.4%, DM: 5.6%				
			Smoking: 43.8%, IHD: 38.2%, CVA: NR, CKD: NR				
			Elective: 0%, Emergency: 100%				
			Aortic pathology: AAA				

Study objectives:			Long-term survival and QOL after EVAR and open AAA repair (EVAR vs. open AAA repair vs. general population)				
Lederle [18]	EVAR	P	*EVAR*	Yes	SF-36, EQ-5D VASC	Yes	80%
2009	n = 444		Male: 99.3%, Age: 70, HTN: NR, DM: 22.5%				
	OR		Smoking: 38.3%, IHD: 39.2%, CVA: 15.1%, CKD: 31.5%				
	n = 437		Elective: 100%, Emergency: 0%				
			Aortic pathology: AAA				
			Open AAA repair				
			Male: 99.5%, Age: 71, HTN: NR, DM: 22.9%				
			Smoking: 44.2%, IHD: 42.3%, CVA: 16%, CKD: 31.1%				
			Elective: 100%, Emergency: 0%				
			Aortic pathology: AAA				
Study objectives:			Compare early postoperative outcomes after EVAR and open AAA repair (preoperative vs. postoperative, EVAR vs. open AAA repair)				
Kurz [61]	EVAR	R	Male: 91%, Age: 71.5, HTN: 67%, DM: 14%	Yes	NHP	Yes	57.1%
2010	n = 270		Smoking: 71%, IHD: 66%, CVA: 16%, CKD: NR				
			Elective: 100%, Emergency: 0%				
			Aortic pathology: AAA				
Study objectives:			QOL after EVAR in octogenarians compared to younger patients (Older vs. younger patients)				
DeRango [62]	EVAR	P	*EVAR*	Yes	SF-36	Yes	76%
2011	n = 173		Male: 95%, Age: 69, HTN: 74%, DM: 16%				
	Surveillance		Smoking: 58%, IHD: 36%, CVA: 11.5%, CKD: 7.1%				
	n = 166		Elective: 100%, Emergency: 0%				
			Aortic pathology: AAA				
			Surveillance				
			Male: 97%, Age: 68.8, HTN: 76%, DM: 11%				
			Smoking: 53%, IHD: 42%, CVA: 19%, CKD: 9%				
			Elective: 100%, Emergency: 0%				
			Aortic pathology: AAA				

(continued)

Table 15.1 (continued)

Original studies—abdominal aorta							
Author / **Year**	**Patients**	**Study design**	**Patient demographics**	**Validated QOL instrument**	**QOL instruments used**	**Follow-up method reported**	**Response rate**
Study objectives:			QOL after EVAR or surveillance in subthreshold aneurysms (EVAR vs. surveillance, preoperative vs. postoperative)				
Kisis [63]	EVAR	P	*EVAR*	Yes	SF-36	Yes	100%
2012	n = 20		Male: 85%, Age: 70, HTN: NR, DM: 15%,				
	OR		Smoking: NR, IHD: 50%, CVA: 5%, CKD: 5%				
	n = 20		Elective: 100%, Emergency: 0%				
			Aortic pathology: AAA				
			Open AAA repair				
			Male: 80%, Age: 67, HTN: NR, DM: 10%,				
			Smoking: NR, IHD: 40%, CVA: 0%, CKD: 10%				
			Elective: 100%, Emergency: 0%				
			Aortic pathology: AAA				
Study objectives:			QOL after EVAR and open AAA repair (preoperative vs. postoperative, EVAR vs. open AAA repair)				
Lederle [12]	EVAR	P	*EVAR*	Yes	SF-36	Yes	85%
2012	n = 444		Male: 99%, Age: 69.6, HTN: 78.2%, DM: 22.5%				
	OR		Smoking: 38.3%, IHD: 39.2%, CVA: 15.1%, CKD: 31.5%				
	n = 437		Elective: 100%, Emergency: 0%				
			Aortic pathology: AAA				
			Open AAA repair				
			Male: 96%, Age: 70.5, HTN: 75.5%, DM: 22.9%				
			Smoking: 44.2%, IHD: 42.3%, CVA: 16.0%, CKD: 31.1%				
			Elective: 100%, Emergency: 0%				
			Aortic pathology: AAA				

Study objectives:			Long-term morbidity and mortality after EVAR vs. open AAA repair (EVAR vs. open AAA repair)				
Pol [64]	EVAR	P	<80 years old	Yes	EQ-5D VASC	Yes	82.1%
2012	<80 years old		Male: 91%, Age: 70.1, HTN: 77%, DM: 20%,				
	n = 926		Smoking: 56%, IHD: 54%, CVA: 12%, CKD: 14.2%				
	EVAR		Elective: 100%, Emergency: 0%				
	>80 years old		Aortic pathology: AAA				
	n = 274		>80 years old				
			Male: 86.5%, Age: 83.3, HTN: 73.1%, Chol: 55.1%, DM: 15.1%				
			Smoking: 24.6%, IHD: 55.5%, CVA: 16.8%, CKD: NR				
			Elective: 100%, Emergency: 0%				
			Aortic pathology: AAA				
Study objectives:			30-day outcome and QOL after EVAR in octogenarians (preoperative vs. postoperative, EVAR vs. open AAA repair)				
AJAX [65]	EVAR	P	*EVAR*	Yes	SF-36	Yes	77%
2014	n = 57		Male: 86%, Age: 74.9, HTN: 23%, DM: 4%				
	OR		Smoking: 40%, IHD: 28%, CVA: NR, CKD: 2%				
	n = 59		Elective: 0%, Emergency: 100%				
			Aortic pathology: AAA				
			Open AAA repair				
			Male: 85%, Age: 74.5, HTN: 17%, DM: 2%				
			Smoking: 34%, IHD: 24%, CVA: NR, CKD: 3%				
			Elective: 0%, Emergency: 100%				
			Aortic pathology: AAA				
Study objectives:			Cost effectiveness and utility of EVAR compared to open AAA repair for ruptured AAA (EVAR vs. open AAA repair)				
Klocker [66]	EVAR	R	Male: NR, Age: NR, HTN: NR, DM: NR,	Yes	SF-12	No	NR
2014	n = 138		Smoking: NR, IHD: NR, CVA: NR, CKD: NR				
			Elective: NR, Emergency: NR				
			Aortic pathology: Descending thoracic aneurysm, dissection, trauma				

(continued)

Table 15.1 (continued)

Original studies—abdominal aorta

Author Year	Patients	Study design	Patient demographics	Validated QOL instrument	QOL instruments used	Follow-up method reported	Response rate
Study objectives:			Incidence of left arm ischemia, function, quality of life after TEVAR (left subclavian coverage vs. no coverage)				
Pol [67]	EVAR	P	<80 years old	Yes	EQ-5D VASC	Yes	67.9%
2014	<80 years old		Male: 90.4%, Age: 70.1, HTN: 75.9%, DM: 19.9%				
	n = 973		Smoking: 56.5%, IHD: 53%, CVA: 11.7%, CKD: 13.9%				
	EVAR		Elective: 100%, Emergency: 0%				
	>80 years old		Aortic pathology: AAA				
	n = 290		>80 years old				
			Male: 86.2%, Age: 83.3, HTN: 73.9%, DM: 19.9%				
			Smoking: 24.6%, IHD: 55.2%, CVA: 15.9%, CKD: 20.1%				
			Elective: 100%, Emergency: 0%				
			Aortic pathology: AAA				
Study objectives:			QOL after EVAR in octogenarians (<80 years old vs. >80 years old, preoperative vs. postoperative)				
De Bruin [68]	EVAR	P	*EVAR*	Yes	SF-36, EQ-5D VASC	Yes	70%
2016	n = 173		Male: 93%, Age: 70.7, HTN: 58.4%, DM: 10.4%				
	OR		Smoking: 63.6%, IHD: 41%, CVA: NR, CKD: 7.5%				
	n = 178		Elective: 100%, Emergency: 0%				
			Aortic pathology: AAA				
			Open AAA repair				
			Male: 90%, Age: 69.6, HTN: 54.5%, DM: 9.6%				
			Smoking: 54.5%, IHD: 47.2%, CVA: NR, CKD: 9%				
			Elective: 100%, Emergency: 0%				
			Aortic pathology: AAA				

Study objectives:			Long-term QOL after EVAR and open AAA repair (preoperative vs. postoperative, EVAR vs. open AAA repair)				
Peach [69]	EVAR	R	*EVAR*	Yes	AneurysmDQOL	Yes	66.3%
2016	n = 103		Male: 86.4%, Age: 76.6, HTN: NR, DM: NR,		AneurysmSRQ		
	OR		Smoking: NR, IHD: NR, CVA: NR, CKD: NR		AneurysmTSQ		
	n = 69		Elective: 100%, Emergency: 0%				
			Aortic pathology: AAA				
			Open AAA repair				
			Male: 97%, Age: 72.7, HTN: NR, DM: NR				
			Smoking: NR, IHD: NR, CVA: NR, CKD: NR				
			Elective: 100%, Emergency: 0%				
			Aortic pathology: AAA				
Study objectives:			QOL, symptoms, satisfaction assessed using AAA specific measures (preoperative vs. postoperative, EVAR vs. open AAA repair)				
IMPROVE [25]	EVAR	P	*EVAR*	Yes	EQ-5D VASC	Yes	78%
2017	n = 316		Male: 78%, Age: 76.7, HTN: NR, DM: NR				
	OR		Smoking: NR, IHD: NR, CVA: NR, CKD: NR				
	n = 297		Elective: 0%, Emergency: 100%				
			Aortic pathology: AAA				
			Open AAA repair				
			Male: 79%, Age: 76.7, HTN: NR, DM: NR				
			Smoking: NR, IHD: NR, CVA: NR, CKD: NR				
			Elective: 0%, Emergency: 100%				
			Aortic pathology: AAA				
Study objectives:			Midterm clinical outcomes and cost effectiveness of EVAR vs. open AAA repair for ruptured AAA (preoperative vs. postoperative, EVAR vs. open AAA repair)				
Kato [70]	EVAR	P	*EVAR*	Yes	SF-8	Yes	64%
2017	n = 25		Male: 96%, Age: 76, HTN: NR, DM: 28%,				
	OR		Smoking: 8%, IHD: NR, CVA: NR, CKD: 28%				
	n = 30		Elective: 100%, Emergency: 0%				
			Aortic pathology: AAA				
			Open AAA repair				
			Male: 93%, Age: 72.8, HTN: NR, DM: 17.7%				
			Smoking: 23.3%, IHD: NR, CVA: NR, CKD: 30%				
			Elective: 100%, Emergency: 0%				
			Aortic pathology: AAA				

(continued)

Table 15.1 (continued)

Original studies—abdominal aorta							
Author / **Year**	**Patients**	**Study design**	**Patient demographics**	**Validated QOL instrument**	**QOL instruments used**	**Follow-up method reported**	**Response rate**
Study objectives:			QOL changes after EVAR and open AAA repair (preoperative vs. postoperative, EVAR vs. open AAA repair)				
Yildirim [71]	EVAR	R	*EVAR*	Yes	SF-36	Yes	72.4%
2017	n = 45		Male: 93%, Age: 76.4, HTN: NR, Chol: NR, DM: NR				
			Smoking: NR, IHD: NR, CVA: NR, CKD: NR				
			Elective: 0%, Emergency: 100%				
			Aortic pathology: AAA				
			Open AAA repair				
			Male: 86%, Age: 71.4, HTN: NR, Chol: NR, DM: NR				
			Smoking: NR, IHD: NR, CVA: NR, CKD: NR				
			Elective: 0%, Emergency: 100%				
			Aortic pathology: AAA				
Study objectives:			Long-term QOL after EVAR and open AAA repair for ruptured AAA (EVAR vs. open AAA repair vs. general population)				
Akbulut [72]	EVAR	P	*EVAR*	Yes	SF-36	No	NR
2018	n = 68		Male: 87%, Age: 67, HTN: NR, DM: 31%,				
	OR		Smoking: 83%, IHD: 63%, CVA: 5%, CKD: 31%				
	n = 39		Elective: 100%, Emergency: 0%				
			Aortic pathology: AAA				
			Open AAA repair				
			Male: 89%, Age: 67, HTN: NR, DM: 31%,				
			Smoking: 80%, IHD: 53%, CVA: 5%, CKD: 24%				
			Elective: 100%, Emergency: 0%				
			Aortic pathology: AAA				
Study objectives:			QOL after EVAR and open AAA repair (preoperative vs. postoperative, EVAR vs. open AAA repair)				

Original studies—thoracic aorta

Author Year	Patients	Study design	Patient demographics	Validated QOL instrument	QOL instruments used	Follow-up method reported	Response rate
Dick [73]	TEVAR	R	*TEVAR*	Yes	SF-36, HADS	Yes	78%
2008	n = 58		Male: 83%, Age: 68.8, HTN: 79%, DM: 15%				
	OR		Smoking: 50%, IHD: 35%, CVA: NR, CKD: NR				
	n = 78		Elective: 52%, Emergency: 48%				
			Aortic pathology: Thoracic aortic dissection/ aneurysm				
			Open descending thoracic aortic repair				
			Male: 84%, Age: 61.6, HTN: 76%, DM: 4%				
			Smoking: 57%, IHD: 49%, CVA: NR, CKD: NR				
			Elective: 80%, Emergency: 20%				
			Aortic pathology: Thoracic aortic dissection/ aneurysm				
Study objectives:			Long-term postoperative QOL after TEVAR or open repair for descending thoracic aortic diseases (TEVAR vs. open repair, TEVAR or open repair vs. general population)				
Dick [74]	Elective	R	*Elective TEVAR*	Yes	SF-36, HADS	Yes	70%
2009	TEVAR		Male: 85%, Age: 71, HTN: 78%, DM: 22%,				
	n = 29		Smoking: 63%, IHD: 59%, CVA: NR, CKD: 30%				
	Emergent		Elective: 100%, Emergency: 0%				
	TEVAR		Aortic pathology: Thoracic aortic dissection/ aneurysm				
	n = 29		*Emergency TEVAR*				
			Male: 80%, Age: 67, HTN: 80%, DM: 8%,				
			Smoking: 36%, IHD: 8%, CVA: NR, CKD: 16%				
			Elective: 0%, Emergency: 100%				
			Aortic pathology: Thoracic aortic dissection/ aneurysm				

(continued)

Table 15.1 (continued)

Author / Year	Patients	Study design	Patient demographics	Validated QOL instrument	QOL instruments used	Follow-up method reported	Response rate
Original studies—thoracic aorta							
Study objectives:			Postoperative QOL after elective or emergent TEVAR for descending thoracic aortic diseases (Elective TEVAR vs. emergent TEVAR vs. general population)				
McBride [75]	TEVAR	R	Male: 70%, Age: 46.7, HTN: NR, DM: NR	Yes	SF-12	Yes	NR
2015	n = 82		Smoking: NR, IHD: NR, CVA: NR, CKD: NR				
			Elective: 0%, Emergency: 10.0%				
			Aortic pathology: Blunt thoracic aortic injury				
Study objectives:			Long-term QOL and return to normal activities after TEVAR with or without left subclavian artery coverage				
Meltzer [76]	TAA	P	*Endovascular TAA repair*	Yes	SF-36	No	NR
2017	n = 22		Male: 77%, Age: 75.1, HTN: 90.9%, DM: 18%				
			Smoking: 23%, IHD: 31%, CVA: 9%, CKD: 23%				
			Elective: NR, Emergency: NR				
			Aortic pathology: TAA				
Study objectives:			Patient experience, emotional wellbeing, QOL after endovascular thoracoabdominal aneurysm repair (preoperative vs. postoperative)				
Bi [77]	TEVAR	P	*TEVAR*	Yes	SF-36	No	97%
2018	n = 40		Male: 88%, Age: 80.9, HTN: 58%, DM: 3%				
			Smoking: 53%, IHD: 5%, CVA: NR, CKD: NR				
			Elective: NR, Emergency: NR				
			Aortic pathology: Type B dissection				
Study objectives:			Midterm outcome and QOL after endovascular repair of Type B aortic dissection (preoperative vs. postoperative)				
Reviews							
Peach [46]		Review	Total studies: 23, Total patients in studies on QOL: 6904				
2012							
Study objectives:			Review evidence on health status changes after EVAR or open AAA repair				
			Hypothesise that EVAR patients have better short term QOL while open AAA repair patients have better long term QOL				
Coughlin [43]		Review	Total studies: 16, Total patients in studies on QOL: 4620				
2013							

Study objectives:			Short and midterm QOL after EVAR and open AAA repair
Propper [47] 2013		Review	Total studies: 4, Total patients in studies on QOL: 3674
Study objectives:			Long-term outcome after EVAR
Kayssi [45] 2015		Review	Total studies: 5, Total patients in studies on QOL: 2108
Study objectives:			Differences in short and long term QOL after EVAR compared to open AAA repair
Jarral [44] 2016		Review	Total studies: 30, Total patients in studies on QOL: 4746
Study objectives:			QOL after intervention on thoracic aorta
Badger [23] 2017		Review	Total studies: 4; Total patients in studies on QOL: 868
Study objectives:			Advantages and disadvantages of EVAR vs. open AAA repair for ruptured AAA
Shan [36] 2019		Review	Total studies: 13; Total patients in studies on QOL: 1272
Study objectives:			QOL after EVAR and open AAA repair in elderly patients

HTN hypertension, *Chol* hypercholesterolemia, *DM* diabetes mellitus, *IHD* ischemic heart disease, *CVA* cerebrovascular disease, *CKD* chronic kidney disease, *NR* not recorded, *AAA* abdominal aortic aneurysm, *R* retrospective, *P* prospective, *QOL* quality of life, *AneurysmDQOL* aneurysm-dependent QOL questionnaire, *AneurysmSRQ* aneurysm symptom rating questionnaire, *Aneurysm TSQ* aneurysm treatment satisfaction questionnaire, *SF-36* medical outcomes 36-item short-form health survey, *SF-12* medical outcomes 12-item short-form health survey, *NHP* Nottingham health profile, *EQ-5D VASC* EuroQOL 5-dimensions, *OR* open AAA repair, *EVAR* endovascular AAA repair

Table 15.2 Quality of life results in included studies

Author Year		Procedure	Follow-up time	Perioperative mortality	Major perioperative complications	Survival at time of QOL assessment
Original studies—abdominal aorta						
Lloyd [48]		EVAR	Pre-op, 6 months	EVAR: 8.8%	NR	EVAR: 82%
2000		Open AAA repair		Open AAA repair: 4.2%		Open AAA repair: 90%
	Key findings:	Most SF-36 domains maintained at preoperative levels				
		Significant worsening of physical function at 6 months for both EVAR and open AAA repair compared to pre-op				
		No significant difference between open AAA repair and EVAR at 6 months across all SF-36 domains				
Malina [49]		EVAR	Pre-op, 5, 30, 90 days	EVAR: 4.8%	NR	EVAR: 95%
2000		Open AAA repair		Open AAA repair 4.8%		Open AAA repair: 95%
	Key findings:	Total NHP scores had an initial Day 5 decline after both open AAA repair and EVAR, but improved to better than baseline at 3 months post-op				
		No difference between open AAA repair and EVAR at any time point in all NHP domains				
		Functional status worse in some domains after open AAA repair compared to EVAR at 1 month, but no difference at 3 months				
		EVAR patients perceive follow-up to be more difficult, open AAA repair patients found the recovery difficult				
Aquino [50]		EVAR	Pre-op. 1 week, 4 weeks, 8 weeks, 52 weeks	EVAR: 0%	EVAR: 0%	EVAR: 96%
2001		Open AAA repair		Open AAA repair: 0%	Open AAA repair: 0%	Open AAA repair: 92%
	Key findings:	At 1 week post-op, physical function, social function, role physical, vitality worse than pre-op for both EVAR and open AAA repair. Open AAA repair had more severe decline				
		All domains return to baseline at 4 weeks after EVAR, and 8 weeks after open AAA repair				
		All domains maintained up to 1 year				
		All domains similar between EVAR and open AAA repair at 1 year				
Arko [51]		EVAR	<6 months, >6 months	EVAR: 0.7%	EVAR: 10.5%	EVAR: 82%
2003		Open AAA repair		Open AAA repair: 3.6%	Open AAA repair: 9.2%	Open AAA repair: 96%
	Key findings:	At 3 months, 95% of EVAR patients felt completely recovered compared to 75% of open AAA repair				
		32 days to fully recovery after EVAR, 99 days for open AAA repair				
		5% after EVAR felt decreased activity level, 23% for open AAA repair				
		No significant difference in functional outcome after 6 months between EVAR and open AAA repair				
		No difference in ambulation, independent living, employment status before and after either treatment				
Lederle [52]		Surveillance	Pre-op, 6-monthly to 8 years	Surveillance: 2.6%	NR	Surveillance: 78.4%
2003		Open AAA repair		Open AAA repair: 3.0%		Open AAA repair: 74.9%

Table 15.2 (continued)

Original studies—abdominal aorta						
Author **Year**		**Procedure**	**Follow-up time**	**Perioperative mortality**	**Major perioperative complications**	**Survival at time of QOL assessment**
	Key findings:	All SF-36 scores declined over 8 year follow-up, physical health more than mental health, particularly after 2 years				
		No significant difference between surveillance and open AAA repair in most domains				
		Impotence was more common in open repair group				
		Maximum activity level similar between groups up to 5 years, thereafter open AAA repair group declined faster				
Ballard [53]		EVAR	Pre-op, 3 weeks, 4 months, 1 year	EVAR: 0%	EVAR: 4.5%	EVAR: 95%
2004		Open AAA repair		Open AAA repair: 0%	Open AAA repair: 9.3%	Open AAA repair: 98%
	Key findings:	After EVAR, PCS significantly worse at 3 weeks, almost baseline at 4 months, baseline by 1 year				
		After EVAR, MCS slightly worse at 3 weeks, slightly better at 4 months and 1 year				
		EVAR patients report average of 5.47 weeks to return to preoperative functional status				
		No difference in PCS or MCS for EVAR compared to open AAA repair at any time point				
		Return to functional status similar for both groups				
Lottman [54]		EVAR	Pre-op, 1 month, 3 months	EVAR: 2%	NR	NR
2004		Open AAA repair		Open AAA repair: 5%		
	Key findings:	At 1 month post-op, both EVAR and open patients had a decline in role and physical health domains and function compared to baseline, but these returned to baseline at 3 months				
		At 1 month post-op, open patients had worse QOL than EVAR in role limitations, physical functioning, pain and level of usual activities. At 3 months, no difference between EVAR and open AAA repair				
Prinssen [55]		EVAR	Pre-op, 3 weeks, 6 weeks, 3 months, 6 months, 12 months	EVAR: 0%	NR	EVAR: 95%
2004		Open AAA repair		Open AAA repair: 0%		Open AAA repair: 89%
	Key findings:	3 weeks: Open repair had a significant decrease compared to baseline level on six of the eight SF-36 domains. EVAR group showed a significant decrease on five of the domains of the SF-36				
		6 weeks: EVAR group showed a significant decrease on five of the domains of the SF-36. The EVAR group had three of the five decreased domains return to baseline				
		3 months: Both groups recovered at least to baseline level on all domains. Significant increase in both groups on mental health				
		1 year: Open repair group showed a significantly higher QOL than the baseline level on three of the eight SF-36 domains. All other domains maintained at baseline. EVAR group showed a significant increase in mental health				
		EuroQOL: Significant decrease at 3 weeks. Both groups showed a completely recovery to baseline at 6 weeks				
		After 6 months, open AAA repair patients have superior QOL compared to EVAR				

(continued)

Table 15.2 (continued)

Original studies—abdominal aorta						
Author / **Year**		**Procedure**	**Follow-up time**	**Perioperative mortality**	**Major perioperative complications**	**Survival at time of QOL assessment**
EVAR-2 [16] 2005		EVAR	Pre-op, 0–3 months, 3–12 months, 12–24 months	7.8%	33%	NR
	Key findings:	0–3 months:				
		• EQ-5D VASC score similar				
		• SF-36 PCS slightly decreased				
		• SF-36 MCS similar				
		3–12 months:				
		• EQ-5D VASC score superior to preoperatively				
		• SF-36 PCS slightly improved compared to 0–3 months				
		• SF-36 MCS slightly worse compared to 0–3 months				
		12–24 months:				
		• EQ-5D VASC score plateaus and remains superior to preoperatively				
		• SF-36 PCS continues to improve but still slightly worse than preoperatively				
		• SF-36 MCS becomes similar to preoperatively				
EVAR-1 [56] 2005		EVAR	Pre-op, 0–3 months, 3–12 months, 12–24 months	EVAR: 1.7%	EVAR: 35%	EVAR: 58%
		Open AAA repair		Open AAA repair: 4.7%	Open AAA repair: 8%	Open AAA repair: 58%
	Key findings:	EQ-5D VASC and SF-36 scores similar across all time points after EVAR				
		After open AAA repair, physical health and EQ-5D VASC score decreased at 0–3 months, but returned to baseline afterwards				
		Physical health domains worse at 0–3 months for open AAA repair compared to EVAR, but results similar by 12–24 months				
Soulez [57] 2005		EVAR	Pre-op, 1 month, 3 months, 6 months, 12 months, 24 months	EVAR: 0%	EVAR: NR	EVAR: NR
		Open AAA repair		Open AAA repair: 0%	Open AAA repair: NR	Open AAA repair: NR
	Key findings:	No difference between open AAA repair and EVAR groups at all time points on SF-36 and Karnofsky score				
		Initial decline in SF-36 scores at 1 month, returned to baseline at 3 months				
		QOL maintained more after open surgery than EVAR at 2 years				
Vogel [58] 2005		EVAR	Pre-op, 0–3 months, 3–12 months	EVAR: 0%	EVAR: NR	EVAR: NR
		Open AAA repair		Open AAA repair: 3.2%	Open AAA repair: NR	Open AAA repair: NR
	Key findings:	Physical and mental health scores significantly better after EVAR compared to open AAA repair at 3 months. No difference after 6 months				
		Decrease in pre-op QOL at 3 months in both EVAR and open AAA repair, but all return to baseline				
Aljabri [59] 2006		EVAR	Pre-op, 1 week, 6 months	0%	30.2%	91%
	Key findings:	QOL deteriorates at 1 week and 1 month after both EVAR and open AAA repair. QOL returns to baseline at 6 months				
		Significant decrease in average SF-36 score at 1-week post-operatively, but by 6 months returns to baseline				
		QOL improves sooner after EVAR, but mean SF-36 score better after open AAA repair compared to EVAR at 6 months				

Table 15.2 (continued)

Original studies—abdominal aorta						
Author / **Year**		**Procedure**	**Follow-up time**	**Perioperative mortality**	**Major perioperative complications**	**Survival at time of QOL assessment**
Dick [60]		EVAR	58 ± 24 months	EVAR: 4.4%	EVAR: NR	EVAR: 72.1%
2008		Elective OR		Elective OR: 0.4%	Elective OR: NR	Elective OR: 79%
		Emergency OR		Emergency OR: 10.1%	Emergency OR: NR	Emergency OR: 77.5%
	Key findings:	All groups have good long-term QOL and all similar				
		All groups have similar QOL to a general population				
Lederle [18]		EVAR	Pre-op, 1 year, 2 years	EVAR: 0.5%	EVAR: 4.1%	EVAR: 93%
2009		Open AAA repair		Open AAA repair: 3%	Open AAA repair: 4.6%	Open AAA repair: 90%
	Key findings:	SF-36 and EQ-5D VASC scores are maintained 1 and 2 years, with similar levels to baseline in both mental and physical health				
		No significant difference between EVAR and open AAA repair				
Kurz [61]		EVAR	Median 34 months	<80 years old: 0%	<80 years old: NR	<80 years old: 100%
2010				>80 years old: 0%	>80 years old: NR	>80 years old: 92%
	Key findings:	Patients >80 years old have similar postoperative scores in pain, sleep, emotional reaction, energy, and social isolation domains compared to patients <80 years old				
		Physical abilities were significant worse in those >80 years old				
DeRango [62] 2011		EVAR	Pre-op, 6 months, >1 year	0.6%	3.4%	85.5%
	Key findings:	At 6 months, mean SF-36 scores increased in EVAR group, but stayed the same in surveillance group				
		Physical domains worsened in surveillance group at 6 months				
		Mental health domains improved in EVAR group at 6 months				
		At >1 year, both mental health and physical health domains were worse compared to baseline after EVAR or surveillance				
		EVAR had better physical and mental health domains at 6 months compared to surveillance, but similar at 1 year				
Kisis [63]		EVAR	Pre-op, 1 month, 1 year	EVAR: 0%	EVAR: NR	EVAR: NR
2012		Open AAA repair		Open AAA repair: 0%	Open AAA repair: NR	Open AAA repair: NR
	Key findings:	At 1 month, almost all SF-36 domains better in EVAR group compared to open repair group				
		At 1 year, mainly physical health domains better in EVAR group compared to open repair				
		After EVAR, PCS and MCS remains similar at 1 month and 1 year.				
		After open repair, PCS and MCS deteriorate 1 month, and are almost back to baseline at 1 year				
Lederle [12]		EVAR	Pre-op, 1 month, 6 months, 12 months, yearly to 8 years	EVAR: 0%	EVAR: 4.1%	EVAR: 67.1%
2012		Open AAA repair		Open AAA repair: 3.0%	Open AAA repair: 4.6%	Open AAA repair: 66.6%
	Key findings:	No significant difference between EVAR and open AAA repair groups at all time points in SF-36 PCS and EQ-5D VASC scores				
		Age related decline in QOL over long term follow-up in all domains				
		SF-36 MCS maintained up to 6 years. Open repair appears more durable than EVAR				

(continued)

Table 15.2 (continued)

Original studies—abdominal aorta						
Author / **Year**		**Procedure**	**Follow-up time**	**Perioperative mortality**	**Major perioperative complications**	**Survival at time of QOL assessment**
Pol [64] / 2012		EVAR	Pre-op, discharge, 30-days	<80 years old: 1.3%	<80 years old: 3.7%	<80 years old: 98.7%
				>80 years old: 1.5%	>80 years old: 5.5%	>80 years old: 98.5%
	Key findings:	Patients >80 years old have worse scores in all EQ-5D VASC domains of mobility, self-care, usual activities, pain, and anxiety/depression at discharge				
		Mental health is similar or better at discharge in both groups				
		At 30 days, mobility, self-care and usual activities are improving, but still less than baseline. Pain and anxiety/depression are similar or slightly better				
		Patients >80 years of age recover slower than younger patients in all health domains, with worse mobility, self-care and usual activities, and similar pain and anxiety/depression				
		No difference in overall health state between age groups				
AJAX [65] / 2014		EVAR	30 days, 3 months, 6 months	EVAR: 21%	EVAR: 32%	EVAR: 72%
		Open AAA repair		Open AAA repair: 25%	Open AAA repair: 37%	Open AAA repair: 69%
	Key findings:	No difference between EVAR or open AAA repair after rupture on SF-36 and EQ-5D VASC				
Pol [67] / 2014		EVAR	Pre-op, discharge, 1 year	<80 years old: 0%	<80 years old: 9.9%	<80 years old: 93.8%
				>80 years old: 0%	>80 years old: 16.3%	>80 years old: 88.3%
	Key findings:	Patients >80 years old did not have significant change in EQ-5D VASC index scores at discharge and 1 year postoperatively				
		Mobility, self-care, usual activities, and pain/discomfort scores were worse at discharge and improved by 1 year to almost baseline				
		Anxiety/depression score was improved at discharge and sustained to 1 year.				
		After 1 year, patients >80 years old still experience problems with mobility, self-care and usual activity compared to younger patients, with a slower recovery				
		Overall health care perception was worse in elderly patients at 1 year, but EQ-5D VASC index was similar				
De Bruin [68] / 2016		EVAR	Pre-op, 3 weeks, 6 weeks, 3 months, 6 months, 12 months, every 6 months to 60 months	EVAR: 1.2%	EVAR: 3.5%	EVAR: NR
		Open AAA repair		Open AAA repair: 4.6%	Open AAA repair: 10.9%	Open AAA repair: NR
	Key findings:	Initial postoperative decline in QOL after both EVAR and open AAA repair, worse after open repair				
		Physical functioning better with EVAR in first 6 weeks				
		QOL after both EVAR and open AAA repair returns to baseline between 6 weeks and 3 months				
		After 3 months, open AAA repair is superior to EVAR especially in mental health domains				
		QOL is maintained in both groups after initial decline				
Peach [69] / 2016		EVAR	Pre-op, 6 weeks, 3 months, 6 months, 12 months, >12 months	NR	NR	NR

Table 15.2 (continued)

Original studies—abdominal aorta

Author Year		Procedure	Follow-up time	Perioperative mortality	Major perioperative complications	Survival at time of QOL assessment
	Key findings:	AneurysmDQOL:				
		• Trend to worse QOL by 12 months, but after 12 months is superior to baseline, but not statistically significant				
		• Friend/social life, doing things for others, household tasks, overall health, feelings about the future and physical discomfort are greatest contributors to negative QOL				
		AneurysmSRQ:				
		• Similar level of symptoms at 6 months				
		• Fewer symptoms at 12 months				
		• After 12 months symptoms become more prevalent to affect QOL				
		AneurysmTSQ:				
		• At 6 months, <10% patients report dissatisfaction				
		• At 12 months, 15% patients report length of stay or side effects causing dissatisfaction				
		• After 12 months, >15% had dissatisfaction due to scan results and 10% were dissatisfied due to need for long-term follow-up				
		Symptoms became progressively worse after EVAR, whereas impact on QOL was worse after open AAA repair				
IMPROVE [25]		EVAR	0–36 months	EVAR: 35.4%	EVAR: NR	EVAR: 43%
2017		Open AAA repair		Open AAA repair: 37.4%	Open AAA repair: NR	Open AAA repair: 38%
	Key findings:	Average EQ-5D VASC scores better after EVAR in the first year, but by 3 years similar in both groups				
Kato [70]		EVAR	Pre-op, 1 month, 6 months, 12 months	EVAR: 0%	EVAR: 12%	EVAR: 96%
2017		Open AAA repair		Open AAA repair: 0%	Open AAA repair: 0%	Open AAA repair: 100%
	Key findings:	After EVAR, PCS worsened at 1 month, but was continually improving after until 12 months. MCS improves steadily until 12 months.				
		After open AAA repair, PCS and MCS decreased 1 month and gradually improved 3–6 months				
		Minimal difference in all domains when comparing EVAR and open AAA repair				
Yildirim [71]		EVAR	46 months	EVAR: 20%	EVAR: 64%	EVAR: NR
2017		Open AAA repair		Open AAA repair: 34.7%	Open AAA repair: 72%	Open AAA repair: NR
	Key findings:	Physical functioning, mental health, role emotional similar to general population in both groups				
		At long-term follow-up open AAA repair has either a significant or trend towards superior QOL in all domains compared to EVAR				
Akbulut [72]		EVAR	30 ± 20 months	EVAR: NR	EVAR: NR	EVAR: 71%
2018		Open AAA repair		Open AAA repair: NR	Open AAA repair: NR	Open AAA repair: 87%
	Key findings:	At 1 month, EVAR group had better SF-36 scores in all domains compared to open AAA repair. No difference at 6 and 12 months				
		EVAR patients maintained their QOL from 1 month onwards, whereas open AAA repair patients took longer to regain preoperative levels				

(continued)

Table 15.2 (continued)

Original studies—thoracic aorta						
Author / **Year**		**Procedure**	**Follow-up time**	**Perioperative mortality**	**Major perioperative complications**	**Survival at time of QOL assessment**
Dick [73]		TEVAR	34 ± 18 months	TEVAR: 8%	TEVAR: NR	TEVAR: 73%
2008		Open thoracic repair		Open thoracic repair: 9%	Open thoracic repair: NR	Open thoracic repair: 83%
	Key findings:	No difference between TEVAR and open repair in all SF-36 domains and on HADS				
		Overall physical and mental health domains similar to general population after open repair				
		PF, RP, VT worse after TEVAR compared to general population, but other domains similar				
Dick [74]		Emergency TEVAR	27–31 months	Emergency TEVAR: 12%	Emergency TEVAR: NR	Emergency TEVAR: 70%
2009		Elective TEVAR		Elective TEVAR: 4%	Elective TEVAR: NR	Elective TEVAR: 72%
	Key findings:	SF-36 scores similar after emergency and elective TEVAR				
		QOL is worse in both groups compared to a general population				
		Mental health on SF-36 and HADS score similar to general population				
Klocker [66] / 2014		TEVAR	4 ± 4 months	NR	NR	57%
	Key findings:	Patency of the left subclavian artery does not affect SF-36 PCS and MCS				
		Overall traumatic aortic injury patients had better SF-36 scores compared to other indications				
McBride [75] / 2015		TEVAR	3.5 ± 2 years	1.2%	NR	93%
	Key findings:	Left subclavian artery coverage didn't affect PCS, but MCS better after coverage				
		Left upper limb extremity symptoms and ability to return to activities same between both groups				
Meltzer [76] / 2017		Endovascular repair TAAA	Pre-op, 1 month, 6 months, 12 months	4.5%	NR	NR
	Key findings:	PCS and MCS scores as well as 6 out of 8 domains individual domains worse at 1 month, but by 6 months all domains returned to baseline levels				
		Patients with complications had worse PCS and MCS				
Bi [77] / 2018		TEVAR	0–4 months, 27 ± 7 months	2.5%	NR	95%
	Key findings:	Physical health domains had significant improvements at the first follow-up, and was maintained until the second follow-up at levels better than baseline				
		Mental health domains were preserved throughout follow-up				
Reviews						
Peach [46]	Key findings:	QOL deteriorates in the first few weeks after both EVAR and open AAA repair. QOL returns to baseline at 4 weeks after EVAR and takes longer after open AAA repair. By 2–3 months QOL has returned to baseline				
2012		QOL continues to be similar or better than baseline at 4–6 months				
		No significant difference between EVAR and open AAA repair after this point				
		Open AAA repair may have a more durable effect with longer term follow-up				
Coughlin [43]	Key findings:	Significant deterioration in SF-36 PCS at 12 months after both EVAR and open AAA repair compared to baseline				
2013		MCS starts to recover by 3 months, and returns to baseline at 12 months in both groups				
		No difference between EVAR and open AAA repair groups on PCS or MCS				

Table 15.2 (continued)

Original studies—thoracic aorta						
Author					**Major**	**Survival at**
Year		**Procedure**	**Follow-up time**	**Perioperative mortality**	**perioperative complications**	**time of QOL assessment**
Propper [47]	Key findings:	QOL declines initially after both EVAR and open AAA repair				
2013		Recovery is more rapid after EVAR				
		Longer term durability of QOL better after open AAA repair compared to EVAR				
Kayssi [45]	Key findings:	SF-36 general health scores higher for EVAR at 3, 6, and 12 months postoperatively.				
2015		SF-36 physical functioning scores higher for EVAR at 6 months, not at 12 months				
		SF-36 social functioning scores higher for EVAR at 12 months				
		SF-36 PCS and MCS not significantly different				
		EVAR has better EQ-5D VASC score at 3, 6, and 12 months, but not at 24 months of follow-up				
Jarral [44]	Key findings:	Minimal data				
2016		No clear difference in QOL between TEVAR and open repair				
Badger [23]	Key findings:	Not enough studies to draw conclusion on QOL				
2017						
Shan [36]	Key findings:	QOL declines in the early postoperative period after EVAR in elderly patients				
2019		Physical health and function take up to 3 months to return to baseline				
		Mental health domains experience improvement as early as 4–6 weeks				
		Physical health domains recover slower than younger patients				
		Excellent patient satisfaction				

NR not recorded, *AAA* abdominal aortic aneurysm, *QOL* quality of life, *AneurysmDQOL* aneurysm-dependent QOL questionnaire, *AneurysmSRQ* aneurysm symptom rating questionnaire, *Aneurysm TSQ* aneurysm treatment satisfaction questionnaire, *SF-36* medical outcomes 36-item short-form health survey, *SF-12* medical outcomes 12-item short-form health survey, *NHP* Nottingham health profile, *EQ-5D VASC* EuroQOL 5-dimensions; *QOL* quality of life, *PCS* physical component summary, *MCS* mental health component summary, *OR* open AAA repair; *EVAR* endovascular AAA repair

after EVAR in elderly patients have been shown to be worse compared to younger patients as is expected, but this increased risk is thought to be acceptable given the prolongation of life [78]. A recent review describes maintained QOL outcomes after EVAR and open AAA repair in patients older than 75 years of age [36]. There is an expected postoperative decline in QOL after EVAR, with rapid recovery of mental health domains by 4–6 weeks. Physical health domains take longer to recover at up to 3 months. Importantly, patient are able to achieve and maintain their preoperative QOL up to at least 1 year.

Thoracic Aorta (Five Studies) [73–77]

Evidence on TEVAR in thoracic aortic pathology is very limited and in general poorly reported. Four studies did not report on or differentiate between elective and emergency intervention [73, 74, 76, 77], two studies mixed aneurysmal disease and dissection [73, 74], two studies reported early outcomes [76, 77], and only one study had specific follow-up time points [76]. These are significant issues that make interpretation of QOL outcomes difficult.

Physical and mental health domains appear to be preserved at follow-up of up to 2 years after an initial decline in physical health domains, presumably due to postoperative recovery. One study suggests there may even be an improvement in physical health domains. At follow-up of up to 3 years, QOL is similar after elective or emergent TEVAR and also similar between TEVAR and open repair. Though overall QOL is reported to be worse compared to the general population, mental health may be similar. In contrast, the literature reports patients with chronic untreated TBAD have a similar overall QOL and functional status as a normal population [79]. One should not interpret this as a negative outcome of TEVAR because those who are medically treated generally have increased risk of long-term aortic related morbidity and mortality. In addition, those who are untreated have a worse perception of their own health due to the anxiety of untreated disease [79, 80].

Utility of Quality of Life Tools

Importance of Quality of Life Assessment and PROMS

QOL and PROMS have become more important in aortic intervention because there is an increasing understanding about the differences between the needs of patient and patient-centred outcomes as opposed to what surgeons perceive as important [81].

A recent review by the Australian Commission on Safety and Quality in Health Care has identified some key aspects of PROMS and QOL [33]. QOL and PROMS are used because patients are the best judges of the effect on their QOL and function. This allows a patient centered model of care and helps improve the quality and safety of various treatments. The effectiveness of different treatments can therefore be more accurately determined.

It is only recently that QOL outcomes have been formally reviewed [23, 36, 43–47]. The primary purpose of any aortic intervention for aneurysms or dissection is to prevent aortic-related mortality. While the technical outcomes of intervention are important, this still needs to be balanced against the postoperative QOL the patient is likely to experience. This is especially important with prophylactic aortic procedures where the patient may be asymptomatic prior to intervention. For example, if intervention achieved the aim of prolonging life, it may not have been worthwhile if as a result of the procedure the patient was bedridden and requiring full time nursing home care. In contrast, diseases which cause consistent symptoms are much more likely to derive significant improvement in QOL from intervention. Therefore, it is a positive outcome if baseline QOL is achieved and maintained after intervention, in addition to the survival benefit. This is largely supported by studies on EVAR. In particular, QOL should not necessarily be expected to improve after revascularisation, particularly for previously asymptomatic patients. When aneurysms are ruptured, intervention is a life or death decision. In these patients, QOL is a less important immediate consideration, but is an important long-term outcome indicator.

Need for Further Research

There are several key issues identified from previous QOL studies that should be addressed in future studies.

Firstly, there is an obvious lack of evidence on QOL outcomes after TEVAR and any complex endovascular intervention on the thoracic, abdominal, or thoracoabdominal aorta. These are procedures that are increasingly performed and becoming mainstream. There are also specific stent technologies, graft types and adjuncts to improve procedural success in specific anatomical set ups. However, the impact of these on QOL outcomes have not been investigated.

Secondly, there is a clear lack of evidence on the use of currently available QOL and PROM instruments in aortic intervention. It is only recently that disease-specific aortic QOL instruments are being developed [69, 82]. Further work is required as previously utilised QOL instruments are not necessarily validated for use in aortic pathology and intervention [83]. Aortic-specific QOL instruments would provide useful measures of change in QOL [35], with the ultimate goal of only using validated instruments for aortic intervention.

Thirdly, there needs to be a standardised set of results that are reported to facilitate objective assessment with meta-analyses. Ideally a standardised common instrument should be used by all studies. QOL data should be expressed as mean ± standard deviation and results given at pre-determined follow-up time points including baseline and final follow-up, rather than a range or median of variable follow-up time points.

Fourthly, there was a relatively low response rate in previously conducted studies. High response rates are compulsory to minimise bias.

Finally, the factors that influence QOL outcomes needs to be explored. In particular, the effect of comorbidities, frailty and disability on QOL outcomes is underappreciated. The burden of comorbidities is a risk factor for frailty, which in turn predisposes to disability [84]. This is because frailty causes decreased reserve and less ability to deal with adverse outcomes [84]. Comorbidities, frailty and disability are therefore separate entities. They are important because they are increasingly prevalent with an ageing population, who are increasingly offered intervention. In addition, procedural outcomes such as endoleak and the need for reintervention are important. This is the Achilles heel of endovascular intervention for aortic aneurysms and their effect on QOL is still to be elucidated.

With implementation of these guidelines, important and clinically relevant information would be obtained. This information provides improved patient-focused outcomes data which facilitates improved quality of care to patients and more accurate analysis of the effectiveness of an intervention. In addition, perhaps the greatest benefit will be its use in policy making, cost-effectiveness analysis, and ultimately resource allocation.

The logistical challenges remain in the design of an instrument which is simple and thorough enough for patients to participate in, as well as the data collection which needs to be consistent and accurate without significant loss to follow-up. QOL after aortic intervention can also be easily overlooked especially where the procedure in performed in an emergent setting. The importance of this aspect of treatment is often underestimated as the traditional teaching heavily emphasises the importance of technical outcomes as the marker of treatment success. Changing this paradigm will take time and efforts to educate the health sector before it becomes part of routine practice.

Effect of Other Outcomes on Quality of Life and Proms

In order assess the relevance of QOL outcomes, the reported morbidity and mortality in the studies that report QOL should be known. Any patients who do not participate in QOL assessment or are lost to follow-up are more likely to have a worse QOL due to a greater burden of comorbidities and physical impairments [36, 85]. Post-operative complications and death will result in incomplete follow-up. According to previous guidelines, a response rate of >85% (loss to follow-up <15%) is considered ideal [86]. This response rate is only reported or achieved in eight studies in the literature [12, 49, 52, 54, 56, 60, 63, 77]. Described QOL outcomes may be overestimated. It is therefore important to assess the both the response rates to identify risk of bias, and also the technical outcomes to put the QOL outcomes into perspective.

Statistical techniques to deal with missing data have been developed to resolve issues such as mentioned above. This includes multiple imputation which is a statistical method of dealing with missing data by combining the results of several different possible data sets [87]. There are particular biases that occur as a result of the missing data, depending on the reason why the data is missing. Multiple imputation may be helpful in both epidemiological studies and randomised controlled trials, but there are potential pitfalls that warrant input from a statistician [87, 88]. Future studies may benefit from incorporation of this technique.

The reported mortality rates after elective and ruptured EVAR are 0–8.8% (mostly <5%) [12, 16, 18, 48–64, 67, 68, 70] and 20–35.4% [25, 65, 71], respectively. These are greater than expected with contemporary practice in high volume centres, especially for elective intervention. This suggests that QOL outcomes could be even better than reported where perioperative complications are lower. After endovascular intervention on the thoracic aorta, mortality ranges from 4% to 12%, though with poor differentiation between elective and emergency procedures and the pathology involved [73–77].

Fig. 15.1 Conclusions

Conclusions

1. QOL and PROMS are critical in contemporary outcomes assessment after endovascular aortic aneurysm repair.
2. EVAR patients can expect to have positive QOL outcomes in the short to medium term.
3. Evidence is greatly limited in TEVAR and complex endovascular aneurysm repair.
4. Future studies are needed to improve methods of QOL assessment and evaluate factors that affect QOL outcomes.

Fifteen studies reported total major complication rates after EVAR [12, 16, 18, 50, 51, 53, 56, 59, 62, 64, 65, 67, 68, 70, 71]. However, the range is variable (0–64%) because the definition of major complications varies. No studies report total morbidity rates after endovascular interventions on the thoracic aorta. Overall, the effect of perioperative morbidity and complications on QOL outcomes and PROMS remains unclear. Given the relatively low incidence of complications in experienced centres, it may not be possible to demonstrate a statistically significant impact. However, clinically it would be prudent to avoid complications which have adverse impacts on both QOL and the cost-effectiveness of the procedure.

Conclusion

QOL and PROMS are the new frontier of outcomes assessment after endovascular aortic intervention (Fig. 15.1). Currently available evidence demonstrates that EVAR patients can expect to have positive QOL outcomes in the short to medium term, especially in the elective setting. It is clear that evidence is greatly limited in TEVAR. Furthermore, there is little to no evidence on QOL after more complex endovascular interventions on either the thoracic, abdominal, or thoracoabdominal aorta. There is a need for more investment in this field with further research conducted with suggestions provided. This information provides improved patient-focused outcomes data which facilitates improved quality of care to patients and more accurate analysis of the effectiveness of an intervention. In addition, perhaps the greatest benefit will be its use in policy making, cost-effectiveness analysis, and ultimately resource allocation.

References

1. Cosford PA, Leng GC. Screening for abdominal aortic aneurysm. Cochrane Database Syst Rev. 2007;2:CD002945.
2. Vallabhaneni SR. Final follow-up of the Multicentre Aneurysm Screening Study (MASS) randomized trial of abdominal aortic aneurysm screening. Br J Surg. 2012;99(12):1649–56.
3. Ashton HA, Gao L, Kim LG, Druce PS, Thompson SG, Scott RA. Fifteen-year follow-up of a randomized clinical trial of ultrasonographic screening for abdominal aortic aneurysms. Br J Surg. 2007;94(6):696–701.
4. Forsdahl SH, Singh K, Solberg S, Jacobsen BK. Risk factors for abdominal aortic aneurysms: a 7-year prospective study: the Tromso Study, 1994-2001. Circulation. 2009;119(16):2202–8.
5. Lederle FA, Johnson GR, Wilson SE, Littooy FN, Krupski WC, Bandyk D, et al. Yield of repeated screening for abdominal aortic aneurysm after a 4-year interval. Aneurysm Detection and Management Veterans Affairs Cooperative Study Investigators. Arch Intern Med. 2000;160(8):1117–21.
6. Olsson C, Thelin S, Stahle E, Ekbom A, Granath F. Thoracic aortic aneurysm and dissection: increasing prevalence and improved outcomes reported in a nationwide population-based study of more than 14,000 cases from 1987 to 2002. Circulation. 2006;114(24):2611–8.
7. Isselbacher EM. Thoracic and abdominal aortic aneurysms. Circulation. 2005;111(6):816–28.
8. Clouse WD, Hallett JW Jr, Schaff HV, Spittell PC, Rowland CM, Ilstrup DM, et al. Acute aortic dissection: population-based incidence compared with degenerative aortic aneurysm rupture. Mayo Clin Proc. 2004;79(2):176–80.
9. Sidloff D, Stather P, Dattani N, Bown M, Thompson J, Sayers R, et al. Aneurysm global epidemiology study: public health measures can further reduce abdominal aortic aneurysm mortality. Circulation. 2014;129(7):747–53.

10. Adar R, Cohen E, Kreitler S. Carotid endarterectomy for symptom-free stenosis: the patient's point of view. Cardiovasc Surg. 1994;2(5):582–5.
11. De Bruin JL, Baas AF, Buth J, Prinssen M, Verhoeven EL, Cuypers PW, et al. Long-term outcome of open or endovascular repair of abdominal aortic aneurysm. N Engl J Med. 2010;362(20):1881–9.
12. Lederle FA, Freischlag JA, Kyriakides TC, Matsumura JS, Padberg FT Jr, Kohler TR, et al. Long-term comparison of endovascular and open repair of abdominal aortic aneurysm. N Engl J Med. 2012;367(21):1988–97.
13. Lederle FA, Kyriakides TC, Stroupe KT, Freischlag JA, Padberg FT Jr, Matsumura JS, et al. Open versus endovascular repair of abdominal aortic aneurysm. N Engl J Med. 2019;380(22):2126–35.
14. Prinssen M, Verhoeven EL, Buth J, Cuypers PW, van Sambeek MR, Balm R, et al. A randomized trial comparing conventional and endovascular repair of abdominal aortic aneurysms. N Engl J Med. 2004;351(16):1607–18.
15. Greenhalgh RM, Brown LC, Kwong GP, Powell JT, Thompson SG, EVAR trial participants. Comparison of endovascular aneurysm repair with open repair in patients with abdominal aortic aneurysm (EVAR trial 1), 30-day operative mortality results: randomised controlled trial. Lancet. 2004;364(9437):843–8.
16. EVAR trial participants. Endovascular aneurysm repair and outcome in patients unfit for open repair of abdominal aortic aneurysm (EVAR trial 2): randomised controlled trial. Lancet. 2005;365(9478):2187–92.
17. Lovegrove RE, Javid M, Magee TR, Galland RB. A meta-analysis of 21,178 patients undergoing open or endovascular repair of abdominal aortic aneurysm. Br J Surg. 2008;95(6):677–84.
18. Lederle FA, Freischlag JA, Kyriakides TC, Padberg FT Jr, Matsumura JS, Kohler TR, et al. Outcomes following endovascular vs open repair of abdominal aortic aneurysm: a randomized trial. JAMA. 2009;302(14):1535–42.
19. Li B, Khan S, Salata K, Hussain MA, de Mestral C, Greco E, et al. A systematic review and meta-analysis of the long-term outcomes of endovascular versus open repair of abdominal aortic aneurysm. J Vasc Surg. 2019;70(3):954–69 e30.
20. Reimerink JJ, Hoornweg LL, Vahl AC, Wisselink W, van den Broek TA, Legemate DA, et al. Endovascular repair versus open repair of ruptured abdominal aortic aneurysms: a multicenter randomized controlled trial. Ann Surg. 2013;258(2):248–56.
21. Investigators IT, Powell JT, Sweeting MJ, Thompson MM, Ashleigh R, Bell R, et al. Endovascular or open repair strategy for ruptured abdominal aortic aneurysm: 30 day outcomes from IMPROVE randomised trial. BMJ. 2014;348:f7661.
22. Desgranges P, Kobeiter H, Katsahian S, Bouffi M, Gouny P, Favre JP, et al. Editor's choice - ECAR (Endovasculaire ou Chirurgie dans les Anevrysmes aorto-iliaques Rompus): a French randomized controlled trial of endovascular versus open surgical repair of ruptured aorto-iliac aneurysms. Eur J Vasc Endovasc Surg. 2015;50(3):303–10.
23. Badger S, Forster R, Blair PH, Ellis P, Kee F, Harkin DW. Endovascular treatment for ruptured abdominal aortic aneurysm. Cochrane Database Syst Rev. 2017;5:CD005261.
24. Sweeting MJ, Balm R, Desgranges P, Ulug P, Powell JT, Ruptured Aneurysm Trialists. Individual-patient meta-analysis of three randomized trials comparing endovascular versus open repair for ruptured abdominal aortic aneurysm. Br J Surg. 2015;102(10):1229–39.
25. Investigators IT. Comparative clinical effectiveness and cost effectiveness of endovascular strategy v open repair for ruptured abdominal aortic aneurysm: three year results of the IMPROVE randomised trial. BMJ. 2017;359:j4859.
26. Abraha I, Romagnoli C, Montedori A, Cirocchi R. Thoracic stent graft versus surgery for thoracic aneurysm. Cochrane Database Syst Rev. 2016;6:CD006796.
27. Alsawas M, Zaiem F, Larrea-Mantilla L, Almasri J, Erwin PJ, Upchurch GR Jr, et al. Effectiveness of surgical interventions for thoracic aortic aneurysms: a systematic review and meta-analysis. J Vasc Surg. 2017;66(4):1258–68 e8.
28. Rocha RV, Friedrich JO, Elbatarny M, Yanagawa B, Al-Omran M, Forbes TL, et al. A systematic review and meta-analysis of early outcomes after endovascular versus open repair of thoracoabdominal aortic aneurysms. J Vasc Surg. 2018;68(6):1936–45 e5.
29. Brunkwall J, Kasprzak P, Verhoeven E, Heijmen R, Taylor P, Trialists A, et al. Endovascular repair of acute uncomplicated aortic type B dissection promotes aortic remodelling: 1 year results of the ADSORB trial. Eur J Vasc Endovasc Surg. 2014;48(3):285–91.
30. Brunkwall J, Lammer J, Verhoeven E, Taylor P. ADSORB: a study on the efficacy of endovascular grafting in uncomplicated acute dissection of the descending aorta. Eur J Vasc Endovasc Surg. 2012;44(1):31–6.
31. Nienaber CA, Rousseau H, Eggebrecht H, Kische S, Fattori R, Rehders TC, et al. Randomized comparison of strategies for type B aortic dissection: the INvestigation of STEnt Grafts in Aortic Dissection (INSTEAD) trial. Circulation. 2009;120(25):2519–28.
32. Nienaber CA, Kische S, Rousseau H, Eggebrecht H, Rehders TC, Kundt G, et al. Endovascular repair of type B aortic dissection: long-term results of the randomized investigation of stent grafts in aortic dissection trial. Circ Cardiovasc Interv. 2013;6(4):407–16.
33. Williams KSJ, Morris D, Grootemaat P, Thompson C. Patient-reported outcome measures: literature review. Sydney, NSW: Healthcare ACoSaQi; 2016.
34. Testa MA, Simonson DC. Assessment of quality-of-life outcomes. N Engl J Med. 1996;334(13):835–40.
35. Urbach DR. Measuring quality of life after surgery. Surg Innov. 2005;12(2):161–5.
36. Shan L, Saxena A, Goh D, Robinson D. A systematic review on the quality of life and functional status after abdominal aortic aneurysm repair in elderly patients

with an average age older than 75 years. J Vasc Surg. 2019;69(4):1268–81.
37. Machin M, Ulug P, Pandirajan K, Bown MJ, Powell JT. Towards a core outcome set for abdominal aortic aneurysm: systematic review of outcomes reported following intact and ruptured abdominal aortic aneurysm repair. Eur J Vasc Endovasc Surg. 2021;61(6):909–18.
38. Peach G, Romaine J, Holt PJ, Thompson MM, Bradley C, Hinchliffe RJ. Quality of life, symptoms and treatment satisfaction in patients with aortic aneurysm using new abdominal aortic aneurysm-specific patient-reported outcome measures. Br J Surg. 2016;103(8):1012–9.
39. Ware JE Jr, Sherbourne CD. The MOS 36-item short-form health survey (SF-36). I. Conceptual framework and item selection. Med Care. 1992;30(6):473–83.
40. Lewis G, Wessely S. Comparison of the general health questionnaire and the hospital anxiety and depression scale. Br J Psychiatry. 1990;157:860–4.
41. WHO. WHOQOL-BREF. Geneva: WHO; 1996. https://www.who.int/mental_health/publications/whoqol/en/.
42. Wiklund I. The Nottingham Health Profile--a measure of health-related quality of life. Scand J Prim Health Care Suppl. 1990;1:15–8.
43. Coughlin PA, Jackson D, White AD, Bailey MA, Farrow C, Scott DJ, et al. Meta-analysis of prospective trials determining the short- and mid-term effect of elective open and endovascular repair of abdominal aortic aneurysms on quality of life. Br J Surg. 2013;100(4):448–55.
44. Jarral OA, Kidher E, Patel VM, Nguyen B, Pepper J, Athanasiou T. Quality of life after intervention on the thoracic aorta. Eur J Cardiothorac Surg. 2016;49(2):369–89.
45. Kayssi A, DeBord Smith A, Roche-Nagle G, Nguyen LL. Health-related quality-of-life outcomes after open versus endovascular abdominal aortic aneurysm repair. J Vasc Surg. 2015;62(2):491–8.
46. Peach G, Holt P, Loftus I, Thompson MM, Hinchliffe R. Questions remain about quality of life after abdominal aortic aneurysm repair. J Vasc Surg. 2012;56(2):520–7.
47. Propper BW, Abularrage CJ. Long-term safety and efficacy of endovascular abdominal aortic aneurysm repair. Vasc Health Risk Manag. 2013;9:135–41.
48. Lloyd AJ, Boyle J, Bell PR, Thompson MM. Comparison of cognitive function and quality of life after endovascular or conventional aortic aneurysm repair. Br J Surg. 2000;87(4):443–7.
49. Malina M, Nilsson M, Brunkwall J, Ivancev K, Resch T, Lindblad B. Quality of life before and after endovascular and open repair of asymptomatic AAAs: a prospective study. J Endovasc Ther. 2000;7(5):372–9.
50. Aquino RV, Jones MA, Zullo TG, Missig-Carroll N, Makaroun MS. Quality of life assessment in patients undergoing endovascular or conventional AAA repair. J Endovasc Ther. 2001;8(5):521–8.
51. Arko FR, Hill BB, Reeves TR, Olcott C, Harris EJ, Fogarty TJ, et al. Early and late functional outcome assessments following endovascular and open aneurysm repair. J Endovasc Ther. 2003;10(1):2–9.
52. Lederle FA, Johnson GR, Wilson SE, Acher CW, Ballard DJ, Littooy FN, et al. Quality of life, impotence, and activity level in a randomized trial of immediate repair versus surveillance of small abdominal aortic aneurysm. J Vasc Surg. 2003;38(4):745–52.
53. Ballard JL, Abou-Zamzam AM, Teruya TH, Bianchi C, Petersen FF. Quality of life before and after endovascular and retroperitoneal abdominal aortic aneurysm repair. J Vasc Surg. 2004;39(4):797–803.
54. Lottman PE, Laheij RJ, Cuypers PW, Bender M, Buth J. Health-related quality of life outcomes following elective open or endovascular AAA repair: a randomized controlled trial. J Endovasc Ther. 2004;11(3):323–9.
55. Prinssen M, Buskens E, Blankensteijn JD, DREAM trial participants. Quality of life endovascular and open AAA repair. Results of a randomised trial. Eur J Vasc Endovasc Surg. 2004;27(2):121–7.
56. EVAR trial participants. Endovascular aneurysm repair versus open repair in patients with abdominal aortic aneurysm (EVAR trial 1): randomised controlled trial. Lancet. 2005;365(9478):2179–86.
57. Soulez G, Therasse E, Monfared AA, Blair JF, Choiniere M, Elkouri S, et al. Pain and quality of life assessment after endovascular versus open repair of abdominal aortic aneurysms in patients at low risk. J Vasc Interv Radiol. 2005;16(8):1093–100.
58. Vogel TR, Nackman GB, Crowley JG, Bueno MM, Banavage A, Odroniec K, et al. Factors impacting functional health and resource utilization following abdominal aortic aneurysm repair by open and endovascular techniques. Ann Vasc Surg. 2005;19(5):641–7.
59. Aljabri B, Al Wahaibi K, Abner D, Mackenzie KS, Corriveau MM, Obrand DI, et al. Patient-reported quality of life after abdominal aortic aneurysm surgery: a prospective comparison of endovascular and open repair. J Vasc Surg. 2006;44(6):1182–7.
60. Dick F, Grobety V, Immer FF, Do DD, Savolainen H, Carrel TP, et al. Outcome and quality of life in patients treated for abdominal aortic aneurysms: a single center experience. World J Surg. 2008;32(6):987–94.
61. Kurz M, Meier T, Pfammatter T, Amann-Vesti BR. Quality of life survey after endovascular abdominal aortic aneurysm repair in octogenarians. Int Angiol. 2010;29(3):249–54.
62. De Rango P, Verzini F, Parlani G, Cieri E, Romano L, Loschi D, et al. Quality of life in patients with small abdominal aortic aneurysm: the effect of early endovascular repair versus surveillance in the CAESAR trial. Eur J Vasc Endovasc Surg. 2011;41(3):324–31.
63. Kisis K, Krievins D, Naskovica K, Gedins M, Savlovskis J, Ezite N, et al. Quality of life after endovascular abdominal aortic aneurysm repair: nellix sac-anchoring endoprosthesis versus open surgery. Medicina. 2012;48(6):286–91.
64. Pol RA, Zeebregts CJ, van Sterkenburg SM, Reijnen MM, Investigators E. Thirty-day outcome and quality

of life after endovascular abdominal aortic aneurysm repair in octogenarians based on the Endurant Stent Graft Natural Selection Global Postmarket Registry (ENGAGE). J Vasc Surg. 2012;56(1):27–35.
65. Kapma MR, Dijksman LM, Reimerink JJ, de Groof AJ, Zeebregts CJ, Wisselink W, et al. Cost-effectiveness and cost-utility of endovascular versus open repair of ruptured abdominal aortic aneurysm in the Amsterdam Acute Aneurysm Trial. Br J Surg. 2014;101(3):208–15.
66. Klocker J, Koell A, Erlmeier M, Goebel G, Jaschke W, Fraedrich G. Ischemia and functional status of the left arm and quality of life after left subclavian artery coverage during stent grafting of thoracic aortic diseases. J Vasc Surg. 2014;60(1):64–9.
67. Pol RA, Zeebregts CJ, van Sterkenburg SM, Ferreira LM, Goktay Y, Reijnen MM, et al. Outcome and quality of life after endovascular abdominal aortic aneurysm repair in octogenarians. J Vasc Surg. 2014;60(2):308–17.
68. de Bruin JL, Groenwold RH, Baas AF, Brownrigg JR, Prinssen M, Grobbee DE, et al. Quality of life from a randomized trial of open and endovascular repair for abdominal aortic aneurysm. Br J Surg. 2016;103(8):995–1002.
69. Peach G, Romaine J, Wilson A, Holt PJ, Thompson MM, Hinchliffe RJ, et al. Design of new patient-reported outcome measures to assess quality of life, symptoms and treatment satisfaction in patients with abdominal aortic aneurysm. Br J Surg. 2016;103(8):1003–11.
70. Kato T, Tamaki M, Tsunekawa T, Motoji Y, Hirakawa A, Okawa Y, et al. Health-related quality of life prospectively evaluated by the 8-item short form after endovascular repair versus open surgery for abdominal aortic aneurysms. Heart Vessel. 2017;32(8):960–8.
71. Yildirim H, van Lammeren GW, Unlu C, van Dongen EP, van de Mortel RH, de Vries JP. Long-term outcome and quality of life after ruptured abdominal aortic aneurysm repair. Vascular. 2018;26:231.
72. Akbulut M, Aksoy E, Kara I, Cekmecelioglu D, Koksal C. Quality of life after open surgical versus endovascular repair of abdominal aortic aneurysms. Braz J Cardiovasc Surg. 2018;33(3):265–70.
73. Dick F, Hinder D, Immer FF, Hirzel C, Do DD, Carrel TP, et al. Outcome and quality of life after surgical and endovascular treatment of descending aortic lesions. Ann Thorac Surg. 2008;85(5):1605–12.
74. Dick F, Hinder D, Immer FF, Savolainen H, Do DD, Carrel TP, et al. Thoracic endovascular aortic repair: impact of urgency on outcome and quality of life. Eur J Cardiothorac Surg. 2009;35(1):96–103.
75. McBride CL, Dubose JJ, Miller CC III, Perlick AP, Charlton-Ouw KM, Estrera AL, et al. Intentional left subclavian artery coverage during thoracic endovascular aortic repair for traumatic aortic injury. J Vasc Surg. 2015;61(1):73–9.
76. Meltzer AJ, Connolly PH, Ellozy S, Schneider DB. Patient-reported quality of life after endovascular repair of thoracoabdominal aortic aneurysms. Ann Vasc Surg. 2017;44:164–70.
77. Bi Y, Chen H, Yu Z, Ren J, Han X. Clinical outcomes and quality of life in patients with Stanford type B aortic dissection after endovascular repair. Heart Surg Forum. 2018;21(5):E382–E6.
78. Han Y, Zhang S, Zhang J, Ji C, Eckstein HH. Outcomes of endovascular abdominal aortic aneurysm repair in octogenarians: meta-analysis and systematic review. Eur J Vasc Endovasc Surg. 2017;54(4):454–63.
79. Winnerkvist A, Brorsson B, Radegran K. Quality of life in patients with chronic type B aortic dissection. Eur J Vasc Endovasc Surg. 2006;32(1):34–7.
80. Chaddha A, Kline-Rogers E, Braverman AC, Erickson SR, Jackson EA, Franklin BA, et al. Survivors of aortic dissection: activity, mental health, and sexual function. Clin Cardiol. 2015;38(11):652–9.
81. Powell JT, Ambler GK, Svensjo S, Wanhainen A, Bown MJ. Beyond the AAA guidelines: core outcome sets to make life better for patients. Eur J Vasc Endovasc Surg. 2019;57(1):6–7.
82. Suckow BD, Schanzer AS, Hoel AW, Wyers M, Marone LK, Veeraswamy RK, et al. A novel quality of life instrument for patients with an abdominal aortic aneurysm. Eur J Vasc Endovasc Surg. 2019;57(6):809–15.
83. Duncan R, Essat M, Jones G, Booth A, Buckley Woods H, Poku E, et al. Systematic review and qualitative evidence synthesis of patient-reported outcome measures for abdominal aortic aneurysm. Br J Surg. 2017;104(4):317–27.
84. Fried LP, Tangen CM, Walston J, Newman AB, Hirsch C, Gottdiener J, et al. Frailty in older adults: evidence for a phenotype. J Gerontol A Biol Sci Med Sci. 2001;56(3):M146–56.
85. Shan L, Shan J, Saxena A, Robinson D. Quality of life and functional status after carotid revascularisation: a systematic review and meta-analysis. Eur J Vasc Endovasc Surg. 2015;49(6):634–45.
86. Wright RW, Brand RA, Dunn W, Spindler KP. How to write a systematic review. Clin Orthop Relat Res. 2007;455:23–9.
87. Sterne JA, White IR, Carlin JB, Spratt M, Royston P, Kenward MG, et al. Multiple imputation for missing data in epidemiological and clinical research: potential and pitfalls. BMJ. 2009;338:b2393.
88. Jakobsen JC, Gluud C, Wetterslev J, Winkel P. When and how should multiple imputation be used for handling missing data in randomised clinical trials - a practical guide with flowcharts. BMC Med Res Methodol. 2017;17(1):162.

16 QOL and PROMS in Catheter Ablation of Cardiac Arrhythmia

Kathleen L. Withers, Helen Morgan, and Mauro Lencioni

Introduction

Percutaneous ablation of cardiac arrhythmias is a relatively safe and effective method for the treatment of sustained and paroxysmal heart rhythm disorders. It has evolved from open heart excision surgery that was used 60 years ago to directly ablate the AV junction, via the use of focused high-voltage energy burns to produce scar tissue in the targeted region without damage to surrounding tissues and structures. The use of surgical cryoablation developed during the 1970s [1], and in 1981, the first successful catheter ablation was performed using DC ablation in a candidate who was unsuitable for surgical ablation, ultimately leading to a decision to treat him with a catheter ablation [2]. Despite earlier experimental work using radiofrequency ablation, it was not until the late 1980s that its safety and efficacy was established [2] with catheter cryoablation subsequently coming into use in the 2000s [3]. Over the last decade catheter ablation has been used increasingly to treat even complex arrhythmias, predominantly using radiofrequency and cryo-energy delivered through flexible catheters [4]. The success of these operations is highly dependent on the technical skill of the surgeon and experience in selecting patients that are likely to benefit from this treatment.

There are three broad categories of indications for catheter ablation: (1) definitive treatment of supraventricular tachycardia that includes nodal re-entrant, nodal dependant and focal arrhythmia substrates, (2) reduction in arrhythmia burden in symptomatic atrial fibrillation that is poorly controlled on anti-arrhythmic medication and (3) definitive treatment of ventricular tachycardia in normal hearts or in structural heart disease where medication has failed in the latter [5, 6]. Technological advances in the field of AF ablation over the last ten years have made this procedure feasible and this in term has driven demand. Currently in the UK, catheter ablation for atrial fibrillation (AF) accounts for approximately 50% of these procedures [7].

A number of new advances are currently being cited as potentially further improving management of patients with cardiac arrhythmias [8, 9], with strategies including electroporation (pulsed-field ablation), and ultra-low temperature cryoablation being investigated. While the benefits of ultra-low cryoablation are still awaited [10],

K. L. Withers (✉)
Cedar, Cardiff and Vale University Health Board, Cardiff Medicentre, Cardiff, UK
e-mail: Kathleen.withers@wales.nhs.uk

H. Morgan
Cedar, Cardiff University, Cardiff Medicentre, Cardiff, UK
e-mail: MorganHE1@cardiff.ac.uk

M. Lencioni
University Hospitals Birmingham NHS Foundation Trust, Birmingham, UK
e-mail: mauro.lencioni@uhb.nhs.uk

T. Athanasiou et al. (eds.), *Patient Reported Outcomes and Quality of Life in Cardiovascular Interventions*,
https://doi.org/10.1007/978-3-031-09815-4_16

studies using pulsed field ablation have shown it to be a safe and durable option [11]. However, quality of life outcomes have yet to be reported for this treatment strategy.

While atrial fibrillation is a major cause of stroke and heart failure [12], the vast majority of cardiac arrhythmias are not life threating but are responsible for considerable morbidity. Paroxysmal SVT's produce anxiety due to the unpredictable initiation of attacks and disabling symptoms during episodes of arrhythmia. Sustained arrhythmias manifest with chronic, less dramatic but equally disabling symptoms [13–15].

Treatment is thus aimed at symptom control rather than risk reduction [16] as supported by a number of recent guidelines [17–19]. Additionally it is well recognised that there is a strong link between cardiac arrhythmias and anxiety and depression [20, 21], further exacerbating the detrimental effect on quality of life in this patient group. It is therefore essential that treatment success is measured not only by objective parameters but also considers the patients view, as changes in symptoms and quality of life (QoL) are areas which are best assessed by patients themselves. Due to this, the use of Patient Reported Outcome Measures (PROMs) in patients with cardiac arrhythmias has grown significantly in recent years as their potential to measure effectiveness of care in this group has been recognised. This is reflected in the increasing support for their use both in routine use and in clinical trials, as illustrated by the recent international Task Force for quality indicators in atrial fibrillation publication which recommends their use, as developed with groups including the European Heart Rhythm Association (EHRA) of the European Society of Cardiology (ESC), the Heart Rhythm Society (HRS), the Asia Pacific Heart Rhythm Society (APHRS), and the Latin-American Heart Rhythm Society (LAHRS) [22]. Similarly, the International Consortium for Health Outcomes Measurement (ICHOM) atrial fibrillation group have developed a set of suggested outcome measures for use in patients with AF [23]. These include clinical and procedural outcomes such as complications and long term consequences of the disease as well as suggested PROMs tools and their timings.

PROM tools in combination with clinical assessment are ideal at assessing effectiveness of arrhythmia treatment. At the clinical level, both patient and operator are able to quantify baseline health and quality of life issues and to review treatment outcome, while published PROMs outcomes can allow patients to make informed decisions about treating centres. Clinicians are also able to use PROM data to refine their selection criteria, offering treatment to patients that are most likely to improve their QoL as well as setting patient treatment expectations. Aggregated PROM outcomes are useful at national level, used by commissioners to determine the value of the treatment and plan future investment. This is increasingly important as growing financial pressures on health service provision means it is essential that the care provided is both effective and economically efficient. Using PROMs in these varied ways can drive improvement in treatment quality and ultimately patient care.

As with other clinical areas, both generic PROMs tools and condition specific tools have been utilised to collect data from this patient group [5, 24, 25]. This chapter provides an overview of the tools which have been used to measure health related quality of life in studies involving patients treated with percutaneous catheter ablation in arrhythmia care.

Search Strategy

A literature search was performed using EMBASE (Ovid); Medline (Ovid) including Medline in Process and Medline Epub Ahead of Print; Scopus (Elsevier); and Web of Science (Science Citation Index). The search strategies used a range of free text terms and, where applicable, subject headings to describe cardiac arrhythmia, catheter ablation and tools used to measure quality of life and patient-reported-outcome measures in patients treated with catheter ablation. The Medline search strategy is available as supplementary material (Appendix). The search period was from 1st January 2010 to

18th December 2021 and limited to English language publications.

Inclusion and Exclusion Criteria

Studies in English which reported HRQoL in adults treated with catheter ablation for any cardiac arrhythmias were included. Studies involving surgical approaches such as Cox-Maze procedures and thorascopic ablation, and studies focusing on patients with implantable devices were excluded as these will be dealt with in other chapters. Studies where the primary diagnosis was not arrhythmia and those using experimental techniques were also excluded. Due to the large number of studies available, this review focuses on those studies reporting disaggregated health related quality of life data at baseline and post ablation only.

Data Extraction

Relevant articles were independently identified by two reviewers and conflicts discussed to reach agreement. Full texts were reviewed to identify whether they met the inclusion criteria. As for previous chapters the information extracted included the following: author and year of publication; study intent; total number of patients; age and gender of patients; length of follow up; instruments used and baseline and follow up patient reported outcome data.

Quality Scoring

A quality assessment of the included studies was not conducted for this overview.

Results

Selected Studies and Their Objectives

The literature search identified 718 studies. Where abstracts and full text publications were available, only the full text paper was selected. Where more than one full text manuscript was available from a single study, all were included as part of the review into factors impacting on quality of life, but data extraction was limited to one paper. Ultimately, 77 papers reporting on 74 studies were selected for review. Kloosterman et al. [26] and Picini et al. [27] both reported on the same study, as did Andrade et al., Samuel et al., and Yao et al. [28–30]. For expediency, where study details are reported below, only Kloosterman et al. [26] and Andrade et al. [28] will be referenced. The data extracted from all identified studies is available to view in Table 16.1.

The studies identified included a total of 20,118 patients with the largest study comprising 2008 patients and the smallest 31 patients. Where the time period was specified the included studies enrolled or followed up patients between the years 1999 and 2020. The majority (n = 38; 51.35%) of the studies were conducted in Europe, including 4 from the UK. Others originated from Asia (n = 15; 20.27%), and North America (n = 9; 12.16%), while a further 12 studies (16.22%) were inter-continental.

The included studies comprised twenty randomised trials [28, 36, 43, 57, 60–63, 65, 66, 74, 81, 84, 85, 88, 89, 93–96], and another six were studies of patients on clinical registries [32, 34, 50, 51, 55, 67]. There were four retrospective studies [68, 69, 97, 98] while the remaining forty-four-studies consisted of prospective cohorts of patients [26, 31, 33, 35, 37–42, 44–49, 52–54, 56, 58, 59, 64, 70–73, 75–80, 82, 83, 86, 87, 90–92, 99–102].

Sixty studies focused only on patients treated for atrial fibrillation (AF) alone [26, 28, 32–39, 41, 43, 45–47, 50–58, 60–62, 64–69, 71, 73–76, 78–81, 84–91, 93–102] while two studies included patients with AF and other types of arrhythmia: Mohanty et al. [63] included patients with co-existent AF and atrial flutter while Evans et al. [48] was a PROMs validation study which enrolled patients with a broad range of arrhythmia substrates including AF, atrioventricular nodal reentry tachycardia (AVNRT), atrial flutter, accessory pathway and ventricular tachycardia.

Table 16.1 Data from identified studies

Paper	Study intent	age	sex = female n (%)	other relevant demographics (race, employment, obesity, diabetes, physical activity, smoking, alcohol, no leisure physical activity)	Total no. of patients	No of patients in Ablation arm reporting QoL data	Follow-up (months)	Instrument(s)
Amir et al. [31]	To compare symptom burden and the quality of life before and 6 months after ablation	43.06 (17–74)	19 (61.3)	Observational, single-centre, cohort study conducted in Indonesia from January through December 2019. Treating patient's refractory to anti-arrhythmic with low-burden premature ventricular complexes	31	31	6	ASTA
Andrade et al. [28]	To evaluate the impact of contact force–guided radiofrequency ablation versus cryoballoon ablation on quality of life and health care utilization	NR	NR	CIRCA-DOSE multicentre prospective parallel-group, single-blinded RCT with blinded endpoint conducted at 8 clinical centres in Canada. 346 patients with paroxysmal AF refractory to at least 1 Class I or III AAD randomized in a 1:1:1 ratio to: (1) contact force–guided point by-point RF ablation (CF-RF); (2) short 2-min cryoballoon ablation duration (CRYO-2); and (3) standard 4-min cryoballoon ablation duration (CRYO-4). (Secondary analysis reported by Samuel et al. [29] and Yao et al. [30]	346	115 CF-RF 115 CRYO-2 115 CRYO-4	12	AFEQT; EQ-5D-3L

Bai et al. [32]	To investigate the impact of a single RF ablation (RFA) on QoL in atrial fibrillation (AF) patients with low stroke risk.	After matching: 61.82 ± 8.90 in RFA group 62.42 ± 10.52 in non-RFA group	After matching: 27 (36.49) RFA group 55 (37.16) non-RFA group	Nine hundred AF patients with low CHADS2 score from the Chinese Atrial Fibrillation Registry prospectively enrolled between 2011 and 2013. After a propensity score matching a cohort of 222 patients was constructed with 74 in the RFA group and 148 in the non-RFA group	222	44	6	AFEQT
Barmano et al. [99]	Exploration of predictors of improvement in arrhythmia specific symptoms and HRQoL following RF ablation for AF	60.5 ± 10.2	56 (29)	Observational study with data from SMURF study, single centre in Sweden. Patients with first RFA ablation for AF prospectively enrolled between Jan 2012 and April 2014	192	192	12	ASTA; HADS: SF-36
Berger et al. [33]	To explore the relationship between documented AF recurrences and QoL in patients following PVI	55.4 ± 8.9	20 (25)	Dutch population, consecutive patients prospectively enrolled between 1st Jan 2008 and 31st Dec 2010. Patients with recurrence of AF (n = 52) compared to those with no recurrence	99	99	12	SF-36

(continued)

Table 16.1 (continued)

Paper	Study intent	age	sex = female n (%)	other relevant demographics (race, employment, obesity, diabetes, physical activity, smoking, alcohol, no leisure physical activity)	Total no. of patients	No of patients in Ablation arm reporting QoL data	Follow-up (months)	Instrument(s)
Biviano et al. [34]	To quantify the healthcare utilization and quality of life benefits of catheter ablation for AF, for patients ≥65 years compared to patients <65 years	71.1 older group 53.6 younger group	284 (38.6)	Analysis uses data from US patients with AF already prospectively enrolled in a prospective observational registry. 381 patients aged <65 years; 355 patients aged 65+ years. Mean age of older group was 71.1 (SD 4.9) years. Mean of Younger group 53.6 (SD 9.1) years. Older group = fewer males; higher rates of anticoagulation usage, hypertension, TIA, CAD, higher CHADS2 risk scores	736	462	12	AFEQT
Bjorkenheim et al. [35]	To evaluate the use of an AF-specific and a generic patient-reported outcomes instrument during continuous rhythm monitoring 2 years after AF ablation	57 ± 9	23 (40)	Scandinavian AF patients prospectively enrolled between 2009 and 2013	57	54	24	AF6; SF-36;
Blandino et al. [100]	To compared the efficacy, safety, and QoL impact of catheter ablation versus antiarrhythmic drugs (AAD) in elderly patients with persistent AF.	75 ± 5 ablation group 76 ± 5 AAD group	44 (29) ablation group 73 (28) AAD group	A prospective study of consecutive patients with persistent AF. Elderly patients aged ≥70: Group A 153 patients treated with ablation; Group B 259 patients treated with AAD. Enrolled between Jan 2005 and Jan 2009	412	153	60	SF-36

Blondstrom-Lundqvist et al. [36]	To assess quality of life with catheter ablation vs antiarrhythmic medication at 12 months in patients with atrial fibrillation	55.8 (10.6) ablation group 56.3 (8.9) AAD group	21 (26.6) ablation group 14 (18.4) AAD group	Patients in Sweden and Finland, enrolled between July 2008 and Sept 2017 on the CAPTAF RCT Trial—Patients with AF treated with Pulmonary vein isolation ablation (n = 79) or antiarrhythmic drugs (n = 76).	155	79	12	SF-36
Boersma et al. [93]	To prospectively assess the population, indications, and outcomes using second-generation phased radiofrequency (RF) ablation (pulmonary vein ablation catheter GOLD) in a global examination of standard-of-care use for the treatment of paroxysmal and persistent atrial fibrillation	60.6 ± 10.9	341 (32.4)	The GOLD AF Registry was a prospective, observational, multi-centre, registry with 40 worldwide sites in France, Germany, Greece, Hungary, Italy, the Netherlands, Poland, Portugal, Spain, Switzerland, UK, Georgia, Israel, and South Korea. Enrolled patients between 2015 and 2017. It included adults (≥18 years old) with PAF, persistent AF (PersAF), or LS PersAF who underwent a phased RF ablation. Patients followed up in person or by telephone.	1054	943	12	AFEQT
Boveda et al. [37]	To report long term outcomes after single PVI ablation in persistent AF patients (CRYO4PERSISTENT AF Trial)	61.8 ± 10.5	26 (25.7)	A prospective, multicentre, single-arm trial in Germany, France and Greece including patients with AF enrolled between Dec 2014 and May 2016	101	101	12	SF-36

(continued)

Table 16.1 (continued)

Paper	Study intent	age	sex = female n (%)	other relevant demographics (race, employment, obesity, diabetes, physical activity, smoking, alcohol, no leisure physical activity)	Total no. of patients	No of patients in Ablation arm reporting QoL data	Follow-up (months)	Instrument(s)
Buist et al. [94]	QoL in patients treated with Catheter ablation (CA) or minimally invasive thoracoscopic PVI and left atrial appendage ligation (MIPI) for AF	57	NR (22)	Single centre RCT enrolled between 2007 and 2013. Patients with symptomatic paroxysmal or early persistent AF	52	25	12 (QoL available to 6 months)	SF-36
Bulkova et al. [38]	To compare QoL after catheter ablation for longstanding persistent AF (LSPAS) compared to paroxysmal AF (PAF) using EQ5D-3L	57 ± 10 (PAF group); 59 ± 9 (LSPAF group)	86 (33% PAF); 27 (21% LSPAF)	261 patients with PAF; 126 with LSPAF. Patients prospectively followed with consecutive enrolment between Jan 2007 and July 2009	387	387	36	EQ5D-3 L
Bulkova et al. [39]	To assess QoL, socioeconomic parameters, and costs of conventional therapy in patients treated by catheter ablation for AF.	58 ± 10	41 (26)	Consecutive patients with AF enrolled in 2007 and prospectively followed up for 2 years. Patients may be a subset of Bulkova et al. [39]	160	160		EQ5D
Cabanas-Grandio et al. [40]	Long term QoL after cavotricuspid isthmus ablation for atrial flutter	64.4 (SD 10.6)	17 (18.1)	Patients with atrial flutter. QoL data standardised and normalised for Spanish population. Consecutively enrolled between Jan 2003 and May 2005, with prospective follow up.	94	94	75	SF-36

Carnlof et al. [41]	To investigate the HRQOL issues in severe symptomatic AF patients before and after pulmonary vein isolation	53 ± 9	10 (25)	Patients at the Karolinski University Hospital, Sweden enrolled between March 2004 and December 2007. 40 patients in study arm, 36 with QoL pre and post matched at baseline to a control group. HRQoL issues assessed in severe symptomatic AF before and after PVI, with control group, prospective follow up	40	36	6 to 18 (data recorded in 12 month extraction table)	SF-36
Carnlof et al. [42]	To assess symptoms, HRQOL and functional impairment before and six months after ablation using a patient and gender perspective, in patients with paroxysmal supraventricular tachycardia (PSVT),	54 ± 15	109 (51)	A prospective study of consecutive patients with paroxysmal SVT at the Karolinski University Hospital, Sweden enrolled between Feb 2013 to May 2015. Outcomes compared by gender: 208 women	214	214	6	SF-36; Symptom Checklist (data not reported for Symptom checklist as disaggregated pre-post ablation data not available)
Chun et al. [95]	Report on the safety and efficacy of cryoballoon ablation for the treatment of AF within a single registry	61 ± 12	106 2 (36.3)	Patient registry including those with paroxysmal AF (PAF) or persistent AF (PsAF) were treated with cryoballoon catheter according to routine practices at 93 sites across 36 countries. 78.7% of patients had PAF. Inclusion, patients with 12 month follow up during the period May 2016–Jan 2020	1440	1213	12	EQ-5D-3L

(continued)

Table 16.1 (continued)

Paper	Study intent	age	sex = female n (%)	other relevant demographics (race, employment, obesity, diabetes, physical activity, smoking, alcohol, no leisure physical activity)	Total no. of patients	No of patients in Ablation arm reporting QoL data	Follow-up (months)	Instrument(s)
Das et al. [43]	Comparing QoL in patients with single AF ablation versus re-isolation regardless of symptoms	61.5 (IQR 55.8 68.0)	38 (47)	A single centre United Kingdom randomised study with consecutively enrolled patients with paroxysmal AF. 40 patients in each arm: 40 single procedure, 40 repeat procedure	80	80	12	AFEQT
Domeyer et al. [44]	To (1) translate, culturally adapt, and preliminarily validate the arrhythmia-specific Umea22 (U22) questionnaire and (2) assess the impact of radiofrequency (RF) ablation and medical treatment on the quality of life of patients with supraventricular tachycardias (SVTs).	46.55 ablation pts 43.55 AAD pts	57 (57) ablation 21 (52.5) AAD	Prospective study of Greek patients with SVT (AVNRT and AVRT), enrolled between Oct 2016 and April 2017. 100 patients treated with ablation 40 with AAD. Age of ablation patients = 46.55 ± 11.4; age of AAD patients 43.55 ± 11.18	140	100	3	SF-36; U22
Du et al. [45]	To assess the clinical outcomes and health-related quality of life of ablation therapy in a real world setting	NR	NR	A prospective non-randomised single centre study. Chinese population. 469 patients enrolled: Following matching—151 in the ablation group (75 with paroxysmal AF, 76 with persistent AF) and 318 in the drug group (162 with paroxysmal AF and 156 with persistent AF)	469	133	9	SF-36; AFEQT

Duytschaever et al. [101]	To determine the longer-term impact of optimized CA on atrial tachyarrhythmia burden by using an insertable cardiac monitor.	62 ± 8	40 (38)	A Belgian prospective, patient-controlled study (CLOSE to CURE), enrolled patients from July 2016. Patients with paroxysmal AF implanted with an ICM 65 days before PVI ablation	105	97	24	AF symptom checklist; SF-36
Efremidis et al. [46]	To investigate associations of pre-ablative QoL and stress parameters with AF ablation outcomes, as well as possible changes in QoL, anxiety, and depression parameters after ablation.	56.9 ± 12.2	23 (40.4)	Prospectively evaluated consecutive Greek patients with symptomatic, drug refractory paroxysmal AF who underwent left atrial ablation	57	57	6	Beck Depression Inventory (BDI): SF36; State-Trait Anxiety Inventory (STAI);
Essebag et al. [47]	To investigate the effect of AF-ablation success and atrial fibrillation burden (AFB) on QOL measures.	57.30 ± 10.80	68 (29.6)	Two ablation strategies including multipolar duty cycled phased RF ablation (PVAC, Medtronic Inc.) and traditional point-by-point RF catheter ablation. Patients enrolled between 2012 and 2017 at six tertiary centres.	230	217	12	AFEQT; CCS-SAF; SF12
Evans et al. [48]	To investigate long-term efficacy of cardiac ablation for symptomatic arrhythmia by gathering generic and arrhythmia-related QoL data using patient-reported outcome measures before and after ablation	62.04 ± 11.83	150 (43.6)	Prospectively evaluated consecutive patients in an observational UK study, enrolled between March 2013 and August 2014. Includes patients with varied arrythmia substrates including AF/AVNRT/Atrial Flutter	390	390	12	Cardiff Cardiac Ablation PROM; EQ-5D-5L

(continued)

Table 16.1 (continued)

Paper	Study intent	age	sex = female n (%)	other relevant demographics (race, employment, obesity, diabetes, physical activity, smoking, alcohol, no leisure physical activity)	Total no. of patients	No of patients in Ablation arm reporting QoL data	Follow-up (months)	Instrument(s)
Farkowski et al. [49]	To describe gender-related differences in clinical presentation, radiofrequency ablation outcomes, and healthcare resource utilization in a group of patients with AVNRT and AVRT.	44.9 ± 13.4 women 44.5 ± 14.4 men	23 (36)	Single centre prospective study of patients in Poland with AVNRT or AVRT. Data available by gender	64	64	2	EQ-5D-3L; PPAQ
Fiala et al. [50]	To identify the factors associated with global functional improvement after successful RF catheter ablation of long standing persistent atrial fibrillation (LSPAF)	59 + 9 restored sinus rhythm at follow up 61 + 8 AF/AT at follow up	35 (20.5%) restored sinus rhythm at follow up 10 (32.3%) AF/AT at follow up	203 consecutive patients from a single centre prospective registry with long-standing persistent atrial fibrillation (LSPAF) treated with an index ablation between July 2006 and December 2011. Data for 171 with restored sinus rhythm at 12 month follow up, 31 with AT/AF at 12 month follow up.	202	202	12	EQ5D
Fichtner et al. [102]	To prospectively assess different aspects of short- and long-term quality of life (QoL) after catheter ablation for AF.	57 ± 10	NR (26)	Prospective study of consecutive patients enrolled at a German centre between July 2004 and August 2006. 46 patients with persistent AF; 87 patients with paroxysmal AF	133	133	48+	AF severity scale; AF symptom checklist; Illness Intrusiveness; Major depression inventory; Sleep and Vegetative disorder; WHO 5-Wellbeing Index; Vital Exhaustion

Fujisawa et al. [51]	The association between a family history (FHx) of AF and patient-reported symptom burden and perception towards treatment.	Family history of AF = 63.3 ± 10.9 No family history of AF = 67.3 ± 11.2	Family history of AF = 57 (27.9) No family history of AF = 309 (28.6)	A retrospective analysis of 1514 newly diagnosed and referred patients with AF recorded on a multicentre Japanese registry between 2012 and 2015. At their initial visit, patients provided information about their family history of AF, and the presence or absence of AF in their parents, siblings, and children.	1514	510 patients with ablation and QoL data (99 with a family history of AF, 411 with no family history of AF)	12	AFEQT
Gupta et al., [52]	Analysis of healthcare utilisation and quality of life (QOL) outcomes, measured association between QOL and atrial fibrillation (AF) burden and factors associated with lack of QOL improvement	61.4 ± 10.0	129 (39.2)	CLOSE-guided ablation was performed in 329 consecutive patients (age 61.4 years, 60.8% male) with drug-refractory PAF in 9 European countries. Patients enrolled between Jan 2017 and March 2018	329	305	12	AFEQT; EQ-5D-5L
Haman et al. [53]	To conduct a single centre study with long term follow up of patients with paroxysmal AF	57	131 (43)	Consecutive Czeck patients enrolled between April 2004 and August 2012, with prospective follow-up, with paroxysmal, persistent or longstanding persistent AF. 489 ablation procedures in 303 AF patients. Paroxysmal = 157 patients; persistent (duration 1-12 months) = 94 patients; longstanding persistent (>12 months) = 52 patients	303	NR	24	EQ5D

(continued)

Table 16.1 (continued)

Paper	Study intent	age	sex = female n (%)	other relevant demographics (race, employment, obesity, diabetes, physical activity, smoking, alcohol, no leisure physical activity)	Total no. of patients	No of patients in Ablation arm reporting QoL data	Follow-up (months)	Instrument(s)
Hoglund et al. [54]	The use of U22 to measure symptom improvement following AF ablation	58	27 (26)	Patients treated with left atrial catheter ablation for paroxysmal and persistent AF at a Swedish centre between 2006 and 2011 with prospective follow up. 52 paroxysmal; 52 non-paroxysmal. All first time ablations	105	105	≈ 10 (data entered at 9 month cells)	SF-36; subset of U22
Ikemura et al. [55]	To examine baseline and 1-year HRQoL outcomes of patients with atrial fibrillation after CA in daily practice	64 (56–70)	261 (23.8)	A registry-based cohort study designed to recruit patients with atrial fibrillation newly referred to 11 hospitals, with data from 1097 consecutive registry patients with atrial fibrillation who underwent CA between 2012 and 2019.	1097	1021	12	AFEQT
Inagaki et al. [56]	To clarify the effectiveness of durable PVI in improving the QOL of patients with AF	66.3 ± 9.5	31 (26.1)	153 consecutive AF patients (paroxysmal AF, n = 133; persistent AF, n = 20) who underwent PVI between October 2014 and December 2017 at the Tokyo Metropolitan Hiroo Hospital were enrolled	119	119; 93 without recurrence, 26 with recurrence	12	AFQLQ

Jain et al. [97]	To evaluate the effect of cryoballoon ablation on long term QoL (STOP-AF study)	NR	NR	A multicentre observational trial at sites in the USA and Canada. Patients with drug refractory symptomatic paroxysmal AF. Post hoc analysis of prospectively collected data	335	335	36	SF-12
Kanda et al. [57]	To investigate the QoL change after persistent AF ablation and the differences between the PVI-alone strategy and the PVI plus strategy	NR	NR	The EARNEST-PVI trial was a multi-centre RCT comparing clinical outcomes of pulmonary vein isolation (PVI) alone and more intensive ablation in addition to PVI including complex fractionated atrial electrogram (CFAE) and linear ablation (PVI plus) in patients with persistent AF	222	222	12	SF-36
Kato et al. [58]	To compare the changes in QOL after extended PVI between patients with Persistent AF (PerAF) and paroxysmal AF (PAF).	65.5 (9.5)	14 (23.3)	Consecutive patients with PAF and PerAF who developed no AF recurrence 6 months after their first PVI from April 2014 to April 2016 were enrolled and QoL data collected prospectively. 38 patients with Paroxysmal AF; 22 with persistent AF	60	60	6	SF-36

(continued)

Table 16.1 (continued)

Paper	Study intent	age	sex = female n (%)	other relevant demographics (race, employment, obesity, diabetes, physical activity, smoking, alcohol, no leisure physical activity)	Total no. of patients	No of patients in Ablation arm reporting QoL data	Follow-up (months)	Instrument(s)
Kesek et al. [59]	To evaluate U22 in a well-defined group of patients with paroxysmal supraventricular tachycardia, undergoing an intervention with a distinct end-point and a high success rate	AP group = 43.9 (17.9); AVNRT group = 57.1 (14.0)	32 (50.8)	Swedish patients undergoing ablation for accessory pathway and atrioventricular nodal re-entrant tachycardia between April 2006 and May 2008. Prospective HRQoL data available for 63 patients: SVTA (accessory pathway (AP) = 26 patients; atrioventricular nodal re-entrant tachycardia (AVNRT) = 37 patients	141	63	≈7 months (data entered at 6 months)	SF-36; subset of U22
Kloosterman et al. [26]	To study sex-differences in efficacy and safety of atrial fibrillation (AF) ablation	Overall = 64 (58–70) Females = 66 (60-72) Males = 63 (57-69)	209 (33)	AXAFA-AFNET 5 trial was a prospective, multicentre (Europe and America), study comparing continuous non-vitamin K antagonist apixaban therapy to vitamin K antagonist therapy in patients undergoing first AF ablation. All patients had symptomatic non-valvular AF, a clinical indication for catheter ablation on continuous anticoagulant therapy, and at least one established stroke risk factor. This analysis population included all patients from the AXAFA-AFNET 5 trial population who were randomized and underwent catheter ablation	674	633	3	EQ-5D-5L; SF12

Kuck et al. [60]	To assess outcome parameters that are important for the daily clinical management of patients using key secondary analyses. Specifically, reinterventions, rehospitalizations, and QoL were examined in this randomized trial of cryoballoon vs. RFC catheter ablation (FIRE and ICE Trial)	NR	NR	Subset of the FIRE and ICE RCT including patients with drug refractory symptomatic paroxysmal AF. 374 patients treated with cryoballoon ablation; 376 treated with RFC	750	525	30 (disaggregated QoL data presented up to 12 months)	ED5D-3L; SF-12
Lo et al. [61]	To demonstrate that RF ablation with a magnetic sensor enabled optical contact force sensing ablation catheter was safe and effective for the treatment of drug refractory, recurrent symptomatic persistent atrial fibrillation.	65.4 ± 10.1	(30.9)	Patients with recurrent symptomatic persistent atrial fibrillation	223	NR	15	EQ-5D-5L
Mantovan et al. [62]	To Compare 3 ablations strategies for high burden paroxysmal/persistent atrial fibrillation (AF): complex fractionated electrogram ablation (CFE), pulmonary vein isolation (PVI), or a combined approach (PVI with CFE).	57 ± 10	26 (26)	The STAR AF Randomised multicentre study of patients undergoing first time ablation for high burden paroxysmal or persistent AF. AF was classified as high-burden paroxysmal in 64 patients (64%) and persistent in 36 patients (36%).Patients randomized to PVI (n = 32), CFE (n = 34), and PVI with CFE (n = 34)	100	100	12	SF-36

(continued)

Table 16.1 (continued)

Paper	Study intent	age	sex = female n (%)	other relevant demographics (race, employment, obesity, diabetes, physical activity, smoking, alcohol, no leisure physical activity)	Total no. of patients	No of patients in Ablation arm reporting QoL data	Follow-up (months)	Instrument(s)
Mohanty et al. [63]	To examine the impact of different ablation strategies on atrial fibrillation (AF) recurrence and quality of life in coexistent AF and atrial flutter (AFL)	63 ± 8 group 1 a 61 ± 11 group 1 b 62 ± 9 group 2	NR (22) group 1a NR (28) group 1b NR (24) group 2	APPROVAL Study - A prospective, randomised, single blind multicentre study with centres in Italy and the USA. Consecutive patients enrolled between Jan 2009 and Sept 2011. 360 enrolled patients with documented coexistent AF and AFL were blinded and randomized to 2 groups: Group 1 (182 patients) where 58 patients had AF + AFL ablation (group 1a) and 124 had AF ablation only Group 1b). Group 2 (178 patients): only AFL was ablated by achieving bidirectional isthmus conduction block. QoL data presented for total of Group 1 and Group 2	360	360	12	BDI; HADS; SF-36; STAI
Mohanty et al.[64]	To report impact of catheter ablation on exercise performance, QoL and symptom perception in asymptomatic longstanding persistent AF (LSP-AF)	62 ± 13	NR (29)	Prospective single centre, single arm centre. Consecutive patients undergoing first catheter ablation or asymptomatic LSP-AF. 25 patients experienced recurrence, 21 of these were symptomatic	61	61	12	SF-36

Morillo et al. [65]	To compare radiofrequency ablation with antiarrhythmic drugs in treating patients with paroxysmal AF as a first-line therapy	56.3 (9.3) ablation group 54.3 (11.7) AAD group	15 (22.7) ablation group 16 (26.2) AAD group	RCT of 127 treatment naïve patients with paroxysmal AF treated at 16 centres in Europe and North America, enrolled between July 2006 and Jan 2010. 66 patients treated with ablation; 61 treated with anti-arrhythmia drugs	127	66	24	EQ5D
Mortsell et al. [66]	Single cryoballoon (CB) application per vein for pulmonary vein isolation (PVI) compared to the standard approach of two consecutive CB applications in patients with atrial fibrillation (AF) for long-term efficacy and safety	61.9 ± 9.08 single cryo 68.3 ± 10.0 routine	21 (30.04) single cryo 16 (22.9) routine	Prospective single centre randomised study of patients with symptomatic AF. 69 patients treated with single cryoablation; 70 with routine cryoablation. Patients enrolled between Nov 2014 and March 2016	139	139	12	EQ5D-5L; SSQ
Nakajima [67]	To understand whether use of catheter ablation would lead to better QOL in comparison to antiarrhythmic drugs	NR	NR	An observational and multicentre outpatient-based AF Japanese registry. Patients with persistent AF divided into four groups; those who underwent catheter ablation and maintained sinus rhythm; patients who underwent catheter ablation and had non-sinus rhythm at the 1 year follow-up; patients who maintained sinus rhythm by AAs; and patients who did not undergo catheter ablation or AA treatment	1040	432	12	AFEQT

(continued)

Table 16.1 (continued)

Paper	Study intent	age	sex = female n (%)	other relevant demographics (race, employment, obesity, diabetes, physical activity, smoking, alcohol, no leisure physical activity)	Total no. of patients	No of patients in Ablation arm reporting QoL data	Follow-up (months)	Instrument(s)
Onishi et al. [68]	To examine the effect of CA for asymptomatic AF patients	NR	NR	Retrospective analysis of patients with asymptomatic persistent AF treated at Tenri hospital. Unclear if any cross over with Onishi et al. [69]	79	79	12	AFQLQ
Onishi et al. [69]	To assess the improvement of QOL and long-term prognosis after CA of asymptomatic persistent AF	62.9 ± 8.6	5 (11.1)	A retrospective single-centre study with patients undergoing an initial RF ablation CA of AF in Tenri Hospital (Japan) from January 2012 to March 2014.	259	45	12	AFQLQ
Papiashvili et al. [70]	To investigate effects of catheter ablation on HRQoL related to age, gender and type pf paroxysmal supraventricular tachycardia	49.31 ± 15.29	50 (71)	Consecutive patients with AVNRT/AVRT or Atrial Tachycardia, enrolled between July 2016 and April 2017 and prospectively followed up. Results compared by gender, age and SVT type	70	70	3	SF36; State-Trait Anxiety Inventory (STAI)
Pavlovic et al. [71]	To present the impact of pulmonary vein isolation (PVI) using CBA compared to AAD therapy on symptom recurrence and QoL	Ablation (n = 107) = 50.5 (13.1) AAD (n = 111) = 54.1 (13.4)	Ablation group = 31 (29) AAD group = 39 (35.1)	A multicentre (Europe, Argentina and Australia), prospective, open blind-endpoint, controlled randomized (1:1) study evaluating PVI using CBA vs AAD therapy in patients with symptomatic paroxysmal AF	218	107	12	AFEQT: SF-36

Pezawas et al. [98]	To determine if PVI for paroxysmal or non-paroxysmal AF increases HRQoL	58 ± 11	NR (27)	A retrospective analysis of patients scheduled for PVI in Vienna between 2009 and 2013 with a diagnosis of paroxysmal, persistent or longstanding AF. SF12 available for 163 patients regarding 187 PVI procedures	229	163	≥12	SF-12
Piccini et al. [27] N.B. Same study population as Kloosterman et al. [26]	To investigate changes in quality of life (QoL), cognition and functional status according to arrhythmia recurrence after atrial fibrillation (AF) ablation	Overall = 64 (58–70)	174 (33.6%)	AXAFA–AFNET 5 enrolled patients scheduled for a de novo/first AF ablation with at least one established stroke risk factor (age > 65 years, heart failure, hypertension, diabetes or prior stroke). For the purpose of this analysis, the study population included all patients from the AXAFA trial population who were randomised, underwent catheter ablation and had available baseline and follow-up QoL data. N.B. Sub group of Kloosterman et al.	518	518	3	EQ-5D-5L; SF12
Pytkowski et al. [72]	To evaluate the HRQoL of patients with structurally normal hearts undergoing elective RF ablation (RFA) of ventricular tachycardia (VT) or premature ventricular contractions (PVC's).	45.5 ± 14.2	34 (NR)	Single centre prospective cohort of patients with symptomatic drug refractory ventricular arrhythmia. 23 patients with VT; 21 with PVCs. Patients enrolled between 1999 and 2004	44	44	3	SF-36

(continued)

Table 16.1 (continued)

Paper	Study intent	age	sex = female n (%)	other relevant demographics (race, employment, obesity, diabetes, physical activity, smoking, alcohol, no leisure physical activity)	Total no. of patients	No of patients in Ablation arm reporting QoL data	Follow-up (months)	Instrument(s)
Raine et al. [73]	To assess the effect of catheter ablation on AF symptoms and QoL	57 ± 10 years	22 (27)	Consecutive patients scheduled for their first ablation, with prospective follow up: 44 patients with Paroxysmal AF; 36 patients with persistent AF	80	80	3	AFEQT; SF-36
Reynolds et al. [74]	To assess effects of catheter ablation and antiarrhythmic drugs (AAD) on QoL in patients with paroxysmal AF	55.5 ± 9.4 ablation group 55.8 ± 13.1 AAD group	32 (31) ablation group; 21 (37) AAD group	A prospective, randomised multicentre trial for patients with paroxysmal AF not controlled by drugs. 103 patients in ablation group; 56 patients in AAD group	159	103	3	SF-36; AF Symptom checklist
Risom et al. [75]	To assess outcomes at 12 and 24 months after participation in a multidisciplinary cardiac rehabilitation program plus usual care compared with usual care alone for patients treated for atrial fibrillation with catheter ablation	59	26%	Consecutive patients from 2 Danish university hospitals treated with ablation for AF were screened. Patients were randomized 1:1 to comprehensive cardiac rehabilitation plus usual care vs usual care stratified by age and type of AF	210	210 (105 in cardiac rehabilitation group; 105 in usual care group)	24	AFEQT; HADS; SF-36
Samuel et al. [29] N.B. Same study population as Andrade et al. [28], Yao et al. [30]	To determine the association between change in AF burden and quality of life in the year following ablation	60(52-66 IQR)	115 (33.3)	A secondary analysis of the CIRCA-DOSE study ([28]; [30]). Patients enrolled between Sept 2014 and July 2017	346	115 CF-RF 115 CRYO-2 115 CRYO-4	12	AFEQT; EQ-5D-3L

Sang et al. [76]	To assess if depression, anxiety, and QoL improve after catheter ablation in patients with paroxysmal AF	55.9 ± 6.1 in ablation group 57.2 ± 5.4 in AAD group	27 (32.9) in ablation group 26 (30.9) in AAD group	Consecutive patients with a primary diagnosis of symptomatic paroxysmal AF enrolled between Feb 2009 and Jan 2010 for prospective review. 84 patients included in antiarrhythmic drug (AAD) group; 82 patients in ablation group	166	82	12	Self-Rating Anxiety Scale (SAS); Self-Rating Depression Scale (SDS); SF-36. No disaggregated follow-up data available for SDS or SAS scales
Seara et al. [77]	To measure HRQoL changes in patients with typical atrial flutter following catheter ablation with results standardised and normalised to the Spanish population	64 ± 11	18 (18.9)	Consecutive Spanish patients with Atrial Flutter referred between Jan 2003 and March 2005, with prospective follow up	95	95	12	SF-36
Spertus et al. [78]	To develop and validate the AFEQT in patients with AF in a 6 centre prospective study	62.1 ± 12	91 (42.5)	A multicentre prospective study of patients with paroxysmal, persistent, longstanding persistent or permanent AF recruited in Canada and the US between Aug 2008 and July 2009. Three groups in study. Before and after treatment QoL presented here for two groups: Group 1—pharmacological change in therapy following baseline assessment (n = 66; mean age 66; 32 females); Group 2—ablation after baseline assessment (n = 76; mean age 60.1; 27 females)	219	76	3	AFEQT; SF-36; AF Severity Scale; EQ-5D; Symptom Checklist (SCL) Score

(continued)

Table 16.1 (continued)

Paper	Study intent	age	sex = female n (%)	other relevant demographics (race, employment, obesity, diabetes, physical activity, smoking, alcohol, no leisure physical activity)	Total no. of patients	No of patients in Ablation arm reporting QoL data	Follow-up (months)	Instrument(s)
Steinberg et al. [79]	To identify patients who experience large improvements in HRQoL; to understand patient factors associated with large improvements in HRQoL; and to describe interval interventions and outcomes among these patients with large improvements in HRQoL	74.0 (67.0–81.0)	300 (47.2%)	The ORBIT-AF registry is a national, US prospective cohort study of outpatients with AF, enrolled from June 2010 to August 2011. The study was managed and coordinated by the Duke Clinical Research Institute	2008	636	12	AFEQT
Su et al. [80]	To assess the safety and efficacy of PVI using the cryoballoon catheter to treat patients with persistent AF	65 ± 9	49 (29.7)	Patients with drug refractory symptomatic PsAF were enrolled into the STOP Persistent AF trial (US, Canada and Japan) between March 2017 and July 2018. 165 patients were treated by cryoballoon PVI, and 145 completed the required 12-month follow up follow-up schedule	165	165	12	AFEQT; SF-12
Terricabras et al. [81]	To evaluate whether the procedural outcome of ablation for AF is associated with quality of life (QOL) measures	60 (SD 9)	115 (21)	Secondary analysis of the STAR AF II RCT, patients enrolled at 35 centres in Europe, Canada, Australia, China, and Korea from November 2010 to July 2012	549	549	18	EQ-5D-3L; SF-36

Timmers et al. [82]	Evaluation of the impact of catheter ablation for ventricular extrasystoles (VES) in structurally normal hearts on quality of life (QOL) and symptomatology	49 ± 22	26 (70.3)	Single centre Belgian study enrolling patients with ventricular extrasystoles between 2016 and 2019	37	37	12	SF-36; MASQ
Walfridsson et al. [83]	To evaluate the impact of RFA on HRQOL in patients with paroxysmal supraventricular tachycardia (PSVT)	48.3 ± 16.3	91 (52)	Prospective design with consecutive patients with AVNRT or PSVT treated at a single centre in Sweden. Age and gender matched to Swedish population	176	156	12	EQ-5D-3L; SF-36
Walfridsson et al. [96]	To assess long-term effect on HRQoL of radiofrequency ablation (RFA) vs. antiarrhythmic drug therapy (AAD) as first-line treatment for patients with PAF (sub study of the MANTRA-PAF) trial, and symptom burden at 12 and 24 months	56 ± 9 RFA group; 54 ± 10 AAD group	46 (32) RFA group 42 (28) AAD group	A Swedish multicentre prospective RCT including patients with PAF. 146 patients treated with RFA; 148 treated with AAD.	294	146	24	SF-36; EQ5D-3L; ASTA
Wazni et al. [84]	To evaluate the change in quality of life (QoL) and symptoms after first-line CBA vs AAD therapy	60.4 ± 11.2 (Ablation group) 61.6 ± 11.2 (AAD group)	41 (39.4) Ablation group 42 (42.4) AAS group	Part of the STOP-AF Study. Patients with symptomatic AF not previously receiving rhythm control therapy were randomized to AAD (class I or III) or CBA	203	104	12	AFEQT; EQ-5D-5L

(continued)

Table 16.1 (continued)

Paper	Study intent	age	sex = female n (%)	other relevant demographics (race, employment, obesity, diabetes, physical activity, smoking, alcohol, no leisure physical activity)	Total no. of patients	No of patients in Ablation arm reporting QoL data	Follow-up (months)	Instrument(s)
Wilber et al. [85]	To determine the efficacy of catheter ablation compared with antiarrhythmic drug therapy (ADT) in treating symptomatic paroxysmal AF	55.7 (95% CI, 54.1-57.4)	NR(33.5)	Prospective multicentre randomised study with sites in the USA, Europe, Canada and Latin America involving patients with symptomatic AF who had not improved with at least 1 drug. 167 patients with paroxysmal AF:106 patients treated with catheter ablation; 61 treated with AAD. Patients enrolled between Oct 2004 and Oct 2007	167	106	9 (QoL data reported only at 3 months)	AF Symptom Checklist; SF-36
Wokhlu et al. [86]	To determine the relationship between AF ablation efficacy, QoL, and AF-specific symptoms at 2 years	55.9 ± 0.3	98 (18)	Consecutive patients with symptomatic AF treated at a single US centre. Patients prospectively followed between Dec 2001 and July 2006 and data collected prospectively until March 2008.323 patients with 2 year QoL follow up	502	323	24	SF-36
Wozniak-Skowerska et al. [87]	To assess the long-term influence of circumferential pulmonary vein ablation (CPVA) on QoL in patients with AF	54.2 ± 9	7 (21)	Prospective study. Data available for patients with and without recurrence of AF	33	33	12	SF-36

Wu et al. [88]	To compare the effects of RFCA and pharmacotherapy on the prognosis of patients with persistent and long standing AF	64.1 ± 11.3 Overall 64.8 ± 12.6 Ablation group 64.4 ± 13.6 Pharmacotherapy group	109 (33.3) Ablation group 118 (36.8) Pharmaco-therapy group	From 2012 to 2014, 648 patients with persistent AF (PAF) or longstanding persistent AF LS-PAF) were enrolled in a multicentre RCT. 267 (41.2%) patients had PAF and 381 (58.8%) had LS-PAF	648	327	60	SF-36
Wynn et al. [89]	To assess the impact of additional linear ablation lines compared to PVI alone	61.9 ± 0.5	42 (32)	Prospective multicentre UK based RCT of patients with persistent AF or sustained paroxysmal AF with risk FACTORS for atrial substrate. 64 patients treated with PVI only; 66 with PVI and additional linear ablation lines	130	122	12	AFEQT; SF-36
Xu et al. [90]	To evaluate QoL after circumferential pulmonary vein isolation (CPVI) compared with antiarrhythmic drug therapy (ADT) in treating AF.	61.5 ± 10.1 CPVI group: 60.9 ± 13.7 ADT group	CPVI = 21; ADT =22	Prospectively enrolled patients with AF: 66 patients treated with CPVI; 57 treated with ADT	123	66	6	SF-36
Yagishita et al. [91]	To assess the QoL, exercise performance, and plasma B-type natriuretic peptide levels following catheter ablation in patients with asymptomatic AF.	60.4 ± 9.2	7 (21)	Consecutively enrolled patients with asymptomatic persistent AF, prospective follow up	34	34	6	SF-36

(continued)

Table 16.1 (continued)

Paper	Study intent	age	sex = female n (%)	other relevant demographics (race, employment, obesity, diabetes, physical activity, smoking, alcohol, no leisure physical activity)	Total no. of patients	No of patients in Ablation arm reporting QoL data	Follow-up (months)	Instrument(s)
Yao et al. [30] N.B. Same study population as Andrade et al. [28], Samuel et al. [29]	to evaluate sex-specific differences in atrial fibrillation (AF) presentation and catheter ablation outcomes in the prospective, multicentre, randomized CIRCA-DOSE study	Females = 60.9 ± 9.1 Males = 57.7 ± 10.3	115 (33)	A secondary analysis of the CIRCA-DOSE study [28]; Samuel et al. [29]	346	115 CF-RF 115 CRYO-2 115 CRYO-4	12	AFEQT; EQ-5D-3L
Yildirim et al. [92]	To assess the QoL and anxiety in patients with Paroxysmal supraventricular tachycardia (PSVT) and the influence of RF ablation (RFA) treatment on these parameters	44.08 ± 11.12	28 (56)	Turkish study with consecutive patients with newly diagnosed paroxysmal supraventricular tachycardia (AVNRT/AVRT). Demographics provided for 50 patients in the ablation study group. These were age and sex matched with healthy individuals. No comparative data provided for WHOQOL domains	100	50	3	STAI; WHOQOL-BREF

Most of the remaining studies included patients with other types of supraventricular tachycardias (SVTs), with AVNRT and atrioventricular re-entrant tachycardia (AVRT) being most common but also including patients with atrial tachycardia, accessory pathways, and Wolf Parkinson White [42, 44, 49, 59, 70, 83, 92]. Three studies [31, 72, 82] included patients with ventricular arrhythmias including premature ventricular contractions (PVC's) and ventricular tachycardia. Two studies [40, 77] only included patients with atrial flutter.

Tools Used

A large number and variety of quality of life measures were used within the studies, with twenty seven different tools used. These broadly fit into three categories of generic health and quality of life PROMs tools; tools examining depression and anxiety, or sleep and exhaustion (i.e. mental wellbeing); and arrhythmia specific measures. The tools used and regularity of inclusion within the selected studies is detailed in Table 16.2.

Thirty nine studies used only one tool, while twenty six studies used two and the others used three or more, with one [102] using 7 different patient reported QoL measures. Within the identified studies, generic tools were widely used, particularly the SF-36 (used in 41 studies) and the EQ. 5D (used in 19 studies), three other generic tools were also used: the SF-12 in six studies, and the WHOQOL-BREF and Illness Intrusiveness scale each used in a single study.

Table 16.2 Tools, category and frequency of use in the included studies

Tool Name	Category of tool	No of studies using tool
AF6—Atrial Fibrillation 6	Arrhythmia specific	1
AFEQT—Atrial Fibrillation Effect on Quality-of-Life	Arrhythmia specific	19
AFSC—AF Symptom Checklist	Arrhythmia specific	4
AFSS—AF Severity Scale	Arrhythmia specific	2
ASTA—Arrhythmia-specific questionnaire in tachycardia & arrhythmia	Arrhythmia specific	3
AFQLQ—AF-specific QOL questionnaire	Arrhythmia specific	3
BDI—Beck Depression Inventory Scale	Mental wellbeing	2
C-CAP—Cardiff Cardiac Ablation PROM	Arrhythmia specific	1
CCS-SAF—Canadian Cardiovascular Society Severity of Atrial Fibrillation	Arrhythmia specific	1
EQ5D (EQ5D-5L and EQ5D-3L)	Generic	19
HADS—Hospital Anxiety and Depression Scale	Mental wellbeing	3
II—Illness Intrusiveness	Generic	1
MASQ—Modified arrhythmia-specific questionnaire	Arrhythmia specific	1
MDI—Major Depression Inventory	Mental wellbeing	1
PPAQ—patient perception of arrhythmia questionnaire	Arrhythmia specific	1
SAS—Self-rating Anxiety scale	Mental wellbeing	1
SCL—Symptom Checklist	Arrhythmia specific	2
SDS—Self-rating depression scale	Mental wellbeing	1
SF-12—Short Form 12	Generic	6
SF-36—Short Form 36	Generic	41
SVD—Sleep & Vegetative Disorder	Mental wellbeing	1
SSQ—Symptom Severity Questionnaire	Arrhythmia specific	1
STAI—Stait-Trait and anxiety inventory	Mental wellbeing	4
U22	Arrhythmia specific	3
Vital Exhaustion	Mental wellbeing	1
WHO-5 Wellbeing Index	Mental wellbeing	1
WHOQOL-BREF—World Health Organisation Quality of Life Scale	Generic	1

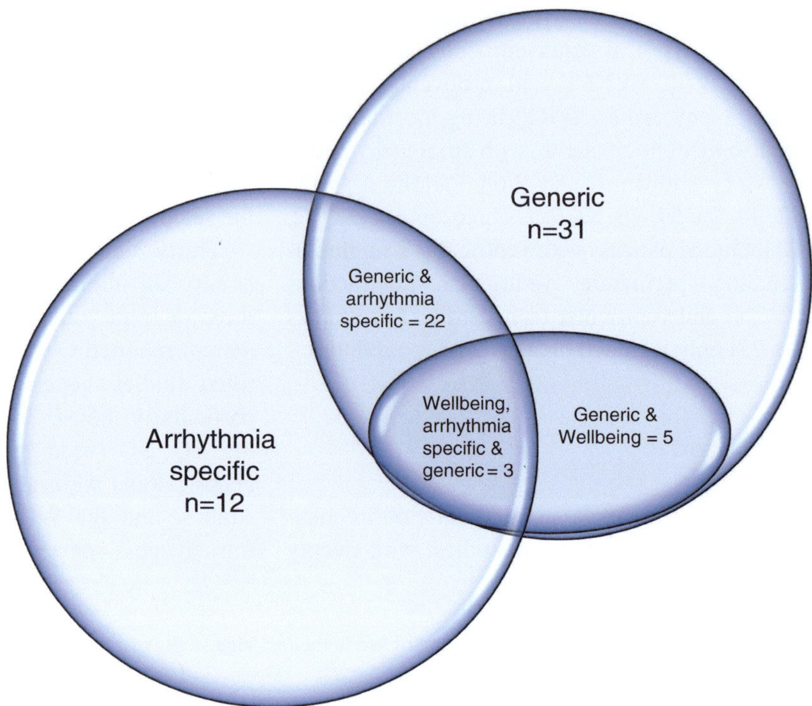

Fig. 16.1 Summary of tool use

Twelve studies did not use a generic quality of life tool at all [31, 32, 34, 43, 51, 55, 56, 67–69, 79, 93]. The combinations of tools used is illustrated in Fig. 16.1.

The most commonly used wellbeing tool was the State—Trait Anxiety Inventory (STAI) which was used in four studies. The Hospital Anxiety and Depression Scale (HADS) and Beck Depression Inventory (BDI) were both used in two studies while the Major Depression Inventory, Self-rating Anxiety scale; Self-Rating Depression Scale Sleep & Vegetative Disorder survey; Vital Exhaustion tool and WHO-5 Wellbeing Index were all used in a single study.

Eleven different arrhythmia specific HRQoL measures were used, the most commonly used of which was the AFEQT (19 studies). The AF symptom checklist was used in 4 studies and the U22, ASTA, and AFQLQ were each used in three. The AS severity scale, and SCL were all used in two studies while the remainder (AF6; C-CAP, CCS-SAF, MASQ, PPAQ, and SSQ) were used in 1 study each. Notably, the inclusion of patient reported outcome measures appears to have increased in the last three years, as detailed in Fig. 16.2.

All of the included studies reported baseline HRQoL and the length of follow up ranged from 2 months [49] to 75 months [40].

Comparative Studies

Twenty-six of the studies compared different treatment strategies [28, 32, 36, 43–45, 57, 60, 62, 63, 65–67, 71, 74–76, 78, 84, 85, 88–90, 94, 96, 100]. Buist et al. [94] compared catheter ablation to minimally invasive thoracoscopic pulmonary vein isolation and left atrial appendage (MIPI) in a study of 52 patients. They found that both treatment options resulted in an improvement in quality of life measures which were maintained at 24 months, although the patients treated with catheter ablation reported significantly fewer physical problems and bodily pain at three months post treatment compared to those treated with MIPI. In their 2015 publication, Bai et al. [32] described selected patients on the Chinese Atrial Fibrillation Register with a low stroke risk who had completed the AFEQT at baseline and six-months, matching 74 patients treated with radiofrequency ablation (RFA) to

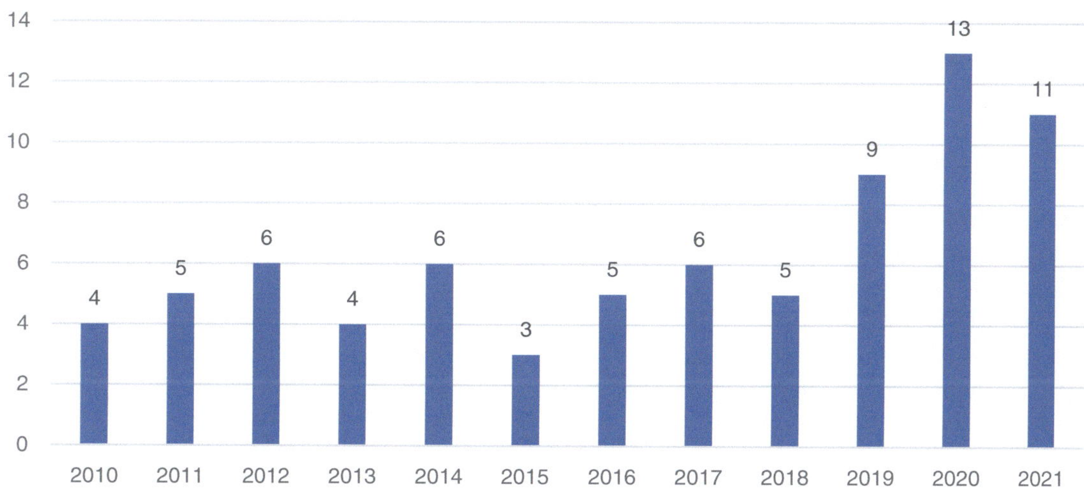

Fig. 16.2 Numbers of identified papers reporting disaggregated QoL data per year

148 who had not received RFA (treatment not specified for this group). QoL improved at six months for both groups with RFA showing only small superiority over no ablation treatment. However, as noted by the authors, patients who moved from the non-ablation to the ablation group were excluded which may result in some study bias.

While Blandino et al. [100] reported better quality of life outcomes and superior rhythm maintenance in those treated with catheter ablation, they also found that treatment with CA increased the risk of embolic complications in elderly patients, particularly those who had suffered a previous transient ischaemic attack or stroke.

Catheter Ablation Versus Anti-arrhythmic Drugs

Fifteen comparative studies [36, 44, 45, 65, 67, 71, 74, 76, 78, 84, 85, 88, 90, 96, 100] including a total of 4811 patients reported HRQoL in patients treated with catheter ablation (CA) compared to patients taking anti-arrhythmic drugs (AAD), with Spertus et al. [78], carrying this comparison out as part of a PROM validation exercise for AFEQT. These studies found that patients treated with CA reported better post treatment quality of life than those treated with AAD, with the exception of Morillo et al. [65] which reported that quality of life was improved in both groups with no significant difference between the two. However, they did find that ablation resulted in a lower rate of arrhythmia recurrence than AAD treatment [65].

Comparative Studies of Different Ablation Strategies

Eight of the studies [28, 43, 57, 60, 62, 63, 66, 89] compared different ablation strategies, using HRQoL as one of their outcome measures. Das et al. [43] compared patients treated with a single pulmonary vein isolation procedure using radiofrequency ablation with those treated with a second re-isolation procedure after two months regardless of symptoms. This study found that patients treated with the re-isolation procedure had improved freedom from recurrence, arrhythmia burden and quality of life than those treated with the standard single procedure.

Mortsell et al. [66] assessed patients treated with cryoballoon (CB) CA, comparing standard treatment of two consecutive CB applications with a single CB application in a randomised trial of 139 patients. Freedom from AF and quality of life following treatment was the same for both groups, however, as well as a shorter treatment time in the single CB arm (99.4 ± 33.3 min vs. 118.4 ± 34.3 min) there was a lower complication rate in the single CB group. A randomised study of 750 patients by Kuck et al. [60] directly compared cryoballoon and radiofrequency ablation in a randomised controlled trial (RCT) to demonstrate non-inferiority of CB ablation. The results suggested that while quality of life outcomes were improved in both groups, those treated with CB had significantly fewer repeat ablations, direct-current cardioversions, all-cause and cardiovascular rehospitalisation during the follow-up period. Another multicentre RCT measured the effect of using of additional linear ablation lines compared to PVI alone, finding that the additional lines increased procedural time and radiation dose but provided no extra clinical benefit to PVI alone. Another study of patients with co-existent atrial fibrillation and atrial flutter randomised patients to receive AF ablation, atrial flutter ablation or ablation of both [63]. Patients treated with atrial flutter ablation alone had higher recurrence and lower QoL than those treated with AF ablation or ablation of both arrhythmia substrates.

Reporting on the Substrate and Trigger Ablation for Reduction of Atrial Fibrillation (STAR AF) trial, Mantovan et al. [62] compared three treatment strategies, randomising patients to receive complex fractionated electrogram ablation (CFE), PVI, or a combined approach (PVI with CFE). Procedural outcomes varied between the treatment groups with the combined PVI and CFE group having the highest freedom from arrhythmia at one year (88%) and CFE alone the lowest (38%). However, all three groups showed significant improvements in physical and mental health following ablation irrelevant of the ablation strategy, including in many of those patients with arrhythmia recurrence, although recurrence was a predictor of worse QoL outcomes. Andrade et al. [28] assessed the quality of life outcomes and healthcare utilization in 346 patients with paroxysmal AF treated with either contact force–guided radiofrequency ablation or cryoballoon ablation. There were no significant differences between the two groups, with both arms showing significant improvement in HRQoL and reduced numbers of cardioversions and emergency department visits. Kanda et al. [57] reported on an RCT with 222 patients which compared the clinical outcomes of pulmonary vein isolation (PVI) alone with more intensive ablation in addition to PVI, including complex fractionated atrial electrogram and linear ablation (PVI plus). Although there was a significant improvement in QoL in both groups, the PVI plus group showed greater improvements than the PVI alone group.

Between Group Comparisons

While other studies did not set out to compare ablation against other treatment options, some did have a comparative nature. Both Bulkova et al. [38] and Kato et al. [58] compared changes in QoL after PVI between patients treated for persistent atrial fibrillation and those with paroxysmal AF. While these studies found that both patient groups reported some improvements, the patients treated for persistent AF had greater improvements in quality of life than those treated for paroxysmal AF. In their 2015 study, Walfridsson et al. [83] sought to compare patients treated with radiofrequency ablation for paroxysmal supraventricular tachycardia with a normal population, finding that HRQoL scores were similar 1 year after treatment. Risom et al. [75] assessed 210 patients who participated in post ablation cardiac rehabilitation with those managed with standard care only. While there was no between group difference in the mortality or hospital admissions, a lower proportion of the patients in the cardiac rehabilitation group had high levels of anxiety than in the standard care group.

Anxiety and Depression

Perhaps unsurprisingly due to the number of PROMs tools used within the studies linked to anxiety and depression, and the link between arrhythmia and anxiety, seven of the studies involving a total of 1178 patients closely focused on collecting patient reported anxiety and depression data within their QoL outcomes [46, 63, 70, 76, 92, 99, 102]. While improved health and quality of life related to successful ablation was reported in all of these studies, interestingly in a small study of 41 patients Efremidis et al. [46] found that patients with higher baseline anxiety and depression were linked to higher recurrence rates.

Exercise Performance

Changes in exercise performance were measured by Mohanty et al. [64] and Yagishita et al. [91] in studies of patients with asymptomatic persistent AF treated with catheter ablation. These studies, including a total of 95 patients, both found that successful ablation improved quality of life and exercise performance.

Healthcare Utilisation

Five studies focused closely on both QoL improvements and resource utilisation. Biviano et al. [34] was a multicentre registry study including over 700 patients treated for paroxysmal AF and sought to identify differences in QoL and healthcare utilisation between younger and older cohorts (≥65 vs. <65 years). This study found that QoL improvements were similar between the two groups, with healthcare cost lower or not significantly different for older patients. Similar outcomes were assessed by Farkowski et al. [49], however this study of 82 patients focused on differences between genders following catheter ablation for RFA for AVNRT or AVRT. While there were no differences in healthcare resource use or HRQoL, women did report higher severity of symptoms than men at the two-month follow up. Quality of life, socioeconomic parameters and costs of conventional therapy were assessed in a 2012 study by Bulkova et al. [39] in a study of 160 AF patients who were followed up for two years post ablation. As well as seeing significant improvements in quality of life, decreased hospital bed days and incapacity, there was a three-fold reduction in costs of conventional therapy (e.g. examination costs, cardioversion, antiarrhythmic drugs etc.) following ablation. Reduction in costs and improvement in quality of life were also reported by Gupta et al. [52] in a study of 329 patients treated with guided ablation where a 42% reduction in cardiovascular hospitalisations was recorded. Similarly, Lo et al. [61] recorded a 55% reduction in annualised event rates of cardiovascular healthcare utilisation in a study of 223 patients treated with RF ablation.

Cryoballoon Ablation

As well as the studies by Andrade et al. [28], Kuck et al. [60] and Mortsell et al. [66] previously detailed, Boveda et al., Chun et al. [95], Jain et al. [97], and Su et al. [37, 80, 95, 97] also reported on studies assessing QoL following cryoballoon ablation. Boveda et al. [37] treated 101 patients with persistent AF, with findings indicating 61% procedural success at 12 months together with significant reductions in symptoms and an improvement in quality of life. Similar results were reported by Jain et al. [97] in their study of 335 patients treated with cryoballoon ablation for paroxysmal AF, and Su et al. [80] who reported 54.8% freedom from AF and significant QoL improvements in a study of 165 patients with persistent AF. Andrade et al. [28] reported a significant improvement in HRQoL and decrease in cardioversions, emergency department visits and hospitalisations following both cryoballoon ablation and contact force–guided radiofrequency ablation.

Cavotricuspid Isthmus Ablation

As noted, studies by Seara et al. [77] and Cabanos-Grandios et al. [40] focused on patients with atrial flutter treated with cavotricuspid isthmus ablation. These both reported improvements in QoL, however there are a number of similarities within the two studies which suggest that the same patient cohort may be included by both authors, with Cabanas-Grandio reporting data after a longer follow up period. At over six years after ablation, predictors of long term QoL included recurrence of atrial flutter, basal QoL history of diabetes mellitus and AF.

Predictors of Success

Two of the included studies [50, 99] specifically explored the factors predictive of CA success. Barmano et al. [99] identified several factors affecting outcomes in patients with AF treated with CA including gender, diabetes, heart failure, left atrial volume and frequency of AF attacks prior to ablation. In a study of patients with long-standing persistent atrial fibrillation Fiala et al. [50] found that younger male patients gained most benefit, while delayed or non-improved left atrial appendage outflow reduced post-ablation functional improvement.

Other Study Aims

Four studies identified [35, 44, 54, 78] collected data as part of PROM validation or evaluation studies, although QoL data for the patients treated with catheter ablation is also available from these.

Predictors of Poor Quality of Life

Although few studies set out specifically to identify the predictors of success, many authors did report on factors which influenced poor quality of life with 60 of the 77 papers identifying predictors of poor quality of life. These were mainly linked to recurrence of arrythmia following ablation / non-maintenance of sinus rhythm (reported in 27 papers), high or continued arrhythmia burden (reported in 15 papers), and non-ablation treatment (e.g. AAD therapy, reported in 11 papers). Other authors reported a range of factors including gender (reported in eight papers), age, low baseline QoL, depression and anxiety, warfarin use, family history of AF, and co-morbidities including prior stroke, obesity, and diabetes. Figure 16.3 is a Venn diagram illustrating predictors of poor outcomes as reported in the included texts.

Limitations of the Included Studies

A large number of tools were used in the studies and this may mean that comparison across studies is difficult. This is particularly true when the outcome measures used were not validated tools, and others were collecting and reporting data as part of a validation study meaning that they may not be robust and reliable. Some of the studies were very small and in some cases quality of life data was reported at just two or three months post ablation. A "blanking period" of three months is often referred to following ablation for atrial fibrillation, and is the time period during which early recurrence of arrhythmias can occur due to transient inflammatory pro-arrhythmic changes. While some of the studies reporting at 3 months or less included other arrhythmia substrates, results for AF patients utilising data collected before this time may be misleading depending on the window of PROMs collection. Additionally, a number of included studies are from authors within the same institution and there is a possibility that some of the studies have presented data on the same patients, leading to double reporting. Only a small number of RCTs were included and many studies were single cohort. Registry data although arguably providing meaningful "real world" feedback, does come with its own limitations, specifically lack of standardised treatment protocols and thus inevitable variation in treatment.

As for any other field, Patient Reported Outcome Measures are subjective and can be influenced by many variables including method of collection, and intentional/unintentional clinician bias.

Critique of the Different Tools Available

The benefits of using generic tools such as the EQ5D and SF-36 as discussed previously include

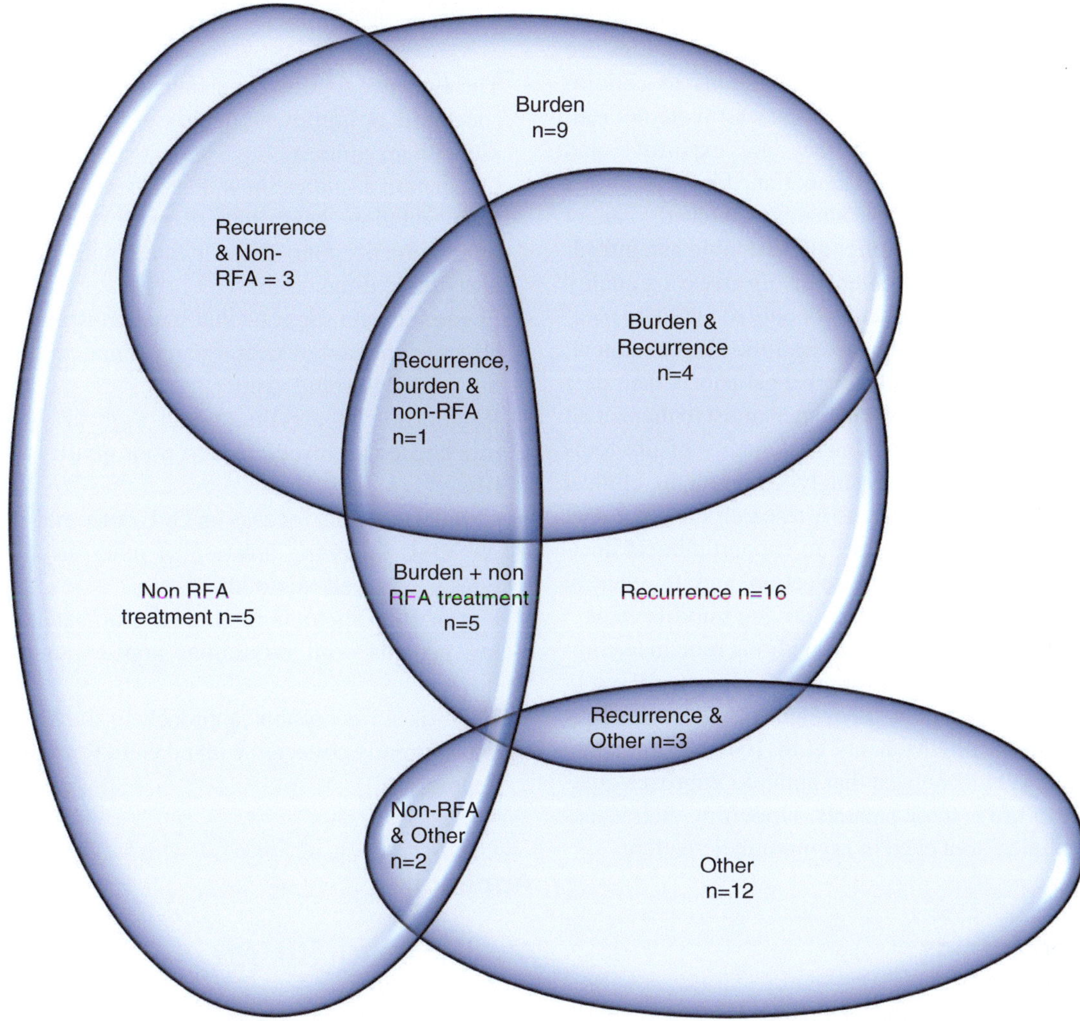

Fig. 16.3 Predictors of poor Quality of Life

the ability to compare between different conditions and also, in some cases, the added benefit of supporting economic evaluations. However, often for arrhythmia patients they are too insensitive to measure the full impact of cardiac arrhythmias on patient quality of life, and similarly unable to measure the benefits of treatment including ablation.

As is the case for other disorders, the use of more sensitive condition specific PROMs tools provides the ability to ensure that all aspects of the condition which are relevant to arrhythmia patients are explored. However, as this group of studies suggests, there is a wide range of potential tools available and currently there appears to be no consensus on a preferred tool, although AFEQT was the most widely used. The additional use of measures of anxiety and depression within the included studies reflects the suggested link between arrhythmias and anxiety, and may serve to identify issues that may otherwise be missed in this patient group.

Comparison to Other Outcomes

Clinical outcomes as traditionally measured via mortality, morbidity and clinical complications are crude and in reality assess failure and not success. In many hospitals, patients are not seen post-ablation procedure and therefore success is assumed and only patients with difficulties are seen at a later stage. Investigations to confirm whether ablation has been successful are not routine, and in addition they are expensive and resource intensive, an important factor in an era where resources are already stretched. Patient reported outcomes offer an accessible and affordable method of comprehensively assessing quality of life before treatment, not only to facilitate measurement of clinical success following treatment, but also to more fully involve patients in their care and to understand what matters most to them at all stages of their treatment. As quality of life tools are becoming increasingly common in clinical practice and not just as a research tool, the data they collect can be used to support clinical decision making, patient selection and to identify good practice, potentially driving improvement.

Some patients with arrhythmia remain asymptomatic despite their diagnosis. However, even in these groups there is evidence as supported by the studies by Mohanty et al. [64] and Yagishita et al. [91] to suggest that ablation improves quality of life in these patients, supporting their use as a clinical tool even in asymptomatic patients.

Conclusions

As the focus of catheter ablation is often to reduce or abolish symptoms it seems that HRQoL tools are an ideal measure of procedural success. The studies included in this overview suggest that it has a high success rate with good outcomes that are maintained during long-term follow up. These outcomes compare favourably to anti-arrhythmia drug therapy which has been the traditional mainstay of treatment. Several ablation strategies were also considered by these studies in different arrhythmia types, all with good clinical and patient outcomes.

The use of anxiety and depression tools may reflect an area of health and quality of life which is not covered by some generic or condition specific tools. Those collecting HRQoL data from patients with arrhythmia should be aware of this aspect of health and ensure it is not overlooked.

In summary, the studies identified suggest:

- The evidence suggests that catheter ablation is successful at improving quality of life in people with arrythmias
- Comparative studies show that patients treated with ablation have better quality of life improvements than those treated with anti-arrhythmic drugs
- Economic data suggests that ablation is a cost effective method of treating arrythmia, reducing related hospital visits
- Recurrence of arrythmia and high arrythmia burden are predictors of poor quality of life
- Clinical trial data focuses on QoL outcomes in AF, QoL following ablation of other arrythmias is less well reported
- Use of PROMs tools in clinical trials including patients with arrythmias appears to be increasing
- There is no consistent approach to the QoL data currently collected with no Gold Standard approach

Appendix

Medline Search Strategy

1. exp. Arrhythmias, Cardiac/
2. arrhythmia*.tw.
3. ((atrial or ventricular) adj1 fibrillation).tw.
4. ((atrial or ventricular) adj1 flutter).tw.
5. (tachycardia or bradycardia or tachyarrhythmia or bradyarrhythmia).tw.
6. ("sick sinus syndrome" or tachybrady).tw.
7. ("heart block" or "atrioventricular block" or "AV block").tw.
8. AVNRT.tw.
9. ((long or short) adj QT).tw.
10. "Wolff-Parkinson-White syndrome".tw.
11. "atrial premature complexes".tw.
12. ("carotid sinus syndrome" or "carotid sinus hypersensitivity").tw.
13. (cardiac adj5 channelopath*).tw.
14. ("QT syndrome*" or LQTS or SQTS).tw.
15. 1 or 2 or 3 or 4 or 5 or 6 or 7 or 8 or 9 or 10 or 11 or 12 or 13 or 14

16. Catheter Ablation/
17. Radiofrequency Ablation/
18. High-Intensity Focused Ultrasound Ablation/
19. ablation techniques/
20. laser therapy/
21. exp. Arrhythmias, Cardiac/su [Surgery]
22. (catheter adj5 (ablat* or isolat*)).tw.
23. (transcatheter adj5 (ablat* or isolat*)).tw.
24. (atrial adj5 ablat*).tw.
25. (electric* adj5 ablat*).tw.
26. ((radiofrequency or RF) adj5 ablat*).tw.
27. (ccryosurg* or cryoablat*).tw.
28. cauteri*.tw.
29. (laser adj5 ablat*).tw.
30. "pulmonary vein isolation*".tw.
31. "high intensity focused ultrasound".tw.
32. or/16-31
33. (HR-PRO or HRPRO or HRQL or HRQoL or QL or QoL or "health index*" or "health indices" or "health profile*").tw.
34. ("quality of life" adj2 (assessment* or index or indices or instrument or instruments or measure or measures or questionnaire* or profile or profiles or scale or scales or score or scores or status or survey or surveys)).tw.
35. Health Status/
36. (patient adj reported adj outcome*).tw.
37. HeartQoL.tw.
38. ("Atrial Fibrillation Effect on QualiTy-of-Life" or AFEQT).tw.
39. ("Quality of Life questionnaire for Patients with Atrial Fibrillation" or AF-QOL18).tw.

References

1. Gallagher JJ, Anderson RW, Kasell J, Rice JR, Pritchett EL, Gault HJ, et al. Cryoablation of drug-resistant ventricular tachycardia in a patient with a variant of scleroderma. Circulation. 1978;57(1):190–7.
2. Scheinman MA, Rutherford JD. The development of cardiac arrhythmia ablation. Circulation. 2017;135(13):1191–3.
3. Jin ES, Wang PJ. Cryoballoon ablation for atrial fibrillation: a comprehensive review and practice guide. Korean Circ J. 2018;48(2):114–23.
4. Morady F. Radio-frequency ablation as treatment for cardiac arrhythmias. N Engl J Med. 1999;340(7):534–44.
5. Calkins H, Gliklich RE, Leavy MB, Piccini JP, Hsu JC, Mohanty S, et al. Harmonized outcome measures for use in atrial fibrillation patient registries and clinical practice: endorsed by the Heart Rhythm Society Board of Trustees. Heart Rhythm. 2019;16(1):e3–e16.
6. Katritsis DG, Boriani G, Cosio FG, Hindricks G, Jais P, Josephson ME, et al. European Heart Rhythm Association (EHRA) consensus document on the management of supraventricular arrhythmias, endorsed by Heart Rhythm Society (HRS), Asia-Pacific Heart Rhythm Society (APHRS), and Sociedad Latinoamericana de Estimulacion Cardiaca y Electrofisiologia (SOLAECE). Europace. 2017;19(3):465–511.
7. HQIP. National audit of cardiac rhythm management devices and ablation—2016–17 report. 2019.
8. Ramirez FD, Reddy VY, Viswanathan R, Hocini M, Jaïs P. Emerging technologies for pulmonary vein isolation. Circ Res. 2020;127(1):170–83.
9. Verma MS, Terricabras M, Verma A. The cutting edge of atrial fibrillation ablation. Arrhythmia Electrophysiol Rev. 2021;10(2):101.
10. De Potter TJ, Boersma LV. Ultra-low temperature cryoablation: the coolest innovation EP has been waiting for? J Cardiovasc Electrophysiol. 2021;32(3):578–9.
11. Reddy VY, Dukkipati SR, Neuzil P, Anic A, Petru J, Funasako M, et al. Pulsed field ablation of paroxysmal atrial fibrillation: 1-year outcomes of IMPULSE, PEFCAT, and PEFCAT II. Clin Electrophysiol. 2021;7(5):614–27.
12. Kirchhof P, Benussi S, Kotecha D, Ahlsson A, Atar D, Casadei B, et al. 2016 ESC Guidelines for the management of atrial fibrillation developed in collaboration with EACTS. Eur Heart J. 2016;37(38):2893–962.
13. Withers KL, White J, Carolan-Rees G, Patrick H, O'Callaghan P, Murray S, et al. Patient reported outcome measures for cardiac ablation procedures: a multicentre pilot to develop a new questionnaire. Europace. 2014;16(11):1626–33.
14. Withers KL, Wood KA, Carolan-Rees G, Patrick H, Lencioni M, Griffith M. Living on a knife edge-the daily struggle of coping with symptomatic cardiac arrhythmias. Health Qual Life Outcomes. 2015;13:86.
15. Thrall G, Lane D, Carroll D, Lip GY. Quality of life in patients with atrial fibrillation: a systematic review. Am J Med. 2006;119(5):448.e1–19.
16. Aliot E, Botto GL, Crijns HJ, Kirchhof P. Quality of life in patients with atrial fibrillation: how to assess it and how to improve it. Europace. 2014;16(6):787–96.
17. Lane DA, Aguinaga L, Blomstrom-Lundqvist C, Boriani G, Dan GA, Hills MT, et al. Cardiac tachyarrhythmias and patient values and preferences for their management: the European Heart Rhythm Association (EHRA) consensus document endorsed by the Heart Rhythm Society (HRS), Asia Pacific Heart Rhythm Society (APHRS), and Sociedad Latinoamericana de Estimulacion Cardiaca y Electrofisiologia (SOLEACE). Europace. 2015;17(12):1747–69.
18. Andrade JG, Verma A, Mitchell LB, Parkash R, Leblanc K, Atzema C, et al. 2018 Focused Update

of the Canadian Cardiovascular Society Guidelines for the Management of Atrial Fibrillation. Can J Cardiol. 2018;34(11):1371–92.

19. Kirchhof P, Benussi S, Kotecha D, Ahlsson A, Atar D, Casadei B, et al. 2016 ESC Guidelines for the management of atrial fibrillation developed in collaboration with EACTS. Eur J Cardiothorac Surg. 2016;50(5):e1–e88.
20. Fu Y, Shen X, Huang W. Association between depression and risk of triggering ventricular arrhythmias: a meta-analysis. Int J Clin Pharmacol Ther. 2019;57(6):306–14.
21. Ismail H, Coulton S. Arrhythmia care co-ordinators: their impact on anxiety and depression, readmissions and health service costs. Eur J Cardiothorac Surg. 2016;15(5):355–62.
22. Arbelo E, Aktaa S, Bollmann A, D'Avila A, Drossart I, Dwight J, et al. Quality indicators for the care and outcomes of adults with atrial fibrillation: task force for the development of quality indicators in atrial fibrillation of the European Heart Rhythm Association (EHRA) of the European Society of Cardiology (ESC): developed in collaboration with the Heart Rhythm Society (HRS), the Asia Pacific Heart Rhythm Society (APHRS), and the Latin-American Heart Rhythm Society (LAHRS). EP Europ. 2021;23(4):494–5.
23. Seligman WH, Das-Gupta Z, Jobi-Odeneye AO, Arbelo E, Banerjee A, Bollmann A, et al. Development of an international standard set of outcome measures for patients with atrial fibrillation: a report of the International Consortium for Health Outcomes Measurement (ICHOM) atrial fibrillation working group. Eur Heart J. 2020;41(10):1132–40.
24. Kotecha D, Ahmed A, Calvert M, Lencioni M, Terwee CB, Lane DA. Patient-reported outcomes for quality of life assessment in atrial fibrillation: a systematic review of measurement properties. PLoS One. 2016;11(11):e0165790-e.
25. Steinberg BA, Dorian P, Anstrom KJ, Hess R, Mark DB, Noseworthy PA, et al. Patient-reported outcomes in atrial fibrillation research. Results Clinicaltrial Anal. 2019;5(5):599–605.
26. Kloosterman M, Chua W, Fabritz L, Al-Khalidi HR, Schotten U, Nielsen JC, et al. Sex differences in catheter ablation of atrial fibrillation: results from AXAFA-AFNET 5. Europace. 2020;22(7):1026–35.
27. Piccini JP, Todd DM, Massaro T, Lougee A, Haeusler KG, Blank B, et al. Changes in quality of life, cognition and functional status following catheter ablation of atrial fibrillation. Heart. 2020;106(24):1919–26.
28. Andrade JG, Macle L, Verma A, Deyell MW, Champagne J, Dubuc M, et al. Quality of life and health care utilization in the CIRCA-DOSE study. JACC Clin Electrophysiol. 2020;6(8):935–44.
29. Samuel M, Khairy P, Champagne J, Deyell MW, Macle L, Leong-Sit P, et al. Association of atrial fibrillation burden with health-related quality of life after atrial fibrillation ablation: substudy of the cryoballoon vs contact-force atrial fibrillation ablation (CIRCA-DOSE) randomized clinical trial. JAMA Cardiol. 2021;6(11):1324–8.
30. Yao RJR, Macle L, Deyell MW, Tang L, Hawkins NM, Sedlak T, et al. Impact of female sex on clinical presentation and ablation outcomes in the CIRCA-DOSE study. JACC Clin Electrophysiol. 2020;6(8):945–54.
31. Amir M, Rabby RA, Kabo P, Setiadji R. The short-term post-ablation outcome of patients with low-burden premature ventricular complexes. Iran Heart J. 2021;22(4):25–33.
32. Bai Y, Bai R, Wu JH, Zhang T, Liu N, Shi XB, et al. Differences in quality of life between atrial fibrillation patients with low stroke risk treated with and without catheter ablation. J Am Heart Assoc. 2015;4(9):e002130.
33. Berger WR, Krul SP, van der Pol JA, van Dessel PF, Conrath CE, Wilde AA, et al. Documented atrial fibrillation recurrences after pulmonary vein isolation are associated with diminished quality of life. J Cardiovasc Med. 2016;17(3):201–8.
34. Biviano AB, Hunter TD, Dandamudi G, Fishel RS, Gidney B, Herweg B, et al. Healthcare utilization and quality of life improvement after ablation for paroxysmal AF in younger and older patients. PACE. 2017;40(4):391–400.
35. Bjorkenheim A, Brandes A, Magnuson A, Chemnitz A, Edvardsson N, Poci D. Patient-reported outcomes in relation to continuously monitored rhythm before and during 2 years after atrial fibrillation ablation using a disease-specific and a generic instrument. J Am Heart Assoc. 2018;7(5):e008362.
36. Blomstrom-Lundqvist C, Gizurarson S, Schwieler J, Jensen SM, Bergfeldt L, Kenneback G, et al. Effect of catheter ablation vs antiarrhythmic medication on quality of life in patients with atrial fibrillation: the CAPTAF randomized clinical trial. JAMA. 2019;321(11):1059–68.
37. Boveda S, Metzner A, Nguyen DQ, Chun KRJ, Goehl K, Noelker G, et al. Single-procedure outcomes and quality-of-life improvement 12 months post-cryoballoon ablation in persistent atrial fibrillation: results from the multicenter CRYO4PERSISTENT AF trial. JACC Clin Electrophysiol. 2018;4(11):1440–7.
38. Bulkova V, Fiala M, Havranek S, Simek J, Sknouril L, Januska J, et al. Improvement in quality of life after catheter ablation for paroxysmal versus long-standing persistent atrial fibrillation: a prospective study with 3-year follow-up. J Am Heart Assoc. 2014;3(4):e000881.
39. Bulkova V, Fiala M, Wichterle D, Haman L, Chovancik J, Havranek S, et al. Quality of life and costs of conventional therapy in patients treated by catheter ablation for atrial fibrillation. Cor Vasa. 2012;54(6):e421–e7.
40. Cabanas-Grandio P, Garcia-Seara J, Gude F, Martinez-Sande JL, Fernandez-Lopez XA, Gonzalez-Juanatey JR. Assessment of long-term quality of life after cavotricuspid isthmus ablation

for typical atrial flutter. Health Qual Life Outcomes. 2014;12(1):47.
41. Carnlof C, Insulander P, Pettersson PH, Jensen-Urstad M, Fossum B. Health-related quality of life in patients with atrial fibrillation undergoing pulmonary vein isolation, before and after treatment. Eur J Cardiovasc Nurs. 2010;9(1):45–9.
42. Carnlof C, Iwarzon M, Jensen-Urstad M, Gadler F, Insulander P. Women with PSVT are often misdiagnosed, referred later than men, and have more symptoms after ablation. Scand Cardiovasc J. 2017;51(6):299–307.
43. Das M, Wynn GJ, Saeed Y, Gomes S, Morgan M, Ronayne C, et al. Pulmonary vein re-isolation as a routine strategy regardless of symptoms: the PRESSURE randomized controlled trial. JACC Clin Electrophysiol. 2017;3(6):602–11.
44. Domeyer PR, Giannakidou SC, Kyriakou P, Katsari V, Antoniadis AP, Lagos IK, et al. Impact of radiofrequency ablation and antiarrhythmic medications on the quality of life of patients with supraventricular tachycardias: preliminary validation of the greek version of the Umea22 (U22) questionnaire. Biomed Res Int. 2018;2018:3059478.
45. Du X, Guo L, He X, Jia Y, Wu J, Long D, et al. A comparison of the real world effectiveness of catheter ablation and drug therapy in atrial fibrillation patients in a Chinese setting. BMC Cardiovasc Disord. 2017;17(1):204.
46. Efremidis M, Letsas KP, Lioni L, Giannopoulos G, Korantzopoulos P, Vlachos K, et al. Association of quality of life, anxiety, and depression with left atrial ablation outcomes. Pacing Clin Electrophysiol. 2014;37(6):703–11.
47. Essebag V, Azizi Z, Alipour P, Khaykin Y, Leong-Sit P, Sarrazin JF, et al. Relationship between quality of life and burden of recurrent atrial fibrillation following ablation: CAPCOST multicentre cohort study. Europace. 2020;22(7):1017–25.
48. Evans JM, Withers KL, Lencioni M, Carolan-Rees G, Wood KA, Patrick H, et al. Quality of life benefits from arrhythmia ablation: a longitudinal study using the C-CAP questionnaire and EQ5D. Pacing Clin Electrophysiol. 2019;42(6):705–11.
49. Farkowski MM, Pytkowski M, MacIag A, Golicki D, AliceWood K, Kowalik I, et al. Gender-related differences in outcomes and resource utilization in patients undergoing radiofrequency ablation of supraventricular tachycardia: results from patients' perspective on radiofrequency catheter ablation of AVRT and AVNRT study. Europace. 2014;16(12):1821–7.
50. Fiala M, Bulkova V, Sknouril L, Nevralova R, Toman O, Januska J, et al. Functional improvement after successful catheter ablation for long-standing persistent atrial fibrillation. Europace. 2017;19(11): 1781–9.
51. Fujisawa T, Kimura T, Kohsaka S, Ikemura N, Katsumata Y, Miyama H, et al. Symptom burden and treatment perception in patients with atrial fibrillation, with and without a family history of atrial fibrillation. Heart Vessel. 2021;36(2):267–76.
52. Gupta D, Vijgen J, Potter T, Scherr D, Van Herendael H, Knecht S, et al. Quality of life and healthcare utilisation improvements after atrial fibrillation ablation. Heart. 2021;107(16):1296–302.
53. Haman L, Dostalova H, Parizek P. Catheter ablation for atrial fibrillation-single center experience. Cor Vasa. 2012;54(6):e369–e74.
54. Hoglund N, Ronn F, Tollefsen T, Jensen SM, Kesek M. U22 protocol as measure of symptomatic improvement after catheter ablation of atrial fibrillation. Ups J Med Sci. 2013;118(4):240–6.
55. Ikemura N, Spertus JA, Kimura T, Katsumata Y, Fujisawa T, Ueda I, et al. Baseline and postprocedural health status outcomes in contemporary patients with atrial fibrillation who underwent catheter ablation: a report from the Japanese outpatient registry. J Am Heart Assoc. 2021;10(18):e019983.
56. Inagaki D, Fukamizu S, Tokioka S, Kawamura I, Kitamura T, Hojo R, et al. Quality of life improvements by durable pulmonary vein isolation in patients with atrial fibrillation. J Cardiovasc Electrophysiol. 2020;31(8):2013–21.
57. Kanda T, Masuda M, Inoue K, Furukawa Y, Hirata A, Egami Y, et al. Differences in quality of life improvement with pulmonary vein isolation alone vs. more extensive ablation of persistent atrial fibrillation: insights from the EARNEST-PVI trial. Eur Heart J. 2021;42(Suppl 1):512.
58. Kato M, Miake J, Ogura K, Iitsuka K, Okamura A, Tomomori T, et al. Different effects of pulmonary vein isolation on quality of life between patients with persistent and paroxysmal atrial fibrillation. Int Heart J. 2019;60(6):1328–33.
59. Kesek M, Ronn F, Tollefsen T, Hoglund N, Naslund U, Jensen SM. Symptomatic improvement after catheter ablation of supraventricular tachycardia measured by the arrhythmia-specific questionnaire U22. Ups J Med Sci. 2011;116(1):52–9.
60. Kuck KH, Furnkranz A, Chun KRJ, Metzner A, Ouyang F, Schluter M, et al. Cryoballoon or radiofrequency ablation for symptomatic paroxysmal atrial fibrillation: reintervention, rehospitalization, and quality-of-life outcomes in the FIRE and ICE trial. Eur Heart J. 2016;37(38):2858–65.
61. Lo MY, Mansour M, Nair DG, Calkins H, Reddy VY, Colley BJ, et al. B-Po04-203 cardiovascular healthcare utilization in persistent atrial fibrillation patients ablated with a contact force catheter. Heart Rhythm. 2021;18(8 Suppl):S361.
62. Mantovan R, Macle L, De Martino G, Chen J, Morillo CA, Novak P, et al. Relationship of quality of life with procedural success of atrial fibrillation (AF) ablation and postablation af burden: substudy of the STAR AF randomized trial. Can J Cardiol. 2013;29(10):1211–7.
63. Mohanty S, Mohanty P, Di Biase L, Bai R, Santangeli P, Casella M, et al. Results from a single-blind, randomized study comparing the impact of differ-

ent ablation approaches on long-term procedure outcome in coexistent atrial fibrillation and flutter (approval). Circulation. 2013;127(18):1853–60.

64. Mohanty S, Santangeli P, Mohanty P, Biase LD, Holcomb S, Trivedi C, et al. Catheter ablation of asymptomatic longstanding persistent atrial fibrillation: impact on quality of life, exercise performance, arrhythmia perception, and arrhythmia-free survival. J Cardiovasc Electrophysiol. 2014;25(10):1057–64.
65. Morillo CA, Verma A, Connolly SJ, Kuck KH, Nair GM, Champagne J, et al. Radiofrequency ablation vs antiarrhythmic drugs as first-line treatment of paroxysmal atrial fibrillation (RAAFT-2) a randomized trial. JAMA. 2014;311(7):692–9.
66. Mortsell D, Malmborg H, Lonnerholm S, Jansson V, Blomstrom-Lundqvist C. Acute and long-term efficacy and safety with a single cryoballoon application as compared with the standard dual application strategy: a prospective randomized study using the second-generation cryoballoon for pulmonary vein isolation in patients with symptomatic atrial fibrillation. Europace. 2018;20(10):1598–605.
67. Nakajima K. Improvement in quality of life in patients that underwent catheter ablation for persistent atrial fibrillation. J Arrhyth. 2019;35(Suppl 1):77.
68. Onishi N, Oi M, Jinnai T, Kaitani K, Harita T, Nishiuchi S, et al. Effect of rhythm control therapy for asymptomatic atrial fibrillation. Eur Heart J. 2020a;41(Suppl 1):i44.
69. Onishi N, Kyo S, Oi M, Jinnai T, Kuroda M, Shimizu Y, et al. Improvement in quality of life and cardiac function after catheter ablation for asymptomatic persistent atrial fibrillation. J Arrhyth. 2020b;37(1):11–9.
70. Papiashvili G, Tabagari-Bregvadze N, Brugada J. Impact of radiofrequency catheter ablation on health-related quality of life assessed by the Sf-36 questionnaire in patients with paroxysmal supraventricular tachycardia. Georgian Med News. 2018:54–7.
71. Pavlovic N, Chierchia GB, Velagic V, Hermida JS, Healey S, Arena G, et al. Initial rhythm control with cryoballoon ablation vs drug therapy: impact on quality of life and symptoms. Am Heart J. 2021;242:103–14.
72. Pytkowski M, Maciag A, Jankowska A, Kowalik I, Kraska A, Farkowski MM, et al. Quality of life improvement after radiofrequency catheter ablation of outflow tract ventricular arrhythmias in patients with structurally normal hearts. Acta Cardiol. 2012;67(2):153–9.
73. Raine D, Langley P, Shepherd E, Lord S, Murray S, Murray A, et al. Effect of catheter ablation on quality of life in patients with atrial fibrillation and its correlation with arrhythmia outcome. Open Heart. 2015;2(1):e000302.
74. Reynolds MR, Walczak J, White SA, Cohen DJ, Wilber DJ. Improvements in symptoms and quality of life in patients with paroxysmal atrial fibrillation treated with radiofrequency catheter ablation versus antiarrhythmic drugs. Circ Cardiovasc Qual Outcomes. 2010;3(6):615–23.
75. Risom SS, Zwisler AD, Sibilitz KL, Rasmussen TB, Taylor R, Thygesen LC, et al. Cardiac rehabilitation for patients treated for atrial fibrillation with ablation has long-term effects: 12-and 24-month follow-up results from the randomized copenheart (RFA) trial. Arch Phys Med Rehabil. 2020;101(11):1877–86.
76. Sang CH, Chen K, Pang XF, Dong JZ, Du X, Ma H, et al. Depression, anxiety, and quality of life after catheter ablation in patients with paroxysmal atrial fibrillation. Clin Cardiol. 2013;36(1):40–5.
77. Seara JG, Gude F, Cabanas P, Sande JLM, Lopez XF, Elices J, et al. Quality of life differences in patients with typical atrial flutter following cavotricuspid isthmus ablation. Revista Espanola De Cardiologia. 2011;64(5):401–8.
78. Spertus J, Dorian P, Bubien R, Lewis S, Godejohn D, Reynolds MR, et al. Development and validation of the Atrial Fibrillation Effect on QualiTy-of-life (AFEQT) questionnaire in patients with Atrial Fibrillation. Circ Arrhythm Electrophysiol. 2011;4(1):15–25.
79. Steinberg BA, Holmes DN, Pieper K, Allen LA, Chan PS, Ezekowitz MD, et al. Factors associated with large improvements in health-related quality of life in patients with atrial fibrillation: results from ORBIT-AF. Circ Arrhythm Electrophysiol. 2020;13(5):e007775.
80. Su WW, Reddy VY, Bhasin K, Champagne J, Sangrigoli RM, Braegelmann KM, et al. Cryoballoon ablation of pulmonary veins for persistent atrial fibrillation: results from the multicenter STOP Persistent AF trial. Heart Rhythm. 2020;17(11):1841–7.
81. Terricabras M, Mantovan R, Jiang CY, Betts TR, Chen J, Deisenhofer I, et al. Association between quality of life and procedural outcome after catheter ablation for atrial fibrillation: a secondary analysis of a randomized clinical trial. JAMA Netw Open. 2020;3(12):e2025473.
82. Timmers L, Vervaet P, Goethals P, De Pooter J, Vanheuverswyn F, Van de Velde E, et al. Quality of life and symptoms in patients selected for ablation of ventricular extrasystoles: a prospective study. J Interv Card Electrophysiol. 2021; https://doi.org/10.1007/s10840-021-01092-x.
83. Walfridsson U, Walfridsson H, Arestedt K, Stromberg A. Impact of radiofrequency ablation on health-related quality of life in patients with paroxysmal supraventricular tachycardia compared with a norm population one year after treatment. Heart Lung. 2011;40(5):405–11.
84. Wazni O, Dandamudi G, Sood N, Hoyt R, Tyler J, Durrani S, et al. Quality of life after the initial treatment of atrial fibrillation with cryoablation versus drug therapy. Heart Rhythm. 2021;16:16.
85. Wilber DJ, Pappone C, Neuzil P, De Paola A, Marchlinski F, Natale A, et al. Comparison of antiarrhythmic drug therapy and radiofrequency

catheter ablation in patients with paroxysmal atrial fibrillation: a randomized controlled trial. JAMA. 2010;303(4):333–40.
86. Wokhlu A, Monahan KH, Hodge DO, Asirvatham SJ, Friedman PA, Munger TM, et al. Long-term quality of life after ablation of atrial fibrillation. the impact of recurrence, symptom relief, and placebo effect. J Am Coll Cardiol. 2010;55(21):2308–16.
87. Wozniak-Skowerska IM, Skowerski MJ, Hoffmann A, Nowak S, Faryan M, Kolasa J, et al. Quality of life in patients with paroxysmal atrial fibrillation after circumferential pulmonary vein ablation. Kardiol Pol. 2016;74(3):244–50.
88. Wu G, Huang H, Cai L, Yang Y, Liu X, Yu B, et al. Long-term observation of catheter ablation vs. pharmacotherapy in the management of persistent and long-standing persistent atrial fibrillation (CAPA study). Europace. 2021;23(5):731–9.
89. Wynn GJ, Panikker S, Morgan M, Hall M, Waktare J, Markides V, et al. Biatrial linear ablation in sustained nonpermanent AF: results of the substrate modification with ablation and antiarrhythmic drugs in nonpermanent atrial fibrillation (SMAN-PAF) trial. Heart Rhythm. 2016;13(2):399–406.
90. Xu Y, Sharma D, Du F, Li G, Xu G. Comparison of circumferential pulmonary vein isolation and antiarrhythmic drug therapy in patients with atrial fibrillation. Cardiol Ther. 2012;1(1):1–7.
91. Yagishita A, Yamauchi Y, Sato H, Yamashita S, Hirao T, Miyamoto T, et al. Improvement in the quality of life and exercise performance in relation to the plasma B-type natriuretic peptide level after catheter ablation in patients with asymptomatic persistent atrial fibrillation. Circ J. 2017;81(4):444–9.
92. Yildirim O, Yontar OC, Semiz M, Erdem A, Canan F, Yontar G, et al. The effect of radiofrequency ablation treatment on quality of life and anxiety in patients with supraventricular tachycardia. Eur Rev Med Pharmacol Sci. 2012;16(15):2108–12.
93. Boersma L, Koźluk E, Maglia G, De Sousa J, Grebe O, Eckardt L, et al. Paroxysmal and persistent atrial fibrillation ablation outcomes with the pulmonary vein ablation catheter GOLD duty-cycled phased radiofrequency ablation catheter: quality of life and 12-month efficacy results from the GOLD Atrial Fibrillation Registry. Europace. 2020;22(6):888–96.
94. Buist TJ, Adiyaman A, Beukema RJ, Smit JJJ, Delnoy PPHM, Hemels MEW, et al. Quality of life after catheter and minimally invasive surgical ablation of paroxysmal and early persistent atrial fibrillation: results from the SCALAF trial. Clin Res Cardiol. 2020;109(2):215–24.
95. Chun KRJ, Okumura K, Scazzuso F, Keun On Y, Kueffer FJ, Braegelmann KM, et al. Safety and efficacy of cryoballoon ablation for the treatment of paroxysmal and persistent AF in a real-world global setting: results from the Cryo AF Global Registry. J Arrhyth. 2021;37(2):356–67.
96. Walfridsson H, Walfridsson U, Cosedis Nielsen J, Johannessen A, Raatikainen P, Janzon M, et al. Radiofrequency ablation as initial therapy in paroxysmal atrial fibrillation: results on health-related quality of life and symptom burden. The MANTRA-PAF trial. Europace. 2014;17(2):215–21.
97. Jain SK, Novak PG, Sangrigoli R, Champagne J, Dubuc M, Adler SW, et al. Sustained quality-of-life improvement post-cryoballoon ablation in patients with paroxysmal atrial fibrillation: results from the STOP-AF post-approval study. Heart Rhythm. 2020;17:485–91.
98. Pezawas T, Ristl R, Schukro C, Schmidinger H. Health-related quality of life changes in patients undergoing repeated catheter ablation for atrial fibrillation. Clin Res Cardiol. 2016;105(1):1–9.
99. Barmano N, Charitakis E, Karlsson JE, Nystrom FH, Walfridsson H, Walfridsson U. Predictors of improvement in arrhythmia-specific symptoms and health-related quality of life after catheter ablation of atrial fibrillation. Clin Cardiol. 2019;42(2):247–55.
100. Blandino A, Toso E, Scaglione M, Anselmino M, Ferraris F, Sardi D, et al. Long-term efficacy and safety of two different rhythm control strategies in elderly patients with symptomatic persistent atrial fibrillation. J Cardiovasc Electrophysiol. 2013;24(7):731–8.
101. Duytschaever M, De Pooter J, Demolder A, El Haddad M, Phlips T, Strisciuglio T, et al. Long-term impact of catheter ablation on arrhythmia burden in low-risk patients with paroxysmal atrial fibrillation: the CLOSE to CURE study. Heart Rhythm. 2020;17(4):535–43.
102. Fichtner S, Deisenhofer I, KindsmUller S, Dzijan-Horn M, Tzeis S, Reents T, et al. Prospective assessment of short- and long-term quality of life after ablation for atrial fibrillation. J Cardiovasc Electrophysiol. 2012;23(2):121–7.

Patient Reported Outcomes and Quality of Life following Percutaneous and Surgical Intervention for Subclavian Artery Disease

17

Lydia Hanna and Richard Gibbs

Introduction

Subclavian artery disease describes a condition whereby a high-grade stenosis in the subclavian artery (SA) narrows the vessel wall (subclavian artery stenosis, SAS [Fig. 17.1a]). SAS occurs in 2% of the general population and 7% of patients who have peripheral arterial disease (PAD) [1]. The presence of PAD is associated with a fivefold increase risk of having SAS. Other risk factors include smoking, hypertension and lower level of high-density lipoprotein (HDL) cholesterol [1]. SAS is also associated with increased total mortality, cardiovascular disease mortality and an increased risk of cerebrovascular ischaemic events [2].

More than 90% of SAS cases are the result of steno-occlusive atherosclerotic plaque. Other causes include arteritis, inflammation, radiation exposure, compression syndromes, fibromuscular dysplasia, and neurofibromatosis [1]. The Left SA (LSA) is three-times more likely to be affected by flow-limiting disease than any of the other supra-aortic vessels due to the acute angle between the origin of the LSA and ascending aorta that can lead to increased flow turbulence and atherogenesis [3, 4].

While most patients are asymptomatic, a haemodynamically significant stenosis in the SA can compromise flow to the axillary, vertebral and internal mammary artery and may eventually result in reversal of blood flow known as 'steal' phenomenon, leading to end-organ ischaemia in downstream tissues (Tables 17.1 and 17.2). Broadly speaking, management centres around best medical therapy with an antiplatelet and a statin to reduce disease progression and cardiovascular risk profile for all patients.

Intervention is reserved for symptomatic patients and for asymptomatic patients undergoing planned surgical bypasses that require preservation of inflow (eg LIMA grafts) [5, 6]. Endovascular intervention involves percutaneous transluminal angioplasty (PTA) and stent insertion whereby wires and catheters are used to cross the lesion, followed by dilatation of the lesion with a balloon and insertion of a stent to maintain patency (Fig. 17.1b) [7]. Surgical revascularisation consists of bypassing the lesion with a prosthetic graft that connects the carotid artery to a more distal and healthy part of the subclavian artery (carotid-subclavian bypass, CSB, Fig. 17.1c). Other less commonly used bypasses include axillo-axillary, carotid-axillary or carotid-carotid bypass. The subclavian artery can also be surgically disconnected from the arch and anastomosed onto the carotid artery (subclavian

L. Hanna · R. Gibbs (✉)
Department of Surgery and Cancer, Imperial College London, London, UK

Imperial Vascular Unit, Imperial College London Healthcare NHS Trust, London, UK
e-mail: l.hanna@imperial.ac.uk; r.gibbs@imperial.ac.uk

T. Athanasiou et al. (eds.), *Patient Reported Outcomes and Quality of Life in Cardiovascular Interventions*, https://doi.org/10.1007/978-3-031-09815-4_17

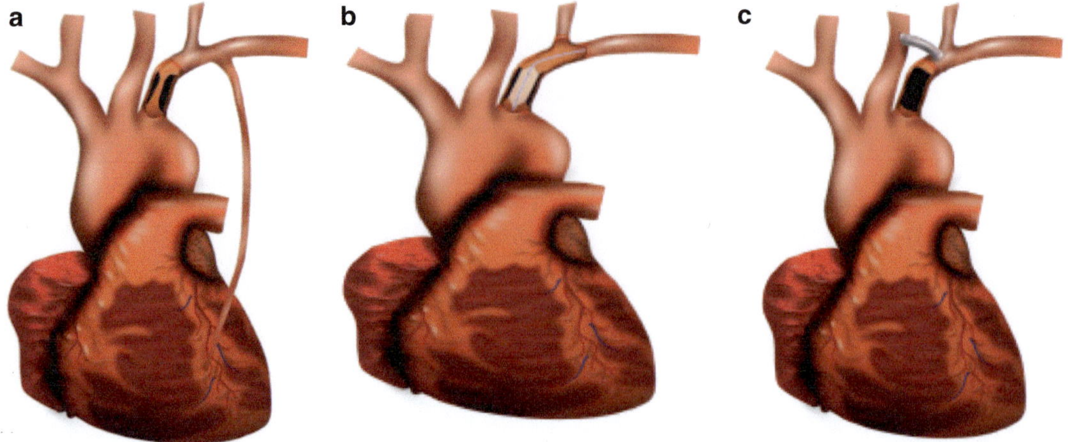

Fig. 17.1 (**a**) Stenosis in subclavian artery. (**b**) Balloon angioplasty. (**c**) Carotid-subclavian artery bypass

Table 17.1 Grades of severity of vertebral artery haemodynamic disturbance in subclavian

- Grade I (pre-subclavian steal): reduced antegrade vertebral flow
- Grade II (intermittent/partial/latent): alternating flow—antegrade flow in the diastolic phase and retrograde flow in the systolic phase
- Grade III (permanent/advanced): permanent retrograde vertebral flow

Table 17.2 Clinical features of Subclavian artery Stenosis (SAS)

Upper limb ischaemia
Arm claudication (pain and fatigue on exertion)
Cool
Paraesthesia
Digital necrosis
Vertebrobasilar symptoms
'Drop attacks'
Diplopia
Dizziness
Tinnitus
Hearing loss
Coronary symptoms
Angina
Myocardial infarction
Heart failure

artery transposition, SCT)) thereby avoiding a prosthetic graft [8, 9].

The 2017 European Society of Cardiology in collaboration with the European Society of Vascular Surgery Guidelines state that in symptomatic patients, both revascularisation options should be considered [5]. Most intervention studies report high technical and clinical success as their end-points with both techniques [10, 11], but it is imperative to also understand the physical, psychological and social impact of these interventions to determine if a minimally invasive intervention offers higher risk patients further advantage in terms of patient-centred outcomes.

This chapter aims to undertake a systematic appraisal of the literature regarding quality of life (QOL) and patient related outcome measures (PROMS) following percutaneous and surgical intervention of subclavian artery disease.

Material and Methods

Search Strategy

This study was performed in accordance with the guidelines for the 'Preferred Reporting Items for Systematic reviews and Meta-Analyses' (PRISMA) [12]. A systematic search of OVID, Embase and Pubmed databases was undertaken up to March 2020 using the following search terms: ('quality of life' or 'patient related outcomes') AND ('subclavian artery disease or stenosis or occlusion or steal') AND ('percutaneous' or 'endovascular' or 'angioplasty' or 'stent' or 'surgery' or 'bypass'). Reference lists of selected papers were also hand searched to check for suitable articles.

Inclusion and Exclusion Criteria

Studies in English reporting QOL and PROMS outcomes with validated tools in adults undergoing intervention percutaneous and surgical revascularisation of the subclavian artery for SAS were included Subclavian artery disease:material and methods. Studies focusing on management of steal symptoms or upper limb ischaemia in relation to traumatic injury or because of LSA coverage during thoracic aortic endovascular repair (TEVAR), were excluded. Studies reporting outcomes for SAS in addition to disease of other supra-aortic vessels were included only if the outcomes for SAS could be extracted.

Outcomes of Interest and Data Extraction

Two reviewers (LH and RG) first screened titles and abstracts Subclavian artery disease:material and methods, and papers of interest were retrieved and reviewed to check if they met the above criteria. A consensus was reached if discrepancies were observed. Data was extracted according to an agreed proforma and included author, year of publication, surgical center location, research type, period of data collection, intervention (percutaneous vs surgical revascularisation), number of subjects, key patient characteristics as reported by authors, QOL/PROMS instrument used, data of preoperative and postoperative QOL/PROMS assessment, follow-up period, follow-up completion rates, key non-QOL/PROMS outcomes as reported by authors.

Quality Scoring

The methodological quality of included studies was assessed using scoring system based on a standardized checklist of 10 items. Studies scoring ≥8 were considered to be of 'high quality', a score in the range 5–7 'moderate quality' and <5 'poor quality' [13, 14].

Results

Selected Studies

The literature search identified 1831 manuscripts. The abstracts for all identified studies were reviewed. Despite this only one study met the inclusion criteria (Fig. 17.2) [15].

Studies Focusing on Percutaneous Intervention

Only one study met the inclusion criteria. Qureshi et al. [15] investigated the short-term treatment effects of percutaneous intervention on QOL of patients with stenotic disease affecting the supra-aortic vessels using pre and postoperative European Quality of Life Five Dimension Five Level Scale (EQ-5D-5L) and the European Quality of Life Visual Analog Scale (EQ-VAS). Angioplasty and/or stent placement was undertaken in ten patients, but only two patients underwent intervention in the right SA for a combination of left hemiparesis, vertigo, ataxia, nausea, and vomiting. Both patients reported improvements following intervention, defined as a difference of at least 0.074 or more in the EQ-5D utility index and an improvement of 10 points or greater on EQ-VAS.

Studies Focusing on Surgical Revascularization

The search strategy did not identify any manuscripts that formally assessed QOL using PROMs following surgical revascularization.

Quality of Included Studies

According to the checklist, the only included study scored a 4.

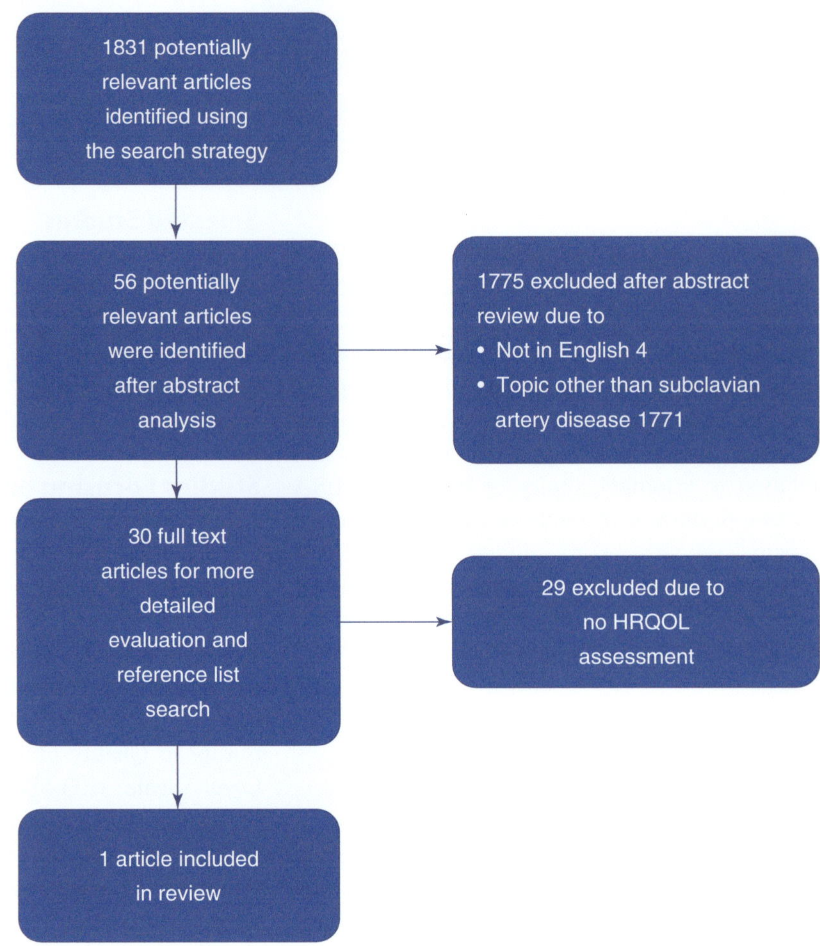

Fig. 17.2 Search Strategy. HRQOL: health related quality of life

Discussion

This study attempted to identify articles that report health related quality of life or patient related outcomes measures in patients who have undergone percutaneous and surgical revascularisation of subclavian artery disease. Despite a systematic and thorough search through the major databases, there is a significant lack of patient reported outcome measures for this group of patients. Overall, the search identified only one study that investigated the impact of the disease and subsequent intervention on the quality of life from a patients' perspective. This observational study however is limited to the experience of only two patients with SAS who underwent percutaneous intervention together with preoperative and 1 month post-procedure assessment with the EQ-5DL and VAS QOL validated tools [15]. While the short follow-up period in this study also prevents an understanding of long-term outcomes, the results overall suggest an improvement in health-related outcomes following endovascular management of SAS. There were no QOL/PROMs studies in patients undergoing surgical revascularisation and there were no comparator studies measuring PROMs between surgical revascularisation and PTA. Similarly, there were no articles exploring the predictors of impaired HRQoL in the management of subclavian artery stenosis. In Fig. 17.3, we have attempted to summarise these potential predictors.

More detailed evaluation of the articles retrieved in the search revealed that most of the

Potential predictors of impaired HRQoL in the management of subclavian Artery Stenosis	
Patient-related	**Procedure-related**
• Increasing Age • Co-morbidities • Higher degree of stenosis • Lack of collateral circulation (incomplete Circle of Willis) • Previous surgery • Symptomatic disease and steal Syndrome	• Procedural complications (eg. Stroke) • Poor technical success • Need for re-do procedures/surgery • Lack of resolution of symptoms despite intervention

Fig. 17.3 Potential predictors of impaired HRQOL in the management of subclavian artery stenosis

published studies in this area focused on 'procedural success' through reporting of 'technical success', 'patency rates' of restenosis or re-occlusion, and difference of blood pressure between the upper limbs post-treatment. Health assessment was mainly through more traditional outcomes such as mortality, morbidity (periprocedural complications and in particular, neurological deficit), survival analysis and 'clinical success' (symptom improvement or recurrence). Aside from the latter, these outcomes differ considerably from patient-related outcomes as they provide data detectable only by clinicians.

While the reporting of 'clinical success' is somewhat dependent on the patient's perception of their health status before and after treatment, it fails to capture the effect this has on their functional, emotional and social status that may in turn impact activities of daily living and quality of life. An assessment of these outcomes can only reliably be obtained from patients with validated tools that serve to standardise the interview and data reporting process. This subsequently allows the efficacy of a treatment to be determined for a cohort of patients affected by the same disease process, and for an individual patient by comparison of patient reported data before and after treatment. Furthermore, a patient who has complete resolution of symptoms may still experience impairment in any of the above domains and therefore experience a poor quality of life.

While surgical revascularisation is considered the gold standard treatment of occlusive disease of the subclavian artery, PTA revascularisation of the subclavian artery, like most minimally invasive endovascular procedures is generally considered the less invasive option for elderly co-morbid patients, without any clear evidence of the direct benefit this has for patients. The high technical and clinical success, that can be obtained with both interventions, in addition to their similar adverse profile [8, 9, 16–22], provides further need for the use of additional patient-centred outcomes to enable informed and individualised decision making for both clinicians and patients.

Due to the paucity of data in this setting, useful insights can be gained from studies comparing open and endovascular interventions in other revascularisation procedures. For instance, a randomised study comparing QOL in patients undergoing open infrarenal aneurysm repair to endovascular aneurysm repair (EVAR) has demonstrated significant health-related quality of life benefits with EVAR in comparison to open repair. The lessened surgical insult of EVAR is thought to account for the significantly improved physical functioning, role limitation, vitality, and pain scores on SF-36 questionnaires, and significantly better scores on the EuroQoL Usual Activities item [22]. Furthermore, there appears to be a faster recovery of postoperative HRQOL scores to baseline with EVAR than open repair [23]. Conversely, a comparative observational study has found no difference in perceived HRQOL between EVAR and open repair and has attributed this to the necessary need for surveillance and reintervention during a patient's lifetime [24].

Similarly, in carotid artery revascularisation, the CREST (Carotid Revascularization Endarterectomy Versus Stenting Trial) and SAPPHIRE (Stenting and Angioplasty with Protection in Patients at High Risk of Endarterectomy) have both demonstrated that patients undergoing CAS had better HRQOL for measures of overall physical function, pain and driving, and fewer limitations relating to eating and neck discomfort using the SF-36 EuroQol (EQ-5D), during early post-operative period, which the authors attribute to the less invasive nature of CAS. Furthermore, health status at 1-year was impaired among those who experienced periprocedural stroke in comparison to those who did not, an event that occurred most commonly following CAS [25, 26].

The implication of the findings in this review are significant when considering individual patient preferences. On the one hand, some patients may value the quicker physical recovery and immediate comfort of minimally invasive interventions, whereas others may place greater value on the long-term impact of impact of continued hospital visits for ongoing surveillance, likely need for reintervention, and procedure specific periprocedural complications and health related sequalae. QOL assessment tools provide a unique opportunity to identify which domains of QOL are perceived to be most important to individuals affected by a certain disease process, and those domains most likely to be affected following (open and minimally invasive) intervention to develop preventative strategies and to better support the needs of patients [27].

Conclusion

There is a significant lack of literature that measures PROMs in percutaneous and surgical revascularisation for subclavian artery disease. At this time, this data is critically needed to quantitatively highlight those issues of greatest importance to patients that may affect their quality of life following these interventions.

References

1. Labropoulos N, Nandivada P, Bekelis K. Prevalence and impact of the subcla- vian steal syndrome. Ann Surg. 2010;252:166–70.
2. Aboyans V, Kamineni A, Allison MA, McDermott MM, Crouse JR, Ni H, Szklo M, Criqui MH. The epidemiology of subclavian stenosis and its association with markers of subclinical atherosclerosis: the Multi-Ethnic Study of Atherosclerosis (MESA). Atherosclerosis. 2010;211:266–70.
3. Shadman R, Criqui MH, Bundens WP, Fronek A, Denenberg JO, Gamst AC, McDermott MM. Subclavian artery stenosis: prevalence, risk factors, and association with cardiovascular diseases. J Am Coll Cardiol. 2004;44:618–23.
4. Zimmerman NB. Occlusive vascular disorders of the upper extremity. Hand Clin. 1993;9:139–50.
5. Aboyans V, Ricco JB, Bartelink ML, Björck M, Brodmann M, Cohner T, Collet JP, Czerny M, De Carlo M, Debus S, Espinola-Klein C. 2017 ESC guidelines on the diagnosis and treatment of peripheral arterial diseases, in collaboration with the European Society for Vascular Surgery (ESVS). Kardiologia Polska (Polish Heart Journal). 2017;75:1065–160.
6. Rogers JH, Calhoun RF. Diagnosis and management of subclavian artery stenosis prior to coronary artery bypass grafting in the current era. J Card Surg. 2007;22:20–5.
7. Brountzos EN, Malagari K, Kelekis DA. Endovascular treatment of occlusive lesions of the subclavian and innominate arteries. Cardiovasc Intervent Radiol. 2006;29:503–10.
8. van de Weijer MA, Vonken EJ, de Vries JP, Moll FL, Vos JA, de Borst GJ. Technical and clinical success and long-term dura- bility of endovascular treatment for atherosclerotic aortic arch branch origin obstruction: evaluation of 144 procedures. Eur J Vasc Endovasc Surg. 2015;50:13–20.
9. Wang KQ, Wang ZG, Yang BZ, Yuan C, Zhang WD, Yuan B, Xing T, Song SH, Li T, Liao CJ, Zhang Y. Long-term results of endovascular therapy for proximal subclavian arterial obstructive lesions. Chin Med J. 2010;123:45–50.

10. Song L, Zhang J, Li J, Gu Y, Yu H, Chen B, Guo L, Wang Z. Endovascular stenting vs. extrathoracic surgical bypass for symptomatic subclavian steal syndrome. J Endovasc Ther. 2012;19(1):44–51.
11. Ozdemir-VAN Brunschot DM, Reijnen MM, VAN Oostayen JA, Schultze Kool LJ, VAN DER Vliet JA. Endovascular versus surgical revascularization in proximal subclavian artery obstruction. J Cardiovasc Surg. 2016;57(5):640–5.
12. Liberati A, Altman DG, Tetzlaff J, Mulrow C, Gotzsche PC, Ioannidis JP, et al. The PRISMA statement for reporting systematic reviews and metaanalyses of studies that evaluate health care interventions: explanation and elaboration. Ann Intern Med. 2009;151:W65–94.
13. Mols F, Vingerhoets AJ, Coebergh JW, van de Poll-Franse LV. Quality of life among long-term breast cancer survivors: a systematic review. Eur J Cancer. 2005;41:2613–9.
14. Baig K, Harling L, Papanikitas J, Attaran S, Ashrafian H, Casula R, et al. Does coronary artery bypass grafting improve quality of life in elderly patients? Interact Cardiovasc Thorac Surg. 2013;17:542–53.
15. Qureshi AI, Saleem MA, Naseem N, Wallery SS. Effect of endovascular treatment on quality of life in patients with recurrent symptoms associated with vertebral, subclavian, or innominate arterial stenosis. J Vasc Interv Neurol. 2018;10(1):7–13.
16. Galyfos GC, Kakisis I, Maltezos C, Geroulakos G. Open versus endovascular treatment of subclavian artery atherosclerotic disease. J Vasc Surg. 2019;69:269–79.
17. Farina C, Sterpetti AV, Schultz RD, Feldhaus RJ, Davenport K. Extrathoracic and transthoracic management of vascular disease of the aortic arch branches: a 16-year experience. Ann Thorac Surg. 1989;47:580–5.
18. Özdemir-VAN Brunschot DM, Reijnen MM, VAN Oostayen JA, Kool LJS, VAN DER Vliet JS. Endovascular versus surgical revascularization in proximal subclavian artery obstruction. J Cardiovasc Surg. 2013;57:640–5.
19. Burihan E, Soma F, Iared W. Angioplasty versus stenting for subclavian artery stenosis. Cochrane Database Syst Rev. 2011;10:CD008461.
20. Klitfod L, Jensen LP. Treatment of chronic upper limb ischaemia is safe and results are good. Dan Med J. 2014;61:A4859.
21. Chatterjee S, Nerella N, Chakravarty S, Shani J. Angioplasty alone versus angioplasty and stenting for subclavian artery stenosisda systematic review and meta-analysis. Am J Ther. 2013;20:520–3.
22. Lottman PE, Laheij RJ, Cuypers PW, Bender M, Buth J. Health-related quality of life outcomes following elective open or endovascular AAA repair: a randomized controlled trial. J Endovasc Ther. 2004;11(3):323–9.
23. Aquino RV, Jones MA, Zullo TG, Missig-Carroll N, Makaroun MS. Quality of life assessment in patients undergoing endovascular or conventional AAA repair. J Endovasc Ther. 2001;8:521–8.
24. Malina M, Nilsson M, Brunkwall J, Ivancev K, Resch T, Lindblad B. Quality of life before and after endovascular and open repair of asymptomatic AAAs: a prospective study. J Endovasc Ther. 2000;7:372–9.
25. Cohen DJ, Stolker JM, Wang K, et al. CREST Investigators. Health-related quality of life after carotid stenting versus carotid endarterectomy: results from CREST (Carotid Revascularization Endarterectomy Versus Stenting Trial). J Am Coll Cardiol. 2011;58(15):1557–65.
26. Stolker JM, Mahoney EM, Safley DM, Pomposelli FB Jr, Yadav JS, Cohen DJ. SAPPHIRE Investigators. Health-related quality of life following carotid stenting versus endarterectomy: results from the SAPPHIRE (Stenting and Angioplasty with Protection in Patients at HIgh Risk for Endarterectomy) trial. JACC Cardiovasc Interv. 2010;3(5):515–23.
27. Black N. Patient reported outcome measures could help transform healthcare. BMJ. 2013;346:f167.

18 QoL and PROMS Following Percutaneous and Surgical Intervention for Renal Artery Disease

Ankur Thapar and Phillip Puckridge

Isolated renal artery intervention is performed in adults mainly for atherosclerosis and fibromuscular dysplasia. Indications for treatment include acute ischaemic nephropathy, transplant renal artery stenosis and multi-drug resistant severe hypertension, particularly in the setting of a solitary functioning kidney.

The authors searched Pubmed from inception to 15 November 2019 using the keywords "renal artery" and "angio*" or "stent*" or "surgery" or "endarterectomy" or "bypass" or "reimplantation". This resulted in quality of life data from three studies.

In atherosclerotic disease a single randomised controlled trial of medical therapy with or without renal artery angioplasty showed no difference in quality of life over a 12 month follow-up period. An age and gender matched cross-sectional survey of different patients pre and post renal artery stenting reported higher physical scores on the SF-36 instrument between the groups, with a key driver being the side effects experienced with antihypertensive medications. A single arm cross-sectional study evaluated quality of life and wellbeing 5 years post stenting. There was no control group, however reasonable quality of life and wellbeing scores were recorded. There was no data on quality of life for surgical correction of atherosclerotic renal artery stenosis.

In fibromuscular dysplasia there was no data on quality of life, however multiple case series suggest that hypertension is curable in 30–50% of patients.

In conclusion there is limited data on the quality of life benefits for intervention for atherosclerotic renal artery stenosis, unless dialysis is imminent. In fibromuscular dysplasia, angioplasty has a higher chance of curing hypertension and thus avoiding the side effects of long-term polypharmacy.

Future studies should focus on patient reported outcomes in patients with fibromuscular dysplasia or those with a solitary kidney.

Renal artery intervention is performed in adults for 3 main pathologies, namely atherosclerosis, fibromuscular dysplasia (FMD) and aneurysmal disease. In addition it is performed as part of the treatment of complex aortic pathologies such as type B dissection and thoracoabdominal aortic aneurysm. This chapter will focus on two commonly treated isolated renal pathologies, namely atherosclerosis and FMD.

Renal artery stenosis is found in upto 32% of hypertensive patients [1]. Key indications for

A. Thapar (✉)
Mid and South Essex NHS Foundation Trust, Essex, UK

Anglia Ruskin University, Cambridge, UK
e-mail: a.thapar@nhs.net

P. Puckridge
Department of Vascular and Endovascular Surgery, Flinders Medical Centre, Adelaide, SA, Australia
e-mail: Phillip.puckridge@sa.gov.au

T. Athanasiou et al. (eds.), *Patient Reported Outcomes and Quality of Life in Cardiovascular Interventions*, https://doi.org/10.1007/978-3-031-09815-4_18

treatment include a >60% stenosis in the following settings [2, 3]:

- Acute ischaemic nephropathy with normal kidney size, especially with a solitary functioning kidney from plaque rupture
- non-anastomotic, transplant renal artery stenosis
- multi-drug resistant severe hypertension (sBP>180 mmHg)
- acute kidney injury leading to flash pulmonary oedema and the requirement for imminent dialysis
- fibromuscular dysplasia with poorly controlled hypertension

Quality of life outcomes are important as the condition is asymptomatic until its late stages and is detected through either hypertension, declining renal function, or on imaging. This field has been revolutionised by the introduction of percutaneous angioplasty and stenting, performed under local anaesthetic (Fig. 18.1a, b) [4]. This has largely superseded the older techniques of aortic endarterectomy, aorto, ilio, spleno or hepatorenal artery bypass and renal artery reimplantation (auto-transplantation). These are still used in selected cases and in the paediatric population. In addition, new drug therapies to manage renal artery stenosis have emerged such as ACE and ARB2 inhibitors, that target the renin-angiotensin-aldosterone axis, the primary driver in renovascular hypertension. A small subset of patients experience deteriorating renal function when these drugs are commenced. These patients may also be considered for renal artery intervention.

The American Heart Association recommends collection of quality of life information in new renal artery revascularisation trials [5]. This can be performed using the generic SF-36 or Euro-QoL instruments.

Search Strategy

Pubmed was searched from inception to 15 November 2019 using the keywords “renal artery” and “angio*” or “stent*” or “surgery” or “endar-

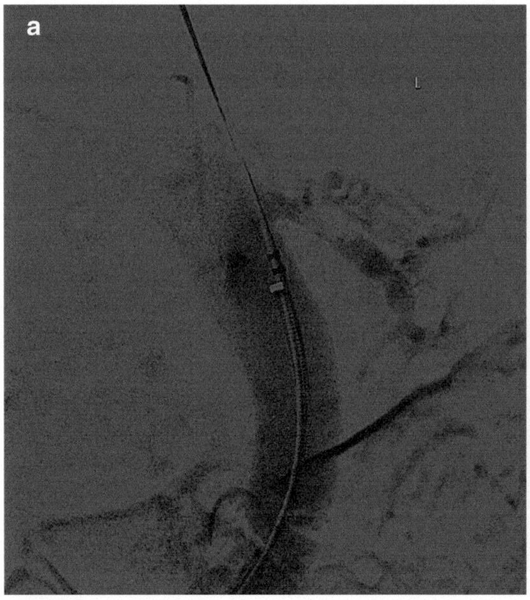

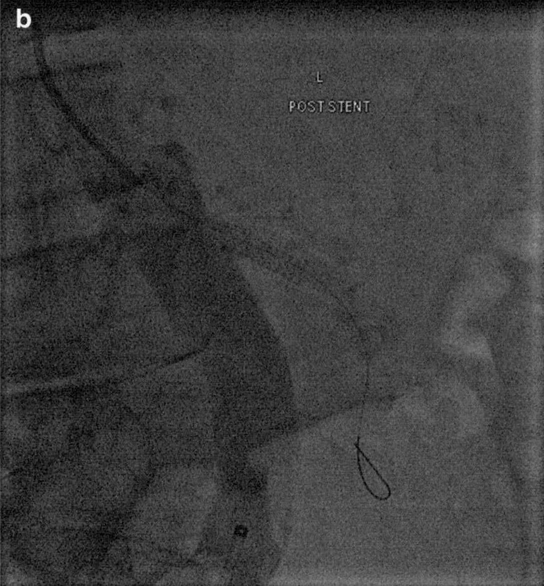

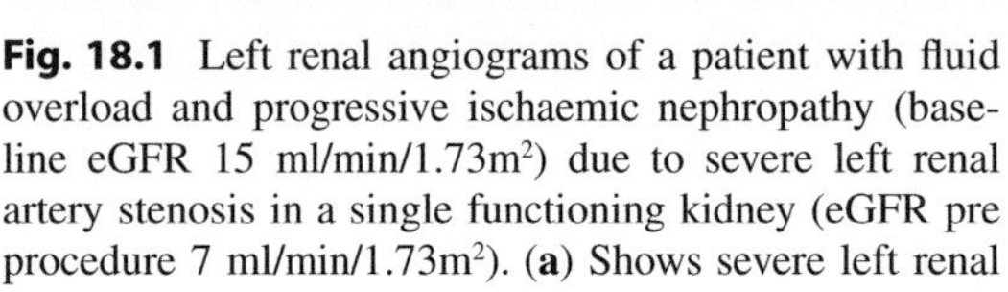

Fig. 18.1 Left renal angiograms of a patient with fluid overload and progressive ischaemic nephropathy (baseline eGFR 15 ml/min/1.73m^2) due to severe left renal artery stenosis in a single functioning kidney (eGFR pre procedure 7 ml/min/1.73m^2). (**a**) Shows severe left renal artery stenosis. (**b**) Shows appearances post left 6 × 18 mm Abbott Herculink Elite bare metal stent (GFR post-procedure 48 ml/min/1.73 m^2). The patient avoided long-term dialysis

terectomy" or "bypass" or "reimplantation", using the limits of human studies in English. Studies were required to focus on adults undergoing primary treatment for renal artery stenosis, fibromuscular dysplasia or transplant renal artery stenosis. Case reports, studies with <10 patients, letters and review articles were excluded. Renal denervation studies were not considered, as they focussed on hypertension not renal artery stenosis. Concomitant renal stenting for aortic aneurysm, renal aneurysm, renal transplant, mid-aortic syndrome or trauma was excluded as the outcome of these pathologies were more likely to influence quality of life. Studies that presented quality of life or PROMs were included in the final analysis.

Search Results

Please see PRISMA diagram (Fig. 18.2).

Atherosclerotic Renal Artery Stenosis: Endovascular Trials

Seven published randomised controlled trials were found that reported on endovascular treatment for hypertensive patients with atherosclerotic renal artery stenosis [6–12]. One trial was unpublished. Inclusion criteria from these trials required equipoise between medical therapy and intervention, namely that patients did not have

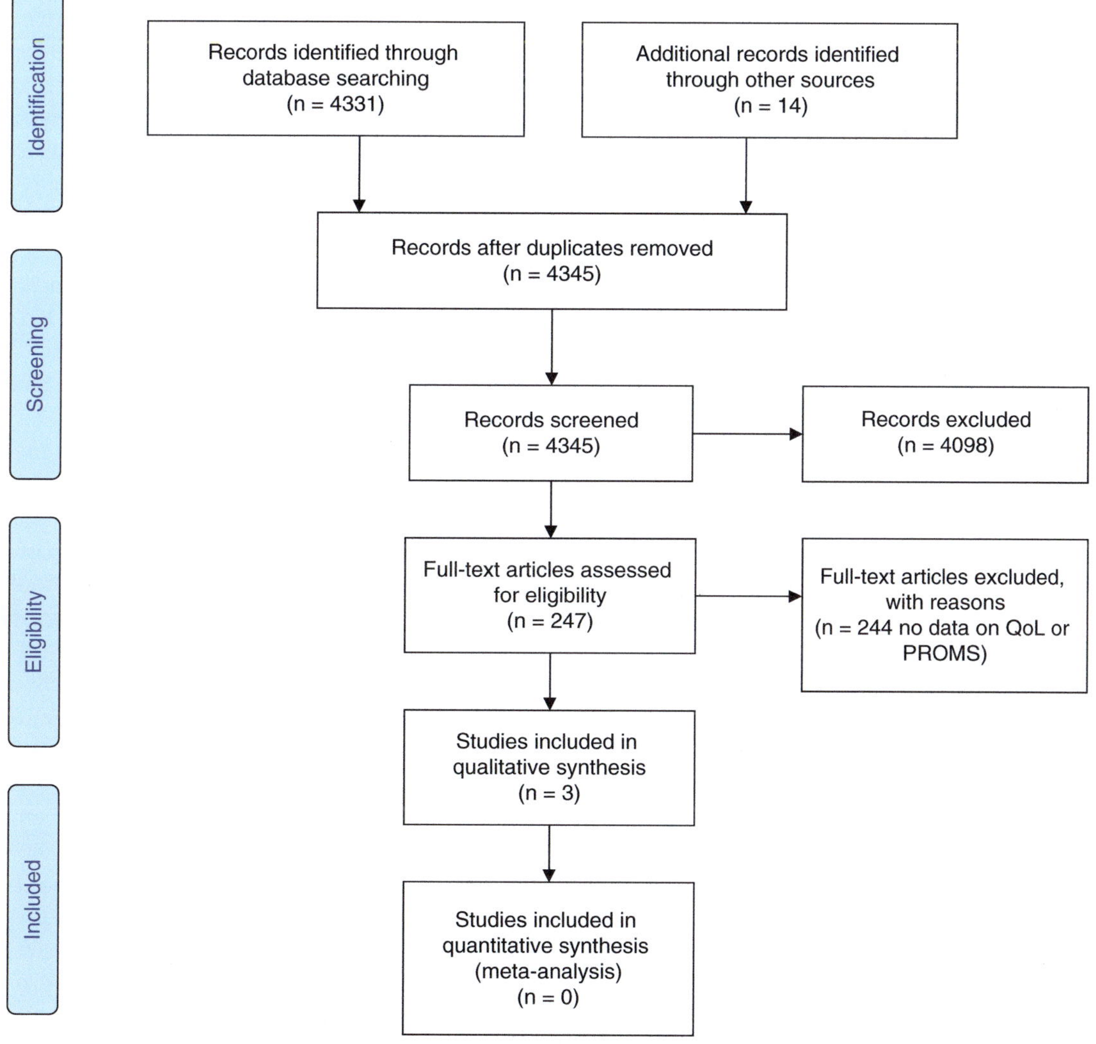

Fig. 18.2 PRISMA diagram

	Randomisation	Allocation concealment	Blinding of participants/ clinicians	Blinded assessment	Outcome data completeness	Reporting of results
ASTRAL	✓	✓	×	?	✓	✓
CORAL	✓	✓	×	✓	✓	✓
DRASTIC	✓	✓	×	?	✓	✓
EMMA	?	✓	×	✓	✓	✓
RADAR	?	?	×	?	?	?
SNRASCG	?	?	×	✓	✓	✓
STAR	✓	✓	×	?	✓	✓

Fig. 18.3 Risk of bias assessment of randomised controlled trials in renal artery angioplasty or stenting [13]. Key ✓ = low risk of bias, ? = unknown, × = high risk of bias

rapidly deteriorating or severely impaired renal function or severe hypertension. Most trials excluded patients with a single functional kidney. Only one trial reported quality of life outcomes [6] and none presented patient reported outcomes. No clinically important difference in blood pressure or renal function was reported in a meta-analysis of these trials [13].

The risk of bias was assessed using the Cochrane Collaboration method (Fig. 18.3). A single trial documented quality of life outcomes [10]: the assessors were unblinded and there was a 22/50 (44%) rate of crossover from medical to surgical treatment for three drug resistant diastolic hypertension (>95 mmHg) or a 0.2 mg/dl elevation in serum creatinine concentration. These angioplastied patients were analysed in an intention-to-treat fashion, which may negate effects seen between the medical and angioplasty groups.

Quality of Life Outcomes in Atherosclerotic Renal Artery Stenting

Quality of life outcomes were examined in a 106 patient sub-study of the DRASTIC randomised controlled trial [14]. Quality of life was reported at baseline and 3 and 12 months after renal artery angioplasty. Instruments used were the Hypertension specific physical symptoms questionnaire, along with the generic EURO-QoL and the MOS General Health Survey. There were no significant differences at any time point up to 12 months using any of these scales. Importantly crossover patients were excluded from this analysis. Crossover patients had uncontrolled hypertension and received an unplanned angioplasty for hypertensive complications or worsening renal function. This represents a potential group where there may be clinical or quality of life benefits to angioplasty which were masked by the trial analysis. This would be particularly important if they suffered side effects from introduction of a fourth drug or if they commenced dialysis. For example, deterioration from stage 4 to stage 5 chronic kidney disease is particularly associated with "role-emotional" impairment to perform work and mental composite summary scores [15].

Two additional non-randomised studies examined quality of life after renal artery stenting.

The first was a cross-sectional US study examining age and gender matched pre (n-30) and post-stenting (n = 56) groups [16]. The participants all received the SF-36 questionnaire, physical distress symptom index, social participation index, life satisfaction index, work performance and satisfaction index and sleep dysfunction scale. The only significant finding between those that had received a stent was that their physical component SF-36 score was higher (37 SD ± 9 stented versus 31 SD ± 9 non-stented). The key drivers were the number of antihypertensive medications, in particular the use of alpha-adrenergic antagonists. This study was a partially matched cross-sectional study and had a substantial risk of bias from unknown confounders. In addition, baseline quality of life was unknown in the stented patients (Table 18.1).

Table 18.1 Key messages

In the only randomised controlled trial of renal artery angioplasty for multidrug resistant hypertension there was no difference in generic or hypertension specific quality of life at 1 year
Patients who have a solitary kidney and who can avoid dialysis stand the most to gain from renal intervention
In young patients with fibromuscular dysplasia hypertension can be cured in a large proportion with renal artery angioplasty but pre and post procedure quality of life data are needed
There is no data on quality of life before and after surgery for renal artery stenosis

Table 18.2 Activity levels 5 years post renal artery angioplasty for hypertension [16]

Activity level	% of patients
Indoor activity	7
Short outdoor walking	38
Unrestricted physical activity	36
Active physical training	12
Active physical exercise training	7

The second was a cross-sectional study of 81 Swedish patients who had undergone renal angioplasty (± selective stenting) 5 years earlier [17]. These patients self-rated their activity level 1 (indoor activity only)–5 (jogging 3 times/week) (see Table 18.2). In addition they self-rated their physical, social and mental wellbeing on a 5 point Likert scale (see Fig. 18.4).

These data suggested reasonable physical functioning scores after renal artery stenting and good mental and social scores. This study did not have a control group and participants were highly selected on the basis of longevity and perceived benefit of stenting. Therefore it is difficult to comment on the benefit of the intervention itself, as patients who were receiving ongoing medical treatment may over time have also seen quality of life benefits. Again baseline quality of life was unknown in this study.

Atherosclerotic Renal Artery Stenosis: Surgical Trials

There were 2 randomised controlled trials of surgery for renal artery stenosis. Neither trial included quality of life or PROMs.

The first was a pilot randomised trial of surgery (mainly trans-aortic endarterectomy, n = 25) versus angioplasty and selective stenting (n = 25) [18]. This trial showed no significant difference in blood pressure reduction or mortality. However there appeared to be a small benefit in terms of renal function in the endovascular group. This study was unblinded with small numbers with important differences such as a higher number of solitary kidneys in the endovascular arm, which may have explained the benefits in renal function seen in this group.

The second trial was again a pilot study of surgery (again mainly transaortic endarterectomy, n = 29) versus angioplasty (n = 29) [19]. This trial showed no significant difference in blood pressure reduction or renal function between the two strategies at 2 years. In this trial it was noted that 14% of patients in the angioplasty group came to surgery and 21% required a second angioplasty. This trial was also unblinded, with small numbers.

Fibromuscular Dysplasia: Endovascular

This non-inflammatory, non-atherosclerotic disease of medium sized arteries, responds extremely well to angioplasty alone. No randomised controlled trials were found for the treatment of renal FMD. In a recent meta-analysis of case series, one-third of hypertensive patients were cured with renal artery angioplasty [20]. The cure rate is proportionate to age, with patients in their 20s approaching cure rates of 50%.

Fibromuscular Dysplasia: Surgery

There were no randomised controlled trials of surgery in FMD. There were 4 case series specifically reporting outcomes in renal FMD. The first single centre case series consisted of 40 patients with severe uncontrolled hypertension [21]. These patients received mainly aortorenal great saphenous vein bypass. Eleven patients had a significant complication which delayed hospital stay and one returned to theatre for haemorrhage control. There were no deaths upto a mean of 29 months follow up. One third of patients were cured of hypertension, with younger patients more likely to be cured.

The second case series was of 26 patients receiving again mainly aorto-renal bypass [22]. The median intensive care stay was 2 days. Primary patency of the reconstructions was 89% at 2 years. 10% of patients experienced a significant complication extending hospital stay. Again one-third of patients were cured of hypertension in this case series.

The third case series reported 28 patients with severe uncontrolled hypertension treated mainly with aortorenal bypass with either vein or internal iliac artery as a conduit [23]. There was a 3% restenosis rate and 97% of patients had improved blood pressure at follow up.

The fourth case series reported 72 patients treated for hypertension or chronic kidney disease, mainly with kidney ex-vivo renal arterial reconstruction and autotransplantation [24]. Patients were followed a mean of 11 years. Immediate surgical complications including

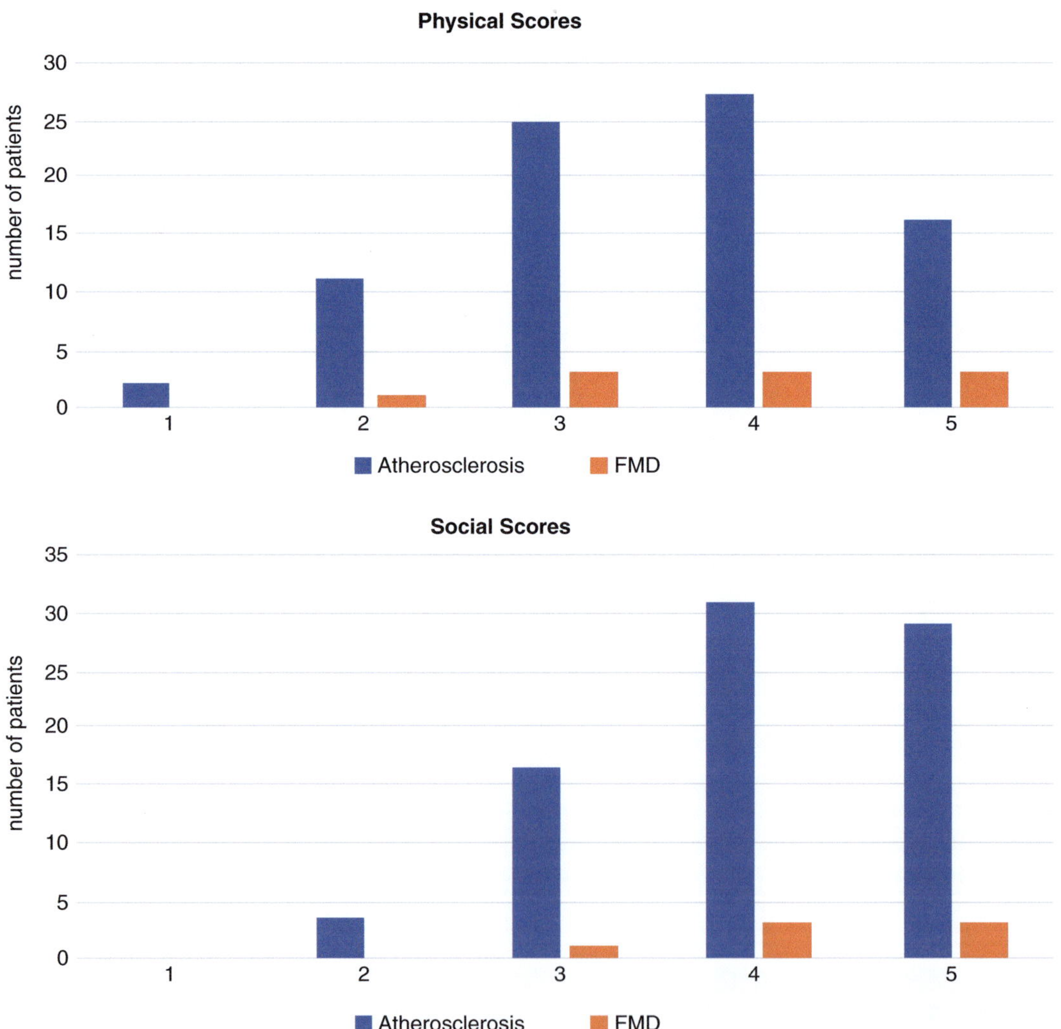

Fig. 18.4 Self- reported physical, social and mental well-being scores in 88 patients (81 atherosclerosis, 7 fibromuscular dysplasia [FMD]) treated with renal artery angioplasty at 5 year follow up [17]. Scores range from 1 = very poor to 5 = very good

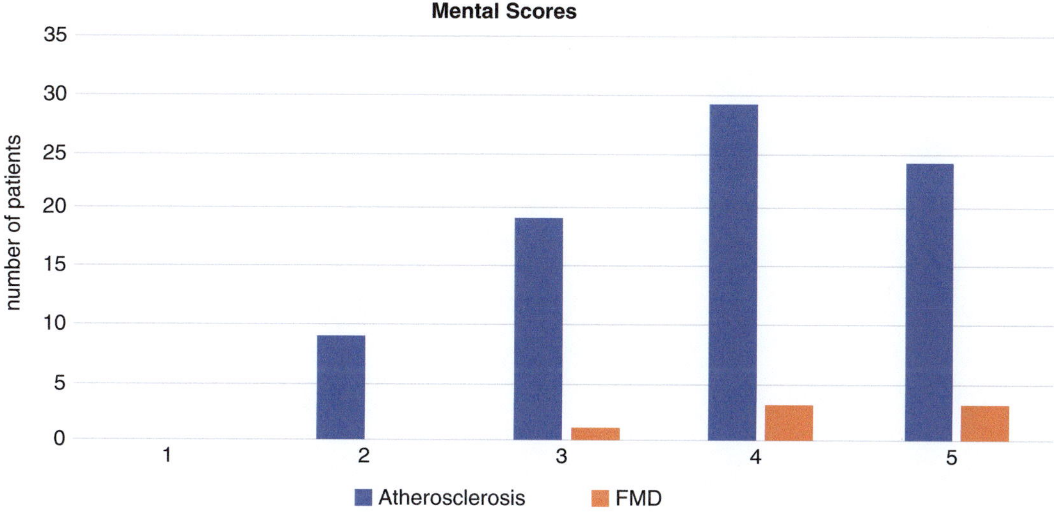

Fig. 18.4 (continued)

arterial thrombosis occurred in 2%. Mean blood pressure was 176/108 mmHg pre-operatively versus 146/89 mmHg post-operatively. Mean eGFR was 59 ml/min/1.73m^2 pre-operatively versus 78 ml/min/1.73m^2 post-operatively.

Quality of Life in Fibromuscular Dysplasia

There was one study, described earlier that reported outcomes in 7 highly selected FMD patients treated with renal angioplasty for hypertension at 5 years [17]. This reported outcomes that were slightly better, or at least comparable to those with atherosclerotic renal artery stenosis (see Fig. 18.4). In addition, 5 year survival was 100% in FMD versus 83% for those with atherosclerosis. Again no baseline measurements or control group was available for comparison.

Effect of Regular Dialysis on Quality of Life

It is clear that in general terms there is very limited evidence for quality of life benefits for patients with renal artery stenosis. However, in the setting of imminent dialysis, there may still be quality of life benefits to successful renal artery revascularisation, if dialysis can be averted. Quality of life on dialysis has been examined in a large scale cross-sectional study, using the Karnofsky performance scale and the Global Score of Sickness Impact [25]. This demonstrated that 26% of those on either haemo or peritoneal dialysis had a severe quality of life impairment (Global SSIP >20 or <60 on Karnofsky scale). Areas of life particularly effected were work, recreation and pastimes, home management and sleep and rest.

Effects of Procedural Complications on Quality of Life

There are no quality of life data on open surgery but it is clear that a laparotomy and intensive care stay will have a larger impact on short term quality of life than local anaesthetic daycase percutaneous renal artery intervention.

In large endovascular series the rate of haemodialysis in the post-procedure period was 2% (usually due to renal infarction from emboli) [26]. Restenosis occurred in 21% of patients at one year, however not all of these required reintervention [27].

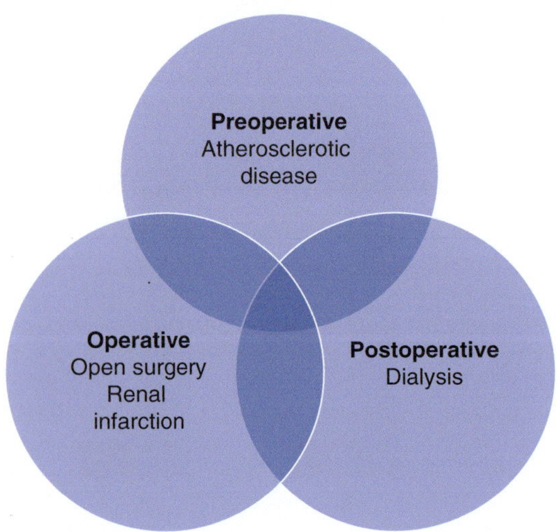

Fig. 18.5 Negative quality of life predictors following treatment of renal artery stenosis

Conclusion

There is limited quality of life data post renal artery intervention. Factors affecting quality of life post-revascularisation are summarised in Fig. 18.5. Key messages are summarised in Table 18.1. The only randomised comparison of quality of life outcomes after renal artery angioplasty and selective stenting for renovascular hypertension showed no quality of life differences up to one year. There is no data for primary stenting or surgery. However important messages were that side effects of multiple anti-hypertensive drugs, negatively impact quality of life as does commencing dialysis. Social and mental functioning scores in selected patients treated with stenting were good 5 years post-procedure, however studies providing similar data for medically managed control patients are lacking. Quality of life and survival in fibromuscular dysplasia are poorly studied but appear at least as good if not better than in atherosclerotic disease and around a third of FMD patients are cured of hypertension.

An important gap in the literature is the comparison of quality of life of patients with fibromuscular dysplasia or a solitary kidney managed with revsacularisation or medication alone. These patients are not studied in trials. Avoidance of dialysis and the complications of severe hypertension (e.g. stroke) are the potential key quality of life benefits for renal artery intervention.

References

1. Davis RP, Pearce JD, Craven TE, Moore PS, Edwards MS, Godshall CJ, et al. Atherosclerotic renovascular disease among hypertensive adults. J Vasc Surg [Internet]. 2008;50(3):564–70. https://doi.org/10.1016/j.jvs.2009.03.062.
2. Parikh SA, Shishehbor MH, Gray BH, White CJ, Jaff MR. Core curriculum SCAI expert consensus statement for renal artery stenting appropriate use. Catheter Cardiovasc Interv. 2014;84:1163–71.
3. ESC Task Force. 2017 ESC Guidelines on the Diagnosis and Treatment of Peripheral Arterial Diseases, in collaboration with the European Society for Vascular Surgery (ESVS) Document covering atherosclerotic disease of extracranial carotid Endorsed by : the European Stro. EHJ. 2018;39:763–821.
4. Blum U, Bernd K, Flugel P, Gabelmann A, Lehnert T, Buitrago-Tellez C, et al. Treatment of ostial renal-artery stenoses with vascular endoprostheses after unsuccessful balloon angioplasty. NEJM. 1997;336(7):459–65.
5. Rundback JH, Sacks D, Kent KC, Cooper C, Jones D, Murphy T, et al. Guidelines for the reporting of renal artery revascularization in clinical trials. Circulation. 2002;106:1572–85.
6. Bax L, Woittiez AJ, Kouwenberg HJ, Buskens E. Stent placement in patients with atherosclerotic renal artery stenosis and impaired renal function. Ann Intern Med. 2019;150(12):840–8.
7. Webster J, Marshall F, Abdalla M, Dominiczak A, Edwards R, Isles CG, et al. Randomised comparison of percutaneous angioplasty vs continued medical therapy for hypertensive patients with atheromatous renal artery stenosis. J Hum Hypertens. 1998;15(5):329–35.
8. ASTRAL Investigators. Revascularization versus medical therapy for renal-artery stenosis. NEJM. 2009;361(20):1953–62.
9. Investigators C. Stenting and medical therapy for atherosclerotic renal-artery disease. NEJM. 2014;370(1):13–22.
10. Investigators D. The effect of balloon angioplasty on hypertension. NEJM. 2000;342(12):1007–14.
11. Chatellier G, Darne B, Raynaud A. Blood Pressure Outcome of Angioplasty in Atherosclerotic renal artery stenosis: a randomized controlled trial. Hypertension. 1998;31:823–9.
12. Zeller T, Krankenberg H, Erglis A, Blessing E, Fuss T, Scheinert D, et al. A randomized, multi-center, prospective study comparing best medical treatment

versus best medical treatment plus renal artery stenting in patients with hemodynamically relevant atherosclerotic renal artery stenosis (RADAR) – one-year results of a pre-maturely terminated study. Trials. 2017:1–9.
13. Jenks S, Se Y, Br C. Balloon angioplasty, with and without stenting, versus medical therapy for hypertensive patients with renal artery stenosis (Review). Cochrane Database Syst Rev. 2014;2014:CD002944.
14. Krijnen P, Van Jaarsveld BC, Hunink MGM, Habbema JDF. The effect of treatment on health-related quality of life in patients with hypertension and renal artery stenosis. J Hum Hypertens. 2005;9:467–70.
15. Pagels AA, Söderkvist BK, Medin C, Hylander B, Heiwe S. Health-related quality of life in different stages of chronic kidney disease and at initiation of dialysis treatment. Health Qual Life Outcomes. 2012;10(71):1–11.
16. Kennedy DJ, Burket MW, Khuder SA, Cooper CJ. Quality of life improves after renal artery stenting. Biol Res Nurs. 2006;8(2):129–37.
17. Jensen G, Annerstedt M, Klingenstierna H, Herlitz H, Hellström M, Jensen G, et al. Survival and quality of life after renal angioplasty: a five-year follow-up study. Scand J Urol Nephrol. 2009;43:236–41.
18. Balzer KM, Pfeiffer T, Rossbach S, Voiculescu A, Mödder U, Godehardt E, et al. Prospective randomized trial of operative vs interventional treatment for renal artery ostial occlusive disease (RAOOD). J Vasc Surg [Internet]. 2009;49(3):667–75. https://doi.org/10.1016/j.jvs.2008.10.006.
19. Weibull H, Bergqvist D, Bergentz S. Percutaneous transluminal renal angioplasty versus surgical reconstruction of atherosclerotic renal artery stenosis : a prospective randomized study. J Vasc Surg. 1993;18(5):841–52.
20. Trinquart L, Mounier-vehier C, Sapoval M, Gagnon N. Efficacy of revascularization for renal artery stenosis caused by fibromuscular dysplasia a systematic review and meta-analysis. Hypertension. 2010;56:525–32.
21. Anderson CA, Hansen KJ, Benjamin ME. Renal artery fibromuscular dysplasia : results of current surgical therapy. J Vasc Surg. 1995;22:207–16.
22. Carmo M, Bower TC, Mozes G, Nachreiner RD, Textor SC, Hoskin TL, et al. Surgical management of renal fibromuscular dysplasia: challenges in the endovascular era. Ann Vasc Surg. 2004;19(2):208–17.
23. Torsello G, Sandmann W, Szabo Z, Stolze T, Grabensee B. Reconstructive vascular surgery for hypertension in renal vascular dysplasia. Cardiology. 1985;72:30–2.
24. Mokos I, Krhen I, Ribic N, Marekovic Z. Long-term outcome after surgical kidney revascularization for fibromuscular dysplasia and atherosclerotic renal artery stenosis. J Urol. 2004;171:1043–5.
25. Moreno F, Gomez JML, Jofre R, Valderrabano F, Gonzalez L, Gorriz JL, et al. Quality of life in dialysis patients. A Spanish multicentre study. Nephrol Dialy Transplan. 1996;11:125–9.
26. Ivanovic V, McKusick M, Johnson MC III, Sabater EA, Andrews JC, Breen JF, et al. Renal artery stent placement: complications at a single tertiary care center. JVIR. 2003;14(2):217–24.
27. Lederman RJ, Mendelsohn FO, Santos R, Phillips HR, Stack RS, Crowley JJ, et al. Primary renal artery stenting: characteristics and outcomes after 363 procedures. Am Heart J. 2001;142(2):314–23.

19 Health-Related Quality of Life Outcomes for Endovascular and Open Surgical Interventions in Aortoiliac and Femoropopliteal Steno-Occlusive Arterial Disease

Jimmy Kyaw Tun, Stefan Lam,
Mohammed Rashid Akhtar, and Ounali Jaffer

Abbreviations

ABPI	Ankle-brachial pressure index
BMT	Best medical therapy
CD-TLR	Clinically-driven target lesion revascularisation
CERAB	Covered endovascular repair of aortic bifurcation
CLTI	Critical limb-threatening ischaemia
DCB	Drug-coated balloon
DES	Drug-eluting stent
EQ	EuroQoL
HRQOL	Health-related quality of life
ICQ	Intermittent claudication questionnaire
MCID	Minimal clinically important difference
OCT	Optical coherence tomography
PAD	Peripheral arterial disease
PAQ	Peripheral arterial questionnaire
PTA	Percutaneous transluminal angioplasty
QALY	Quality-adjusted life year
RCT	Randomised controlled trial
SF	Short form
SFA	Superficial femoral artery
SET	Supervised exercise therapy
WIQ	Walking impairment questionnaire

J. K. Tun · M. R. Akhtar · O. Jaffer (✉)
Department of Interventional Radiology, Royal London Hospital, Barts Health NHS Trust, London, UK
e-mail: jimmy.kyawtun@nhs.net; mohammedrashid.akhtar@nhs.net; ounali.jaffer@nhs.net

S. Lam
Barts and the London School of Medicine & Dentistry, Queen Mary University of London, London, UK
e-mail: stefan.lam@nhs.net

Introduction

There is an impending epidemic in peripheral arterial disease (PAD), largely due to an aging population and increased rates of obesity and diabetes, with the condition currently prevalent in 5.6% of the adult population worldwide.

Sufferers of PAD often experience a decreased quality of life and reduced functional independence. The symptoms experienced depend on disease severity and range from limited walking distance in claudicants, to rest pain and tissue loss with risk of major amputation in those with critical limb-threating ischaemia (CLTI) [1]. The quality of life in those with PAD is often further degraded by concomitant related disorders including hypertension, dyslipidaemia, diabetes and nephropathy [2].

T. Athanasiou et al. (eds.), *Patient Reported Outcomes and Quality of Life in Cardiovascular Interventions*,
https://doi.org/10.1007/978-3-031-09815-4_19

There is an ever-increasing armamentarium available for lower limb revascularisation, particularly in terms of endovascular treatment with the advent of drug-coated balloons (DCB) and drug-eluting stents (DES) to atherectomy and lithotripsy; but these innovations also come with significantly increased costs. It is therefore necessary to evaluate both clinical effectiveness and health economics of these interventions. Conventionally, studies evaluating lower limb interventions have focused on physician-orientated outcome measures such as technical success (e.g. successful revascularisation of an occluded artery), patency rates, ankle-brachial pressure index (ABPI), freedom from clinically-driven target lesion revascularisation (CD-TLR) and freedom from amputation [1]. However, these measures alone do not take into account the patient's perspective. For instance, vascular clinicians generally consider major amputation to be an adverse outcome in PAD, yet it has been shown that health-related quality of life (HRQOL) can improve following major amputations [3]. A systematic review comparing primary amputations and revascularisation in CLTI found insufficient evidence to support one treatment over another in terms of HRQOL outcomes [4].

There is an increasing recognition for the need to evaluate HRQOL outcomes for intervention in PAD to take into account the patient's perspective to better inform treatment decisions [5]. This is emphasised by the use of quality-adjusted life years (QALYs) by the National Institute for Health and Clinical Excellence (NICE) for health technology assessment. In order to generate QALYs, health utilities (or HRQOL weights) are needed. As such, the measure is reliant on both the quality and the quantity of the life lived in order to determine health outcomes and therefore health economics.

The focus of this study is to present a systematic review of the current evidence of HRQOL outcomes in relation to endovascular and open surgical treatment of aortoiliac and femoropopliteal steno-occlusive disease. A review of the evidence for intervention in infrapopliteal disease is presented in Chap. 20.

Materials and Methods

Search Strategy

This systematic review was conducted according to PRISMA (Preferred Reporting Items for Systematic Reviews and Meta-Analyses) guidelines. The initial search strategy focused on identifying papers based on specific interventions (e.g. iliac angioplasty, aortoiliac bypass graft). However, on manual review of the references of several key systematic reviews, it was evident that this search strategy omitted some relevant papers. Therefore, a much broader search strategy was employed as follows.

A systematic search using Embase (Including Embase Classic) (1947 to February 2020), Medline (1946 to February 2020) and PsycINFO (1950 to February 2020) was conducted. The search terms used were as follows: "quality of life" AND ("peripheral arterial disease" OR "peripheral vascular disease" OR "intermittent claudication" OR "critical limb ischaemia" OR "critical limb ischemia").

Inclusion and Exclusion Criteria

Studies published in the English language reporting HRQOL outcomes in adults undergoing invasive intervention—i.e. both open and endovascular surgery—for steno-occlusive disease in the aortoiliac and femoropopliteal segments were sought. Although the primary focus of this review was to evaluate the outcomes of invasive interventions, studies comparing non-invasive treatments such as supervised exercise therapy (SET) and best medical treatment (BMT) to invasive interventions were also included.

Studies were only included if they presented results specific to an anatomical segment. Papers which included patients treated across a range of anatomical segments were excluded if outcome data specific to an anatomical segment (aortoiliac or femoropopliteal) was not available. If the study included distal (below knee) intervention and/or distal bypass surgery, then these were also excluded. Studies were excluded if they had less than 6 months follow-up data.

Study Selection and Data Extraction

The broad search criteria yielded an initial extensive list of abstracts. Therefore, one researcher (JKT) performed an initial screening of abstracts to remove articles that were clearly irrelevant. A second stage review of the full texts of the remaining articles was then performed by JKT and MRA and where there was uncertainty or difference in opinion, adjudication was performed by a third reviewer (OJ).

Data obtained included: author, year of publication, study objective, study type, number of patients, study centre location, HRQOL outcomes, follow-up period and completion rates.

The methodological quality of the studies was assessed by SL and MRA using a 10-point scoring system described by Mols et al. [6] Studies scoring ≥8 were considered to be of 'high quality', those scoring between 5 and 7 were deemed to be of a 'moderate quality' and <5 were categorized as 'poor quality' (Appendix).

Results

The literature search initially identified 3284 abstracts (reduced from 4893 following deduplication and limiting to English language studies in adult humans). In total, 89 papers remained after the initial screening process. Two additional studies were added following the review of reference lists of published related systematic reviews. Following the second stage review, 38 papers were included in this study (Fig. 19.1).

Study Objectives, Design and Population

Of the 38 papers selected for review, there were four pairs of papers which reported the longer and shorter term follow-up outcomes of the same studies, and thus were merged for analysis (34 studies in total) [7–14].

The study period ranged from 1993 to 2017, with the majority of included papers published after 2000 (33 out of 34). The clinical study design of the 34 studies included 15 randomised controlled trials (RCTs), 17 prospective cohort studies and two retrospective cohort studies. Eight studies were related to intervention in the aortoiliac segment, 25 studies were related to intervention in the femoropopliteal segment, and one additional paper studied interventions in both the aortoiliac and femoropopliteal segments.

Health-Related Quality of Life Outcome Measures

A total of nine different QOL instruments were used (Table 19.1). Five generic QOL instruments were used including: EuroQol (EQ)-5D-3L, EQ-5D-5L, RAND-36, Short form (SF)-36, SF-12, SF-8. Four disease specific QOL instruments were used including: Walking Impairment Questionnaire (WIQ), Peripheral Arterial Questionnaire (PAQ), VascuQOL and Intermittent Claudication Questionnaire (ICQ).

Many papers reported using the EuroQOL instrument but did not specify which variant was used, e.g. EQ-5D-3L versus EQ-5D-5L.

Studies Focused on Aortoiliac Steno-Occlusive Disease

Nine studies were identified which focused on surgical and/or endovascular interventions for aortoiliac steno-occlusive disease. Details of outcomes are shown in Table 19.2.

One prospective multicentre observational study investigating outcomes of patients who had undergone endovascular intervention (angioplasty and/or stenting) for Rutherford 2–4 aortoiliac disease demonstrated significant improvements in HRQOL outcome at the 12-month follow-up compared to baseline [16].

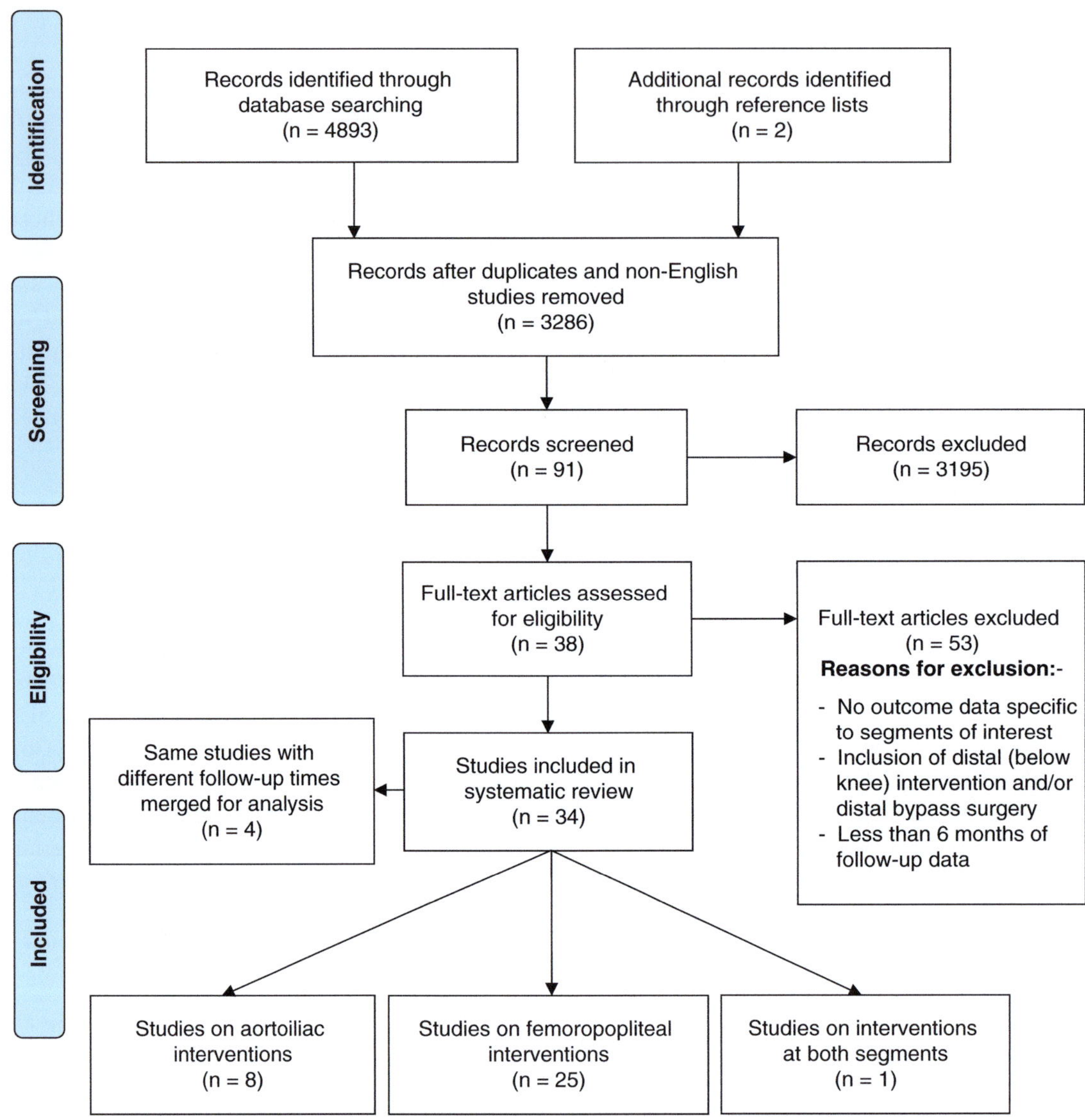

Fig. 19.1 Flow diagram of literature review

A further three multicentre prospective cohort studies specifically investigated the use of primary stenting with bare metal stent for aortoiliac disease [17–19]. All three demonstrated an improvement in HRQOL measures at follow-up.

An RCT published in 2015 compared three treatment arms: BMT, stenting with BMT, and SET with BMT. The study demonstrated that patients who received either stenting or SET had significantly better HRQOL than those whom received BMT alone at both the 6- and 18-month follow-up timepoints [14]. No significant difference in HRQOL outcomes was seen between the SET and stenting group. Another RCT comparing percutaneous transluminal angioplasty (PTA) combined with SET and BMT to BMT combined with SET demonstrated better HRQOL outcomes in the PTA group at 24-month follow-up [22].

Table 19.1 Description of health-related quality of life instruments utilised by included studies

Health-related quality of life (HRQOL) instrument	Description
Short Form Health Survey (SF-36, SF-12, SF-8)	*SF-36*—A 36-item, patient-reported survey of patient health status consisting of eight domains: Vitality, Physical functioning, Bodily pain, General health perceptions, Physical role functioning, Emotional role functioning, Social role functioning and Mental health (summarised physical and mental component scores are also calculated). Each domain is scored on a 0–100 scale, with a lower score representing greater disability.
	SF-12 and SF-8—Shortened versions of SF-36 with 12 and 8 items respectively, evaluating the same eight domains.
Walking Impairment Questionnaire (WIQ)	A subjective measure of patient-reported walking performance in patients with peripheral arterial disease consisting of three domains: Walking distance, Walking speed and Stair-climbing ability (a total mean score is also calculated). Each domain is scored from 0% to 100%, with a lower percentage representing a poorer walking performance.
EuroQol Five Dimensions (EQ-5D)	A self-reported, standardized instrument for measuring generic health status consisting of five dimensions: Mobility, Self-care, Usual activities, Pain/discomfort, and Anxiety/depression—each dimension is rated on a three-level (EQ-5D-3L) or five-level (EQ-5D-5L) scale based on severity. An evaluation of overall health is done on the day of questionnaire completion using a Visual Analogue Scale (EQ-VAS)—this is indicated on a vertical scale from 0 to 100.
RAND 36-item Health Survey (RAND-36)	This instrument utilises the same 36-item questionnaire as SF-36 and evaluates the same eight domains with minor differences in scoring the General health perceptions and Bodily pain scales.
Peripheral Artery Questionnaire (PAQ)	A 20-item, patient-reported peripheral artery disease-specific HRQOL questionnaire consisting of six domains (Physical limitation, Symptoms, Symptom stability, Social limitation, Treatment satisfaction and Quality of life) and a summary score. Each domain is scored on a 0–100 scale, with higher scores indicating less functional limitation, fewer symptoms, better treatment satisfaction, higher social functioning, and better health status.
Vascular Quality of Life Questionnaire (VascuQoL)	*VQ-25*—A 25-item patient-reported peripheral artery disease-specific HRQOL questionnaire consisting of five domains (Activities, Symptoms, Pain, Social life, Emotions) and an overall (mean) score. Each item is scored on a 7-point response scale, with higher scores indicating better HRQOL.
	VQ-6—A 6-item, short form of VQ-25 evaluating the same domains except on a 4-point response scale.
Intermittent Claudication Questionnaire (ICQ)	A 16-item self-administered intermittent claudication-specific HRQOL instrument evaluating severity of pain, limitations on activities of daily living, emotional impact and interference with activities. Each item is assessed on a 5-point adjectival scale and scored between 0 and 100 (0 = worst, 100 = best).

One paper presented a direct comparison of two endovascular procedures within an RCT study design. The trial compared stenting to PTA and demonstrated improvement in HRQOL outcomes in both groups at 24-month follow-up, but no significant difference between the two groups [20]. Of the remaining two papers relating to intervention in the aortoiliac segment, one prospective cohort study demonstrated improved HRQOL measures at 6 months following laparoscopic aorto-bifemoral bypass surgery [15]; while the other retrospective observational study—which compared stenting to aorto-bifemoral bypass surgery—demonstrated no significant difference in HRQOL outcomes between the groups [21]. However, subgroup analysis did reveal significantly improved outcomes in the endovascular group compared to the surgical group in one item of the WIQ questionnaire (difficulty in walking 150 m).

Table 19.2 Studies including interventions on aorto-iliac steno-occlusive disease

Type of intervention / Device type, Brand name (if applicable)	Author (year of publication), Study period, Study type	Study intent/ associated study	Cohort size, study centre(s)	Patient characteristics	Preop HRQOL assessment	Follow-up period	HRQOL instrument(s) used, method of delivery, completion rate	Key outcomes	Main findings related to HRQOL	Quality score
Surgery	Kazmi et al. (2017) [15]	To examine HRQOL in patients operated with laparoscopic aortobifemoral bypass (LABFB) for athero-sclerotic obstruction in aortoiliac segment.	50	Consecutive patients with TASC II D lesions presenting with IC.	Yes	6 months	SF-36	Patients operated with LABFB for Trans-Atlantic Inter-Society Consensus II, type D lesions have substantial and statistically significant improvement in the patients' HRQL.	Statistically significant improvement from baseline was found in all domains as well as in the summary scores. Substantial at 1 month, sustained until 6 month follow-up.	8
	2005–2011		Oslo University Hospital, Sweden	Mean age 62 year, Male 46%			Not stated		The PCS summary scores showed significant improvement at all the postoperative survey time points as compared to the preoperative scores, whereas the MCS scores showed improvement only at 6 months	
	Prospective study			All patients were in Rutherford's category 3, except two patients who were in Rutherford's category 5.			80%		Concomitant operations had a statistically significant negative impact on the physical components of SF-36 (PF, RP).	
									When studying PCS, a positive impact of smoking and a negative impact of concomitant operation and blood loss were found. In case of MCS, only the length of hospital stay had a statistically significant ($p < 0.03$) negative effect on the score, but its magnitude was not substantial (–0.3 points change per day).	

Endovascular (balloon-expandable stent, self-expandable stent, PTA)	Yamauchi et al. (2019) [16]	1-year clinical outcomes of endovascular therapy (EVT) for de novo aortoiliac lesions in patients with symptomatic PAD (Rutherford classification 2, 3 or 4).	893 (1128 limbs)	Mean age of 73 ± 9	No	1 year	WIQ, EQ-5D	1-year data from our ongoing multicentre prospective study indicate acceptable safety and efficacy of aortoiliac EVT, supporting the recent recommendation that EVT can be a first-line treatment for aortoiliac disease.	EQ-5D: All global and domain (utility score, VAS) scores showed improvement at 1 year after EVT (p < 0.001).	5
	2014–2019		64 centres in Japan	83% male			Not stated		WIQ: All global and domain (pain, distance, speed, climbing) scores showed improvement at 1 year after EVT (p < 0.001).	
	Prospective observational study			Rutherford category: 2/3/4 = 42%/51%/7%			Not stated. Use of multiple imputations to generate data for patients lost to follow-up			
				Chronic total occlusion (per limb) = 36%						
				Femoropopliteal lesion (per limb) = 37%						
Stent	Burket et al. (2016) [17]	To evaluate the safety and efficacy of a self-expanding bare-metal nitinol stent (Astron) for the treatment of atherosclerotic lesions in the common and external iliac arteries.	161	The mean age of the evaluable patients was 63.6 years with the majority being male (65.2%). Patient risk factors included hyperlipidemia (77.6%), hypertension (72.7%) and patients that were current smokers (48.4%).	Yes	12 months	WIQ	The MAE rate at 12 months was 2.1% (p < 0.001). The acute procedural success and 30-day clinical success outcomes were both 95%. The primary patency rate at 12 months was 89.8%.	The WIQ PAD specific score, walking distance score, walking speed score and stair climbing score each showed a significant increase from baseline to 12 months (p < 0.001).	7
Self-expandable, bare nitinol stent	2011–2014		30 centres (USA, Canada, Austria)	Common iliac 67%, external iliac 33%			Not stated	The Astron stent system was shown to be safe and effective in the treatment of patients with atherosclerotic disease. The observed MAE rate met the pre-specified performance goal of 15%. The stent demonstrated a high 12-month primary patency rate and showed improvement in quality of life measures.		
	Prospective study			TASC II A/B = 62%/35%			WIQ: 89%			
Astron				De novo 91.3%, moderate/severe calcification 70.8%						

(continued)

Table 19.2 (continued)

Type of intervention Device type, Brand name (if applicable)	Author (year of publication), Study period, Study type	Study intent/ associated study	Cohort size, study centre(s)	Patient characteristics	Preop HRQOL assessment	Follow-up period	HRQOL instrument(s) used, method of delivery, completion rate	Key outcomes	Main findings related to HRQOL	Quality score
Stent	Murphy et al. (2005) [18]	To determine the effect of aortoiliac stent placement on walking ability and health-related quality of life (QOL) for aortoiliac insufficiency in elderly individuals with moderate to severe intermittent claudication.	35 (46 limbs)	Mean age 61.1 (SD 9.5), Male 71%, HTN 54%, DM 14%	Yes	12 months	SF-36, WIQ	Mean ABI significantly improved from 0.64 ± 0.15 to 0.89 ± 0.19 (p < 0.01).	WIQ: significant improvement from baseline in all three dimensions (walking distance, walking speed, and stair climbing).	9
Self-expandable, bare alloy stent/ self-expandable, polyester covered alloy stent/ balloon-expandable bare stainless-steel stent	1996–1999		Rhode Island Hospital, Rhode Island, USA	Stenosis n = 30, chronic arterial occlusions n = 16			Self-administered (optional help from research assistant)	Mean initial claudication duration improved (1.7 ± 1.0 to 4.7 ± 3.3 months) and mean MWD on treadmill test improved (3.3 ± 1.8 to 8.7 ± 4.4 months).	SF-36: Significant improvement from baseline for health dimensions of physical functioning, role physical, bodily pain and vitality; also, physical component scale	
	Prospective study						80%			
Wallstent/ Wallgraft/ Palmaz								No 30-day mortality. Complication rate 9% (n = 3).		
								High technical success (97%).		

Stent	Laird et al. (2019) [19]	To assess the performance of the LIFESTREAM balloon-expandable covered stent for the treatment of iliac artery atherosclerotic lesions.	155	Eligible patients had symptoms of lifestyle-limiting claudication or ischemic rest pain (Rutherford categories 2–4) and de novo or re-stenotic, non-stented lesions (! 50% of the reference vessel diameter) in the iliac artery.	Yes	9 months	WIQ	The primary composite endpoint rate was 16.2% (93.5% confidence interval [CI]: 10.6–23.2%), primary patency was 89.1% (95% CI: 82.6–93.7%), and freedom from TLR was 96%.	The proportion of patients with cumulative improvement from baseline of at least one Rutherford category at the 9-month visit was 90.5% (124 of 137; 95% CI: 84.3–94.9%).	7
Balloon-expandable, ePTFE covered stainless-steel stent	2014–2015		17 centres (Europe, USA, NZ)	Mean age 64 years, Male 69%, HTN 76%, DM 32%			Not stated		WIQ: mean change in total score from baseline 32.1 ± 26.84. Improvements noted in all domains.	
LIFESTREAM	Prospective study			Common iliac 73%, external iliac 27%			88%	The LIFESTREAM balloon-expandable covered stent provided satisfactory 9-month clinical outcomes including a low rate of target lesion revascularization for the treatment of stenotic and occlusive lesions of the iliac arteries.		
				TASC A/B/C and D = 62%/27%/11%						
				Rutherford 2/3/4 = 16%/76%/8%						

(continued)

Table 19.2 (continued)

Type of intervention / Device type, Brand name (if applicable)	Author (year of publication), Study period, Study type	Study intent/ associated study	Cohort size, study centre(s)	Patient characteristics	Preop HRQOL assessment	Follow-up period	HRQOL instrument(s) used, method of delivery, completion rate	Key outcomes	Main findings related to HRQOL	Quality score
Stent versus Angioplasty	Bosch et al. (1999) [20]	To assess the quality of life in patients with iliac artery occlusive disease, we compared primary stent placement versus primary angioplasty followed by selective stent placement in a multicentre randomized controlled trial.	279	All patients with intermittent claudication or critical ischemia caused by stenosis or occlusion in the iliac arteries.	Yes	24 months	RAND-36, EQ-5D	Health-related quality of life improves equally after primary stent placement and primary angioplasty with selective stent placement in the treatment of intermittent claudication caused by iliac artery occlusive disease.	When the two treatments were compared, no significant difference was observed ($p < 0.05$). All measurements showed a significant improvement in the quality of life after treatment ($p < 0.05$).	9
	1993–1996		Six centres in Netherlands	Stent ($n = 143$): Mean age 59, Male 71%; common iliac 70%, external iliac 30%; 80% >50% stenosis			Telephone interview		In both groups, scores of all RAND-36 dimensions showed significant improvement after revascularization. The scores were still significantly higher than before treatment, with the exception of the dimension of general health perception in stent group ($p = 0.20$) and PTA group ($p = 0.09$).	
	Randomised control trial			PTA ($n = 136$): Mean age 60, Male 73%; common iliac 67%, external iliac 33%; 82% >50% stenosis			36%		The effect of treatment was highest for physical functioning, physical role functioning, and bodily pain. Scores on all RAND-36 dimensions were not significantly different between the groups.	
				The treatment groups demonstrated no significant differences with respect to descriptive variables, baseline quality-of-life measures, and baseline clinical measures.					All valuational quality-of-life measures (time trade-off, standard gamble, rating scale, health utilities index, EQ-5D) demonstrated a significant improvement after treatment, with the exception of the standard gamble.	
									The values were not significantly different between the groups.	

Stent versus surgery	Rocha-Neves et al. (2020) [21]	Compare technical, clinical, and economic outcomes between endovascular and aortobifemoral bypass grafting (ABF)/open approaches in patients with type D aortoiliac occlusive disease.	59	Mean age of 65.6 ± 12.2 (endovascular), 62.1 ± 6.5 (ABF)	No	67.84 months (95% CI = 61.85–73.83)	WIQ, EQ-5D-5L	ABF group had higher technical success ($p = 0.001$). Similar limb salvage and patency rates between groups.	WIQ: No statistically significant intergroup differences, except Higher global WIQ pain score in endovascular group ($p = 0.52$) and increased degree of difficulty walking 150 m ($p < 0.001$).	7
Balloon-expandable and self-expandable stents/double-woven synthetic graft	2011–2017	Patients with common femoral artery obstructive disease or aortoiliac aneurysmatic disease were excluded.	Centro Hospitalar de Sao Joao (referral center) and Hospital Padre Americo (regional hospital), Porto, Portugal	Mean Rutherford = 3.3, CLI (n = 4)			Not stated	Shorter length-of-stay and lower hospital expenses in endovascular group, with a similar procedure cost in both groups.	EQ-5D-5L: No statistically significant intergroup differences in individual or index scores	
	Retrospective cohort			Similar characteristics in both groups, except higher proportion of CHF and CKD in endovascular group, and higher proportion of smokers in ABF group			61% of all; 77% of those alive			

(continued)

Table 19.2 (continued)

Type of intervention Device type, Brand name (if applicable)	Author (year of publication), Study period, Study type	Study intent/ associated study	Cohort size, study centre(s)	Patient characteristics	Preop HRQOL assessment	Follow-up period	HRQOL instrument(s) used, method of delivery, completion rate	Key outcomes	Main findings related to HRQOL	Quality score
PTA vs. BMT	Greenhalgh et al. (2008) [22]	Patients with symptoms of stable mild to moderate intermittent claudication (MIMIC) were randomised in two multi-centre trials, for femoropopliteal and aortoiliac arterial disease, to receive either PTA or no PTA against a background of supervised exercise, smoking cessation and best medical therapy and followed up for 24 months.	Femoro-popliteal (FP)—93	FP (PTA, Control: 48, 45)—differences in mean age, IHD and statin use	No	24 months	SF-36	There were significant improvements in both AWD and ICD in the PTA groups for both trials. The adjusted AWD was 38% greater in the PTA group for the femoropopliteal trial (95%; CI 1–90) (p = 0.04) and 78% greater in the PTA group for the aortoiliac trial (95%; CI 0–216) (p = 0.05).	**FP:** No significant intergroup differences in mean physical and mental scores of SF-36.	9
	2003–2006		Aortoiliac (AI)—34	AI (PTA, Control: 19, 15)—no apparent differences			Not stated		**AI:** Significant intergroup differences in mean physical scores of SF-36 in favour of PTA group.	
	Randomised control trial		Nine centres in UK				Femoropop-liteal—86%			
							Aortoiliac—76%			

Stent versus Supervised exercise	Murphy et al. (2015) [14]	To report the longer-term (18-month) efficacy of supervised exercise (SE) compared with stent revascularization (ST) and optimal medical care (OMC) in claudication due to aortoiliac peripheral artery disease [CLEVER study]	111	Adults over 40 years of age with moderate-to-severe claudication that was due to aortoiliac PAD.		6, 18 months	SF-12, WIQ, PAQ	Both SE and ST had better 18-month outcomes than OMC. SE and ST provided comparable durable improvement in functional status and in quality of life up to 18 months. The durability of claudication exercise interventions merits its consideration as a primary PAD claudication treatment.	**6 months**	
	2007–2011		29 centres (USA, Canada)	Randomised into three groups: OMC only, OMC + ST (ST), OMC + SE (SE).			Not stated		The ST group improved more than the OMC group for every QOL measure except the SF-12 mental summary scale and the WIQ stair-climbing scale. The SE group improved more than the OMC group for every scale except SF-12 mental, WIQ pain, WIQ stair climbing, PAQ symptom stability, and PAQ treatment satisfaction. Compared with SE, ST was associated with significantly greater benefit across most of the disease-specific QOL measures but not for the generic scales. The difference between ST and SE for the PAQ overall summary score (14.78 points) exceeded the 8-point difference that has been considered to be clinically meaningful. More patients in the ST group than the SE group reported no claudication symptoms on the WIQ.	
	Randomised control trial			Mean age 64.4 ± 9.5, Male 62%			6 months		**18 months**	
				DM 24%, HTN 85%			89%		There were no baseline differences in quality of life among the treatment groups. At 18 months, improvement in disease-specific scales (WIQ, PAQ) was statistically superior for ST and SE compared with OMC, but ST and SE differed significantly from each other (favouring ST) only for PAQ symptoms, PAQ treatment satisfaction, PAQ quality of life, and PAQ summary.	
				Baseline characteristics of the three study groups were similar.			18 months			
				There were no significant differences in baseline characteristics between the 79 patients who completed the 18-month treadmill test and the 32 patients who did not.			SF-12 Physical: 69%			
							WIQ-pain: 71%			
							WIQ-walking distance: 70%			
							PAQ-physical limitation, symptoms, QoL: 68%			
							PAQ-summary: 69%			

Studies Focused on Femoropopliteal Steno-Occlusive disease

Twenty-six articles were identified which focused on surgical and/or endovascular interventions for femoropopliteal steno-occlusive disease. Details of outcomes are shown in Table 19.3.

A three-arm RCT which evaluated PTA, SET, and a combination of PTA and SET demonstrated some improvement in both generic and disease specific HRQOL measures when compared to baseline, although no significant difference was seen between the three treatment groups [35]. Another two-arm RCT which compared BMT, smoking cessation therapy and SET to BMT, smoking cessation, SET and PTA demonstrated no significant difference in SF-36 scores [22].

Four multicentre prospective cohort studies investigated outcomes of femoropopliteal angioplasty with DCBs, all of which demonstrated improved HRQOL measures when compared to baseline [12, 36, 37, 39]. Two of these were conducted by the same research group studying the effectiveness of a DCB (IN.PACT Admiral, Medtronic) on shorter (<15 cm) and longer (>15 cm) femoropopliteal lesions [12, 36]. An additional cohort study investigating the use of DCB in in-stent restenosis demonstrated a trend towards improvement in HRQOL outcomes, although no statistically significant difference was seen [38].

Five multicentre RCTs compared the use of a specific DCB device to standard PTA (four different DCB devices studied in total). All of the studies demonstrated improved HRQOL measures for both the PTA and DCB treatment groups at 12-month follow-up compared to baseline [7, 40–43]. One of these studies by Rosenfield et al. demonstrated statistically significant better outcomes with DCB when compared to PTA in one item of the HRQOL measures obtained ('Walking distance' item of the WIQ) [40]. No significant difference in HRQOL outcomes between DCB and PTA were found in the other four studies.

In total, eight studies investigated HRQOL outcomes of femoropopliteal artery stenting. One retrospective cohort study and four prospective cohort studies evaluated HRQOL outcomes following self-expanding nitinol bare metal stenting for femoropopliteal disease [30–34]. All studies demonstrated significantly improved HRQOL outcomes when compared to baseline. Of these studies, Han et al. specifically looked at gender difference in HRQOL outcomes post stenting. Although HRQOL measures improved for both men and women, there was less sustainability of HRQOL outcomes for women at 3 years.

Two of the eight studies were multicentre RCTs which compared different stents. One of the studies compared a covered self-expanding nitinol stent to a bare metal self-expanding nitinol stent [28]. Both stents demonstrated poor primary patency rates, however, a sustained improvement in HRQOL scores was demonstrated at 3 years for both groups. The authors did not present a statistical comparison of the HRQOL outcomes between the treatment groups, though the outcomes appear to be similar. The other study compared two different self-expanding bare metal nitinol stents placed in the femoropopliteal segment. No difference was identified in HRQOL outcomes between the two stents at 24 months, but an improvement was seen for each stent compared to the baseline [29].

The final study was a multicentre RCT which compared primary stenting of superficial femoral artery (SFA) lesions to BMT. This demonstrated significant improvement in HRQOL outcomes in the stenting group, but no improvement in the BMT group [9].

Two of the studies identified were RCTs that compared stenting to PTA in the femoropopliteal segment. The first study by Laird et al. demonstrated a significant improvement in HRQOL outcomes at 12 months in both groups [44]. Primary patency was significantly higher in the stent group, but no significant difference in HRQOL measures was seen between the groups. A subgroup analysis of the WIQ scores did, however, find significantly better outcomes with respect to claudication pain in the stent group. The other RCT study by Chalmers et al. also demonstrated improved HRQOL measures post intervention, but no difference between the groups. A significantly worse HRQOL outcome

Table 19.3 Studies including interventions on femoral-popliteal steno-occlusive disease

Type of intervention										
Device type, Brand name (if applicable)	Author (year of publication), Study period, Study type	Study intent/ associated study	Cohort size, Study centre(s)	Patient characteristics	Preop HRQOL assessment	Follow-up period	HRQOL instrument(s) used, Method of delivery, Completion rate	Key outcomes	Main findings related to HRQOL	Quality score
Atherectomy	Rastan et al. (2018) [23]	To report the effectiveness of directional atherectomy for the treatment of popliteal artery occlusive disease [DEFINITIVE LE Trial]	158 (162 procedures)	Mean age 72.0 ± 10.9 years	Yes	12 months	EQ-5D, WIQ	The 1-year primary patency rate was 75.0% (IC patients 78.2% and CLI patients 67.5%, p = 0.118). The freedom from major amputation in both cohorts was 100%.	Rutherford: Overall 3.3 ± 1.2 at baseline to 1.2 ± 1.4 at 1 year (p < 0.001); mean change IC (−1.6 ± 1.1) and CLI (−3.1 ± 1.8)	8
Directional atherectomy catheter	2009–2012		Multicentre (n = 47) (Europe, USA)	82 men (52%)			Not stated	Procedure success (≤30% residual stenosis) was achieved in 84.4% of treated lesions; adjunctive stenting was required in 6 (3.7%) of the 162 lesions.	EQ-5D (VAS): increased from a mean of 64.1 ± 20.1 at baseline to 72.3 ± 17.7 at 1 year (p < 0.001)	
SilverHawk	Prospective study			48 (30%) CLI, 110 (70%) IC			77%		WIQ: walking distance improved in IC cohort only with a mean score of 21.0 ± 23.3 at baseline increasing to 48.7 ± 39.2 at 1 year (p < 0.001).	
				Similar characteristics in the IC and CLI cohorts with the exception of diabetes, which was more common in the CLI patients.						
				Of the patients with IC, the majority had RC 3 ischemia (71, 64.5%), whereas three-quarters of the CLI patients (36, 75%) had ischemic wounds (RC categories 5/6).						

(continued)

Table 19.3 (continued)

Type of intervention Device type, Brand name (if applicable)	Author (year of publication), Study period, Study type	Study intent/ associated study	Cohort size, Study centre(s)	Patient characteristics	Preop HRQOL assessment	Follow-up period	HRQOL instrument(s) used, Method of delivery, Completion rate	Key outcomes	Main findings related to HRQOL	Quality score
Atherectomy	Schwindt et al. (2017) [24]	To evaluate the safety and efficacy of a novel optical coherence tomography (OCT)–guided atherectomy catheter in treating patients with symptomatic femoropopliteal disease [VISION Study]	158 (198 lesions)	Mean age 67.2 ± 10.5 years; 55% men	Yes	6 months	SF-12, VascuQoL	97% (192/198) achieved primary efficacy outcome of technical success (<50% residual diameter stenosis).	Rutherford classification improved in 120/144 (83.3%) from baseline ($p < 0.001$).	8
Optical coherence tomography-guided atherectomy catheter	2014–2015		20 centres (19 USA, 1 Europe)	DM 44%, HTN 91%			Not stated	The composite Major adverse events outcome through 6 months occurred in 25 (16.6%) of 151 subjects.	VascuQol score and SF-12 Physical component score significantly improved from baseline ($p < 0.001$).	
Pantheris	Prospective cohort study			SFA 81%, SFA/Pop 6%, Popliteal 13%			86%	OCT-guided atherectomy for femoropopliteal disease is safe and effective. Additionally, the precision afforded by OCT guidance leads to greater removal of plaque during atherectomy while sparing the adventitia.		

Bypass grafts	Bosma et al. (2012) [25]	Study of long-term QoL and mobility after supragenicular prosthetic femoropopliteal bypass (PTFE vs. Dacron)	140	Consecutive patients presenting with claudication, ischaemic rest pain, gangrene.	No	Mean 84 months	EQ-5D, EQ-VAS, WIQ	Primary outcomes were QOL scores.	Primary bypass occlusion did not affect QOL scores.	7
Prosthetic Dacron and PTFE grafts	1997–2003		Amsterdam and Zoetermeer, Netherlands	PTFE (n = 77), Dacron (n = 63)		(3–135)	Self-administered	Secondary: 5-year, 10-year survival was 58%, 51%.	Bypass patency at the end of follow-up (open [with or without intervention] versus occluded) did not result in significant difference in QOL scores.	
	Prospective observational study			Mean age 66 (37–87)			89% (63/71 survivors)	Bypass failure occurred more frequently in pts treated with a bypass occlusion.	Amputees vs. Non-amputees (WIQ, EQ-5D, EQ-VAS): 0.16, 0.487, 66/0.42, 0.496, 56	
				66% Male				Rutherford runoff score significantly associated with occlusion, but no significant association with graft type.	Dacron (0.49) higher WIQ score than PTFE (0.26). No significant difference in EQ-5D and EQ-VAS.	
				HTN 68%					Male sex was significantly associated with better WIQ, EQ-5D, and EQ-VAS scores.	
				62% no previous intervention					A better WIQ score is significantly associated with a better QoL (p 0.001)	
				Rutherford 1, 2, 3 (58%, 21%, 21%)						
				n = 69 died during follow-up						

(continued)

Table 19.3 (continued)

Type of intervention Device type, Brand name (if applicable)	Author (year of publication), Study period, Study type	Study intent/ associated study	Cohort size, Study centre(s)	Patient characteristics	Preop HRQOL assessment	Follow-up period	HRQOL instrument(s) used, Method of delivery, Completion rate	Key outcomes	Main findings related to HRQOL	Quality score
Stent versus PTA	Chalmers et al. (2013) [26]	To determine whether primary stenting reduces the rate of restenosis compared with balloon angioplasty alone in the endovascular treatment of long superficial femoral artery lesions; and to assess the effect of treatment on quality of life.	150	Patients with SFA occlusion or severe stenosis randomized to either primary stenting with the SMART stent or PTA (with bailout stenting).	Yes	12 months	EQ-5D Utility, EQ-VAS	No significant intergroup differences of restenosis. Fewer TLR in stent group but not statisitically different. No difference in rate of amputation.	Both EQ-5D scoring systems showed generally lower values with increasing disease severity as described by the Rutherford classification.	8
Self-expandable, nitinol stent	2005–2008		17 centres in UK	Stent group (n = 74): Mean age 65.9 ± 9.0; Male 78%; DM 31%; HTN 66%			Not stated	Primary stenting of long lesions in predominantly occluded superficial femoral arteries does not reduce the rate of binary restenosis compared with balloon angioplasty and bailout stenting.	Both sets of scores were similar for both groups of patients at each time point. Both treatment strategies resulted in a marked and statistically significant increase in utility score from baseline to 3 months (p < 0.0001 for both), which was maintained to 12 months, also for both groups.	
Cordis SMART	Randomised control trial			PTA group (n = 76): Mean age 69.8 ± 8.5; Male 86%; DM 38%; HTN 67%			EQ-5D Utility: 75%		Some patients with restenosis had very low scores at 12 months compared with those who did not, as reflected by a much lower 25th percentile (0.15 vs. 0.62 respectively).	
				There were minor imbalances between the two groups, none of which reached statistical significance, apart from age, where patients randomized to PTA were 3.9 years older (p < 0.01).			EQ-VAS: 77%			
				High proportion of vessels being totally occluded (95.9% and 90.8% in the stent and PTA groups, respectively). Stent group had significantly longer occlusions than those randomized to PTA (83.9 ± 46.3 mm vs. 62.8 ± 37.1 mm, p < 0.01); all other baseline lesions characteristics were similar.						

Stent versus PTA	Laird et al. (2010) [44]	Outcomes of Nitinol Stent Implantation Versus Balloon Angioplasty for Obstructive Lesions in the Superficial Femoral Artery and Proximal Popliteal Artery with IC at 12 months (RESILIENT Randomised Trial)	206	2:1 randomization ratio to treatment with either a self-expanding nitinol stent after predilation (n = 134) or PTA (n = 72).	Yes	12 months	SF-8, WIQ	Acute lesion success (30% residual stenosis) was superior for the stent group compared with the angioplasty group (95.8% versus 83.9%; p < 0.01).	Both treatment groups demonstrated a significant improvement in all QOL measures at 6 and 12 months compared with baseline. The baseline SF-8 physical score was 41.0 ± 10.5 (PTA) and 41.4 ± 9.2 (stent). SF-8 increased similarly in both groups (5.9 ± 11.2 versus 5.7 ± 11.2; p < 0.0001 versus baseline). Walking distance score was 22.3 ± 23.2 (PTA) and 22.8 ± 24.2 (stent). Walking distance scores had increased similarly in both groups (29.4 ± 37.4 versus 25.6 ± 34.6; p < 0.0001 versus baseline). Patients in the PTA group reported more claudication pain at 12 months than patients in the stent group (Walking Impairment Questionnaire evaluation, p < 0.009), but there were no other significant differences in QOL measures between treatment groups (*t* test p > 0.05).	8
Self-expandable, bare nitinol stent	2004–2006		24 centres (Europe, USA)	Baseline patient demographics (age, sex, and race) and pre-procedure classification of symptoms (Rutherford category and ankle brachial index) were not significantly different between treatment groups (p < 0.05).			Not stated	Freedom from target lesion revascularization was 87.3% for the stent group compared with 45.1% for the angioplasty group (p < 0.0001).		
LifeStent	Randomised control trial			Pre-existing risk factors were not significantly different between patient groups (p < 0.09), except PTA group had a significantly higher reported prevalence of hypertension than the stent group (p < 0.03).			83%	Duplex ultrasound-derived primary patency at 12 months was better for the stent group (81.3% versus 36.7%; p < 0.0001).		
				Lesion characteristics were similar between the two treatment groups.						

(continued)

Table 19.3 (continued)

Type of intervention: Device type, Brand name (if applicable)	Author (year of publication), Study period, Study type	Study intent/ associated study	Cohort size, Study centre(s)	Patient characteristics	Preop HRQOL assessment	Follow-up period	HRQOL instrument(s) used, Method of delivery, Completion rate	Key outcomes	Main findings related to HRQOL	Quality score
Stent versus bypass	Reijnen et al. (2017) [27]	To compare heparin-bonded endografts with femoropopliteal bypass, including quality of life, using general health and disease-specific questionnaires as well as patency rates.	125	Endoluminal n = 63, Surgical n = 62	Yes	1 month and 12 months	SF-36, WIQ	Heparin-bonded endoluminal bypass for long segment lesions shows promising results (less morbidity, faster recovery, and improvement in quality of life with indistinguishable patency rates at 1 year) compared with surgical bypass.	At 1 month: SF-36 significantly better in endoluminal group (50.2 vs. 37.1; p = 0.011). Overall WIQ scores in IC patients were significantly better in endoluminal group. Endoluminal group showed an earlier improvement too.	10
Heparin-bonded ePTFE endografts/venous and prosthetic bypass grafts	2010–2015		Six centres in Netherlands	Mean age 69, 67			Self-administered (optional help from nurses)		At 12 months: Improvement in most domains of SF-36 in both groups from baseline. No significant differences between groups, except for experienced Health change (endoluminal better).	
	Randomised control trial			Male 73%, 80%			81% (endoluminal), 89% (surgical)		Significant improvement in all WIQ domains in IC patients in both groups from baseline, while stairs domain better in endoluminal group.	
				Rutherford Cat 3 (IC) 62%, 68%						
				No significant differences between groups at baseline in demographics and anatomical details.						
				Similar baseline HRQOL, except worse SF-36 Mental health and higher Health Change in endoluminal group.						

Stent vs. BMT	Lindgren et al. (2018) [9]	Assessment of the 24-month impact of primary stenting with nitinol self-expanding stents compared to best medical treatment (BMT) alone in patients with stable IC due to SFA disease on health-related quality of life (HRQoL).	100	IC patients already on BMT, randomised into Stent (n = 48) or control (n = 52) group.	Yes	12, 24 months	SF-36, EQ-5D, WIQ	ABI and walking distance significantly improved from baseline in both groups.	**12 months:** In the stent group the following SF-36 domains improved: Physical Function, 19 points ($p < .001$); Bodily Pain, 14 points ($p = .001$); General Health, 6 points ($p = .019$); Vitality, 10 points ($p = .004$); Physical Component Summary, 6.5 points ($p < .001$); EQ5D, 0.14 points ($p = .008$); and WIQ 22 points ($p < .001$). They were unchanged in the control group.	10
Self-expandable, nitinol, bare metal stent	2010–2015		Seven Swedish hospitals	Six withdrew consent, two died.			Self-administered	Significantly better WIQ score in stent group.	Walking distance (WD) (from 171 ± 90 to 613 ± 381 m, $p < .001$, in the stent group and from 209 ± 106 to 335 ± 321 m, $p = .012$, in the control group) improved.	
	Randomised control trial			Well matched groups for age, sex, smoking habits, BP, cholesterol, duration of IC, lesion characteristics and HRQOL.			92%		**24 months:** Significantly better SF-36 Physical Component Summary ($p = 0.024$) and physical domain scores such as Physical Function ($p = 0.012$), Bodily Pain ($p = 0.002$), General Health ($p = 0.037$), and EQ5D ($p = 0.010$) were reported in intergroup comparison between the stent and the control group.	
				Mean age in stent (71), control (70)					Stent group improved from baseline in SF-36 PCS score, Physical function, Bodily pain and Vitality.	
									No improvement from baseline in control group.	

(continued)

Table 19.3 (continued)

Type of intervention Device type, Brand name (if applicable)	Author (year of publication), Study period, Study type	Study intent/ associated study	Cohort size, Study centre(s)	Patient characteristics	Preop HRQOL assessment	Follow-up period	HRQOL instrument(s) used, Method of delivery, Completion rate	Key outcomes	Main findings related to HRQOL	Quality score
Stent vs. Stent	Geraghty et al. (2013) [28]	Comparing the long-term outcomes of complex superficial femoral artery disease intervention using the VIABAHN endoprosthesis to those obtained with bare nitinol stent implantation (VIBRANT Trial)	148	Symptomatic complex superficial femoral artery disease (TransAtlantic Inter-Society Consensus I class C and D lesions, accompanied by intermittent claudication or ischemic rest pain.)	Yes	36 months	SF-36, ICQ	Primary patency rates (VIABAHN 24.2% vs. 25.9%; p = 0.392)	ICQ: Declined (improved) post procedure and sustained. VIABAHN improved from 46.6 ± 20.1 (n = 72) to 20.8 ± 19.6 (n = 40). Bare stent improved from 50.1 ± 18.2 (n = 75) to 22.9 ± 21.2 (n = 45).	7
Self-expandable, ePTFE covered nitinol stent/bare nitinol stent	2005–2007		19 centres in USA	Bare stent n = 76, VIABAHN n = 72			Not stated	Stent fractures (VIABAHN 2.6% vs. 50.0%)	SF-36 (physical domain): immediate improvement post procedure and sustained.	
VIABAHN/-	Randomised control trial			Similar demographics and medical history, except VIABAHN significantly older.			ICQ: 57%	Secondary patency rates (VIABAHN 79.5% vs. 89.3%; p = 0.304)	Rutherford: significantly improved from baseline post procedure, then sustained throughout follow-up period.	
				(Male 65%, 63%; Mean age 64, 69; DM 45%, 43%; HTN 76%, 88%)			SF-36: 57%	No procedure-related mortality or amputation.		
							Rutherford: 64%	Similar long-term outcomes in both groups.		

Stent vs. stent	Laird et al. (2018) [29]	To evaluate the safety and effectiveness of the TIGRIS stent for lesions up to 24 cm in the superficial femoral and proximal popliteal arteries (SFA/PPA).	274	Subjects were randomly assigned in a 3:1 ratio to treatment with the TIGRIS stent (n = 197; mean age 66.7 ± 9.28 years; 141 men) or LifeStent (n = 70; mean age 67.9 ± 8.87 years; 49 men).	Yes	24 months	EQ-5D, PAQ	The TIGRIS stent and LifeStent were similarly effective (primary patency, MAE, TLR, procedure success) for the treatment of lesions in the SFA and PPA. The high flexibility and zero fracture rate associated with the TIGRIS stent make this device favourable for use in high-flexion arteries.	QoL measures including EQ-5D, PAQ, and changes in the Rutherford category and ABI/TBI all demonstrated improvement over baseline for subjects in both the study and control arms of the trial with no statistically significant differences for any indicators.	7
Self-expandable nitinol stent interconnected with PTFE/ Self-expandable, bare nitinol stent	2012–2014		36 centres (Europe, USA)	Both groups had >85% current or former smokers and other comorbidities typical of a PAD population. There were more non-whites in the study group.			Not stated		>85% of patients participating in the study demonstrated sustained Rutherford category improvement at 12 and 24 months post procedure.	
TIGRIS/LifeStent	Randomised control trial			For both groups, 44% of lesions were located in the distal SFA or proximal PPA. Both groups also had ~40% occlusions and 50% moderately or severely calcified lesions. Rutherford 2/3/4 = 32%/64%/4% (TIGRIS); 31%/61%/8% (LifeStent)			Rutherford: 73% EQ-5D: 74% PAQ: 73%			

(continued)

Table 19.3 (continued)

Type of intervention Device type, Brand name (if applicable)	Author (year of publication), Study period, Study type	Study intent/ associated study	Cohort size, Study centre(s)	Patient characteristics	Preop HRQOL assessment	Follow-up period	HRQOL instrument(s) used, Method of delivery, Completion rate	Key outcomes	Main findings related to HRQOL	Quality score
Stent	Dippel et al. (2006) [30]	Reporting the technical feasibility and impact on quality of life (QOL) for angioplasty and primary stenting of chronic total occlusion (CTO) of the superficial femoral artery (SFA).	44 (51 limbs)	Mean age 70.3 (SD 9.6), Male 59%	Yes	12 months	WIQ	CFO SFAs can be treated by percutaneous nitinol stenting with a high degree of success (90.2%) that is durable at 12-month follow-up.	The mean pre- and post-intervention WIQ scores were 722 ± 1503 and 8421 ± 5741 ($p < 0.0005$), respectively. The mean delta-WIQ was 7405 (95% CI: 6555–9245).	5
Self-expandable bare nitinol stent	Not stated		Genesis Medical Centre, Davenport, Iowa, USA	HTN 84%, DM 39%			Not stated	Clinically driven target lesion revascularization rate was 11.8%.		
SMART	Retrospective cohort			Rutherford 2 and 3/4 and 5 = 88%/12%			93%	Patients have significant ABI improvement.		
				All lesions were TASC D lesions.						
Stent	Ohki et al. (2017) [31]	The objective of this study was to assess 1-year safety, efficacy, and invasiveness outcomes of endovascular stent grafting of symptomatic long lesions (≥10 cm) in the superficial femoral artery (SFA) as a substitute for above-knee open bypass surgery.	103	74.2 ± 7.0 years old; 17.5% female; 97.1% claudicants	Yes	12 months	VascuQoL	Stent grafting appears to be a safe and less invasive alternative to above-knee bypass surgery, providing 88–92% primary patency at 12 months in long, complex lesions.	VascuQoL score increased from 58.6 ± 15.7% of maximum possible points to 72.9 ± 18.6% between baseline (4.1 ± 1.1 points) and the 12-month follow-up (5.1 ± 1.3 points; $p < .0001$)	7
Self-expandable, ePTFE covered nitinol stent with a Heparin coating	2012–2013		15 centres in Japan	Rutherford 2/3 n = 100, 4/5 n = 3			Not stated	Target vessel revascularization, major amputation, or death did not occur through postoperative 30 days. No life- or limb-threatening intraoperative or perioperative adverse events and no acute limb ischemia cases were observed during follow-up.	Clinical success (improvement of at least one Rutherford class) occurred in 90.9% of 99 subjects with known status at the 12-month end point.	
	Prospective study			Hypertension (88.3%), smoking history (78.6% overall; 28.2% current smokers), dyslipidemia (62.1%), and diabetes mellitus (60.2%).			97%			
VIABAHN				n = 100 at 12 month follow-up—two died, one withdrew consent						

Stent	Garcia et al. (2015) [32]	Wire-Interwoven Nitinol Stent Outcome in the Superficial Femoral and Proximal Popliteal Arteries 12-month Results of the SUPERB Trial	264	Symptomatic peripheral artery disease (lifestyle limiting intermittent claudication or ischemic rest pain (Rutherford–Becker scale 2–4)) undergoing percutaneous treatment of de novo or restenotic lesions of the superficial femoral or proximal popliteal (femoropopliteal) artery.	Yes	12 months	SF-12, PAQ	On the basis of the high primary patency rate, absence of stent fracture, and significant improvements in functional and quality-of-life measures, the Supera stent provides safe and effective treatment of femoropopliteal lesions in symptomatic patients with peripheral artery disease.	Rutherford: Improvement by at least 1 category in 88.7% of patients and by 3 levels in 53.5% of patients at 12 months.	8
Self-expandable, wire-interwoven nitinol stent	2009–2011		46 centres in USA				Not stated		At 6 and 12 months, SF-12 physical score and Peripheral Artery Questionnaire scales improved significantly ($p < 0.001$ for all comparisons except treatment satisfaction, which received a high rating initially and throughout). Mean SF-12 physical score at 12 months increased from baseline by ≈8 points, >3x the minimum threshold considered to be clinically meaningful. Evaluation at 12 months demonstrated 13–35 point improvement in all Peripheral Artery Questionnaire scales; overall summary score increased 32 points, 4× the threshold considered to be clinically important.	
Supera	Prospective cohort study			Mean (±SD) age was 68.7 (±10.0) years; 63.6% were males			Rutherford: 87%			
				HTN 95%, DM 44%			SF-12: 87%			
				Rutherford 2/3/4 = 38%/57%/5%			PAQ-Physical limitation: 78%			
				Proximal/Middle/Distal SFA = 12%/54%/32%			PAQ-Social limitation: 80%			
							PAQ-symptoms, symptom stability, treatment satisfaction, QoL, summary score: 87%			

(continued)

Table 19.3 (continued)

Type of intervention Device type, Brand name (if applicable)	Author (year of publication), Study period, Study type	Study intent/ associated study	Cohort size, Study centre(s)	Patient characteristics	Preop HRQOL assessment	Follow-up period	HRQOL instrument(s) used, Method of delivery, Completion rate	Key outcomes	Main findings related to HRQOL	Quality score
Stent	Bunte et al. (2018) [33]	To evaluate the clinical and health status outcomes of patients undergoing superficial femoral artery (SFA) revascularization for de novo or restenotic femoropopliteal arterial lesions using the Shape Memory Alloy Recoverable Technology (S.M.A.R.T.®) nitinol self-expanding stent through 3 years of follow-up [STROLL study]	250	Mean age 67.7, Male 62%, DM 47%, HTN 89%	Yes	36 months	PAQ, WIQ, SF-12, EQ-5D	In patients undergoing revascularization for moderately complex SFA disease, use of the self-expanding S.M.A.R.T® stent was associated with a high rate of target vessel patency through 3 years and led to substantial and sustained health status benefits.	Baseline health status was significantly impaired on both generic and disease-specific measures. There was a large early gain in reported health status scores on all scales at 1 month, and these benefits over baseline were sustained out to 36 months follow-up with minimal decrement.	8
Self-expandable bare nitinol stent	2008–2010		39 centres in USA	Rutherford 2/3/4 = 46%/51%/3%			Not stated		Overall, the relative improvements were larger in magnitude from baseline using the disease-specific PAQ and WIQ instruments than for the generic SF-12 and EQ-5D health status instruments.	
SMART	Prospective study						100%			

Stent	Han et al. (2016) [34]	This study investigated the effects of gender on the 3-year outcomes of the StuDy for EvalUating EndovasculaR TreAtments of Lesions in the	287	Patients that were at least 18 years old with stenotic, restenotic, or occluded lesions of the superficial femoral artery (SFA) and proximal popliteal arteries with moderate to severe claudication were included.	Yes	36 months	WIQ	Comparable primary, assisted primary and secondary patency rates in women and men.	Women versus men had inferior walking distance scores at presentation (13.6 vs. 25.7, $p < 0.001$), scores were equalized by 2 years (51.6 vs. 60.8, $p < 0.05$); however, 3-year follow-up demonstrated less durable results for women versus men (37.3 vs. 58.8, $p < 0.05$). In addition, women had worse WIQ scores for pain, walking speed, and stair climbing. However, the relative change in scores between men and women were comparable, with both groups seeing similar improvements from baseline for these parameters.	7
Self-expandable, bare nitinol stent	2007–2010		44 centres in USA	Female (n = 97): 71.3 ± 11.2 years; Rutherford 2/3/4 = 30%/65%/5% Male (n = 190): 65.9 ± 9.9 years;			Not stated	Women continue to see clinical improvement after intervention, achieving comparable ABIs and walking distance to men at 2 years. These benefits are diminished at 3-year follow-up with women achieving lower absolute ABI and WIQ parameters compared with men but improved overall compared with scores at presentation.		
EverFlex	Prospective study	Superficial Femoral Artery and Proximal Popliteal By usIng the Protege EverfLex NitInol STent System II (DURABILITY II) trial.		Rutherford 2/3/4 = 44%/51%/5% Women less likely to have hyperlipidemia (79.4% vs. 89.5%), but otherwise, all demographics and preoperative characteristics were comparable between the two groups. More women (64.9%) presented with severe claudication (Rutherford 3) versus men (51.1%, p = 0.03). Men had lesions with more severe degree of calcification than women.			77%			

(continued)

Table 19.3 (continued)

Type of intervention Device type, Brand name (if applicable)	Author (year of publication), Study period, Study type	Study intent/ associated study	Cohort size, Study centre(s)	Patient characteristics	Preop HRQOL assessment	Follow-up period	HRQOL instrument(s) used, Method of delivery, Completion rate	Key outcomes	Main findings related to HRQOL	Quality score
PTA vs. SEP vs. PTA SEP	Mazari et al. (2012) [35]	To compare percutaneous transluminal angioplasty (PTA), a supervised exercise programme (SEP) and combined treatment (PTA plus SEP) for intermittent claudication due to femoropopliteal arterial disease.	178	Randomised into three groups: PTA only (n = 60), SEP only (n = 60), PTA + SEP (n = 58). All given medical treatment.	Yes	12 months	SF-36, VascuQoL	On intergroup analysis, PTA and SEP alone were equally effective in improving clinical outcomes, although the effect was short-lived. PTA plus SEP produced a more sustained clinical improvement, but there was no significant QoL advantage.	A statistically significant improvement was seen in all clinical indicators (resting and post-exercise ABPI, MWD and PRWD) at all time points, including the final endpoint at 1 year in all three treatment arms except post-exercise ABPI in the SEP group.	9
	2002–2007		Academic Vascular Surgical Unit, University of Hull, Hull, UK	Male 60%, Median age 70			Not stated		PTA only: statistically significant improvements in all SF-36 domains and the VascuQol score, except in the vitality (V) domain of SF-36.	
	Randomised control trial			There were no significant differences in demographics, risk factors or clinical and QoL indicators at baseline among the three treatment groups.			81%			
								For patients with intermittent claudication due to femoropopliteal disease, PTA, SEP, and PTA plus SEP were all equally effective in improving walking distance and QoL after 12 months.	SEP only: statistically significant improvements in VascuQol score and in the PF, role limitation emotional (RE) and mental health (MH) domains.	
									PTA + SEP: statistically significant improvements in the VascuQol scores and SF-36 domains for PF, BP and SF.	
									There were no statistically significant differences between the three treatment arms in any other clinical indicator, ISCVS outcomes or QoL indicators at 12 months.	

PTA vs. BMT	Greenhalgh et al. (2008) [22] 2003–2006 Randomised control trial	Patients with symptoms of stable mild to moderate intermittent claudication (MIMIC) were randomised in two multi-centre trials, for femoropopliteal and aortoiliac arterial disease, to receive either PTA or no PTA against a background of supervised exercise, smoking cessation and best medical therapy and followed up for 24 months.	Femoropopliteal (FP): 93 Aortoiliac (AI): 34 Nine centres in UK	FP (PTA, Control: 48, 45)—differences in mean age, IHD and statin use AI (PTA, Control: 19, 15)—no apparent differences	No	24 months	SF-36 Not stated Femoropopliteal: 86% Aortoiliac: 76%	There were significant improvements in both AWD and ICD in the PTA groups for both trials. The adjusted AWD was 38% greater in the PTA group for the femoropopliteal trial (95%; CI 1–90) (p = 0.04) and 78% greater in the PTA group for the aortoiliac trial (95%; CI 0–216) (p = 0.05).	**FP:** No significant intergroup differences in mean physical and mental scores of SF-36. **AI:** Significant intergroup differences in mean physical scores of SF-36 in favour of PTA group.	9

(continued)

Table 19.3 (continued)

Type of intervention Device type, Brand name (if applicable)	Author (year of publication), Study period, Study type	Study intent/ associated study	Cohort size, Study centre(s)	Patient characteristics	Preop HRQOL assessment	Follow-up period	HRQOL instrument(s) used, Method of delivery, Completion rate	Key outcomes	Main findings related to HRQOL	Quality score
DCB	Micari et al. (2013) [36]	To appraise 2-year outcomes after percutaneous treatment of femoropopliteal artery disease with paclitaxel-eluting balloons (PEB).	105	Consecutive patients with Rutherford class 2–4 disease due to femoropopliteal lesions 15 mm long and with 3- to 7-mm reference vessel diameter.	Yes	12, 24 months	EQ-5D	Primary patency was maintained in 71 (72.4%), and major adverse events had occurred in 17 (17.5%). Secondary patency rate was achieved in 89 cases (84.7%).	**12 months**	6
Paclitaxel-eluting balloon	Not stated		Six centres in Italy	Mean age 68 (SD 9), Male 81%, HTN 86%, DM 49%			Not stated	PEBs are associated with favourable functional and clinical outcomes at 2 years in patients with femoropopliteal artery disease requiring percutaneous revascularization.	Rutherford: A significant shift of patients to Rutherford classes (RC) 0 and 1 is observed at 3, 6, and 12 months post-PEB procedure ($p < 0.001$).	
In.Pact Admiral	Prospective study			Rutherford 1/2/3/4 = 1%/27%/65%/7%			12 months: 88%		EQ-5D: The percentage of patients reporting any problem across the five dimensions of health-related quality of life (QOL) was reduced post-PEB procedure ($p < 0.001$ for baseline vs. 3 months, 6 months, and 12 months).	
				SFA/Popliteal = 89%/11%			24 months: 93%		**24 months**	
									Rutherford: Statistically significant improvement in Rutherford Class (RC) from baseline to post procedure maintained.	
									EQ-5D: Significant improvement for mobility, usual activities, pain/ discomfort ($p < 0.001$)	

DCB	Micari et al. (2017) [12]	To appraise 2-year outcomes after percutaneous transluminal angioplasty of long femoropopliteal artery disease using paclitaxel-coated IN.PACT Admiral balloons (PCBs) [SFA-Long study]	105	Consecutive patients with Rutherford class 2–4 disease due to femoropopliteal lesions >15 cm long.	Yes	12, 24 months	EQ-5D	PCBs benefits on primary patency and target vessel revascularization satisfactorily extend over 24 months in patients undergoing percutaneous transluminal angioplasty for symptomatic femoropopliteal disease.	The proportion of asymptomatic (Rutherford class 0) patients increased from 0% at baseline to 51% at 24 months while being 58% at the 12-month follow-up assessment.	6
Paclitaxel-eluting balloon	2012–2014		Six centres in Italy	Mean age 68 ± 9 years; 81.9% men			Not stated	Primary patency rate of 70.4%, with major adverse events rate of 10%.	EQ-5D: At 12 months, there was significant improvement from baseline as well as in walking impairment at 12 months (p = 0.01). This was sustained until 24-month follow-up.	
In.Pact Admiral	Prospective study			Rutherford 2/3/4 and 5 = 28%/62%/10%			89%			
DCB	Chen et al. (2019) [37]	To confirm the safety and effectiveness of the IN.PACT Admiral drug-coated balloon (DCB) as a treatment for de novo and native artery restenotic lesions in the superficial femoral artery (SFA) and/or proximal popliteal artery in Chinese subjects.	143	Mean age 66.8 ± 7.7 years; 75% men	Yes	12 months	EQ-5D, WIQ	Primary safety outcome 99% at 30 days.	Improvement compared with baseline in all outcome metrics (Rutherford category, ankle-brachial index (ABI), WIQ, EQ-5D)	7
Paclitaxel-eluting balloon	2014–2015		15 centres	HTN (73%), DM (46%)			Not stated	High 1-year primary patency estimated 91%.	All Rutherford Cat 4 patients—>Cat 3	
In.Pact Admiral	Prospective study			Rutherford category 2, 3, 4 = 48%, 39%, 13%			EQ-5D 92%	Low rate of CD = TLR 2.9%.		
							WIQ-walking impairment 92%	Consistent with other IN.PACT DCB trials.		
							WIQ-distance, speed, stair climbing 60%			
DCB	Bague et al. (2017) [38]	To assess 18-month outcomes of the paclitaxel eluting balloon (PEB) in patients with femoropopliteal (FP) in-stent restenosis (ISR).	53 (55 limbs)	48 (87%) claudication, 7 (13%) CLI	Yes	12 and 18 months	EQ-5D	At 1 year, the survival rate was 96 ± 2.7% and freedom from TLR and TER were 90.2 ± 4.2% and 85 ± 5%, respectively. Sustained primary and secondary clinical improvements were 78.6 ± 5.7% and 92.0 ± 3.8%, respectively. At 1 year, the primary patency rate was 83.7 ± 5.0%.	Improvement trend, but not significant.	7
Paclitaxel-eluting balloon	2012–2013		Ten centres in France	Mean age 69 (SD 12)			Not stated		The visual analog scale (VAS) score increased from 65.8 ± 14.1 at baseline to 76.2 ± 16.3 at 12 months (p = 0.10) and 72.3 ± 17.7 at 18 months (p = 0.14).	
In.Pact Admiral	Prospective cohort study			Male 79%			94%		At 12 months and 18 months, 77% and 67% of the patients were asymptomatic (Rutherford 0), respectively.	
				HTN 81%, DM (30%)						
				Ten violated protocol. Three died.						

(continued)

Table 19.3 (continued)

Type of intervention Device type, Brand name (if applicable)	Author (year of publication), Study period, Study type	Study intent/ associated study	Cohort size, Study centre(s)	Patient characteristics	Preop HRQOL assessment	Follow-up period	HRQOL instrument(s) used, Method of delivery, Completion rate	Key outcomes	Main findings related to HRQOL	Quality score
DCB	Scheinert et al. (2016) [39]	To report a subanalysis of the German centres enrolling patients in the prospective, global, multicentre, randomized LEVANT 2 pivotal trial (n = 476) (ClinicalTrials.gov identifier NCT01412541) of the Lutonix drug-coated balloon (DCB) for the treatment of femoropopliteal occlusive disease.	126	Randomised into Lutonix DCB (n = 83), PTA (n = 43)	Yes	12 months	EQ-5D, WIQ	12-month primary patency rate was 80% vs. 58% (p = 0.015) and the composite safety endpoint rate was 94% vs. 72% (p = 0.001), respectively. Freedom from TLR was higher for DCBs (96%) vs. PTA (82%, p = 0.012). Major adverse events were similar for both groups. The benefit favouring DCB over PTA was observed in German men and women.	WIQ change from baseline: DCB 29.2 ± 28.9 (n = 71); PTA 21.6 ± 29.5 (n = 33)	8
Paclitaxel-coated balloon	2011–2012		Eight centres in Germany	Demographic, clinical, and lesion characteristics were matched between Lutonix DCB and PTA groups, as were the final percent diameter stenosis (19%) and procedure success (91%).			Not stated		EQ-5D change from baseline: DCB 0.11 ± 0.21 (n = 70); PTA 0.14 ± 0.18 (n = 34)	
Lutonix	Randomised control trial			Mean age 67.1 ± 9.6 years; 63% men			WIQ 83%		Rutherford category was improved at 12 months for 91.2% of DCB patients compared to 78.8% in the PTA group (p = 0.08). Sustained clinical benefit was observed for 85.3% of DCB-treated patients compared with 58.6% for PTA (p < 0.001).	
				Severe calcification was present in 11% of lesions, and 23% were total occlusions.			EQ-5D 83%			
				SFA 92%, Popliteal 8%						
				Rutherford 2/3/4 = 32%, 65%, 3%						

DCB	Rosenfield et al. (2015) [40]	To assess efficacy and safety of Paclitaxel-coated balloon for the treatment of symptomatic femoropopliteal peripheral artery disease (cf. PTA only).	476	Randomised into 2:1 DCB (n = 316): PTA only (n = 160)	Yes	12 months	SF-36, EQ-5D, WIQ	DCB higher primary patency rate at 12 months (65.2% vs. 52.6%, p = 0.02).	SF-36 change from baseline: Physical component DCB 6.0 ± 11.4, PTA 5.4 ± 10.2; no significant change in Mental component	9
Paclitaxel-coated balloon	2011–2012		54 centres (Europe, USA)	Rutherford 2/3/4 = 31%/61%/8%			Not stated	Free from primary safety events was 83.9% DCB, 79.0% PTA (p = 0.005 for noninferiority).	EQ-5D change from baseline: No significant change in both groups	
Lutonix	Randomised control trial			Both groups well-matched at baseline. 42.9% of the patients had diabetes, and 34.7% were current smokers.			100%	There were no significant between-group differences in functional outcomes or in the rates of death, amputation, thrombosis, or reintervention.	WIQ change from baseline: Improved significantly in both groups across all domains. Walking distance showed significant intergroup difference of 9.3 ± 36.5 (95% CI: 1.6–17.0).	
				Mean age 68.2 ± 9.7, Male 63%					Rutherford: −1.9 ± 1.1 (DCB), −1.7 ± 1.1 (PTA)	

(continued)

Table 19.3 (continued)

Type of intervention: Device type, Brand name (if applicable)	Author (year of publication), Study period, Study type	Study intent/ associated study	Cohort size, Study centre(s)	Patient characteristics	Preop HRQOL assessment	Follow-up period	HRQOL instrument(s) used, Method of delivery, Completion rate	Key outcomes	Main findings related to HRQOL	Quality score
DCB vs. PTA	Laird et al. (2015) [7]	Investigate the longer-term outcomes (beyond 1 year) of a paclitaxel-eluting DCB compared to PTA for symptomatic femoropopliteal lesions (Rutherford 2–4) up to 18 cm in length.	331	Randomly assigned in a 2:1 ratio to treatment with DCB (n = 220) or PTA (n = 111)	Yes	12, 24 months	EQ-5D, WIQ	DCB group showed significantly higher primary patency and lower reintervention rates. DCB had a lower overall mortality rate.	**12 months:** EQ-5D change from baseline: No significant difference between treatment groups but trended in favour of DCB.	7
Paclitaxel-eluting balloon	2010–2017	Part of IN.PACT SFA Trial	Multicentre (Europe, USA)	Groups were well matched at baseline with similar demographics, comorbidities, and lesion characteristics (incl. Rutherford)			Not stated	No device or procedure related deaths and no major amputations in either group during follow-up period. No new vessel thrombosis reported.	WIQ: Both groups showed improvement in Walking distance from baseline.	
In.Pact Admiral	Randomised control trial						24 months		**24 months:** Both groups improved from baseline in all assessments.	
							EQ-5D: 80%		EQ-5D: results trended in favour of DCB group	
							WIQ-walking impairment: 79%		WIQ: favoured DCB across all domains, notably walking distance and stair climbing	
							WIQ-walking distance: 48%		Patients treated with DCB achieved these similar levels of quality-of-life improvement despite 58% fewer reinterventions than with PTA.	
							WIQ-walking speed: 48%		With the exception of patients having ischemic rest pain (Rutherford Category 4), all subgroups showed better results with DCB.	
							WIQ-stair climbing: 48%			

DCB vs. PTA	Krishnan et al. (2017) [41]	Pharmacokinetic and clinical outcomes of two studies (ILLUMENATE Pivotal RCT and PK Prospective studies) in Stellarex DCB treatment of femoropopliteal disease.	300	Obstructive SFA or Popliteal lesions with Rutherford Cat 2–4; DCB n = 200, PTA n = 100	Yes	12 months	WIQ, EQ-5D	The data demonstrate superior safety and effectiveness of the Stellarex DCB in comparison with PTA, and plasma levels of paclitaxel fall to low levels within 1 h.	WIQ: 78% improved from baseline patients in both groups. Mean change 20.1 ± 29.4 (n = 176) DCB; 22.5 ± 28.1 (n = 93) PTA	8
Paclitaxel-coated balloon	2013–2015		41 USA, two Austria	Majority Rutherford Cat 3 in both groups.			Not stated		EQ-5D: Mean change 0.10 (55.9% improved) in DCB; 0.04 (53% improved) in PTA	
Stellarex	Randomised control trial			SFA, Pop = 191, 9 (DCB), 191, 9 (PTA)			WIQ 90%		Rutherford: Mean change—1.9 in both groups	
				Higher percentage of men (DCB: 56.0% versus PTA: 64.0%, p = 0.185), patients with diabetes mellitus (DCB: 49.5% versus PTA: 52.0%, p = 0.683), obesity (DCB: 39.5% versus PTA: 30.0%, p = 0.107)			EQ-5D 61% Rutherford 90%		DCB had 46.9% lower TLR rate.	

(continued)

Table 19.3 (continued)

Type of intervention Device type, Brand name (if applicable)	Author (year of publication), Study period, Study type	Study intent/ associated study	Cohort size, Study centre(s)	Patient characteristics	Preop HRQOL assessment	Follow-up period	HRQOL instrument(s) used, Method of delivery, Completion rate	Key outcomes	Main findings related to HRQOL	Quality score
DCB vs. PTA	Steiner et al. (2018) [42]	To evaluate the performance of the Ranger paclitaxel-coated balloon versus uncoated balloon angioplasty for femoropopliteal lesions at 12 months.	105	Patients with symptomatic lower limb ischemia (Rutherford category 2–4) and stenotic lesions in the nonstented femoropopliteal segment.	Yes	12 months	EQ-5D-3L, SF-12V2, WIQ	The DCB group had a greater primary patency rate at 12 months (Kaplan-Meier estimate 86.4% vs. 56.5%), with a significantly longer time to patency failure (log-rank p < 0.001). The estimated freedom from target lesion revascularization rate was 91.2% in the DCB group and 69.9% in the control group at 12 months, with a significantly longer time to reintervention (p = 0.010). No target limb amputations or device-related deaths occurred in either group.	Rutherford: Significant improvement in distribution across Rutherford categories was observed in both the DCB and control groups (Kruskal-Wallis rank sum test p < 0.001 for each group), but the difference between the groups was not statistically significant (p = 0.638).	7
Paclitaxel-coated balloon	2014–2016		Ten centres (Europe)	DCB (n = 71): Mean age 68 ± 8 years, Male 75%, DM 39%, HTN 82%; Proximal/Mid/Distal SFA = 17%/44%/36%			In-office visit		WIQ: Mean total WIQ scores increased from 38 ± 22 at baseline to 66 ± 26 at 6 months and were sustained at 64 ± 28 at 12 months in the DCB group, with a similar increase observed in the control group. The WIQ total scores and parameters of distance, speed, and stair climbing did not differ significantly between the DCB and control groups at any time point.	
Ranger	Randomised control trial			TASC II A/B = 66%/27%			83%		No significant differences in health-related quality of life scores (EQ-5D-3L, SF12v2) were observed between the DCB and control groups.	
				Control (n = 34): Mean age 67 ± 9 years, Male 68%, DM 35%, HTN 76%;						
				Proximal/Mid/Distal SFA = 6%/37%/53%						
				TASC II A/B = 69%/22%						

DCB vs. PTA	Iida et al. (2018) [43]	To assess the safety and effectiveness of the MDT-2113 (IN.PACT Admiral) drug-coated balloon (DCB) for the treatment of de novo and native artery restenotic lesions in the superficial femoral and proximal popliteal arteries vs. percutaneous transluminal angioplasty (PTA) with an uncoated balloon in a Japanese cohort.	100	Randomized (2:1) 100 patients (mean age 73.6 ± 7.0 years; 76 men) to treatment with DCB (n = 68) or PTA (n = 32). Baseline characteristics were similar between the groups, including mean lesion length (9.15 ± 5.85 cm and 8.89 ± 6.01 cm for the DCB and PTA groups, respectively).	Yes	12 months	EQ-5D, WIQ	Results from the MDT-2113 SFA Japan trial showed superior treatment effect for DCB vs. PTA, with excellent patency and low CD-TLR rates. These results are consistent with other IN.PACT SFA DCB trials and demonstrate the safety and effectiveness of this DCB for the treatment of femoropopliteal lesions in this Japanese cohort.	Both treatment groups showed similar improvement from baseline in all functional outcomes assessed, but with no significant intergroup differences.	8
Paclitaxel-eluting balloon	2013–2018		11 centres in Japan				Not stated		EQ-5D: mean change from baseline to 12 months was 0.081 ± 0.149 for DCB vs. 0.095 ± 0.157 for PTA (p = 0.705).	
In.Pact Admiral	Randomised control trial			DCB: Rutherford 2/3/4 = 54%/41%/4%			96%		WIQ: both groups showed similar improvement in walking distance (23.7 ± 37.8 m DCB vs. 8.8 ± 29.8 m PTA; p = 0.156).	
				PTA: Rutherford 2/3/4 = 59%/38%/3%					Despite improvement in functional outcomes in both groups, patients treated with DCB required 77% fewer reinterventions than their PTA-treated counterparts.	

was found in patients who developed lesion restenosis [26].

A prospective cohort study investigating long-term outcomes (up to 10 years) following use of two bypass graft materials (PTFE and Dacron) demonstrated that HRQOL outcomes were not directly correlated to bypass patency in the long term [25]. Higher WIQ scores were observed in the Dacron group but no differences were found in the other HRQOL measures.

A RCT which compared femoropopliteal surgical bypass to primary stenting using a Heparin-bonded covered self-expanding stent demonstrated significantly better HRQOL measures in the endovascular group at early follow-up (1 month) [27]. At 12 months, there was an overall significant improvement in HRQOL measures from baseline in both groups. No significant difference in overall HRQOL measures at 12 months was observed between the two groups; subgroup analysis did demonstrate comparatively better outcomes in the endovascular group for the given HRQOL questionnaire items (Table 19.3).

Two prospective cohort studies which investigated the use of endovascular atherectomy were identified: one using directional atherectomy in the popliteal segment and another using optical coherence tomography (OCT)-guided atherectomy in the femoral and popliteal segments [23, 24]. Both studies demonstrated improved HRQOL outcomes post intervention when compared to baseline.

Quality of Included Studies

The methodological quality of the studies in terms of QOL assessment ranged from 5 to 10 (median = 8) according to the scoring system [6]. Eighteen papers scored 8 or above.

Timing and Completion of Follow-Up

The response rate ranged from 36% to 100%. QOL was a primary outcome measure in six studies and secondary outcome measure in 28 studies. Follow-up period ranged from 6 months to 11 years. Twenty-nine studies had a follow-up period of 2 years or less.

The methods of HRQOL questionnaire administration were as follows: office visit in one study, telephone interview in one study, self-administered in five studies (of which two papers stated the availability of optional help from a research assistant) and unstated in 27 studies.

Discussion

This systematic review provides a current evidence base on HRQOL outcomes following invasive intervention for aortoiliac and femoropopliteal steno-occlusive disease. The range of interventions include PTA, use of DCB, stenting, atherectomy and bypass surgery.

The follow-up period in the majority of studies is short (2 years or less). In general, all interventions, whether endovascular or surgical, in both the aortoiliac and femoropopliteal segment disease resulted in improved HRQOL outcomes in the short term. None of the studies in this review compared the HRQOL outcomes at medium or long-term follow-up to baseline measures.

A study by van Hattum et al. which is not included in this review (as it included patients with crural and pedal bypass surgery) demonstrated a deterioration in HRQOL, particularly in physical parameters, following peripheral bypass surgery in the long term regardless of bypass patency [45]. The HRQOL further worsens in patients who have had a subsequent adverse vascular event. This reflects the fact that PAD is only one manifestation of the more general atherosclerosis disease spectrum and with time these patients' general health and resultant HRQOL is likely to decline. It also stresses the importance of secondary prevention as well as lifestyle and health optimisation. From the perspective of conducting longer term HRQOL research, this study also highlights an issue with measuring HRQOL in PAD patients in that general deterioration is likely to be expected in the long term, particularly in those with multiple risk factors. As such, we feel this should be factored in when measuring effectiveness of an intervention in those with PAD.

There were nine studies which investigated HRQOL outcomes following the use of DCB for SFA disease, all of which demonstrated improved HRQOL outcomes post intervention [8, 12, 36–42]. Five of these were RCTs comparing PTA to various Paclitaxel DCB devices, each with slightly different properties in terms of drug dose and delivery. Only one of these demonstrated a significant difference in an HRQOL outcome (one item in the WIQ) between the two interventions; the rest did not demonstrate any significant difference in HRQOL outcomes. There were, however, significantly higher primary patency and lower reintervention rates in the DCB group in comparison to PTA. The authors in some of these papers posited DCB to be the superior intervention tool compared to PTA, as it achieves the same HRQOL outcomes whilst requiring fewer interventions. However, of concern, a recent and controversial meta-analysis by Katsanos et al. demonstrated an increased risk of mortality amongst patients with intermittent claudication or rest pain treated with Paclitaxel DCBs when compared to PTA [46]. Whilst there is ongoing debate as to whether this observed increased mortality is directly caused by Paclitaxel administration, it does raise serious questions of whether DCBs should be used in such patients, given that there has been no reported significant HRQOL benefit over PTA.

On review of other studies which compared different treatment modalities, they suggest that the improvement seen in terms of patency outcomes does not uniformly translate to HRQOL outcomes. For example, a large multicentre RCT by Laird et al. which compared primary stenting to PTA for SFA disease showed significantly improved freedom from CD-TLR rates, though the HRQOL outcomes are variable. In this study, the stent group had significantly better WIQ scores, however, no significant differences were observed in all other the HRQOL measures evaluated [44]. When comparing invasive revascularisation of a stenosed or occluded vessel over non-invasive approaches, the evidence is also unclear as to which leads to better HRQOL outcomes. One multicentre RCT which compared iliac stenting to SET demonstrated no significant difference in the HRQOL outcomes [14]. Two RCTs by Greenhalgh et al. and Marazi et al. which compared SET to PTA for femoropopliteal disease did not demonstrate any difference in HRQOL outcomes [22, 35]. Interestingly, the study by Greenhalgh also compared iliac PTA to SET which did demonstrate significantly better HRQOL outcomes in the PTA group, though the SET group did still demonstrate significant improvement from baseline. The latter does raise the need to consider what degree of HRQOL improvement one should aim for when deciding on treatment options. For example, a patient may prefer a less invasive treatment to an invasive treatment if it sufficiently improves their HRQOL without the risk of surgical complications. Some studies have been conducted to determine the minimally clinically important difference (MCID) for the VascuQol in PAD patients [47, 48]. Conjin et al. found that an improvement in overall VascuQol score by between 1.19 and 1.66 is clinically relevant to patients. However, to the best of our knowledge, no such studies have been conducted for the other HRQOL tools in this review in relation to PAD. Future studies are required to determine the MCID for any existing or indeed any future tools used to measure HRQOL in PAD. This will allow for a more meaningful interpretation of HRQOL outcomes following PAD intervention.

An interesting finding within this review is that in some of the comparative studies (e.g. stent versus PTA), even if a significant difference in conventional outcomes measures (e.g. patency rate) is seen, there is often no significant difference seen in HRQOL outcomes. No justification for this observation is posited by the studies reviewed, however, there are some possible explanations. First, by taking the study results at face value, it may simply be that clinically the comparative, improved patency rates alone (such as for DCB over PTA) may not directly translate to increased HRQOL outcomes. Second, it is possible that the studies are insufficiently powered to detect a difference in HRQOL between the different interventions. As stated earlier, in most studies, HRQOL was a secondary outcome measure and studies may have only been sufficiently powered to the primary outcome measures (i.e. patency rates). Third, it may be that there are inherent issues with the psychometric properties of the HRQOL tools, resulting in them being insufficiently sensitive or accurate in detecting differences in patient outcomes. As an example, a study evaluating the VascuQoL-6 questionnaire demonstrated poor test-retest reliability (<70%) [49]. A recent in-depth study evaluating VascuQol demonstrated a number of significant flaws including nine 'weak' questionnaire items. On interviewing patients and clinicians, a number of items identified were considered irrelevant to the majority of patients such as Item 2: "*I have been worried that I might injure my leg*"; others were only relevant to a subgroup of PAD patients with CLTI such as Item 17: "*Ulcers or sores on my leg (or foot) have caused me pain or distress*". These findings suggest the need for more robust HRQOL measures which take in to account the symptoms of different types of PAD patients, i.e. claudicants who primarily suffer from limited walking distance and CLTI patients who may have rest pain and tissue loss.

Interestingly, there remains a difference in opinion as to the best tools to measure HRQOL in PAD. Vries et al. compared the disease specific VascuQol to the generic HRQOL questionnaires (SF-36 and EuroQol-5D) and demonstrated that VascuQoL was better at discriminating a large versus a small change in disease severity [50]. Another study by Petersohn et al. of generic HRQOL questionnaires suggested that EQ-5D may be superior to SF-36 and VAS [5]. A recent systematic review by Poku et al. which looked at the properties of seven disease specific and six generic HRQOL tools, did not demonstrate the superiority of one over the other [51]. Whilst a recent consensus paper strongly recommended the inclusion of HRQOL outcomes within a trial design, no expert statement has been published to date which either addresses the issues with the current methods of measuring HRQOL or how best to incorporate them into studies [52]. Given this, further research on how best to measure HRQOL outcomes both for research and clinical practice would seem prudent.

Although the increasing inclusion of HRQOL outcomes in PAD studies is encouraging, a number of issues should first be addressed. As stated, for most of the studies in this review, HRQOL outcomes were included as a secondary outcome measure. As such, these are likely to be insufficiently powered and therefore making interpretation of the results in such instances challenging. The approach to measuring HRQOL outcomes was also highly variable. Most studies did not describe the method of administering the HRQOL questionnaires, e.g. whether it was performed in clinic, via post, and with or without assistance from the research team. However, the method of administration could have an effect on both the validity and reliability of the questionnaire. The rationale for why specific HRQOL questionnaires were used was also not always evident. Many studies used a combination of HRQOL questionnaires. However, when many of these questionnaires were originally designed, they were tested for their psychometric properties as standalone tools. Administering multiple questionnaires in combination may potentially result in unintentional bias. For example, a question in Tool A may inadvertently influence a patient's response to a question in Tool B. Combining questionnaires may also have the inadvertent effect of causing response fatigue due to the increased length of time spent by the respondents [53]. These are some issues that warrant more consideration in future HRQOL studies in PAD. In particular, we argue for the need for a standardised approach to HRQOL assessment in order to improve the quality, consistency and comparability of future studies.

In addition to the issues with measuring HRQOL outcomes in PAD intervention, this review also highlighted some areas relating to the interventions and surgical procedures that require future research. For example, there is no study at present comparing techniques such as covered endovascular repair of aortic bifurcation (CERAB) to conventional aortoiliac bypass. There is also a relative paucity of studies evaluating HRQOL outcomes of surgical bypass compared to the number of endovascular studies.

The reasons for poor HRQOL outcomes following endovascular intervention or surgery remain poorly understood, but are likely complex and multifactorial. Procedure-related outcomes of interventions including failed revascularisation and lesion recurrence may contribute to poor HRQOL outcomes [54, 55]. However, as mentioned, the relationship between primary patency and HRQOL has not been definitively demonstrated. Equally, whilst there is some suggestion that avoidance of major limb amputation by means of revascularisation may lead to improved HRQOL, other studies have demonstrated that HRQOL can significantly improve after amputation because of an elimination of pain, as well as CLTI induced complications such as ulceration and infection [56, 57]. HRQOL outcomes following amputation were also found to be dependent on several patient factors, including family support and age. Patient factors may also contribute to poorer HRQOL outcomes following revascularisation interventions; type D personality (i.e. tendency towards negative affectivity) and baseline frailty have both been demonstrated to be associated with worse HRQOL outcomes [58, 59]. Socioeconomic deprivation has been shown to negatively impact clinical outcomes and may also play a role in HRQOL [60]. Further research to better understand patient-related predictors of poor HRQOL outcomes is necessary to guide appropriate patient selection. An overview of possible predictors of poor HRQOL outcomes following intervention is presented in Fig. 19.2.

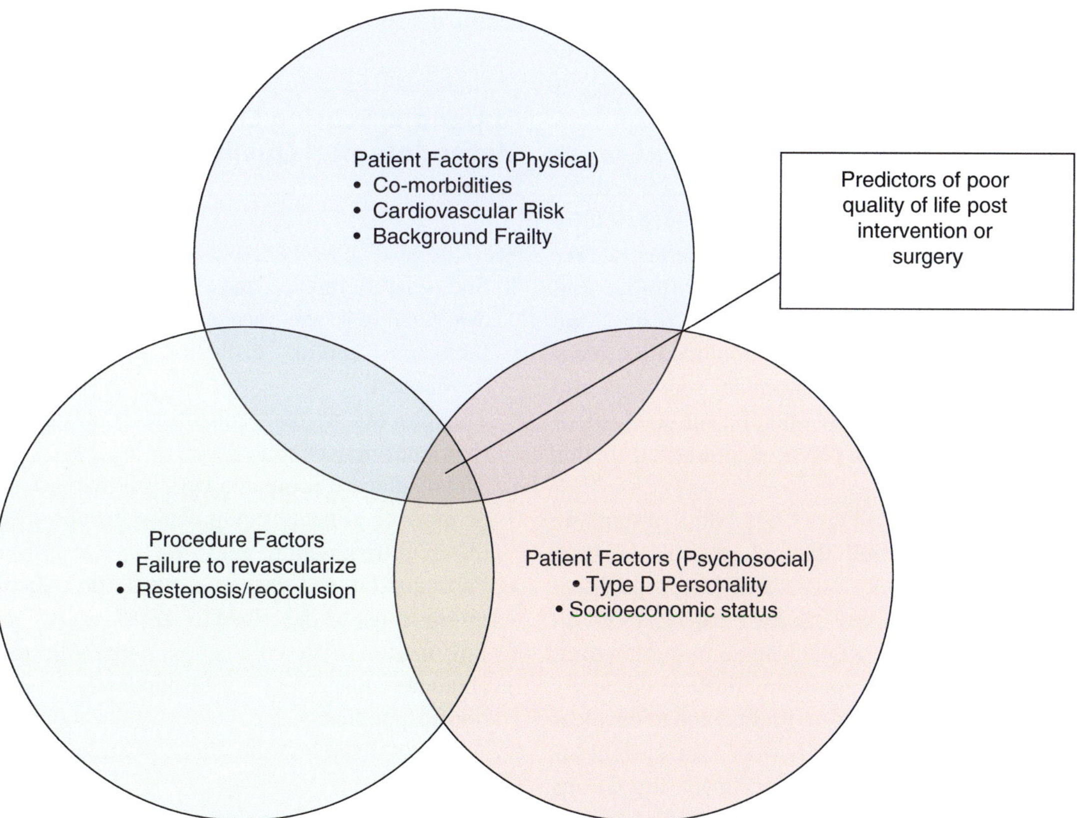

Fig. 19.2 Possible predictors of poor HRQOL outcomes following surgery and intervention for peripheral vascular disease

Fig. 19.3 Highlighted conclusions

Highlighted Conclusions

- There is increasing recognition for the need to assess HRQOL outcomes following invasive interventions for peripheral arterial disease.
- In general, invasive interventions for aortoiliac and femoropopliteal steno-occlusive artery disease can lead to an improvement in HRQOL outcome
- Due to issues with research methodology, the inferences that can be drawn from current research in HRQOL outcomes are limited.
- The approach to measuring HRQOL outcomes in existing studies is inconsistent and highly variable.
- Further research is required to determine how best to measure HRQOL outcomes both for research and clinical practice

Recent developments and trends in conducting "big data" research by mining data collected through routine clinical care may hold great potential for HRQOL research in PAD intervention. Such an approach would provide a large volume of data from real-world practice and may overcome some of the limitations observed in existing RCTs and cohort studies previously mentioned. To facilitate this big data research, it is important for vascular clinicians to adopt evaluation and standardised documentation of HRQOL measures into routine clinical practice.

In this systematic review, we purposefully identified studies which where specific to predefined anatomical segments, i.e. aortoiliac and femoropopliteal. However, as a result, we excluded many studies which included interventions across different anatomical segments and did not provide segment specific sub-analysis of the results; this is a potential limitation to this review.

In conclusion (Fig. 19.3), this systematic review demonstrated that in general, invasive interventions for aortoiliac and femoropopliteal steno-occlusive artery disease can lead to an improvement in HRQOL outcomes. However, the possibility to ascertain further clinically meaningful inferences are limited due to the clear methodological constraints within the current literature. Perhaps the most pertinent limitations are that HRQOL are often secondary outcome measures and therefore likely to lack statistical power; the highly variable selection and use of HRQOL tools also make it impossible to compare outcomes of different studies. To overcome these limitations, adequately powered studies, along with a standardised approach to measuring HRQOL outcomes, is required to improve the quality of future research and allow more patient-centric decision making.

Appendix: Scoring Criteria to Assess Methodological Quality of Included Papers

- Socio-demographic and medical data are described (e.g. age, race, etc.)
- Inclusion and/or exclusion criteria are formulated
- The process of data collection is described (e.g. interview or self-report)
- The results are compared between two groups or more (e.g. healthy population groups with different treatment or age)
- Participation and response rates for patient groups must be described as >75%
- Information is presented about patient/disease characteristics of respondents and non-respondents
- A standardized or valid QOL questionnaire is used
- Results are not only described for QOL but also for the physical, psychological and social domains

- Mean, median, standard deviations or percentages are reported for the most important outcome measures
- Patients signed an informed consent form before study participation

1 point is awarded for each criterion met. Maximum achieveable score = 10.

References

1. Donker J, de Vries J, Ho G, et al. Review: quality of life in lower limb peripheral vascular surgery. Vascular. 2016;24(1):88–95. https://doi.org/10.1177/1708538115578961.
2. Abaraogu UO, Ezenwankwo EF, Dall PM, Seenan CA. Living a burdensome and demanding life: a qualitative systematic review of the patients experiences of peripheral arterial disease. PLoS One. 2018;13(11):e0207456. https://doi.org/10.1371/journal.pone.0207456.
3. Peters CML, de Vries J, Lodder P, et al. Quality of life and not health status improves after major amputation in the elderly critical limb ischaemia patient. Eur J Vasc Endovasc Surg. 2019;57(4):547–53. https://doi.org/10.1016/j.ejvs.2018.10.024.
4. Bosma J, Vahl A, Wisselink W. Systematic review on health-related quality of life after revascularization and primary amputation in patients with critical limb ischemia. Ann Vasc Surg. 2013;27(8):1105–14. https://doi.org/10.1016/j.avsg.2013.01.010.
5. Petersohn S, Ramaekers BLT, Olie RH, et al. Comparison of three generic quality-of-life metrics in peripheral arterial disease patients undergoing conservative and invasive treatments. Qual Life Res. 2019;28(8):2257–79. https://doi.org/10.1007/s11136-019-02166-0.
6. Mols F, Vingerhoets AJJM, Coebergh JW, van de Poll-Franse LV. Quality of life among long-term breast cancer survivors: a systematic review. Eur J Cancer. 2005;41(17):2613–9. https://doi.org/10.1016/j.ejca.2005.05.017.
7. Laird JR, Schneider PA, Tepe G, et al. Durability of treatment effect using a drug-coated balloon for femoropopliteal lesions: 24-month results of IN.PACT SFA. J Am Coll Cardiol. 2015;66(21):2329–38. https://doi.org/10.1016/j.jacc.2015.09.063.
8. Tepe G, Laird J, Schneider P, et al. Drug-coated balloon versus standard percutaneous transluminal angioplasty for the treatment of superficial femoral and popliteal peripheral artery disease: 12-month results from the IN.PACT SFA randomized trial. Circulation. 2015;131(5):495–502. https://doi.org/10.1161/CIRCULATIONAHA.114.011004.
9. Lindgren HIV, Qvarfordt P, Bergman S, Gottsäter A. Swedish Endovascular Claudication Stenting Trialists. Primary stenting of the superficial femoral artery in patients with intermittent claudication has durable effects on health-related quality of life at 24 months: results of a randomized controlled trial. Cardiovasc Interv Radiol. 2018;41(6):872–81. https://doi.org/10.1007/s00270-018-1925-0.
10. Lindgren HI, Pärsson H, Gottsäter A, Bergman S. Patients with intermittent claudication and chronic widespread pain improves in health-related quality of life after invasive but not after noninvasive treatment. Clin Med Insights Cardiol. 2017;11:1179546817747528. https://doi.org/10.1177/1179546817747528.
11. Micari A, Vadalà G, Castriota F, et al. 1-Year results of paclitaxel-coated balloons for long femoropopliteal artery disease: evidence from the SFA-long study. JACC Cardiovasc Interv. 2016;9(9):950–6. https://doi.org/10.1016/j.jcin.2016.02.014.
12. Micari A, Nerla R, Vadalà G, et al. 2-Year results of paclitaxel-coated balloons for long femoropopliteal artery disease: evidence from the SFA-long study. JACC Cardiovasc Interv. 2017;10(7):728–34. https://doi.org/10.1016/j.jcin.2017.01.028.
13. Murphy TP, Cutlip DE, Regensteiner JG, et al. Supervised exercise versus primary stenting for claudication resulting from aortoiliac peripheral artery disease: six-month outcomes from the claudication: exercise versus endoluminal revascularization (CLEVER) study. Circulation. 2012;125(1):130–9. https://doi.org/10.1161/CIRCULATIONAHA.111.075770.
14. Murphy TP, Cutlip DE, Regensteiner JG, et al. Supervised exercise, stent revascularization, or medical therapy for claudication due to aortoiliac peripheral artery disease: the CLEVER study. J Am Coll Cardiol. 2015;65(10):999–1009. https://doi.org/10.1016/j.jacc.2014.12.043.
15. Kazmi SS, Krog AH, Berge ST, Sundhagen JO, Sahba M, Falk RS. Patient-perceived health-related quality of life before and after laparoscopic aortobifemoral bypass. Vasc Health Risk Manag. 2017;13:169–76. https://doi.org/10.2147/VHRM.S134669.
16. Yasutaka Y, Mitsuyoshi T, Yoshiaki S, et al. One-year outcomes of endovascular therapy for aortoiliac lesions. Circ Cardiovasc Interv. 2019;12(1):e007441. https://doi.org/10.1161/CIRCINTERVENTIONS.118.007441.
17. Burket MW, Brodmann M, Metzger C, Tan K, Jaff MR. Twelve-month results of the nitinol Astron stent in iliac artery lesions. J Vasc Interv Radiol. 2016;27(11):1650–1656.e1. https://doi.org/10.1016/j.jvir.2016.06.008.
18. Murphy TP, Soares GM, Kim HM, Ahn SH, Haas RA. Quality of life and exercise performance after aortoiliac stent placement for claudication. J Vasc

Interv Radiol. 2005;16(7):947–53; quiz 954. https://doi.org/10.1097/01.RVI.0000161140.33944.ED.

19. Laird JR, Zeller T, Holden A, et al. Balloon-expandable vascular covered stent in the treatment of iliac artery occlusive disease: 9-month results from the BOLSTER multicenter study. J Vasc Interv Radiol. 2019;30(6):836–844.e1. https://doi.org/10.1016/j.jvir.2018.12.031.
20. Bosch JL, van der Graaf Y, Hunink GM. Health-related quality of life after angioplasty and stent placement in patients with iliac artery occlusive disease. Circulation. 1999;99(24):3155–60. https://doi.org/10.1161/01.CIR.99.24.3155.
21. Rocha-Neves J, Ferreira A, Sousa J, et al. Endovascular approach versus aortobifemoral bypass grafting: outcomes in extensive aortoiliac occlusive disease. Vasc Endovasc Surg. 2020;54(2):102–10. https://doi.org/10.1177/1538574419888815.
22. Greenhalgh RM, Belch JJF, Brown LC, et al. The adjuvant benefit of angioplasty in patients with mild to moderate intermittent claudication (MIMIC) managed by supervised exercise, smoking cessation advice and best medical therapy: results from two randomised trials for stenotic femoropopliteal and aortoiliac arterial disease. Eur J Vasc Endovasc Surg. 2008;36(6):680–8. https://doi.org/10.1016/j.ejvs.2008.10.007.
23. Rastan A, McKinsey JF, Garcia LA, et al. One-year outcomes following directional atherectomy of popliteal artery lesions: subgroup analysis of the prospective, multicenter DEFINITIVE LE trial. J Endovasc Ther. 2018;25(1):100–8. https://doi.org/10.1177/1526602817740133.
24. Schwindt AG, Bennett JG, Crowder WH, et al. Lower extremity revascularization using optical coherence tomography-guided directional atherectomy: final results of the EValuatIon of the PantheriS OptIcal COherence Tomography ImagiNg Atherectomy System for Use in the Peripheral Vasculature (VISION) Study. J Endovasc Ther. 2017;24(3):355–66. https://doi.org/10.1177/1526602817701720.
25. Bosma J, Turkçan K, Assink J, Wisselink W, Vahl AC. Long-term quality of life and mobility after prosthetic above-the-knee bypass surgery. Ann Vasc Surg. 2012;26(2):225–32. https://doi.org/10.1016/j.avsg.2011.05.029.
26. Chalmers N, Walker PT, Belli AM, et al. Randomized trial of the SMART stent versus balloon angioplasty in long superficial femoral artery lesions: the SUPER study. Cardiovasc Interv Radiol. 2013;36(2):353–61. https://doi.org/10.1007/s00270-012-0492-z.
27. Reijnen MMPJ, van Walraven LA, Fritschy WM, et al. 1-Year results of a multicenter randomized controlled trial comparing heparin-bonded endoluminal to femoropopliteal bypass. JACC Cardiovasc Interv. 2017;10(22):2320–31. https://doi.org/10.1016/j.jcin.2017.09.013.
28. Geraghty PJ, Mewissen MW, Jaff MR, Ansel GM, VIBRANT Investigators. Three-year results of the VIBRANT trial of VIABAHN endoprosthesis versus bare nitinol stent implantation for complex superficial femoral artery occlusive disease. J Vasc Surg. 2013;58(2):386–395.e4. https://doi.org/10.1016/j.jvs.2013.01.050.
29. Laird JR, Zeller T, Loewe C, et al. Novel nitinol stent for lesions up to 24 cm in the superficial femoral and proximal popliteal arteries: 24-month results from the TIGRIS randomized trial. J Endovasc Ther. 2018;25(1):68–78. https://doi.org/10.1177/1526602817749242.
30. Dippel E, Shammas N, Takes V, Coyne L, Lemke J. Twelve-month results of percutaneous endovascular reconstruction for chronically occluded superficial femoral arteries: a quality-of-life assessment. J Invasive Cardiol. 2006;18(7):316–21.
31. Ohki T, Kichikawa K, Yokoi H, et al. Outcomes of the Japanese multicenter Viabahn trial of endovascular stent grafting for superficial femoral artery lesions. J Vasc Surg. 2017;66(1):130–142.e1. https://doi.org/10.1016/j.jvs.2017.01.065.
32. Garcia L, Jaff MR, Metzger C, et al. Wire-interwoven nitinol stent outcome in the superficial femoral and proximal popliteal arteries: twelve-month results of the SUPERB trial. Circ Cardiovasc Interv. 2015;8(5):e000937. https://doi.org/10.1161/CIRCINTERVENTIONS.113.000937.
33. Bunte MC, Cohen DJ, Jaff MR, et al. Long-term clinical and quality of life outcomes after stenting of femoropopliteal artery stenosis: 3-year results from the STROLL study. Catheter Cardiovasc Interv. 2018;92(1):106–14. https://doi.org/10.1002/ccd.27569.
34. Han DK, Faries PL, Chung C, et al. Intermediate outcomes of femoropopliteal stenting in women: 3-year results of the DURABILITY II trial. Ann Vasc Surg. 2016;30:110–7. https://doi.org/10.1016/j.avsg.2015.10.005.
35. Mazari FAK, Khan JA, Carradice D, et al. Randomized clinical trial of percutaneous transluminal angioplasty, supervised exercise and combined treatment for intermittent claudication due to femoropopliteal arterial disease. Br J Surg. 2012;99(1):39–48. https://doi.org/10.1002/bjs.7710.
36. Micari A, Cioppa A, Vadalà G, et al. 2-year results of paclitaxel-eluting balloons for femoropopliteal artery disease: evidence from a multicenter registry. JACC Cardiovasc Interv. 2013;6(3):282–9. https://doi.org/10.1016/j.jcin.2013.01.128.
37. Chen Z, Guo W, Jiang W, et al. IN.PACT SFA clinical study using the IN.PACT admiral drug-coated balloon in a Chinese patient population. J Endovasc Ther. 2019;26(4):471–8. https://doi.org/10.1177/1526602819852084.
38. Bague N, Julia P, Sauguet A, et al. Femoropopliteal in-stent restenosis repair: midterm outcomes after paclitaxel eluting balloon use (PLAISIR trial). Eur J Vasc Endovasc Surg. 2017;53(1):106–13. https://doi.org/10.1016/j.ejvs.2016.10.002.

39. Scheinert D, Schmidt A, Zeller T, et al. German center subanalysis of the LEVANT 2 global randomized study of the Lutonix drug-coated balloon in the treatment of femoropopliteal occlusive disease. J Endovasc Ther. 2016;23(3):409–16. https://doi.org/10.1177/1526602816644592.
40. Rosenfield K, Jaff MR, White CJ, et al. Trial of a paclitaxel-coated balloon for femoropopliteal artery disease. N Engl J Med. 2015;373(2):145–53. https://doi.org/10.1056/NEJMoa1406235.
41. Krishnan P, Faries P, Niazi K, et al. Stellarex drug-coated balloon for treatment of femoropopliteal disease: twelve-month outcomes from the randomized ILLUMENATE pivotal and pharmacokinetic studies. Circulation. 2017;136(12):1102–13. https://doi.org/10.1161/CIRCULATIONAHA.117.028893.
42. Steiner S, Willfort-Ehringer A, Sievert H, et al. 12-Month results from the first-in-human randomized study of the ranger paclitaxel-coated balloon for femoropopliteal treatment. JACC Cardiovasc Interv. 2018;11(10):934–41. https://doi.org/10.1016/j.jcin.2018.01.276.
43. Iida O, Soga Y, Urasawa K, et al. Drug-coated balloon vs standard percutaneous transluminal angioplasty for the treatment of atherosclerotic lesions in the superficial femoral and proximal popliteal arteries: one-year results of the MDT-2113 SFA Japan randomized trial. J Endovasc Ther. 2018;25(1):109–17. https://doi.org/10.1177/1526602817745565.
44. Laird JR, Katzen BT, Scheinert D, et al. RESILIENT Investigators. Nitinol stent implantation versus balloon angioplasty for lesions in the superficial femoral artery and proximal popliteal artery: twelve-month results from the RESILIENT randomized trial. Circ Cardiovasc Interv. 2010;3(3):267–76. https://doi.org/10.1161/CIRCINTERVENTIONS.109.903468. Epub 2010 May 18. PMID: 20484101.
45. van Hattum ES, Tangelder MJD, Lawson JA, Moll FL, Algra A. The quality of life in patients after peripheral bypass surgery deteriorates at long-term follow-up. J Vasc Surg. 2011;53(3):643–50. https://doi.org/10.1016/j.jvs.2010.09.021.
46. Konstantinos K, Stavros S, Panagiotis K, Miltiadis K, Dimitrios K. Risk of death following application of paclitaxel-coated balloons and stents in the femoropopliteal artery of the leg: a systematic review and meta-analysis of randomized controlled trials. J Am Heart Assoc. 2018;7(24):e011245. https://doi.org/10.1161/JAHA.118.011245.
47. Conijn AP, Bipat S, Reekers JA, Koelemay MJW. Determining the minimally important difference for the VascuQol Sumscore and its domains in patients with intermittent claudication. Eur J Vasc Endovasc Surg. 2016;51(4):550–6. https://doi.org/10.1016/j.ejvs.2015.12.012.
48. Nordanstig J, Pettersson M, Morgan M, Falkenberg M, Kumlien C. Assessment of minimum important difference and substantial clinical benefit with the vascular quality of life questionnaire-6 when evaluating revascularisation procedures in peripheral arterial disease. Eur J Vasc Endovasc Surg. 2017;54(3):340–7. https://doi.org/10.1016/j.ejvs.2017.06.022.
49. Kumlien C, Nordanstig J, Lundström M, Pettersson M. Validity and test retest reliability of the vascular quality of life Questionnaire-6: a short form of a disease-specific health-related quality of life instrument for patients with peripheral arterial disease. Health Qual Life Outcomes. 2017;15(1):187. https://doi.org/10.1186/s12955-017-0762-1.
50. de Vries M, Ouwendijk R, Kessels AG, et al. Comparison of generic and disease-specific questionnaires for the assessment of quality of life in patients with peripheral arterial disease. J Vasc Surg. 2005;41(2):261–8. https://doi.org/10.1016/j.jvs.2004.11.022.
51. Poku E, Duncan R, Keetharuth A, et al. Patient-reported outcome measures in patients with peripheral arterial disease: a systematic review of psychometric properties. Health Qual Life Outcomes. 2016;14:161. https://doi.org/10.1186/s12955-016-0563-y.
52. Conte MS, Bradbury AW, Kolh P, et al. Global vascular guidelines on the management of chronic limb-threatening ischemia. J Vasc Surg. 2019;69(6S):3S–125S.e40. https://doi.org/10.1016/j.jvs.2019.02.016.
53. Rolstad S, Adler J, Rydén A. Response burden and questionnaire length: is shorter better? a review and meta-analysis. Value Health. 2011;14(8):1101–8. https://doi.org/10.1016/j.jval.2011.06.003.
54. Klevsgård R, Risberg BO, Thomsen MB, Hallberg IR. A 1-year follow-up quality of life study after hemodynamically successful or unsuccessful surgical revascularization of lower limb ischemia. J Vasc Surg. 2001;33(1):114–22. https://doi.org/10.1067/mva.2001.109769.
55. Sabeti S, Czerwenka-Wenkstetten A, Dick P, et al. Quality of life after balloon angioplasty versus stent implantation in the superficial femoral artery: findings from a randomized controlled trial. J Endovasc Ther. 2007;14(4):431–7. https://doi.org/10.1177/152660280701400401.
56. Dua A, Rothenberg KA, Lee JJ, Gologorsky R, Desai SS. Six-month freedom from amputation rates and quality of life following tibial and pedal endovascular revascularization for critical limb ischemia. Vasc Endovasc Surg. 2019;53(3):212–5. https://doi.org/10.1177/1538574418823378.
57. Silva JC, Oliveira VC, Lima P, Correia M, Moreira M, Anacleto G. Change in domains that influence quality of life after major lower limb amputation in patients with peripheral arterial disease. Ann Vasc Surg. 2021;75:179–88. https://doi.org/10.1016/j.avsg.2021.01.082.
58. Aquarius AE, Denollet J, de Vries J, Hamming JF. Poor health-related quality of life in patients with peripheral arterial disease: type D personality and severity of peripheral arterial disease as independent predictors. J Vasc Surg. 2007;46(3):507–12. https://doi.org/10.1016/j.jvs.2007.04.039.

59. van Aalst FM, Verwijmeren L, van Dongen EPA, de Vries JPPM, de Groot E, Noordzij PG. Frailty and functional outcomes after open and endovascular procedures for patients with peripheral arterial disease: a systematic review. J Vasc Surg. 2020;71(1):297–306.e1. https://doi.org/10.1016/j.jvs.2018.12.060.
60. Schoenweger P, Miller F, Cromwell DA, et al. Outcomes of lower limb angioplasty vary by area deprivation in England. Eur J Vasc Endovasc Surg. 2020;60(5):784–5.

Infrapopliteal Arteries (Classical and Percutaneous)

20

Richard Anthony Meena and Olamide Alabi

The Emergence and Importance of QOL and PROMS for Peripheral Artery Disease

Peripheral artery disease (PAD) is defined by chronic, atherosclerotic disease in arterial beds outside of the heart or brain. Arterial occlusive disease of the lower extremities is the third most common manifestation of systemic atherosclerosis behind heart disease and stroke, and this condition affects over ten million cases nationwide and over 200 million people worldwide [1]. Risk factors associated with PAD include multiple standard cardiovascular risk factors including tobacco abuse, diabetes mellitus, hypertension, dyslipidemia, hyperhomocysteinemia, male sex, age, and renal insufficiency. PAD manifests along a clinical spectrum from asymptomatic patients to tissue loss in the foot and carries a significant risk of cardiovascular morbidity and mortality. This condition is associated with three times the average risk of cardiovascular events and mortality [2] and carries a high risk for major amputation with over 185,000 major amputations taking place each year in the United States [3]. The prevalence of PAD in the general population increases dramatically with age [4], and the number of interventions provided to those with PAD has demonstrated a steady increase over time [5].

As more patients with PAD present to vascular specialists for medical attention, the necessity and timing of intervention(s) have become a topic of important inquiry. Lower extremity revascularization is often a temporizing measure because established goals include symptom improvement or resolution, wound healing, and limb preservation; however, there are no curative medical or surgical therapies available to date. Given the significant morbidity associated with vascular interventions and sequelae of potentially poor outcomes, vascular specialists are faced with even more complex decisions when formulating a plan of care for patients with PAD.

Whether or not to intervene on a patient with significant lower extremity PAD can be a difficult decision to make. Traditionally, outcomes such as revascularization patency, readmission, limb loss, and mortality are frequently reported after lower extremity revascularization [6–8]. Although these outcomes are critical metrics to evaluate after operative intervention, for the interventionalist and healthcare system, they do not always embody what the individual patient values most. Therefore, providers have begun to

R. A. Meena · O. Alabi (✉)
Division of Vascular Surgery and Endovascular Therapy, Department of Surgery, Emory University School of Medicine, Atlanta, GA, USA
e-mail: richard.meena@emory.edu; olamide.alabi@emory.edu

T. Athanasiou et al. (eds.), *Patient Reported Outcomes and Quality of Life in Cardiovascular Interventions*,
https://doi.org/10.1007/978-3-031-09815-4_20

Predictors of poor quality of life	
Low or borderline ABI(12)	Wu A, et al.
Tissue loss(13)	Duff S, et al.
Rest pain(13)	Duff S, et al.
Poor cognitive status(14)	Gardner AW, et al.
Lack of therapeutic options(15)	Sprengers RW, et al.

Fig. 20.1 Predictors of poor quality of life in patients with peripheral artery disease

incorporate patient-reported outcome measures (PROMS), including quality of life (QoL) assessments, as part of their decision-making algorithm. In the 1960s and 1970s, clinicians began to use QoL assessments to evaluate the utility of new technologies in patient care [9]. Vascular interventionalists paralleled medicine as a whole in that early QoL metrics centered on cost effectiveness, such as quality-adjusted life years (QALYs). For example, a landmark vascular trial, Asymptomatic Carotid Artery Stenosis (ACAS), was re-analyzed under the scope of QALYs in 1997 [10]. Since 2000, these analyses extend far beyond cost effectiveness and have begun to incorporate patient-reported outcomes as guidance to proceed with and/or defer specific vascular interventions for some patients.

Measuring QoL on a larger scale has been shown to directly impact clinical medicine. Norman et al. demonstrated that minimally important difference estimates for QoL assessments only approach half a standard deviation. Therefore, even small shifts in QoL metrics could significantly impact patient care [11].

Several studies have suggested certain factors that may predispose patients to a lower quality of life in peripheral artery disease (Fig. 20.1). Lower ankle-brachial index alone has been associated with worse patient-reported outcome measures [12]. Chronic limb-threatening ischemia, as defined as rest pain or tissue loss, further has been associated with lower quality of life endpoints [13]. Finally, poor cognitive status in patients with peripheral artery disease may further lead to a worse quality of life [14]. These known risk factors serve as a foundation on which providers can tailor care discussions with their patients.

Assessing QoL and PROMS in Peripheral Artery Disease

In both the intermittent claudication (IC) and chronic limb threatening ischemia (CLTI) populations, intervention has not clearly demonstrated improved or worsened QoL. This is in large part due to the non-binary nature of QoL measurements. As QoL has become an increasingly important topic of research, particularly with such a morbid disease process and overwhelmingly elderly patient population, great strides have been made to qualify these shades of gray, rather than black-and-white, outcomes.

Questionnaires have long been the primary tool used to assess QoL in surgical research, as they allow patients to express their opinions while maintaining a standard form from which researchers can capture data. Created in the late 1980s, the 36-item Short Form Health Survey (SF-36) sought to capture adult patients' perceptions regarding their health and wellbeing. This instrument assesses eight domains, including physical function as it relates to one's health, limitations related to physical and emotional concerns, social functioning, bodily pain, and general and mental health; the instrument has since been validated in the general population and general chronic disease states [16]. The European Quality of Life 5 Dimension scale (EQ-5D) similarly uses domains to assess quality of life in a general population. This tool's prior iteration, the EuroQol instrument, was found to have relatively poor validity when compared to the SF-36 and with evidence of being less sensitive at the ceiling [17]. The instrument was further refined to a five-domain scale, the EQ-5D. EQ-5D domains include assessment of mobility, self-care, usual activities, pain/discomfort, and anxiety/depression. Clearly, patterns can be appreciated when comparing SF-36 and EQ-5D; physical and mental health, as well as "usual activities" and pain, all can be drawn from when assessing general QoL in health care.

Though useful, both SF-36 and EQ-5D are fairly generic tools used to assess a general population regarding QoL. The ability to provide such generalizable results is undoubtedly why these questionnaires have become so useful in health services research. However, it became evident that tools specific to PAD would provide a more appropriate assessment in this population. The Vascular Quality of Life questionnaire (now referred to VascuQoL-25) captures data using a 25 question review of five domains—symptoms, pain, activities, social life, and emotional state—and a 7-point response scale [18]. When comparing the generalized questionnaires and VascuQoL-25 in the assessment of patients suffering from PAD, de Vries et al. suggested that the VascuQoL-25 should become the primary questionnaire when creating any future studies evaluating QoL in PAD given that this instrument provides a better description of the unique struggles vascular patients with chronic conditions experience daily [19].

Over time, it became evident that patient compliance with lengthy questionnaires was not sustainable. In the PREVENT III trial, for example, patient compliance with questionnaires was documented to decline significantly over time, from 92% at the start of the study, to 61% at 3 months, and ultimately to 52% at 1 year [20]. To combat patient fatigue with questionnaires yet still obtaining accurate disease-specific measurements of QoL, these lengthy questionnaires have been modified. VascuQoL-25 has been limited to VascuQoL-6, cutting the length of the questionnaire by nearly 75% [21].

Measurement of QoL in those who suffer from vascular disease is extremely important given associated burden including severe symptoms, high morbidity either from their chronic disease state, risk of limb loss, and/or death, resource utilization from family members and healthcare facilities, and financial costs associated with their care. Over the years, clinicians have struggled with determining the best intervention, if any, for patients suffering from PAD just as investigators have attempted to refine their methods of assessing vascular intervention quality and outcomes. What has traditionally been lacking in the literature is the voice of the patient and what matters most to them and their families. Many have met this charge with beginning to describe and better understand how patients with PAD view the quality of the lives they lead with or without PAD intervention.

QoL and PROMS in Intermittent Claudication (IC)

Patients with IC have a significantly reduced QoL. In a 1995 multicenter study from the Scottish Vascular Audit Group, 201 patients with IC completed SF-36 health status questionnaires and, compared to the general population, had worse QoL in all domains [22]. Severity of disease, defined as walking distance prior to onset of symptoms, was a significant predictor of all parameters except mental and emotional wellbeing, as per QoL evaluations with the SF-36 form. The authors recommended that for IC, the goal should be improved QoL; therefore, use of these QoL assessments in clinical practice (as opposed to just within the confines of research) may assist PAD interventionalists in their decision making with the PAD patient with IC. Malgor et al. published a systematic review compiling data on treatment in patients with intermittent lower extremity claudication symptoms [23]. They concluded that both endovascular and open intervention as well as exercise therapy improved QoL compared to medical management alone. They also acknowledged that procedures can beget complications and many procedures have limited long term durability in this population.

Multiple randomized controlled trials, such as the OBACT trial, MIMIC, and others, have compared the benefit of intervention in the setting of IC and included QoL comparisons in their cohorts [24–26]. The MIMIC trial reviewed 93 patients with IC on best medical therapy and participating in a supervised exercise program [25]. They were enrolled to a treatment arm with percutaneous transluminal angioplasty (PTA) versus no PTA. Using the SF-36, they found that those enrolled in the PTA treatment arm did not demonstrate improvement in QoL compared to no PTA. This was dissimilar to the CLEVER trial in that stent angioplasty conferred an improvement in reported QoL compared to supervised exercise programs [27]. Given IC as the symptomatology at the time of presentation in these studies, the majority of these interventions are targeting vessels above the level of the knee. Thus, while it is important to understand the body of literature regarding QoL effects after lower extremity revascularizations, this is not the focus of this chapter. As well, OBACT, a single center study following patients with IC for 2 years and used the SF-36 as well as CLAU-S (a claudication specific QoL questionnaire), found that patients with IC undergoing early peripheral intervention with medical therapy compared to patients on optimal medical therapy alone, had improved functional, hemodynamic, and QoL outcomes [24].

QoL and PROMS in Chronic Limb-Threatening Ischemia (CLTI)

Chronic limb-threatening ischemia (CLTI) represents the most severe manifestation of lower extremity PAD. The TransAtlantic Inter-Society Consensus for the Management of Peripheral Artery Disease (TASC II) guidelines define as chronic ischemic rest pain or ischemic skin lesions. CLTI is associated with significant morbidity and mortality [2]. Due to the associated burden of high morbidity with or without intervention, high resource utilization, and associated excess healthcare costs, investigators have now begun to look toward patient-reported outcome measures (PROMs) and QoL measures early on when determining an appropriate plan of care for these patients.

Initial studies regarding QoL after LE open surgical bypass reviewed patients' pre- and postoperative functional status. In 1996, Abou-Zamzam et al. reviewed functional status after infrainguinal bypasses [28]. Five hundred thirteen patients in this patient underwent infrainguinal bypass at a single center over 15 years. All included patients had ischemic rest pain or tissue loss and over 90% of the patients reviewed had a distal bypass target below the level of the knee. Of those patients who ambulated with assist devices preoperatively, 97% were found to maintain this level of function at 6 months postoperatively. Independent living status was assessed; of those patients living independently preoperatively, 99% maintained their independence at 6 months after surgery. A similar review of patients with CLTI retrospectively looked at 334 patients who underwent 419 infrainguinal bypasses at two institutions over a 7-year period [29]. Sixty-two percent of these bypasses had a distal target located below the knee. Limb salvage was reported as 85% at 1 year, with only a 6% drop over the course of the next 2 years; however, the authors emphasized that one-quarter of their patients had not achieved wound healing at 1 year, nearly one-fifth had lost ambulatory status, and 5% were no longer living independently. These studies clearly demonstrate the juxtaposition of excellent provider-specific outcomes alongside poor/failing PROMs.

Markers of functional status, including independent living and ambulatory status, are not age-independent, as increasing age certainly impacts both the pathophysiology underlying CLTI and the potential risk of morbidity and mortality with interventions. Pomposelli et al. evaluated octogenarians undergoing open lower extremity arterial revascularization at a single center, with approximately 287 patients undergoing intervention for CLTI, and with 80.6% of those patients having a tibiopedal distal target [30]. Ninety-two percent of patients in this study cohort were ambulatory preoperatively, and after undergoing intervention, roughly one-half required assist devices. Unfortunately, approximately 5% of the patients were non-ambulatory 12 months after their procedures, and less than half were alive at 5 years, emphasizing the importance of risk stratification in a population with increased age, varying levels of function, and high mortality within 5 years. Taylor et al. evaluated 841 patients with CLTI undergoing suprainguinal bypasses, infrainguinal bypasses, and endovascular repair (1000 total operations) [31]. Of note, over 70% of these procedures were infrainguinal and likely with distal targets given the presence of multilevel disease. Overall, 71% of their patients maintained their ambulatory status, and 81% maintained their independent living status at 5 years of follow up.

PREVENT III was a large multicenter trial exploring the use of edifoligide in those who undergo lower extremity bypass for PAD [32]. They also evaluated this cohort of patients with the VascuQoL-25 QoL assessment. PREVENT III explored PROMs in the setting of open surgical lower extremity revascularization for CLTI and the results related to QoL were favorable [20]. The authors reported improved global scoring on the VasculQoL-25 questionnaire from a baseline mean score of 2.8–4.7 at 3 months and 5.1 at 12 months. This QoL improvement was noted to be statistically significant and seen across all domains.

Published in 2005, the BASIL trial explored 452 patients who underwent open or endovascular lower extremity revascularization for "severe limb ischemia" (referring to patients with CLTI) manifesting as ischemic rest pain or tissue loss) and reviewed QoL and PROMS in their analysis utilizing the SF-36, VascuQol-25, and EQ-5D QoL instruments [33]. No difference was found between revascularization methods (bypass surgery versus angioplasty) for amputation-free survival or generic or disease specific health related QoL. Interestingly, though, when the team looked at those patients who lived 2 or more years after randomization, they found that those patients who underwent a bypass operation had improved overall survival and trended toward improved amputation-free survival. A plateau effect was noted after the first 3 months for all generic- and disease-specific health related QoL scores for both bypass and endovascular revascularization types in this cohort.

There are few studies that focus their investigation on quality of life in patients who undergo below-knee interventions via endovascular means. Dua et al. reviewed tibial and pedal endovascular interventions in patients with CLTI [34]. This single center reviewed outcomes after lower extremity endovascular revascularizations that included tibiopedal revascularization between 2016 and 2017. Some of these patients also have more proximal endovascular interventions in the same procedure. They reported low subsequent major amputation rates (4% at 6 months) and no adverse events in 30 days after procedure. Of note, QoL scores improved over time after endovascular tibiopedal revascularization with higher Stark QoL scores at 1, 3, and 6 months post-revascularization. It is important to note that the Stark QoL questionnaire was assessed at every post-procedure visit with high respondent rates likely owing to the fact that the questionnaire contains primarily pictures and minimal words, and it takes, on average, less than 5 min to complete [35]. As well, the multicenter, randomized Comparing Angioplasty and DES in the Treatment of Subjects With Ischemic Infrapopliteal Arterial Disease (ACHILLES) trial reviewed endovascular infrapopliteal interventions for CLTI using either sirolimus eluting stents (SES) or balloon angioplasty (BAP) [36]. QoL was assessed using EQ-5D in the 200 enrolled patients and found improvement in most domains in during the study period. These improvements were noted primarily within the first 6 weeks after revascularization, and notably the domains of self-care and activity did not improve. No significant difference was noted

Conclusions
Peripheral artery disease (PAD) is a serious diagnosis, with associated increased risks of cardiovascular morbidity, mortality, and lower extremity amputation.
While outcomes in PAD are often evaluated on technical terms, patient reported quality of life measures are critical outcomes that need increased emphasis in the literature.
For patients with intermittent claudication, supervised exercise therapy with or without therapeutic intervention appears to confer increased quality of life compared to medical therapy alone.
For patients with chronic limb-threatening ischemia, intervention appears to improve patient reported quality of life measures, without definitive differences in type of revascularization (endovascular versus open).
There is a lack of comparative evidence on new technologies such cutting balloons and drug-eluting balloons and their impact on patient reported quality of life measures.

Fig. 20.2 Summary of conclusions

between the SES group compared to the BAP group, however. This was similar to the multi-center, single blind, randomized, concurrently controlled Lutonix-BTK trial that reviewed paclitaxel coated balloons to BAP for below-the-knee revascularizations [37]. They found no difference between treatment groups in terms of QoL as assessed on the 5Q-ED or the Walking Impairment Questionnaire.

Another interesting cohort that is less well studied regarding QoL are patients with CLTI who have no revascularization options. One study sought to gain more information on this cohort by reviewing 47 patients with no-options CLTI with SF-36 and EQ-5D QoL questionnaires [15]. The authors found that patients with no-option CLTI scored low on all SF-36 domains (Fig. 20.2). Physical-related SF-36 domains remained low when compared to other patients with mild PAD as well as patients with cardiovascular risk factors only. No-option CLTI patients also scored low on the pain and discomfort domains of the EQ-5D.

Limitations/Future Directions

The future of PAD research should shift away from the heavy focus on metrics related to both optimal medical therapy with or without intervention and provider-reported outcomes. As Dr. Tsai addresses in his editorial to the *Journals of American College of Cardiology: Cardiovascular Interventions*, by emphasizing technical aspects more than quality of life metrics, our studies may be highlighting less important end points for the patient [38].

Additionally, as new technologies emerge, particularly in the endovascular space, providers and researchers should assess the technologies' impact on patient-reported outcome measures, not just on technical outcomes. Limited data exist today describing these newer technologies' impact on patient quality of life. One new technology that has emerged for patients with peripheral artery disease is footplate neuromuscular stimulation electrical stimulation (NMES). This technology could potentially augment or replace supervised exercise programs, which often suffer from poor patient compliance. By releasing electrical energy, NMES promotes active muscle contraction in an attempt to aid lower extremity circulation. Early data demonstrate improved patient reported outcome measures for these patients, as calculated from the EQ-5D and Intermittent Claudication Questionnaire assessment [39]. NMES can serve as an example of the importance of using patient-reported outcome measures as a part of the validation algorithm for new technologies.

It is vital that we begin to find the balance of technical measures to patient-reported outcome measures that directly impact the patient's quality of life, whether that be domains such as physical, emotional, and/or mental health or other facets of QoL as assessed by the SF-36, VascuQoL-25, and other generic and disease specific health related QoL instruments. More recent investigations and study design have only begun to scratch the surface. There is a great deal that we can learn by listening to our patients and understanding how they perceive and accept the interventions we offer as well as how those interventions affect their quality of life. This holistic approach is necessary to provide better quality, patient centered care in such a vulnerable patient population (Fig. 20.2).

References

1. Fowkes GF, Rudan D, Rudan I, Aboyans V, Denenberg JO, McDermott MM, et al. Comparison of global estimates of prevalence and risk factors for peripheral artery disease in 2000 and 2010: a systematic review and analysis. Lancet. 2013;382:1329–40.
2. Grenon SM, Vittinghoff E, Owens CD, Conte MS, Whooley M, Cohen BE. Peripheral artery disease and risk of cardiovascular events in patients with coronary artery disease: insights from the Heart and Soul Study. Vasc Med. 2013;18(4):176–84.
3. Owings MF, Kozak LJ. Ambulatory and inpatient procedures in the United States, 1996. Vital Health Stat 13. 1998;139:1–119.
4. Benjamin EJ, Virani SS, Callaway CW, et al. American Heart Association Council on Epidemiology and Prevention Statistics Committee and Stroke Statistics Subcommittee. Heart disease and stroke statistics—2018 update: a report from the American Heart Association. Circulation. 2018;137(12):e67–e492.
5. Rowe VL, Lee W, Weaver FA, Etzioni D. Patterns of treatment for peripheral arterial disease in the United States: 1996-2005. J Vasc Surg. 2009;49(4):910–7.
6. Secemsky EA, Schermerhorn M, Carroll BJ, Kennedy KF, Shen C, Valsdottir LR, et al. Readmissions after revascularization procedures for peripheral arterial disease: a nationwide cohort study. Ann Intern Med. 2018;168(2):93–9.
7. Heikkila K, Loftus IM, Mitchell DC, Johal AS, Waton S, Cromwell DA. Population-based study of mortality and major amputation following lower limb revascularization. Br J Surg. 2018;105(9):1145–54.
8. Mustapha J, Katzen BT, Neville RF, Lookstein RA, Zeller T, Miller LE, et al. Determinants of long-term outcomes and costs in the management of critical limb ischemia: a population-based cohort study. J Am Heart Assoc. 2018;7(16):e009724.
9. Pennacchini M, Bertolaso M, Elvira MM, De Marinis MG. A brief history of the Quality of Life: its use in medicine and in philosophy. La. Clin Ter. 2011;162(3):e99–e103.
10. Cronenwett JL, Birkmeyer JD, Nackman GB, Fillinger MF, Bech FR, Zwolak RM, et al. Cost-effectiveness of carotid endarterectomy in asymptomatic patients. J Vasc Surg. 1997;25(2):298–309.
11. Norman G, Sloan J, Wyrwich K. Interpretation of changes in health-related quality of life: the remarkable universality of half a standard deviation. Med Care. 2003;41(5):582–92.
12. Wu ACJ, Selvin E, Tanaka H, Heiss G, Hirsch AT, Jaar BG, Matsushita K. Lower extremity peripheral artery disease and quality of life among older individuals in the community. J Am Heart Assoc. 2017;6:e004519.
13. Duff SMM, Bhounsule P, Hasegawa JT. The burden of critical limb ischemia: a review of recent literature. Vasc Health Risk Manag. 2019;15:187–208.
14. Gardner AWWS, Montgomery PS, Zhao YD. Effect of cognitive status on exercise performance and quality of life in patients with symptomatic peripheral artery disease. J Vasc Surg. 2016;63(1):98–104.
15. Sprengers RW, Teraa M, Moll FL, Ardine de Wit G, van der Graaf Y, Verhaar MC, et al. Quality of life in patients with no-option critical limb ischemia underlines the need for new effective treatment. J Vasc Surg. 2010;52(4):843–9.
16. Brazier JE, Harper R, Jones NM, O'Cathain A, Thomas KJ, Usherwood T, et al. Validating the SF-36 health survey questionnaire: new outcome measure for primary care. Br Med J. 1992;305:160–4.
17. Brazier J, Jones N, Kind P. Testing the validity of the Euroqol and comparing it with the SF-36 health survey questionnaire. Qual Life Res. 1993;2(3):169–80.
18. Morgan MBG, Crayford SM, Murrin B, Fraser SC. Developing the vascular quality of life questionnaire: a new disease-specific quality of life measure for use in lower limb ischemia. J Vasc Surg. 2001;33(4):679–87.
19. de Vries M, Ouwendijk R, Kessels AG, de Haan MW, Flobbe K, Hunink MGM, et al. Comparison of generic and disease-specific questionnaires for the assessment of quality of life in patients with peripheral arterial disease. J Vasc Surg. 2005;41(12):261–8.
20. Nguyen LL, Moneta GL, Conte MS, Bandyk DF, Clowes AW, Seely BL, et al. Prospective multicenter study of quality of life before and after lower extremity vein bypass in 1404 patients with critical limb ischemia. J Vasc Surg. 2006;44(5):977–83.
21. Nordanstig J, Wann-Hansson C, Karlsson J, Lundstrom M, Pettersson M, Morgan MBF. Vascular Quality of Life Questionnaire-6 facilitates health-related quality of life assessment in peripheral arterial disease. J Vasc Surg. 2014;59:700–7.
22. Pell JP. Impact of intermittent claudication on quality of life. The Scottish Vascular Audit Group. Eur J Vasc Endovasc Surg. 1995;9(4):469–72.
23. Malgor RD, Alahdab F, Elraiyah TA, Rizvi AZ, Lane MA, Prokop LJ, et al. A systematic review of treat-

ment of intermittent claudication in the lower extremities. J Vasc Surg. 2015;61(3 Suppl):54S–73S.
24. Nylaende M, Abdelnoor M, Stranden E, Morken B, Sandbaek G, Risum O, et al. The Oslo balloon angioplasty versus conservative treatment study (OBACT)—the 2-years results of a single centre, prospective, randomised study in patients with intermittent claudication. Eur J Vasc Endovasc Surg. 2007;33(1):3–12.
25. Greenhalgh RM, Belch JJF, Brown LC, Gaines PA, Gao L, Reise JA, et al. The adjuvant benefit of angioplasty in patients with mild to moderate intermittent claudication (MIMIC) managed by supervised exercise, smoking cessation advice and best medical therapy: results from two randomised trials for stenotic femoropopliteal and aortoiliac arterial disease. Eur J Vasc Endovasc Surg. 2008;36(6):680–8.
26. Mazari FAK, Khan JA, Samuel N, Smith G, Carradice D, McCollum PC, et al. Long-term outcomes of a randomized clinical trial of supervised exercise, percutaneous transluminal angioplasty or combined treatment for patients with intermittent claudication due to femoropopliteal disease. Br J Surg. 2017;104(1):76–83.
27. Murphy TP, Cutlip DE, Regensteiner JG, Mohler ER, Cohen DJ, Reynolds MR, et al. Supervised exercise versus primary stenting for claudication resulting from aortoiliac peripheral artery disease: six-month outcomes from the claudication: exercise versus endoluminal revascularization (CLEVER) study. Circulation. 2012;125(1):130–9.
28. Abou-Zamzam AM Jr, Lee RW, Moneta GL, Taylor LM Jr, Porter JM. Functional outcome after infrainguinal bypass for limb salvage. J Vasc Surg. 1997;25(2):287–95.
29. Chung J, Bartelson BB, Hiatt WR, Peyton BD, McLafferty RB, Hopley CW, et al. Wound healing and functional outcomes after infrainguinal bypass with reversed saphenous vein for critical limb ischemia. J Vasc Surg. 2006;43(6):1183–90.
30. Pomposelli FB, Arora S, Gibbons GW, Grykberg R, Smakowski P, Campbell DR, et al. Lower extremity arterial reconstruction in the very elderly: successful outcome preserves not only the limb but also residential status and ambulatory function. J Vasc Surg. 1998;28(2):215–25.
31. Taylor SMKC, Blackhurst DW, Cass AL, Trent EA, Langan EM III, Youkey JR. Determinants of functional outcome after revascularization for critical limb ischemia: an analysis of 1000 consecutive vascular interventions. J Vasc Surg. 2006;44(4):747–56.
32. Conte MS, Lorenz TJ, Bandyk DF, Clowes AW, Moneta GL, Lynn Seely B. Design and rationale of the PREVENT III clinical trial: edifoligide for the prevention of infrainguinal vein graft failure. Vasc Endovasc Surg. 2004;39(1):15–23.
33. Forbes JF, Adam DJ, Bell J, Fowkes FGR, Gillespie I, Raab GM, et al. Bypass versus Angioplasty in Severe Ischaemia of the Leg (BASIL) trial: health-related quality of life outcomes, resource utilization, and cost-effectiveness analysis. J Vasc Surg. 2010;51(5):43S–51S.
34. Dua A, Rothenberg KA, Lee JJ, Gologorsky R, Desai SS. Six-month freedom from amputation rates and quality of life following tibial and pedal endovascular revascularization for critical limb ischemia. Vasc Endovasc Surg. 2019;53(3):212–5.
35. Hardt J. A new questionnaire for measuring quality of life - the Stark QoL. Health Qual Life Outcomes. 2015;13:174.
36. Katsanos K, Spiliopoulos S, Diamantopoulos A, Siablis D, Karnabatidis D, Scheinert D. Wound healing outcomes and health-related quality-of-life changes in the ACHILLES trial: 1-year results from a prospective randomized controlled trial of infrapopliteal balloon angioplasty versus sirolimus-eluting stenting in patients with ischemic peripheral arterial disease. J Am Coll Cardiol Intv. 2016;9(3):259–67.
37. Mustapha JA, Broadman M, Geraghty PJ, Saab F, Settlage RA, Jaff MR, et al. Drug-coated vs uncoated percutaneous transluminal angioplasty in infrapopliteal arteries: six-month results of the Lutonix BTK trial. J Invasive Cardiol. 2019;31(8):205–11.
38. Tsai T. Missing the forest for the trees?: drug-eluting balloon treatment for infrapopliteal disease. J Am Coll Cardiol Intv. 2015;8(12):1623–5.
39. Babber ARR, Onida S, Lane TRA, Davies AH. Effect of footplate neuromuscular electrical stimulation on functional and quality-of-life parameters in patients with peripheral artery disease: pilot, and subsequent randomized clinical trial. Br J Surg. 2020;107(4):355–63.

Quality-of-Life (QOL) and Patient-Reported Outcome Measures (PROMs) Following Intervention for Chronic Venous Disease

21

Kosmas I. Paraskevas, Andrew N. Nicolaides, and George Geroulakos

Introduction

Lower extremity chronic venous disease affects a considerable percentage of the population. Approximately 25 million people in the United States have varicose veins and the annual prevalence of venous thromboembolism (including both deep vein thrombosis and pulmonary embolism) is approximately one million people [1]. Although the majority of patients with lower extremity chronic venous disease are asymptomatic, a number of serious complications can occur, including venous leg ulcers, acute and chronic venous thromboembolism (that can cause pulmonary embolism), chronic thromboembolic pulmonary hypertension and death [2].

A serious and common complication/manifestation of lower extremity chronic venous disease is the formation of venous leg ulcerations. Venous leg ulcers affect approximately 600,000 individuals in the United States and place a burden on patients in terms of quality of life (QoL), pain and social isolation [3, 4]. In addition to the psychosocial consequences of these complications, lower extremity chronic venous disease is associated with high costs, which are estimated between $150 million and $1 billion per year in the United States [3, 4].

The management of chronic venous disease may be conservative/non-invasive and invasive. Graduated compression stockings and a number of venotropic drugs (e.g. flavonoids [e.g. daflon], naftidrofuryl, naftazone, hydroxyethylrutosides [e.g. venoruton], etc.) have been shown to be effective in the control of venous disease (reduction of pain and swelling) [1, 2]. The traditional surgical management (high venous ligation and stripping in combination with ambulatory/transilluminated powered phlebectomies) has been largely replaced by the endovenous techniques (endovenous laser ablation [EVLA], radiofrequency ablation [RFA], liquid/foam/glue sclerotherapy, cyanoacrylate embolization and mechanochemical ablation) [1–3]. A description/comparison of the various techniques available is beyond the scope of this article and is presented in greater detail elsewhere [5].

Non-invasive hemodynamic measurements and ultrasonic anatomic evaluation can be used to objectively assess the effect of intervention on venous insufficiency (such as venous filling index

K. I. Paraskevas · G. Geroulakos (✉)
Department of Vascular Surgery, "Attikon" University Hospital, National and Kapodistrian University of Athens, Athens, Greece
e-mail: g.geroulakos@imperial.ac.uk; ggeroulakos@med.uoa.gr

A. N. Nicolaides
Department of Surgery, University of Nicosia Medical School, Nicosia, Cyprus

T. Athanasiou et al. (eds.), *Patient Reported Outcomes and Quality of Life in Cardiovascular Interventions*, https://doi.org/10.1007/978-3-031-09815-4_21

[as measured by air-plethysmography] that measures the global venous reflux) [1–3]. Besides these objective outcomes, however, there is also the perceived satisfaction/symptom relief as experienced by the patient. Patient-reported outcome measures (PROMs) provide a means by which the impact of varicose veins or their treatments can be measured on the patient's QoL [6]. Several questionnaires have been developed to assess the impact of chronic venous disease and venous leg ulcers. The items in these questionnaires aim to capture the patient's experience using psychometric analyses and to explore their relationship with each and their overall ability to detect change [6]. The effect of venous interventions on quality of life can be assessed by general and specific assessments. Disease-specific quality-of-life instruments can be divided in PROMs and physician-reported outcome measurements.

The reliability of a PROM is its ability to produce the same results when measurements are repeated in populations with similar characteristics [6]. PROMs commonly use more than one item to measure a single dimension that is important to the patient [6]. These items need to be reliable, valid and internally consistent [6]. A brief description of the available PROMs to assess chronic venous disease is presented.

Table 21.1 Available questionnaires with patient-reported outcome measures (PROMs) to assess chronic venous diseases

Questionnaire	Dimensions (number of items)
Freiburg Life Quality Assessment questionnaire [7]	Physical complaints (14), everyday life (10), social life (6), emotional status (9), treatment (4), satisfaction (7), VAS General Health (1), VAS Skin condition (1) and VAS Quality of Life (1)
Specific Quality of life and Outcomes Response—Venous questionnaire [8]	Discomfort, Appearance, Restriction of movements, Risk, Emotional Problems, Physical impact, Psychosomatic impact, Global Score
Chronic Venous Insufficiency Questionnaire (CIVIQ) [9]	Physical repercussions (e.g. standing/squatting/kneeling, walking quickly/climbing stairs, travelling), psychological repercussions (e.g. anxiousness, tiredness, embarrassment), pain repercussions (e.g. pain, interference with work/sleep), social repercussions, overall quality of life score
Aberdeen Varicose Vein Questionnaire [10]	Functional status (physical/social functioning, role limitations attributed to physical/emotional problems), wellbeing (mental health, energy/fatigue, pain), overall evaluation of health (interference with work/leisure, concern)
Venous insufficiency epidemiological and economic study on quality of life [11]	Symptoms (10), limitations in daily activities (9), time of greatest intensity (1), change over the past year (1), psychological impact (5)

VAS visual-analogue scale

PROMs to Assess Chronic Venous Disease

Five questionnaires have been developed for patients with venous leg symptoms or signs, but without ulcers (Table 21.1), namely:

1. **The Freiburg Life Quality Assessment (FLQA) questionnaire** [7]**:** The FLQA consists of 93 items and differentiates between limitations in QoL in seven scales: physical complaints, everyday life, social life, emotional status, treatment, satisfaction and general health [7].
2. **The Specific Quality of life and Outcomes Response—Venous (SQOR-V) questionnaire** [8]**:** This questionnaire consists of 46 items with special attention to the patients' main complaints with relevance for venous disorders [8].
3. **The ChronIc Venous Insufficiency Questionnaire (CIVIQ)** [9]**:** This is a 20-item questionnaire which explores four dimensions: psychological, physical, social functioning and pain [9].
4. **The Aberdeen Varicose Vein Symptom Severity (AVVSS) Score or Aberdeen Varicose Vein Questionnaire (AVVQ)** [10]**:** This questionnaire is devoted exclusively to

the QoL measurement of patients suffering from varicose veins. It includes information on four important health factors: pain and dysfunction, cosmetic appearance, extent of varicosity and complications [10].

5. **The VEnous INsufficiency Epidemiological and Economic Study on Quality of Life (VEINES-QoL)** [11]**:** This is a scientifically sound, patient-reported outcome score that evaluates quality of life and symptoms across a range of conditions (e.g. telangiectasias, varicose veins, edema, skin changes, leg ulcers) in chronic venous disorders of the leg [11].

Besides these five questionnaires, there are another four scales dedicated to patients with venous leg ulcers, namely:

1. **The Venous Leg Ulcer Quality of Life (VLU-QoL) questionnaire** [12]**:** This questionnaire consists of 34 items on three domains: Activities (12 items), Psychological (12 items) and Symptom Distress (10 items). This questionnaire is a useful tool to assess the outcomes of treatment from the patients' point-of-view [12].
2. **The Leg and Foot Ulcer Questionnaire of Hyland (LFUQ)** [13]**:** This questionnaire measures functional limitations and emotional reactions to quantify QoL deficits. Functional limitations and emotional reactions are inter-correlated to evaluate the effect of venous leg ulcers on the patient's global QoL [13].
3. **The Sheffield Preference-based Venous leg Ulcer Questionnaire with five Dimensions (SPVU-5D)** [14]**:** This is a questionnaire consisting of 16 disease-specific items and life-satisfaction questions. It assesses the level of pain and discomfort, as well as the psychological effects of venous ulcerations [14].
4. **The Charing Cross Venous Leg Ulceration Questionnaire (CCVUQ)** [15]**:** This questionnaire assesses four important health domains: social function, domestic activities, cosmetic appearance and emotional status [15].

Finally, the Short Form 36-Item (SF-36) and 12-Item (SF-12) health surveys [6] are tools that assess QoL in association with:

1. **The Venous Clinical Severity Score (VCSS)** [16]**:** VCSS assesses venous disease severity using several characteristics, including pain, varicose veins, edema, pigmentation, inflammation, induration, number and size of ulcers, ulcer duration and use of compression (Table 21.2) [16].
2. **The Clinical, Etiologic, Anatomic, Pathophysiologic (CEAP) score** [17]**:** The CEAP classification for chronic venous disorders was developed in 1994 by an international ad hoc committee of the American Venous Forum. The CEAP classification provides a descriptive classification of chronic venous disease (Table 21.2) [17].

The above-mentioned questionnaires and PROMs have been used to compare the various interventions for the treatment of chronic venous diseases and assess their efficacy from the patient's perspective. A comparison of the various methods used in randomised controlled trials with respect to the QoL of the patient using PROMs is presented in Table 21.3. The different comparisons that have been assessed are presented below.

Table 21.2 Available questionnaires to assess quality-of-life in patients with chronic venous diseases

Questionnaire	Dimensions (number of items)
Venous Clinical Severity Score [16]	Absent/Mild/Moderate/Severe classification in pain, varicose veins, venous edema, skin pigmentation, inflammation, induration, number and size of active ulcers, ulcer duration, compression
Clinical, Etiologic, Anatomic, Pathophysiologic score [17]	Clinical classification (8), Etiologic classification (4), Anatomic Classification (4), Pathophysiologic classification (4)

Table 21.3 A list of all randomized controlled trials, questionnaires used and outcomes

Study (year)	# Limbs	Follow-up (month)	Instrument	Design	Comparison	Outcome
Lurie (2003) [18]	86	4	CIVIQ2-QoL	Prospective multicenter RCT	44 RFA vs. 36 L&S	Global score (72 h): 13.3 (SE: 3.1) vs. −3 (2.3); p < 0.0001 Global score (1 week): 3.7 (2.5) vs. −9.2 (2.3); p < 0.0001
Lurie (2005) [19]	65	24	CIVIQ2-QoL	Prospective multicenter RCT	36 RFA vs. 29 L&S	Global score at 1 and 2 years; p < 0.05
Subramonia (2010) [20]	88	1	AVVSSS	Prospective 2-center RCT	47 RFA vs. 41 L&S	Mean improvement in global QoL score: −9.12 vs. −8.24; p = 0.532
Rasmussen (2013) [21]	580	36	AVVSSS	Prospective 2-center RCT	148 RFA vs. 144 EVLA vs. 144 UGFS vs. 142 L&S	RFA AVVSSS: 18.74 (8.63) to 4.43 (6.58); p < 0.0001 EVLA AVVSSS: 17.97 (9.00) to 4.61 (5.8); p < 0.0001 UGFS AVVSSS: 18.38 (9.07) to 4.76 (5.71); p < 0.0001 L&S AVVSSS: 19.3 (8.46) to 4.00 (4.87); p < 0.0001
Rasmussen (2007) [22]	137	6	VCSS, SF-36, AVVSSS	Prospective 2-center RCT	69 EVLA vs. 68 L&S	EVLA VCSS: from 2.8 (1–8) to 0.4 (0–7); p < 0.001 EVLA L&S: from 2.4 (2–12) to 0.2 (0–2); p < 0.001
Rasmussen (2011) [23]	580	12	VCSS, SF-36, AVVSSS	Prospective 2-center RCT	148 RFA vs. 144 EVLA vs. 144 UGFS vs. 142 L&S	The VCSS, AVVSSS and SF-36 all improved significantly after the procedure (p < 0.001) with no significant difference between them
Christenson (2010) [24]	200	24	VCSS, SF-36, AVVSSS	Prospective single-center RCT	100 L&S vs. 100 EVLA	The VCSS, AVVSSS and SF-36 all improved significantly after each procedure with no significant difference between the groups
Biemans (2013) [25]	223	12	CEAP, CIVIQ, EuroQoL	Prospective 2-center RCT	78 EVLA vs. 77 UGFS vs. 68 L&S	The CIVIQ and EuroQoL improved in all groups at 3 months and showed no significant difference between the groups.
Pronk (2010) [26]	130	12	CEAP, EuroQoL	Prospective single-center RCT	62 EVLA vs. 68 L&S	Although pain scores were higher after EVLA up to Day 14 (p = 0.01), no differences were noted between the procedures at 1 year (p = 0.87)
Flessenkamper (2013) [27]	449	42	CEAP	Prospective multicenter RCT	159 L&S vs. 142 EVLA vs. 148 EVLA + L&S	The CEAP classification improved in all groups already at 2 months and showed no significant difference between the groups.

Table 21.3 (continued)

Study (year)	# Limbs	Follow-up (month)	Instrument	Design	Comparison	Outcome
Mozafar (2014) [28]	65	18	CEAP, AVVSSS	Prospective single-center RCT	30 EVLA vs. 35 L&S	The CEAP classification improved in both groups significantly and showed no between-group difference.
Roopram (2013) [29]	175	1.5	AVVSSS, EuroQoL	Prospective 2-center RCT	118 EVLA vs. 57 L&S	Both groups showed significant improvement ($p < 0.001$) with no between-group difference.
Brittenden (2019) [30]	595	60	AVVSSS, EuroQoL	Prospective multicenter RCT	162 EVLA vs. 219 UGFS vs. 214 L&S	The AVVSSS and EuroQoL improved in all 3 groups and showed no difference between the groups.
Carradice (2011) [31]	280	12	VCSS, SF-36, AVVSSS	Prospective single-center RCT	140 EVLA vs. 140 L&S	The VCSS, SF-36 and AVVSSS improved in both groups with no between-group difference.
Samuel (2013) [32]	106	12	VCSS, SF-36, AVVSSS	Prospective single-center RCT	53 EVLA vs. 53 L&S	The VCSS, AVVSSS and SF-36 improved in all groups with no significant between-group difference
Darwood (2008) [33]	80	3	AVVSSS, VCSS	Prospective single-center RCT	54 EVLA vs. 26 L&S	The VCSS and AVVSSS improved in both groups with no significant between-group difference
Bountouroglou (2006) [34]	60	3	AVVSSS, VCSS	Prospective single-center RCT	30 UGFS vs. 30 L&S	The VCSS and AVVSSS improved in both groups with no significant between-group difference
Campos (2015) [35]	58	12	AVVSSS, VCSS, VDS	Prospective single-center RCT	29 UGFS vs. 29 L&S	The VCSS, VDS and AVVSSS improved in both groups with no significant between-group difference
Shadid (2012) [36]	430	24	VCSS, EuroQoL	Prospective 3-center RCT	230 UGFS vs. 200 L&S	The VCSS and EuroQoL improved in both groups with no significant between-group difference
Michaels (2006) [37]	217	24	SF-36, EuroQoL	Prospective 2-center RCT	160 L&S vs. 57 UGFS	The SF-36 and EuroQoL improved in both groups with no significant between-group difference
Wozniak (2015) [38]	102	36	VCSS	Prospective single-center RCT	52 thermal ablation vs. 50 L&S	The VCSS scores improved significantly ($p < 0.05$) in both groups with no between-group difference
Lattimer (2013) [39]	90	15	AVVSSS, VCSS, STS	Prospective single-center RCT	44 EVLA vs. 46 UGFS	The AVVSSS, VCSS and STS were all reduced from baseline ($p < 0.0005$) with no between-group difference
Shepherd (2015) [40]	110	6	AVVSSS, VCSS	Prospective single-center RCT	54 EVLA vs. 56 RFA	The VCSS and AVVSSS improved in both groups with no significant between-group difference

(continued)

Table 21.3 (continued)

Study (year)	# Limbs	Follow-up (month)	Instrument	Design	Comparison	Outcome
Nordon (2011) [41]	159	3	AVVSSS, EuroQoL	Prospective single-center RCT	80 EVLA vs. 79 RFA	The AVVSSS and EuroQoL improved in both groups with no significant between-group difference
Carradice (2009) [42]	50	12	AVVSSS, VCSS	Prospective single-center RCT	25 EVLA alone vs. 25 EVLA plus phlebectomies	VCSS and AVVSSS were lower in EVLA plus phlebectomies vs. EVLA alone in 3 months (for both, $p < 0.0001$) but at 1 year there were no differences
Liu (2011) [43]	134	60	CEAP	Prospective single-center RCT	74 EVLA vs. 60 EVLA + stab avulsions	There was no difference in pain between groups after Day 5 onwards.
Theivacumar (2008) [44]	68	3	AVVSSS	Prospective single-center RCT	23 EVLA AK vs. 23 EVLA ABK vs. 22 EVLA BK + UGFS	There was significant improvement in AVVSSS ($p < 0.001$) in all groups with no difference between groups at 3 months
van den Boss (2014) [45]	227	3	VCSS, AVVSSS	Prospective single-center RCT	110 EVLA vs. 117 thermal ablation	The VCSS and AVVSSS improved in both groups with no significant between-group difference
Morrison (2015) [46]	222	3	AVVSS, EuroQoL, VCSS	Prospective single-center RCT	108 cyanoacrylate embolization vs. 114 RFA	VCSS, AVVSS and EuroQoL improved significantly ($p < 0.01$) for both procedures with no between-group difference at 3 months.
Gibson (2018) [47]	222	24	AVVSS, EuroQoL, VCSS	Prospective single-center RCT	108 cyanoacrylate embolization vs. 114 RFA	VCSS, AVVSS and EuroQoL improved significantly ($p < 0.01$) for both procedures with no between-group difference at 24 months.

L&S ligation and stripping, *RFA* radiofrequency ablation, *EVLA* endovenous laser ablation, *UGFS* ultrasound-guided foam sclerotherapy, *AVVSSS* Aberdeen varicose vein symptom severity score, *VCSS* venous clinical severity score, *VDS* venous disability score, *STS* saphenous treatment score, *AK* above-knee, *ABK* above-below-knee, *BK* below-knee, *VSDS* venous segmental disease score, *CXVUQ* disease specific ulcer questionnaire

Comparison of Surgical vs. Endovenous Interventions

These include the following comparisons: (a) high ligation and stripping vs. RFA, (b) high ligation and stripping vs. EVLA, (c) high ligation and stripping vs. sclerotherapy, and, (d) high ligation and stripping vs. thermal ablation.

High Ligation and Stripping vs. RFA

One randomised controlled trial (RCT) measured quality of life using the CIVIQ-2 score at baseline, 1-week and 2-year follow-up [18]. There was a marked difference in perceived pain already at 72 h in favour of RFA compared with high ligation and stripping (-1.77 ± 0.6 vs. 2.9 ± 0.7, respectively; $p < 0.0001$). This difference persisted at 1 week postoperatively (−2.4 ± 0.6 vs. 1.2 ± 0.7, respectively; $p < 0.0001$) and was coupled with a significantly better global QOL (pain, physical, social and psychological) score (−9.2 ± 2.3 vs. 3.7 ± 2.5, respectively; $p < 0.0001$) [18]. The differences in pain and global QOL scores disappeared at 3 weeks after treatment, but then surprisingly reappeared in favour of the RFA group at 1 year postoperatively and remained significant at 2 years [19].

Two RCTs compared QoL after RFA vs. surgery using the AVVSS score [20, 21]. The first RCT showed improvement in QoL after both surgery and RFA, with no difference between the two groups [20]. The second RCT similarly showed no difference between the two groups at 3 days, 1 month, 1 year and 3 years [21]. This RCT also reported less pain on the visual analog scale (VAS) in the RFA group at 10 days post-operatively compared with the high ligation and stripping arm [21]. In conclusion, it appears that there may be an early advantage with RFA compared to the traditional open surgery in QoL that in subsequent assessments is no longer measurable.

High Ligation and Stripping vs. EVLA

Three studies including a total of 780 patients compared high ligation and stripping vs. EVLA [22–24]. All three studies used the AVVSS score, the VCSS and several domains of the Medical Outcomes Study Short Form-36 QoL scores [22–24]. The AVVSS score, VCSS and Short Form-36 scores improved after both procedures. None of the studies found any significant difference in any of the clinical severity scores and QoL between groups (Fig. 21.1). Similarly, when the CEAP score was used (n = 4 studies; 867 patients), no difference could be demonstrated at 12 months following the intervention (Fig. 21.2) [25–28]. Another four studies reported AVVSS

Study name	Std diff in means	Lower limit	Upper limit	Z-Value	p-Value
Rasmussen, 2017	0.000	−0.621	0.621	0.000	1.000
Rasmussen, 2011	0.062	−0.293	0.417	0.344	0.731
Christenson, 2010	0.000	−0.281	0.281	0.000	1.000
	0.021	−0.186	0.229	0.201	0.840

Fig. 21.1 Forest plot of long-term VCSS effects for high ligation and stripping vs. EVLA

Study name	Std diff in means	Lower limit	Upper limit	Z-Value	p-Value
Biemans, 2013	0.168	−0.167	0.503	0.984	0.325
Pronk, 2010	0.029	−0.333	0.309	0.155	0.877
Flessenkamper, 2013	0.019	−0.207	0.245	0.163	0.871
Mozafar, 2014	0.090	−0.398	0.577	0.360	0.719
	0.090	−0.096	0.219	0.760	0.447

Fig. 21.2 Forest plot of CEAP effects for high ligation and stripping vs. EVLA

and EuroQoL-5D scores at various time-points post-intervention [25, 29–31]. Once again, disease-specific QoL did not differ between surgery and EVLA up to 5 years post-procedurally [25, 29–31].

Finally, six studies (n = 663 patients) evaluated long-term QoL using the AVVSS score (Fig. 21.3) [23, 24, 28, 31–33]. Like before, after the periprocedural period no long-term difference was found between the two treatment strategies. The early benefits associated with EVLA as demonstrated with PROMs were virtually abolished after the first month following the intervention [23, 24, 28, 31–33].

High Ligation and Stripping vs. Sclerotherapy

Five studies reported VCSSs at various time after high ligation and stripping vs. sclerotherapy [23, 30, 34–36]. One of these studies reported a significant improvement in mean scores from baseline to 1-year follow-up for both sclerotherapy (from 12.26 ± 3.05 to 4.26 ± 3.05, respectively; $p < 0.001$) and surgery (from 12.5 ± 1.64 to 3.39 ± 1.57, respectively; $p < 0.001$), but without any significant difference between groups [35]. Another study reported a significant improvement from baseline to 6-month VCSS scores for both treatment groups (sclerotherapy: from 4.9 ± 2.6 to 1.6 ± 1.7, respectively; $p < 0.001$; surgery: from 5.1 ± 2.5 to 1.4 ± 1.7, respectively; $p < 0.001$) without between-group difference [30]. The other three studies also reported improvements in VCSS scores at different time points [23, 34, 36]. One of these three studies demonstrated an additional improvement in CEAP score, as well [34].

Three of these five studies also reported AVVSS scores at various time points ranging from baseline to 3 years post-intervention [23, 30, 35]. All three studies showed decreased scores at 3 years, thus indicating an improvement in symptoms, but no difference between groups. Finally, three studies (n = 900 patients) explored the long-term change in QoL as measured by EuroQoL-5D (Fig. 21.4) [25, 30, 37]. Once again, these studies did not demonstrate any difference between the two modalities. The early advantage in pain and discomfort with foam sclerotherapy compared with open surgery was abolished completely at 1 month following the procedure.

High Ligation and Stripping vs. Thermal Ablation

Only one study reported VCSS scores after endovenous thermal (steam) ablation (n = 52 patients) vs. high ligation and stripping (n = 50 patients) [38]. This study showed that the mean VCSS scores were reduced from 7.25 to 1.78 in the

Study name	Std diff in means	Lower limit	Upper limit	Z-Value	p-Value
Rasmussen, 2011	−0.058	−0.333	0.216	−0.417	0.677
Carradice, 2011	0.000	−0.255	0.255	0.000	1.000
Christenson, 2010	−0.139	−0.417	0.139	−0.978	0.328
Mozafar, 2014	0.602	0.104	1.101	2.368	0.018
Samuel, 2013	0.188	−0.207	1.583	0.933	0.351
Darwood 2008	0.318	−0.461	1.098	0.800	0.424
	0.063	−0.122	0.247	0.666	0.505

Fig. 21.3 Forest plot of long-term AVVSS score effects for high ligation and stripping vs. EVLA

Study name	Difference in means	Lower limit	Upper limit	Z-Value	p-Value
Brittenden,2014	−0.005	−0.036	−0.026	−0.318	−0.751
Biemans, 2013	−0.040	−0.149	−0.229	−0.414	−0.679
Michales, 2006	−0.030	−0.054	−0.114	−0.720	−0.483
	−0.000	−0.028	−0.029	−0.007	−0.994

Difference in means and 95% CI

−1.00 −0.50 0.00 0.50 1.00

Favors Sclerotherapy Favors Surgery

Fig. 21.4 Forest plot of QoL effects for high ligation and stripping vs. sclerotherapy

endovenous thermal ablation group and from 8.28 to 2.2 in the surgical group (for both interventions, $p < 0.05$), but without any between-group difference in QoL [38]. The conclusion reached was that endovenous thermal ablation is safe and comparable with surgery.

Comparison Between Different Endovascular Interventions

Sclerotherapy vs. EVLA

Three RCTs reported information on QoL following EVLA vs. endovenous foam sclerotherapy [23, 30, 39]. These studies provided AVVSS scores at 6 weeks [30], 3 months [39], 6 months [30], 15 months [39] and 3 years [23] for each group. In one study, there was a statistically significant between-group difference regarding effect size in the adjusted data for AVVSS scores at 6 weeks in favour of the EVLA group ($p = 0.032$) [30]. However, this difference did not persist beyond the 3 months. In another study from the Imperial College, London, UK [39], both the VCSS and AVVSS scores were significantly reduced compared to baseline ($p < 0.0005$), but without any statistical difference between the groups [39].

RFA vs. EVLA

Two RCTs reported AVVSS scores for EVLA vs. RFA [40, 41]. At 6 weeks the mean between-group change of AVVSS scores was 0.2 in the EVLA group and −0.3 in the RFA group [40]. At 3 months the mean within-group change of AVVSS scores was −11.2 in the EVLA group and −10.3 in the RFA group [41]. There was no statistically significant between-group difference ($p = 0.12$), but AVVSS scores improved within each group at 3 months [41].

Despite the lack of difference in AVVSS scores, these studies showed that there was a statistically significant between-group difference with regards to the 10-point VAS pain scores at 7 [41] and 10 [40] days. The first study reporting median pain scores at 7 days showed a statistically significant difference in favor of the RFA group with a median pain score of 13.5 in the EVLA group and 0 in the RFA group ($p = 0.001$) [41]. In the other study, the RFA group similarly reported better improvement in the pain score compared with the EVLA group at 10 days (12.3 vs. −6.3, respectively; $p = 0.01$) [40]. However, with the introduction of the higher frequency laser equipment (1470-nm), there are no longer any differences in pain scores at 3 and 10 days, 1 month and 1 year [48].

RFA Plus Phlebectomies vs. EVLA Plus Phlebectomies

One good-quality RCT [22] (n = 762 patients) reported comparisons of EVLA plus phlebectomies vs. endovenous RFA plus phlebectomies. Patients in the RFA group reported significantly less postoperative pain than those in the EVLA group (Mean ± SD: 1.21 ± 1.72 vs. 2.58 ± 2.41; $p < 0.001$) [23]. The scores improved significantly in both groups from 1 month after the procedure, with no difference between groups thereafter. The mean AVVSS scores at 3 years presented in the RCT did not differ between groups (4.61 vs. 4.43, for the EVLA plus phlebectomies vs. the RFA plus phlebectomies groups, p = not significant) [23]. The same applied to the mean VCSS scores (0.34 vs. 0.44, for the EVLA plus phlebectomies vs. the RFA plus phlebectomies groups, p = not significant) [23].

EVLA vs. EVLA Plus Phlebectomies

Two RCTs compared EVLA vs. EVLA plus phlebectomies [42, 43]. In the first RCT, the VCSS at 3 months was lower with EVLA plus phlebectomies compared with EVLA alone (0 vs. 2, respectively; $p < 0.001$) [42]. The AVVSS scores were also lower for the EVLA plus phlebectomies group at 6 weeks (7.9 vs. 13.5, respectively; $p < 0.001$) and 3 months (2.0 vs. 9.6, respectively; $p = 0.015$). However, there were no differences in either VCSS or AVVSS scores at 1 year [42].

The second RCT reported the number of patients with pain at 1 and 4 weeks for each group [43]. The EVLA alone group reported fewer patients with pain compared with the EVLA plus phlebectomies group at 1 week (11 vs. 22 patients, $p = 0.002$). However, no patients in either group reported pain at 4 weeks [43].

EVLA vs. EVLA Plus Sclerotherapy

One small single-centre RCT from the UK reported a comparison of EVLA above the knee (n = 23 patients) vs. EVLA above and below the knee (n = 23 patients) vs. EVLA above the knee plus foam sclerotherapy (n = 22 patients) [44]. The median AVVSS scores improved significantly in all groups. There was a significant between-group difference in terms of patient satisfaction at 6 weeks in favor of EVLA above the knee plus foam sclerotherapy ($p = 0.015$) [44].

EVLA vs. Thermal Ablation

One RCT reported a comparison of EVLA vs. endovenous thermal (steam) ablation in 237 patients with symptomatic lower extremity chronic venous insufficiency/reflux and varicose veins [45]. Both groups showed improvement in AVVSS scores at 12 weeks postprocedure, but no statistically significant between-group difference was noted [45]. Similarly, VCSS scores improved in both groups but the improvement in between-group comparison was not significant ($p = 0.242$) [45].

Cyanoacrylate Embolization vs. RFA

One multicentre (n = 10) RCT from the U.S. reported a comparison of cyanoacrylate embolization vs. RFA using AVVSS scores on 242 patients with symptomatic lower extremity chronic venous insufficiency/reflux and varicose veins [46]. At 1 month, AVVSS scores improved significantly both in the cyanoacrylate group and in the RFA group, without any statistically significant between-group difference [46]. There was also no difference in postoperative pain between the two groups according to the 10-point VAS score ($p = 0.36$) [46]. In the subsequent report of the 2-year results, there was once again no difference in patients' QoL through 24 months [47].

The conclusion reached was that both cyanoacrylate embolization and RFA of the great saphenous vein are safe and durable up to 2 years [47].

Recurrence Rates Following Different Interventions

A key parameter in selecting the appropriate intervention for the management of lower extremity chronic venous disease is recurrence rates. In the earlier mentioned RCT comparing EVLA vs. RFA vs. ultrasound-guided foam sclerotherapy vs. surgical stripping, there was no difference in varicose vein recurrence rates at 3 years between the procedures (20% vs. 14.9% vs. 19.1% vs. 20.2%, respectively; $p = 0.66$) [21]. There were more patients in the sclerotherapy group presenting with reflux in the groin compared with the other groups ($p = 0.34$) and more reoperations performed in the sclerotherapy group compared with the EVLA, RFA and surgical groups (31.6% vs. 12.5% and 11.1% and 15.5%, respectively; $p < 0.0001$). However, patients undergoing sclerotherapy were only give a single injection of foam and were not seen again [21]. This is an inadequate method to offer foam sclerotherapy, as approximately 20–30% of patients require additional foam in tributaries at 6 weeks to complete their treatment. Nevertheless, the VCSS, SF-36 and AVVSS QoL scores all improved significantly in all the groups with no difference between the various procedures [21].

Other RCTs similarly demonstrated no significant difference in recurrence rates between the various modalities despite a slightly higher incidence of great saphenous vein reflux [39, 49, 50]. Nevertheless, this slightly higher reflux rate was not related to deterioration in QoL indicating that this reflux was largely asymptomatic [39].

The Finnish Venous Study was a randomized trial comparing the effect of ultrasound-guided foam sclerotherapy vs. EVLA with phlebectomies vs. surgery on the QoL of patients receiving treatment for great saphenous varicose veins [49]. It showed significant improvement in AVVSS QoL scores postoperatively in all groups, with no significant differences between them [49]. In contrast, a similar randomized trial from the Netherlands and Belgium [50] demonstrated a significant deterioration in CIVIQ scores in the sclerotherapy group compared with the EVLA group ($p = 0.013$). However, the CIVIQ scores for the conventional surgery group did not differ from those in the EVLA and the sclerotherapy group, and the EuroQoL-5D scores improved equally in all groups [50]. The extended 5-year results of the Finnish Venous Study similarly showed a sustained improvement in AVVSS scores from baseline for all procedures, with no significant difference in terms of QoL between the procedures at 5 years [51].

Conclusions

The effect of several procedures on QoL has been extensively investigated for patients with lower extremity chronic venous disease (Fig. 21.5).

Although no long-term difference is seen in effectiveness between RFA and high ligation and stripping, RFA is associated with less periprocedural pain, faster improvement in symptom scores and QoL. Among patients undergoing endovenous interventions, RFA, EVLA and sclerotherapy all demonstrate improvement in QoL and standardized symptom scores. When compared with patients offered EVLA, those treated with foam sclerotherapy had significantly less periprocedural pain, while patients treated with RFA had significantly less periprocedural pain but also less short-term improvement in VCSS. Patients treated with foam sclerotherapy demonstrate significant improvement in standardized symptom scores and QoL compared with placebo. Similarly, patients treated with high ligation plus stripping demonstrate improved long-term symptoms and QoL compared with those patients managed with compression therapy alone. Endovascular techniques have a sig-

Fig. 21.5 Summary and concluding remarks

Quality-of-life (QOL) and Patient-Reported Outcome Measures (PROMs) following intervention for Chronic Venous Disease

- Venous leg ulcers affect patients in terms of quality-of-life(QoL), pain and social isolation
- Patient-reported outcome measures (PROMs) provide a means by which the impact of varicose veins or their treatments can be measured on the patient's QoL
- PROMs explore several dimensions in patients' QoL, including psychological effects, physical effects, social well-being, pain and cosmetic appearance
- Radiofrequency ablation has an early advantage over high ligation and stripping but this disappears at 3-4 weeks after treatment
- Endovenous laser ablation, thermal ablation and sclerotherapy have no significant difference in PROMs compared with surgery
- There is no difference in varicose vein recurrence rates between any procedures

nificant early improvement of the quality of life in patients who are treated for chronic venous insufficiency compared to open traditional surgery (saphenofemoral ligation and saphenectomy). This early advantage is lost with intermediate and long-term follow-up compared to the quality of life in patients treated with saphenofemoral ligation and long saphenous vein stripping. As the long-term results are comparable irrespective of the technique that is used for the management of the patient, the choice of the intervention will depend on patient's preference, local expertise, the configuration of the varicose vein and the diameter of the saphenous trunk.

References

1. Eberhardt RT, Raffetto JD. Chronic venous insufficiency. Circulation. 2014;130(4):333–46.
2. Kearon C, Akl EA, Comerota AJ, Prandoni P, Bounameaux H, Goldhaber SZ, et al. Antithrombotic therapy for VTE disease: antithrombotic therapy and prevention of thrombosis, 9th edn., American College of Chest Physicians Evidence-Based Clinical Practice Guidelines. Chest. 2012;14(2 Suppl):e419S–96S.
3. Korn P, Patel ST, Heller JA, Deitch JS, Krishnasastry KV, Bush HL, et al. Why insurers should reimburse for compression stockings in patients with chronic venous stasis. J Vasc Surg. 2002;35(5):950–7.
4. Smith JJ, Garratt AM, Guest M, Greenhalgh RM, Davies AH. Evaluating and improving health-related quality of life in patients with varicose veins. J Vasc Surg. 1999;30(4):710–9.
5. Nicolaides AN, Kakkos SK, Baekgaard N, Comerota A, De Maessener M, Eklof B, et al. Management of chronic venous disorders of the lower limbs. Guidelines according to scientific evidence. Part II. Int Angiol. 2020;37:181.
6. Poku E, Aber A, Phillips P, Essat M, Buckley Woods H, Palfreyman S, et al. Systematic review assessing the measurement properties of patient-reported outcomes for venous leg ulcers. BJS Open. 2017;1(5):138–47.
7. Augustin M, Dieterle W, Zschocke I, Brill C, Trefzer D, Peschen M, et al. Development and validation of a disease-specific questionnaire on the quality of life of patients with chronic venous insufficiency. Vasa. 1997;26(4):291–301.
8. Guex JJ, Zimmet SE, Boussetta S, Nguyen C, Taieb C. Construction and validation of a patient-reported outcome dedicated to chronic venous disorders: SQOR-V (specific quality of life and outcome response – venous). J Mal Vasc. 2007;32(3):135–47.
9. Launois R, Reboul-Marty J, Henry B. Construction and validation of a quality of life questionnaire in chronic lower limb venous insufficiency (CIVIQ). Qual Life Res. 1996;5(6):539–54.
10. Garratt AM, Macdonald LM, Ruta DA, Russell IT, Buckingham JK, Krukowski ZH. Toward measurement of outcome for patients with varicose veins. Qual Health Care. 1993;2(1):5–10.
11. Lamping DL, Schroter S, Kurz X, Kahn SR, Abenhaim L. Evaluation of outcomes in chronic venous disorders of the leg: development of a scientifically rigorous, patient-reported measure of symptoms and quality of life. J Vasc Surg. 2003;37(2):410–9.
12. Hareendran A, Doll H, Wild DJ, Moffatt CJ, Musgrove E, Wheatley C, et al. The venous leg ulcer quality of life (VLU-QoL) questionnaire: development and psychometric validation. Wound Repair Regen. 2007;15(4):465–73.
13. Hyland ME, Ley A, Thomson B. Quality of life of leg ulcer patients: questionnaire and preliminary findings. J Wound Care. 1994;3(6):294–8.
14. Palfreyman S. Assessing the impact of venous ulceration on quality of life. Nurs Times. 2008;104:34–7.
15. Smith JJ, Guest MG, Greenhalgh RM, Davies AH. Measuring the quality of life in patients with venous ulcers. J Vasc Surg. 2000;31(4):642–9.

16. Passman MA, McLafferty RB, Lentz MF, Nagre SB, Iafrati MD, Bohannon WT, et al. Validation of Venous Clinical Severity Score (VCSS) with other venous severity assessment tools from the American Venous Forum, National Venous Screening Program. J Vasc Surg. 2011;54(6 Suppl):2S–9S.
17. Eklof B, Rutherford RB, Bergan JJ, Carpentier PH, Gloviczki P, Kistner RL, et al. American Venous Forum International Ad Hoc Committee for Revision of the CEAP Classification. Revision of the CEAP classification for chronic venous disorders: consensus statement. J Vasc Surg. 2004;40(6):1248–52.
18. Lurie F, Creton D, Eklof B, Kabnick LS, Kistner RL, Pichot O, et al. Prospective randomized study of endovenous radiofrequency obliteration (closure procedure) versus ligation and stripping in a selected patient population (EVOLVeS Study). J Vasc Surg. 2003;38(2):207–14.
19. Lurie F, Creton D, Eklof B, Kabnick LS, Kistner RL, et al. Prospective randomised study of endovenous radiofrequency obliteration (closure) versus ligation and vein stripping (EVOLVeS): two-year follow-up. Eur J Vasc Endovasc Surg. 2005;29(1):67–73.
20. Subramonia S, Lees T. Randomized clinical trial of radiofrequency ablation or conventional high ligation and stripping for great saphenous varicose veins. Br J Surg. 2010;97(3):328–36.
21. Rasmussen L, Lawaetz M, Serup J, Bjoern L, Vennits B, Blemings A, et al. Randomized clinical trial comparing endovenous laser ablation, radiofrequency ablation, foam sclerotherapy and surgical stripping for great saphenous varicose veins with 3-year follow-up. J Vasc Surg Venous Lymphat Disord. 2013;1(4):349–56.
22. Rasmussen LH, Bjoern L, Lawaetz M, Blemings A, Lawaetz B, Eklof B. Randomized trial comparing endovenous laser ablation of the great saphenous vein with high ligation and stripping in patients with varicose veins: short-term results. J Vasc Surg. 2007;46(2):308–15.
23. Rasmussen LH, Lawaetz M, Bjoern L, Vennits B, Blemings A, Eklof B. Randomized clinical trial comparing endovenous laser ablation, radiofrequency ablation, foam sclerotherapy and surgical stripping for great saphenous varicose veins. Br J Surg. 2011;98(8):1079–87.
24. Christenson JT, Gueddi S, Gemayel G, Bounameaux H. Prospective randomized trial comparing endovenous laser ablation and surgery for treatment of primary great saphenous varicose veins with a 2-year follow-up. J Vasc Surg. 2010;52(5):1234–41.
25. Biemans AA, Kockaert M, Akkersdijk GP, van den Bos RR, de Maeseneer MG, Cuypers P, et al. Comparing endovenous laser ablation, foam sclerotherapy, and conventional surgery for great saphenous varicose veins. J Vasc Surg. 2013;58(3):727–34.
26. Pronk P, Gauw SA, Mooij MC, Gaastra MT, Lawson JA, van Goethem AR, et al. Randomised controlled trial comparing sapheno-femoral ligation and stripping of the great saphenous vein with endovenous laser ablation (980 nm) using local tumescent anaesthesia: one-year results. Eur J Vasc Endovasc Surg. 2010;40(5):649–56.
27. Flessenkamper I, Hartmann M, Hartmann K, Stenger D, Roll S. Endovenous laser ablation with and without high ligation compared with high ligation and stripping in the treatment of great saphenous varicose veins: initial results of a multicenter randomized controlled trial. Phlebology. 2013;28(1):16–23.
28. Mozafar M, Atgjaee K, Haghighatkhah H, Taheri MS, Tabatabaey A, Lotfollahzadeh S. Endovenous laser ablation of the great saphenous vein versus high ligation: long-term results. Lasers Med Sci. 2014;29(2):765–71.
29. Roopram AD, Lind MY, Van Brussel JP, Terlouw-Punt LC, Birnie E, De Smet AA, et al. Endovenous laser ablation versus conventional surgery in the treatment of small saphenous vein incompetence. J Vasc Surg Venous Lymphat Disord. 2013;1(4):357–63.
30. Brittenden J, Cooper D, Dimitrova M, Scotland G, Cotton SC, Elders A, et al. Five-year outcomes of a randomized trial of treatments for varicose veins. N Engl J Med. 2019;381(10):912–22.
31. Carradice D, Mekako AI, Mazari FA, Samuel N, Hatfield J, Chetter IC. Randomized clinical trial of endovenous laser ablation compared with conventional surgery for great saphenous varicose veins. Br J Surg. 2011;98(4):501–10.
32. Samuel N, Carradice D, Wallace T, Mekako A, Hatfield J, Chetter I. Randomized clinical trial of endovenous laser ablation versus conventional surgery for small saphenous varicose veins. Ann Surg. 2013;257(3):419–26.
33. Darwood RJ, Theivacumar N, Dellagrammaticas D, Mavor AI, Gough MJ. Randomized clinical trial comparing endovenous laser ablation with surgery for the treatment of primary great saphenous varicose veins. Br J Surg. 2008;95(3):294–301.
34. Bountouroglou DG, Azzam M, Kakkos SK, Pathmarajah M, Young P, Geroulakos G. Ultrasound-guided foam sclerotherapy combined with saphenofemoral ligation compared to surgical treatment of varicose veins: early results of a randomised controlled trial. Eur J Vasc Endovasc Surg. 2006;31(1):93–100.
35. Campos W Jr, Torres IO, da Silva ES, Casella IB, Puech-Leao P. A prospective randomized study comparing polidocanol foam sclerotherapy with surgical treatment of patients with primary chronic venous insufficiency and ulcer. Ann Vasc Surg. 2015;29(6):1128–35.
36. Shadid N, Ceulen R, Nelemans P, Dirksen C, Veraart J, Schurink GW, et al. Randomized clinical trial of ultrasound-guided foam sclerotherapy versus surgery for the incompetent great saphenous vein. Br J Surg. 2012;99(8):1062–70.
37. Michaels JA, Campbell WB, Brazier JE, Macintyre JB, Palfreyman SJ, Ratcliffe J, et al. Randomised clinical trial, observational study and assessment of cost-effectiveness of the treatment of varicose

veins (REACTIV trial). Health Technol Assess. 2006;10(3):1–196.
38. Wozniak W, Mlosek RK, Ciostek P. Assessment of the efficacy and safety of steam vein sclerosis as compared to classic surgery in lower extremity varicose vein management. Wideochir Inne Tech Maloinwazyjne. 2015;10(1):15–24.
39. Lattimer CR, Kalodiki E, Azzam M, Makris GC, Somiayajulu S, Geroulakos G. Interim results on abolishing reflux alongside a randomized clinical trial on laser ablation with phlebectomies versus foam sclerotherapy. Int Angiol. 2013;32(4):394–403.
40. Shepherd AC, Ortega-Ortega M, Gohel MS, Epstein D, Brown LC, Davies AH. Cost-effectiveness of radiofrequency ablation versus laser for varicose veins. Int J Technol Assess Health Care. 2015;31(5):289–96.
41. Nordon IM, Hinchliffe RJ, Brar R, Moxey P, Black SA, Thompson MM, et al. A prospective double-blind randomized controlled trial of radiofrequency versus laser treatment of the great saphenous vein in patients with varicose veins. Ann Surg. 2011;254(6):876–81.
42. Carradice D, Mekako AI, Hatfield J, Chetter IC. Randomized clinical trial of concomitant or sequential phlebectomy after endovenous laser therapy for varicose veins. Br J Surg. 2009;96(4):369–75.
43. Liu P, Ren S, Yang Y, Liu J, Ye Z, Lin F. Intravenous catheter-guided laser ablation: a novel alternative for branch varicose veins. Int Surg. 2011;96(4):331–6.
44. Theivacumar NS, Dellagrammaticas D, Mavor AI, Gough MJ. Endovenous laser ablation: does standard above-knee great saphenous vein ablation provide optimum results in patients with above- and below-knee reflux? A randomized controlled trial. J Vasc Surg. 2008;48:173–8.
45. Van den Boss RR, Malskat WS, De Maeseneer MG, de Roos KP, Groeneweg DA, Kockaert MA, et al. Randomized clinical trial of endovenous laser ablation versus steam ablation (LAST trial) for great saphenous varicose veins. Br J Surg. 2014;101(9):1077–83.
46. Morrison N, Gibson K, McEnroe S, Goldman M, King T, Weiss R, et al. Randomized clinical trial comparing cyanoacrylate embolization and radiofrequency ablation for incompetent great saphenous veins (VeClose). J Vasc Surg. 2015;61(4):985–94.
47. Gibson K, Morrison N, Kolluri R, Vasquez M, Weiss R, Cher D, et al. Twenty-four month results from a randomized trial of cyanoacrylate closure versus radiofrequency ablation for the treatment of incompetent great saphenous veins. J Vasc Surg Venous Lymphat Disord. 2018;6(5):606–13.
48. He G, Zheng C, Yu MA, Zhang H. Comparison of ultrasound-guided endovenous laser ablation and radiofrequency for the varicose veins treatment: an updated meta-analysis. Int J Surg. 2017;39:267–75.
49. Venermo M, Saarinen J, Eskelinen E, Vahaaho S, Saarinen E, Railo M, et al. Finnish Venous Study Collaborators. Randomized clinical trial comparing surgery, endovenous laser ablation and ultrasound-guided foam sclerotherapy for the treatment of great saphenous varicose veins. Br J Surg. 2016;103(11):1438–44.
50. van der Velden SK, Biemans AA, De Maeseneer MG, Kockaert MA, Cuypers PW, Hollestein LM, et al. Five-year results of a randomized clinical trial of conventional surgery, endovenous laser ablation and ultrasound-guided foam sclerotherapy in patients with great saphenous varicose veins. Br J Surg. 2015;102(10):1184–94.
51. Vahaaho S, Halmesmaki K, Alback A, Saarinen E, Venermo M. Five-year follow-up of a randomized clinical trial comparing open surgery, foam sclerotherapy and endovenous laser ablation for great saphenous varicose veins. Br J Surg. 2018;105(6):686–91.

Index

T. Athanasiou et al. (eds.), *Patient Reported Outcomes and Quality of Life in Cardiovascular Interventions*,
https://doi.org/10.1007/978-3-031-09815-4

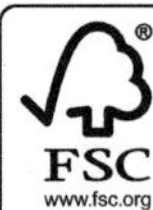

MIX
Papier aus verantwortungsvollen Quellen
Paper from responsible sources
FSC® C105338

If you have any concerns about our products,
you can contact us on
ProductSafety@springernature.com

In case Publisher is established outside the EU,
the EU authorized representative is:
Springer Nature Customer Service Center GmbH
Europaplatz 3, 69115 Heidelberg, Germany

Printed by Libri Plureos GmbH
in Hamburg, Germany